Glaucoma: A Clinician's Guide

Glaucoma: A Clinician's Guide

Edited by Ned Mueller

AMERICAN
MEDICAL PUBLISHERS
www.americanmedicalpublishers.com

American Medical Publishers,
41 Flatbush Avenue,
1st Floor, New York,
NY 11217, USA

Visit us on the World Wide Web at:
www.americanmedicalpublishers.com

ISBN: 978-1-63927-382-9

Cataloging-in-Publication Data

Glaucoma : a clinician's guide / edited by Ned Mueller.
p. cm.
Includes bibliographical references and index.
ISBN 978-1-63927-382-9
1. Glaucoma. 2. Glaucoma--Treatment. 3. Eye--Diseases. 4. Ophthalmologists--Guidebooks.
5. Hospitals, Ophthalmic and aural--Guidebooks. I. Mueller, Ned.

RE871 .G53 2022
617.741--dc23

Table of Contents

Preface

Glaucoma is a group of eye disorders that cause damage to the optic nerve and loss of vision. Some of its symptoms are eye pain, blurred vision, redness of the eye, nausea, etc. Open-angle glaucoma, closed-angle glaucoma and normal-tension glaucoma are a few of its types. Open-angle glaucoma is the most common type. It develops slowly and the drainage angle for fluid within the eye remains open. It results in vision loss and sometimes permanent blindness. Closed-angle glaucoma involves severe eye pain, mid-dilated pupil, blurred vision and nausea. There are certain risk factors for glaucoma. These include increased pressure in eyes, high blood pressure and a family history of the condition. Techniques such as tonometry, ophthalmoscopy, gonioscopy, pachymetry, etc. are used in the diagnosis of glaucoma. Strategies such as surgery, laser treatment and glaucoma medications are available for the management of glaucoma. Laser treatments are usually effective in both open-angle and closed-angle glaucoma. This book explores all the important aspects of glaucoma in the present day scenario. It is a valuable compilation of topics, ranging from the basic to the most complex advancements in the diagnosis and treatment of glaucoma. This book is appropriate for students seeking detailed information in this area as well as for experts.

All of the data presented henceforth, was collaborated in the wake of recent advancements in the field. The aim of this book is to present the diversified developments from across the globe in a comprehensible manner. The opinions expressed in each chapter belong solely to the contributing authors. Their interpretations of the topics are the integral part of this book, which I have carefully compiled for a better understanding of the readers.

At the end, I would like to thank all those who dedicated their time and efforts for the successful completion of this book. I also wish to convey my gratitude towards my friends and family who supported me at every step.

Editor

1

Exploring Eye Movements in Patients with Glaucoma When Viewing a Driving Scene

David P. Crabb[1]*, Nicholas D. Smith[1], Franziska G. Rauscher[1], Catharine M. Chisholm[2], John L. Barbur[1], David F. Edgar[1], David F. Garway-Heath[3]

1 Department of Optometry and Visual Science, City University London, London, United Kingdom, **2** Bradford School of Optometry and Vision Science, University of Bradford, Bradford, United Kingdom, **3** NIHR Biomedical Research Centre for Ophthalmology, Moorfields Eye Hospital NHS Foundation Trust and UCL Institute of Ophthalmology, London, United Kingdom

Abstract

Background: Glaucoma is a progressive eye disease and a leading cause of visual disability. Automated assessment of the visual field determines the different stages in the disease process: it would be desirable to link these measurements taken in the clinic with patient's actual function, or establish if patients compensate for their restricted field of view when performing everyday tasks. Hence, this study investigated eye movements in glaucomatous patients when viewing driving scenes in a hazard perception test (HPT).

Methodology/Principal Findings: The HPT is a component of the UK driving licence test consisting of a series of short film clips of various traffic scenes viewed from the driver's perspective each containing hazardous situations that require the camera car to change direction or slow down. Data from nine glaucomatous patients with binocular visual field defects and ten age-matched control subjects were considered (all experienced drivers). Each subject viewed 26 different films with eye movements simultaneously monitored by an eye tracker. Computer software was purpose written to pre-process the data, co-register it to the film clips and to quantify eye movements and point-of-regard (using a dynamic bivariate contour ellipse analysis). On average, and across all HPT films, patients exhibited different eye movement characteristics to controls making, for example, significantly more saccades ($P<0.001$; 95% confidence interval for mean increase: 9.2 to 22.4%). Whilst the average region of 'point-of-regard' of the patients did not differ significantly from the controls, there were revealing cases where patients failed to see a hazard in relation to their binocular visual field defect.

Conclusions/Significance: Characteristics of eye movement patterns in patients with bilateral glaucoma can differ significantly from age-matched controls when viewing a traffic scene. Further studies of eye movements made by glaucomatous patients could provide useful information about the definition of the visual field component required for fitness to drive.

Editor: Sheng He, University of Minnesota, United States of America

Funding: Nicholas Smith was supported by unrestricted funding from the Moorfields Eye Hospital Special Trustees. The authors acknowledge the UK Department for Transport financial support for the project that secured the HPT data in patients with glaucoma. One of the authors (DGH) has received a proportion of his funding from the Department of Health's National Institute for Health Research Biomedical Research Centre at Moorfields Eye Hospital and the UCL Institute of Ophthalmology. The views expressed in this publication are those of the authors and not necessarily those of the UK Department of Health. The funders had no role in study design, data collection and analysis, decision to publish, or preparation of the manuscript.

Competing Interests: The authors have declared that no competing interests exist.

* E-mail: David.Crabb.1@city.ac.uk

Introduction

Glaucoma is a chronic progressive neuropathy involving the visual pathway: it is the most common cause of irreversible blindness in the world and a leading cause of visual morbidity. Given its chronic progressive nature, the rise in prevalence with age and the increasing longevity of the population, the impact of the disease is substantial and rising.

Automated visual field assessment is the principal functional measurement in the clinical management of patients with glaucoma. However, insight into how visual field defects manifesting at different stages in the disease process impact on patients' everyday visual function is only recently gaining momentum in the research literature. Linking the clinical measurements to what patients can do functionally is important in the management of the condition. For example, there is emerging evidence of glaucomatous patients being at greater risk of falls and accidents, even with relatively modest visual field defects [1,2,3]. There is also evidence of the impact of glaucomatous field defects on self-reported disability [4,5,6,7,8] and, more recently, objective measures in laboratory based studies demonstrate the difficulty patients have with some everyday tasks [9,10]. Glaucoma undoubtedly impacts on an individual when visual field loss causes the removal of a driving licence, and several studies of varying experimental design have shown that certain glaucomatous visual field defects are not compatible with safe driving [1,11,12,13]. The issue of driving with glaucoma is a serious one, with a significant proportion of patients suffering visual loss that results in driving ineligibility, certainly in the UK [14,15]. Moreover, it has been demonstrated that patients perceive this particular potential outcome of their disease to be as serious to them as the long-term risk of blindness [16].

One aspect of visual function in glaucoma that has received little attention is eye movements. It is accepted that patients' perception of the severity of their peripheral visual field loss is influenced by one eye essentially 'filling in' for the other, but very little is known about how eye movements might contribute to any compensatory mechanism for loss of function. It would, for example, be useful to know if glaucoma patients exhibit the same eye movement behaviour as healthy subjects, or maintain the same point of regard when looking at, or interpreting, an everyday scene. This evidence may inform future studies that attempt to relate the severity, extent and location of a visual field defect to what a patient can and cannot do in terms of real life activities, especially driving. It may even provide a basis for incorporating attention to eye movements into visual rehabilitation and coping strategies for the patient with glaucoma.

The Hazard Perception Test (HPT) was introduced as an element of the UK driving licence theory test in 2003 as a measure to encourage appropriate visual scanning of the road or highway and to develop the ability to recognise at the earliest opportunity that a potentially dangerous driving situation might arise. In this context a 'learner driver' is shown a film of a real driving scene, seen from the perspective of the driver, with the task being to detect potential 'hazards': these are defined as something that would make the camera car take evasive action, such as braking for an oncoming cyclist or a pedestrian unexpectedly crossing the road/street. Primarily, it is a useful educational tool allowing learner drivers to encounter 'on road' driving scenes from the safety of a computer monitor. A subject's performance on the HPT is clearly dependent on instruction, prior experience and perception of what represents a driving hazard, and HPT performance in terms of simply detecting a hazard in visually healthy subjects is certainly variable [17]. Previously the HPT, as a simple reaction test to hazards, was investigated as a potential proxy measure for identifying visual defects that would impinge on fitness to drive, and was found to have limited value for this purpose [18]. Whether the HPT is an indicator of subjects' visual strategies when driving under the conditions in which they are most likely to have an accident is open to debate, and is not the subject of this study. Rather, for the purposes of this study, this realistic and relevant visual scenario can be 'played out' on a computer screen allowing for accurate gaze tracking in a controlled laboratory setting, thus making it most suitable for examining the eye movement behaviour of glaucomatous patients compared to control subjects whilst viewing an everyday scene.

The aim of this study is to perform eye tracking on subjects as they simultaneously view a series of HPT film clips to examine the hypothesis that patients with binocular glaucomatous field defects exhibit significant differences in eye movement characteristics to healthy control subjects. Moreover, in the context of visual field defects and fitness to drive, the data can also be used to examine qualitatively how these patients' eye movements relate to the events and hazards in the video sequences.

Materials and Methods

Ethics Statement

The study was approved by the ethics committee of each of the participating institutions where subjects were recruited (Moorfields and Whittington Research Ethics Committee, London; School of Community and Health Sciences Research and Ethics Committee, City University London). All participants were asked about their general health and were excluded if they were on any significant medication (other than that for their glaucoma). Written informed consent, according to the tenets of the Declaration of Helsinki, was obtained prior to examination from each subject. All the data, with patient identifiers removed, were transferred to a secure computer at the university.

Subjects

This study took advantage of some of the data collected as part of a UK Department for Transport (DfT) funded study conducted at City University London, fully reported elsewhere [17,18]. In short, this UK DfT study aimed to examine the agreement between the outcome of conventional visual field tests and proxy measures of driving safety in subjects with binocular paracentral scotoma, resulting from a range of visual disorders, but preserved visual acuity (VA). One experiment in the original study, not performed on all study participants, examined the performance of subjects on the HPT whilst eye movements were simultaneously recorded. Glaucoma patients were recruited from the Central Middlesex Hospital (North West London Hospitals NHS Trust), Moorfields Eye Hospital Trust London and the Fight for Sight Optometry Clinic at City University London. Data from these patients, along with those from a group of visually healthy control subjects, are the subject of this study.

All patients had a clinical diagnosis of glaucomatous optic neuropathy (primary open angle glaucoma) in both eyes and are, therefore, representative of those patients who should undergo further testing to satisfy the visual field requirements for legal fitness to drive in the UK [17,19]. Prior to inclusion in the study, all patients had a full eye examination including central visual fields (24-2 or 30-2 SITA Standard) recorded on a Humphrey Visual Field Analyzer (HFA, Carl Zeiss Meditec, CA, USA). Patients were excluded if they produced unreliable fields at this first visit. VA of at least 6/9 was required in both eyes, with no other significant ocular disease reported other than glaucoma. Visually healthy control subjects were recruited from University staff, centres for the elderly and the University optometry clinic. A full eye examination, including HFA visual fields, was carried out to exclude any abnormality before a volunteer was accepted into the study. A VA of at least 6/9 was required for each eye.

The HPT film clips used in this study have been used elsewhere [20] and consisted of 26 short films (range 40–73 seconds) showing a range of driving environments (e.g. dual-carriageway or divided highway, rural lane, busy urban streets). Each film contained between one and three 'hazardous driving events'. The films were digitised (with a standard mpeg codec running at 25 frames per second) and shown on a 42 inch plasma widescreen monitor (1280 by 1024 pixel resolution) in a rectangle of width 824 mm and height 512 mm. Participants were seated at a chin rest 120 cm from the screen and the image subtended 39° horizontally and 25° vertically. Eye movements were monitored using a SMI Eyelink eye tracker (SensoMotoric Instruments, Teltow, Berlin, Germany) sampling at 250 Hz. The SMI eye tracker has reported spatial accuracy better than 0.5°. Calibration, drift correction, and validation were performed using the algorithms provided by the instrument. In this system, adjustment of the measurements for head position is carried out automatically using detectors in the four corners of the monitor, but a chin rest was also used to stabilise head movements and ensure a constant viewing distance.

Participants were all given the same verbal instructions: that they should look out for events that would cause the camera-car to take evasive action such as braking or evasive steering. They held a response button in their preferred hand, and were instructed to press the button whenever they judged one of these hazards as imminent. This 'press button' performance in the actual hazard detection task was not considered in this study because previous analysis indicated large variability in 'press button' scores and the influence of subject specific definition of what constitutes a hazard [18]. Following calibration of the eye tracker, each subject was shown two introductory films prior to the commencement of data collection, to allow them to familiarise themselves with the task. The film clips were presented in random order with occasional rest periods between films.

Participants were asked to estimate the number of years they had been actively driving. For this study, participants were excluded if they had never held a valid driving licence or had less than 5 years driving experience. Moreover, for this study analysis was restricted to participants that were 50 years of older at the time of the study to ensure that the mean and distribution of age was matched between participants with glaucoma and controls. None of the participants had previously performed the HPT and were therefore naïve to the task.

Analysis

The eye tracker yields an enormous amount of raw data: essentially a trace of 'gaze' recorded as (x,y) coordinates related to the viewing area every 4.2ms for each film. The results from this experiment contained more than six million of these data points. A bespoke application written in Microsoft Visual C# was developed for analysing these time series [21] and this is freely available from the authors; what follows is a short description of the techniques employed in the main analysis.

Eye movements were divided into fixations, saccades and 'smooth pursuits' using a velocity based criterion. One difficulty is correctly separating these movements from the variability in the measurement process. Therefore, a noise removal technique was first applied to the data which filters out highly variable non-physiological measurements (high frequency noise) by taking a window or block of 50 (x,y) coordinate eye gaze positions (around 210ms) and calculates the speed of any eye movement between the positions recorded at time point t and t+1. If more than 75% of the recordings within that window move at 30°/s or more then the whole window is removed from the trace because these measurements are assumed less likely to be physiological movements and are more likely attributed to measurement variability. The window moves along the trace to perform the same procedure on the next 50 samples. On completion, an eight sample median filter is passed over the remaining data to remove or dampen 'low frequency' noise. Blinks (denoted by zero value data), gaze outside the viewing area and other eye tracking failures were identified then removed from the traces. Films in which less than 40% of the recordings remained were discarded to ensure that we were not removing too much data per film, following a previously used protocol [22].

Once the data are filtered, saccades were defined as the proportion of the trace where the velocity of the eye movement is faster than 30°/s. This criterion of 30°/s or higher for identifying saccades is common in eye movement studies and eye tracking instrumentation, since this is considered the upper limit of pursuit eye movement speed.[23,24,25] Any saccade exceeding a duration of 120 ms or is less than 10 ms were excluded from the analysis. In addition saccades that originate or terminate outside the confines of the dimensions of the display of the film (calibration errors) were excluded from the analysis. Fixations were defined as the proportion of the trace where gaze was 'still' and the velocity of the eye movement is less than 1.5°/s. We defined periods of the trace where the speed was greater that 1.5°/s but less that 30°/s to be 'pursuit' movements, where gaze was most likely 'tracking' a moving object in the film. In truth, these pursuit movements are very difficult to quantify even with a sophisticated eye tracker operating at a high frame rate, but we shall refer to them as possible 'smooth pursuits' lacking the stability characteristic of a fixation, but without being fast enough to be classified as a physiological saccade. The algorithm then automatically records the number of fixations, the number of saccades and the number of smooth pursuits per second of film. It also yields average fixation duration (ms), average 'smooth pursuit' duration (ms) and average saccade amplitude (size in degrees). These six summary eye movement parameters were recorded for each film as viewed by each subject.

The experimental design aimed to minimize 'the between subject measurement variability' in the eye movement parameters with all participants viewing the same films, so these were assumed to be the blocks in the experiment. A General Linear Model (GLM) was used to perform univariate analysis of variance (ANOVA) with an unbalanced design (accommodating missing data by the method of median imputation) to assess each of six different eye movement parameters (response variables) using the statistical software package Minitab v.14 (Minitab Inc., Pennsylvania, USA). In this two way ANOVA arrangement, variation in the response variable (each eye movement parameter) was expected to be different across the films and across the subjects, with the null hypothesis of real interest being no difference in the average value for the eye movement parameters between the patients and controls examined (F test on the main factor, participant group, from the ANOVA).

In order to consider the hypothesis that any differences in eye movement characteristics between patients and controls were similar at the time of the hazards compared to sequences of the HPT where no hazards occurred, the films were divided into 'safe' and 'unsafe' segments. One of the authors (NS) carefully reviewed all the films and identified the sequence in the film where the hazard emerged and then ended. The six summary eye movement parameters were calculated for both the 'hazard sequence' and the 'non-hazard' sequence for each film and each participant. The individual differences were then calculated, and these differences were treated as the response variable analysed with a GLM ANOVA. The null hypothesis being no difference in the average value for the eye movement parameters between the patients and controls examined in the two different sequences (F test on the main factor, participant group, from the ANOVA).

A novel 'point of regard' analysis was also implemented. The eye tracking sequence is co-registered to the film sequence with each frame of the film equating to nine eye-tracking samples; a mean of these (x,y) points is defined as the 'point of regard' for that frame. This is repeated for all the control subjects such that each film frame has a sample of 'points of regard' (x,y), one for each control subject, for that particular frame. To quantify the spatial coincidence of the point of regard location for all the control subjects, we calculated the best-fit bivariate contour ellipse (BCE). The BCE area has been previously used to quantify fixation eye movement stability in patients with macular degeneration [22,26,27] and to quantify viewing areas for subjects as they watch movies [28]. For our application we implemented the method as described by Goldstein et al [28] but in a novel development we also plotted the ellipse on each frame of the film [29,30] thus giving a dynamic visual representation of the region of interest for the control subjects. The centre of the BCE represents the mean 'point of regard' of the controls, with the spatial extent of the ellipse being one standard deviation from this centre along two principal axes, theoretically affording 'coverage' of approximately 67% of the 'point of regard' locations in a given frame. The percentage of patients' points of regard falling inside the BCE should be 67% under a null hypothesis that the glaucomatous patients were, on average, viewing the same parts of the driving scene as the visually healthy subjects.

Monocular visual fields for the patients were merged to form an integrated visual field [19,31]: a simulated binocular visual field in which patients' best point-by-point monocular sensitivity is used (PROGRESSOR software: Moorfields Eye Hospital, London, UK/Medisoft Ltd., Leeds, UK). The software application developed in this work then aligns and scales a greyscale of this binocular field of view to the gaze point for each patient; this provides a dynamic illustration of a patient's restricted field of view as the film sequence runs, giving an insight into the difficulty of the task from the patient's perspective.

Results

Data from nine glaucomatous patients and ten age-matched healthy control subjects fulfilled the inclusion criteria used for this study. The mean age of the patients was 67.6 (SD:9.3) years compared to a mean age of 64.4 (SD = 11.4) years for the control subjects (Averages not significantly different; P = 0.52; two sample t-test. Variances not significantly different; P = 0.59; F-test). The self-reported mean number of years actively driving was 29 (SD = 10) and 30 (SD = 12) for the patients and the controls respectively (averages not significantly different; P = 0.86; two sample t-test). The patients had a range of visual field defect severity: average HFA mean defect (MD) was -8.0 (SD = 8.8) dB, -5.4 (SD = 5.7) dB and -8.9 (SD = 8.6) in the right eye, left eye and worse eye, respectively.

A small number of films were missing for the nine patients and ten control subjects because of corrupt data or particularly noisy sequences where more than 60% of the data were removed by the filtering: a threshold used in previous studies.[22] This affected results from one control subject and two glaucomatous patients, but none of these had fewer than 23 films available for analysis. Prior to settling on the numbers for this study, other subjects fulfilling all the other inclusion criteria for the study (2 patients and 2 controls) had several films (more than 12) where a large proportion of data were corrupt, missing, poorly calibrated or had more that 60% removed by the filtering algorithm: these subjects (some of whom had reported difficulty with the task or eye tracking failures) were not included in the final 19 assessed.

Each of the eye movement parameters was assessed in a GLM ANOVA: the departure of the F statistic (on 1 and 25 degrees of freedom) from 1 summarises the extent of a difference in the main factor (patients versus controls) and the P-value refers to the null hypothesis of no effect, or no difference, in that main factor. (No obvious departure from Normality was observed in any of the response variables as assessed by the Kolmogorov-Smirnov test). There was considerable statistical evidence that on average patients made more saccades per second ($P<0.001$; $F_{1,25} = 48.6$; mean increase 15.8%; 95% confidence interval [CI]: 9.2 to 22.4%), more fixations per second ($P<0.001$; $F_{1,25} = 53.4$; mean increase 16.9%; 95% CI: 11.7 to 22.1%) and more smooth pursuits per second ($P<0.001$; $F_{1,25} = 85.3$; mean increase 18.4%; 95% CI: 14.4 to 22.4%) than the control subjects. There was no evidence for a difference in average saccade amplitude ($P = 0.12$; $F_{1,25} = 2.6$) There was evidence of average duration of the fixations being shorter in patients ($P<0.001$; $F_{1,25} = 29.6$; mean difference 16.5%; 95% CI: 10.0 to 23.0%) compared to controls. There was also evidence of the average duration of smooth pursuits being significantly greater in the controls compared to the patients ($P<0.001$; $F_{1,25} = 22.1$; mean difference of 7.4%; 95% CI 3.2 to 11.6%). These results are further illustrated in figure 1: each graph considers a different eye movement parameter, with each point in the graph being the result from each of the 26 films. If the average value for an eye movement parameter for the patients was identical to the controls' then the point would fall exactly on the line of unity. The relative position of the points either below or above this line of unity gives a graphical indication of the magnitude and direction of the experimental effect and illustrates the ANOVA results.

Ten of the films had one hazard, fourteen films had two hazards and two films had three hazards. On average, and across all films, the 'hazardous' sections made up 18% (95% CI: 15 to 21%) of the total film sequence. The difference in each of the six eye movement parameters, for each film and for each subject was calculated then used as the response variable in a GLM ANOVA. As before, the F-statistic on the main factor (patients versus controls) was assessed, with the null hypothesis that there was, on average, no effect across the patients and controls between hazard and non-hazard sequences. There was no such significant effect in any of the eye movements across the main factor ($F_{1,25}$ less than 2.92 and P at least >0.10 in all 6 parameters). For example, the average percentage increase in number of saccades per second for the patients compared to controls was 15.7% during the non-hazard sequence (95% CI: 8.9 to 22.5) and 16.3% (95% CI: 6.2 to 26.4 %) during the hazard sequence. This does not support a hypothesis that differences in eye movement measurements between glaucomatous patients and control subjects became more significant or more exaggerated during the 'hazardous' parts of the film.

The BCE analysis attempted to compare the overall viewing region of the two groups (figure 2 and Audio/Video - S1). The mean number of points of regard that fell in the BCE was calculated for each patient with the overall average for the glaucomatous group being 62.8% (SD 8.3%). This average was clearly not significantly different from the theoretically expected value (67%) generated from the control group ($P = 0.49$; one sample t-test). In some films, this average value was as high as 84.9% and in others as low as 56.1% but there did not seem to be any observed pattern of viewing region in the patients departing from that of the controls being associated with the type of driving scene (e.g. rural, urban, divided highway/dual carriageway). In short, participants tended to view the same overall region of the driving scene whether they were glaucomatous or not, but this was on average, and considering the group as a whole. By using the software developed for this study it was possible to follow the viewing pattern of individual patients as they viewed the different films and compare this view with the pattern from all the control subjects simultaneously. Although difficult to quantify, there were some very revealing examples of individual patients clearly not following the control viewing pattern and unambiguous cases where the patient was unaware of emerging hazards. These examples became more informative when the integrated visual field defect of the patient was superimposed on the films giving a perspective of the patient's 'struggle' with their restrictive binocular central field defect. One of these cases is shown as a montage in figures 3 and as film clips in Audio/Video - S2, Audio/Video - S3.

Discussion

These results provide some new evidence that some characteristics of eye movements in glaucomatous patients with binocular visual field defects are different to those of healthy control subjects when performing the HPT. On average, the patients made more saccades and more fixations than controls. With this task we speculate that patients are, unconsciously or otherwise, making

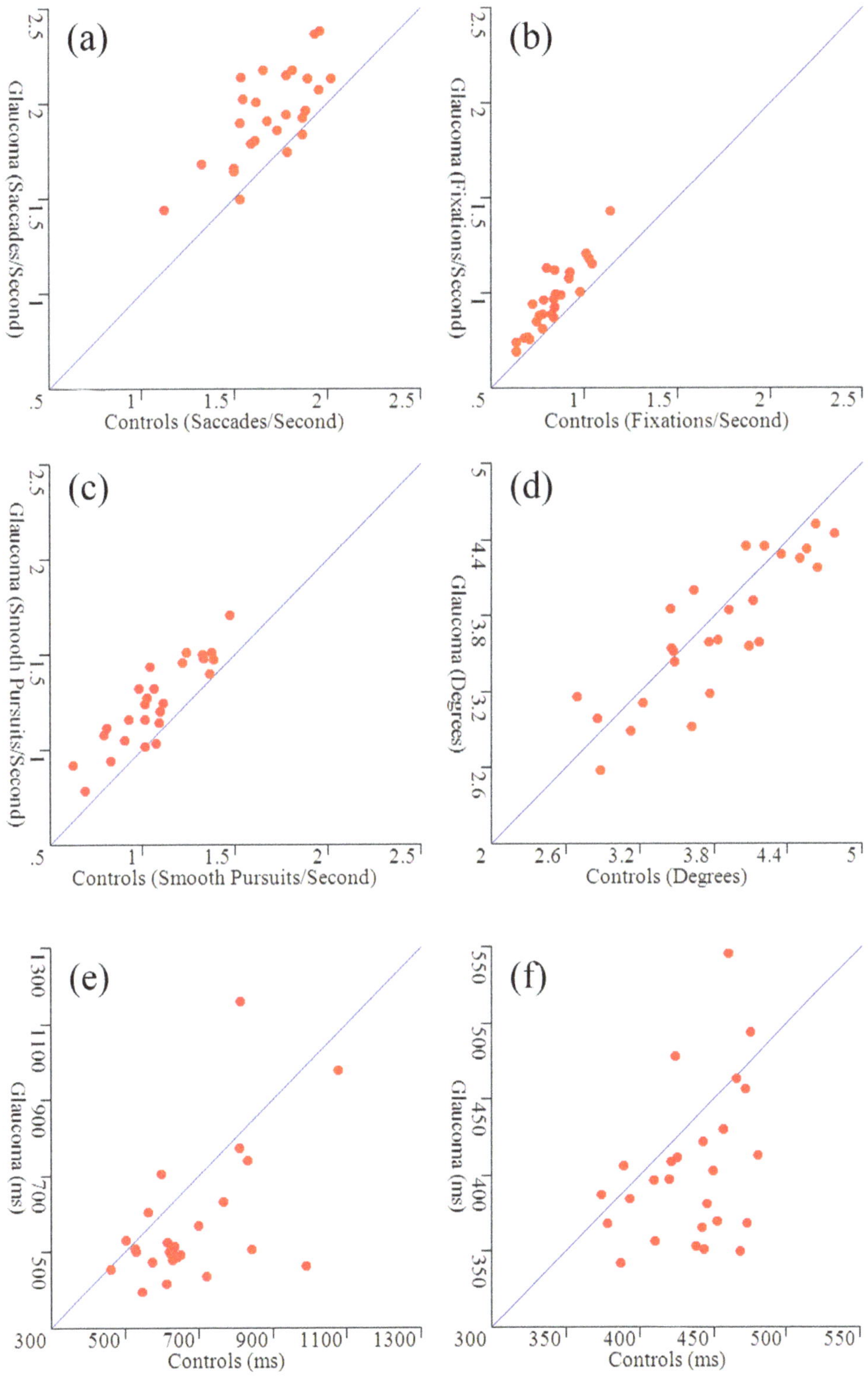

Figure 1. Eye movements for patients and controls. Graphs showing the average response in each eye movement parameter for the patients and the controls with (a) average number of saccades per second; (b) average number fixations per second; (c) number of smooth pursuits per second of film; (d) average saccade amplitude (size in degrees); (e) average fixation duration (ms); and (f) average 'smooth pursuit' duration (ms). Each symbol represents the results from one of the 26 films. If there were no differences in the averages then symbols would fall exactly on the line of unity. For example, (a) indicates that the patients made, on average, more saccades across the films than the control subjects, which illustrates the statistically significant effect found in the GLM ANOVA.

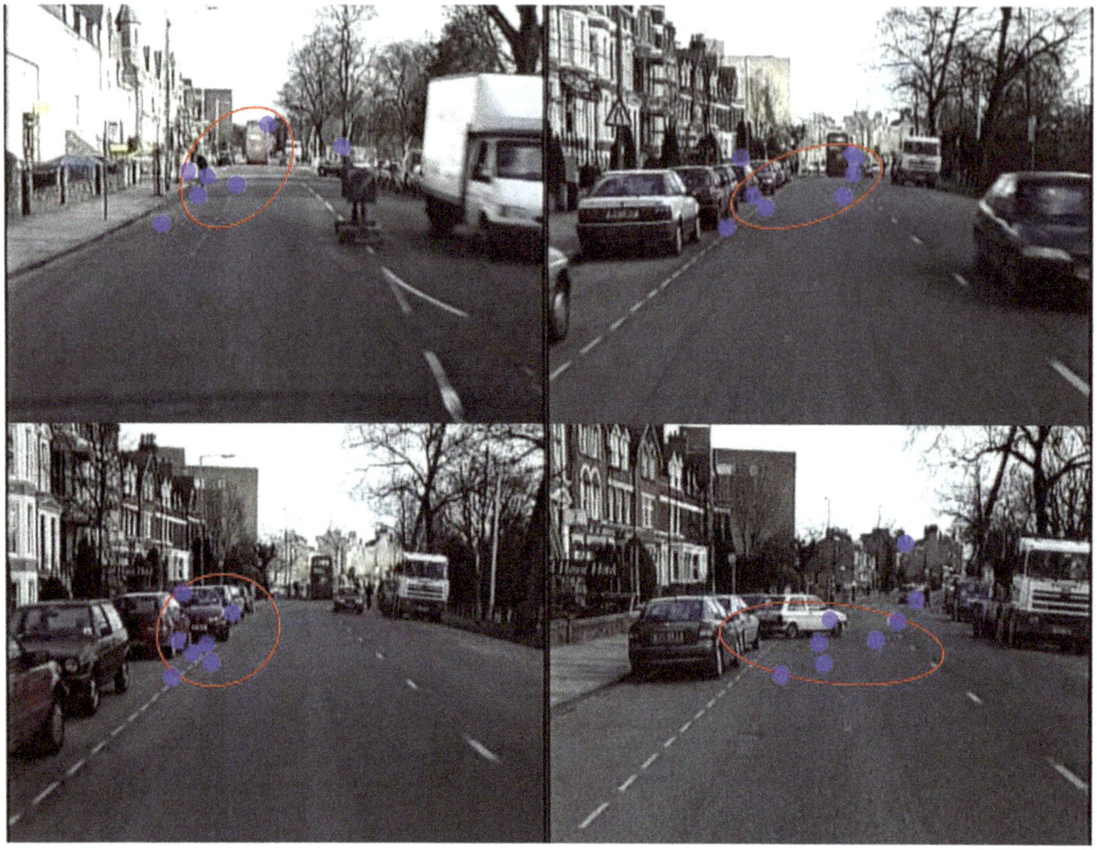

Figure 2. Novel 'Point of Regard' Analysis. Examples of the BCE 'point of regard' analysis superimposed on frames from some of the HPT films. The centre of the red ellipse represents the mean 'point of regard' of the controls with the spatial extent of the ellipse being one standard deviation from this centre along two principal axes, theoretically affording 'coverage' of approximately 67% of the 'point of regard' locations in a given frame. Note how the location and spatial extent of this ellipse changes with each frame of the film as the control subjects' view is drawn to different aspects of the changing road scene. For each frame the number of patients' points of regard (blue symbols) 'captured' by the ellipse can be automatically counted and compared to the expected value under the null hypothesis that the average 'viewing area' is the same in the two groups. Note that not all nine patients are recorded in each frame because of blinks, loss of data, and variable responses. Also, note that in the UK vehicles are driven on the left hand side of the road. See Audio/Video - S1.

more saccades to search the image as a 'compensation' for their restricted field of view. Since a binocular visual field defect reduces the amount of visual information available, this might suggest fewer eye movements [32], but this was not the case when patients were viewing these moving images. Our results also indicate that fixation duration was, on average, shorter with patients compared to controls. In contrast, it has been previously shown that fixation duration increases with the size of absolute central scotomas, but this was in a study using artificial scotomas on healthy subjects and a different task (searching a static image) [32]. Others have shown a reduction in fixation duration when an artificial scotoma is used to block foveal vision. [33]

Whilst most of the eye movement measurements were, on average, different between patients and controls, the BCE analysis indicated that patients were, on average, looking at the same areas as control subjects in the HPT movies. Despite the novelty and computational difficulty of this analysis it is probably too insensitive to the subtle departures in patient gaze as compared to the controls. The BCE area was often relatively large, being poorly estimated with so few controls. Moreover, there was no evidence from this sample to support the idea that eye movements become more or less exaggerated in patients compared to controls during the sequence of the film where a hazard was present or emerging. This temporal analysis suffers from the difficulty of the likely weaker estimates of the eye movement measurements during the hazard sequence because they only make up a smaller percentage of the film sequence. Looking at individual cases viewing individual films is helpful but provides little quantitative information about how the patients differ from a 'normal' viewer. A better post-hoc analysis might mark out areas in the frames that are of interest, perhaps associated with the looming hazards, and then quantify the patient's gaze falling in these areas. Such an analysis would need larger sample numbers than made available for this study to provide an adequate comparison.

Eye movement studies in 'real world' or simulated 'real world' environments have tended to focus on experiments with artificial scotomas or, when carried out in patient groups, with retinitis pigmentosa (RP) [34,35] and age-related macular degeneration (MD) [36]. Few studies have previously examined eye movement behaviour in glaucomatous subjects. An elegant study by Cheong et al [37] examined 'traffic gap' judgement and eye movements in subjects with peripheral visual field loss, including three subjects with glaucoma, as compared to healthy subjects. They reported restricted gaze patterns using the BCE approach but little evidence of difference in saccade amplitudes, or fixation duration. Eye tracking experiments by Geruschat et al [38] demonstrated that on

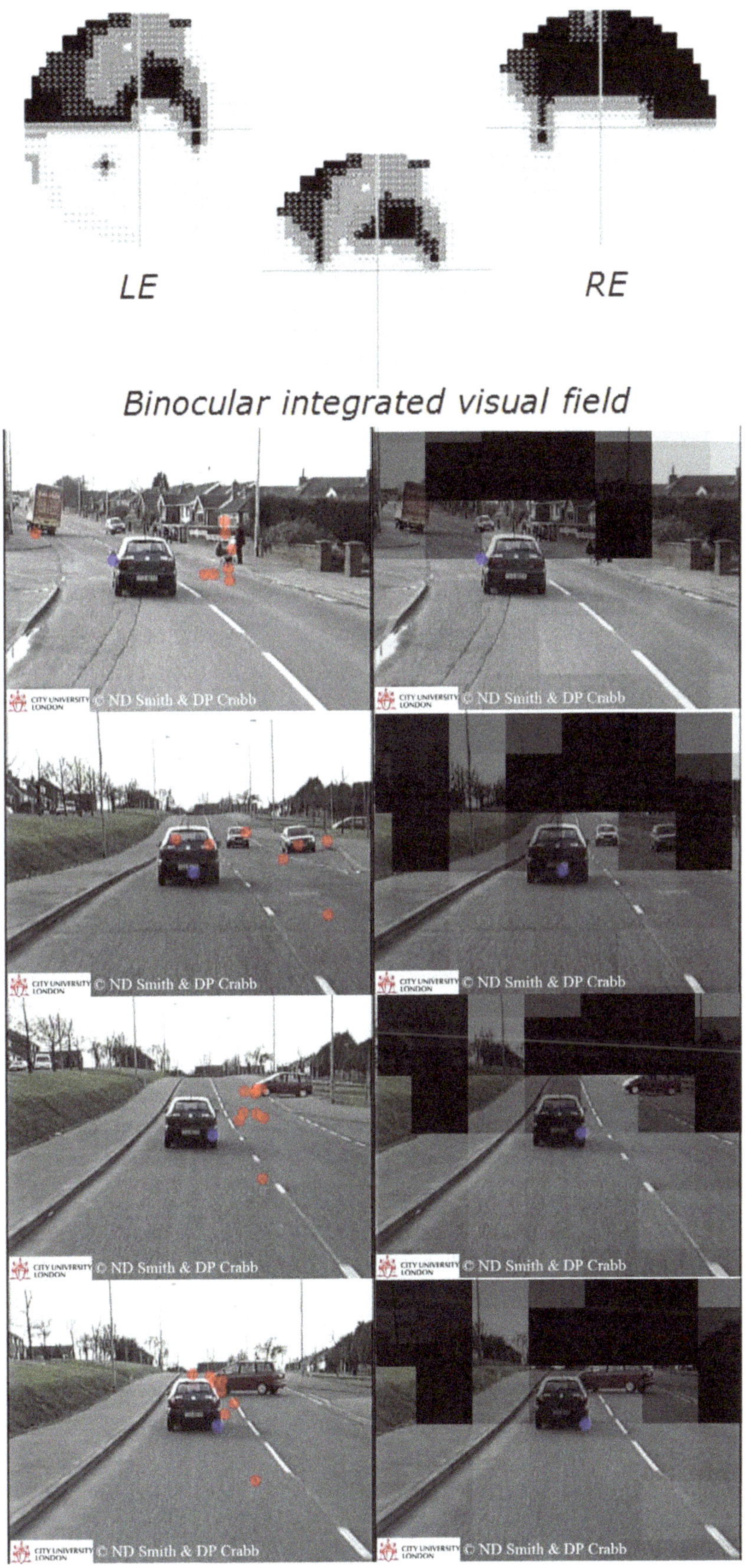

Figure 3. Visual fields, dynamic 'point of regard' and HPT films – example. HFA grayscales for monocular (30-2) and binocular integrated visual fields for one of the participants with bilateral glaucoma. The integrated visual field is scaled and superimposed on the point of regard HPT film

to give a representation of the restricted field of view. The panels show a montage of selected frames from one of the films. In the top frame, whilst most of visually healthy subjects (red symbols) fixate on the pedestrian with a pram/pushchair, seeing them as a potential hazard, the patient (blue symbol) fails to alter their gaze. Similarly in the next frames most of control subjects quickly move their fixation towards the looming hazard of the car hazardously turning on to the main street from the right intersection. Note that in the UK vehicles are driven on the left side of the road. The patient's view of this hazard is masked by their defect and they do not alter their gaze even at the late stage where the camera car 'brakes' to take evasive action (bottom frame). This patient has a binocular visual field that is on the borderline of satisfying the UK guideline for visual field fitness to drive. This montage is shown as a film in Audio/Video - S2 and Audio/Video - S3.

average glaucomatous patients (n = 12) had similar fixation patterns as compared to controls when crossing a street. Coeckelbergh et al [39] measured eye movements on a simple static search task and attempted to relate these to an actual on-road driving test in 50 subjects with field loss, some of whom were glaucomatous (number not given in the study). The number of fixations in the search task increased as a function of the size of the peripheral visual field defect, a finding consistent with our results. They reported some association between fixation duration and severity of central field defect but then indicated that eye movement parameters recorded during a simple static search task did not predict viewing behaviour in the actual task of driving. This is not surprising since gaze patterns are intrinsically related to the specific task: their patterns obtained from a static search task are likely to differ from patterns for a 'driving' task. Indeed eye movement patterns for the latter have been shown to be extremely complex [40].

The HPT was previously studied as a possible surrogate for the UK visual field standard for fitness to drive [18]. The main measurement considered was the press button response which yielded the percentage of hazards missed and the mean hazard response time. The main finding from this study was that the HPT, when using detection and speed of detection of the hazard, was of limited value when used alone in identifying subjects with visual field loss incompatible with current UK driving standards. Our current interest in the HPT is quite different: for the purpose of our current study, the HPT is used as a realistic, dynamic, visually challenging 'scene' whilst eye movements are simultaneously recorded.

As in any case-control study it is prudent to highlight potential confounders. The patients were age-matched to the controls and previous work with the HPT and eye movement analysis in healthy subjects has shown there is little evidence of an age-related difference in HPT performance anyway [41]. It has been previously shown that experienced drivers demonstrate more extensive scanning than the novices in performing the HPT [42,43]. In this study we only included participants that had driven for at least 5 years, and the patient and control groups were almost identically matched for self reported years of driving experience. Participants were excluded from the original study if they were on any 'significant medication' other than that for their glaucoma. Significant medication' included anti-depressants or treatment for diabetes or significant use of β-blocker medication, all of which were deliberately mentioned. However, this was done by self report rather than verification with their general medical practitioner and this might limit the interpretation of the results. Moreover, participants may not have reported use of mild anti-hypertensive or statins or other commonly used drugs in an elderly population. There is, however, no reason to suspect that the glaucomatous group would have had more or less of these participants compared to the age-matched control group.

Other caveats to be considered when interpreting the results from this study include the difficulty in truly identifying and separating the different types of eye movement, especially delineating saccades from smooth pursuits when the participant observes a moving image. This is a challenging task even with modern eye tracking instrumentation. We took the approach of excluding some subjects and removing significant sections of eye movement traces where it was not possible to identify clearly the different movements using an algorithm based on eye movement velocity developed for the purpose. The experiment was not an easy one for some subjects to perform, taking around 30 minutes to view all the film clips, and this probably contributed to the variability in the measurements. Furthermore, the patient group for our study was small, meaning population inference should be treated cautiously, but the sample size was certainly equivalent to those used in many experimental eye movement studies in the literature.

Anecdotally, some patients criticize the current static binocular visual field test (Esterman Test) used to establish legal fitness to drive in the UK for not allowing 'scanning' for a target. An eye movement and HPT task might be useful as a test for visual field restriction and fitness to drive. The set up would benefit from films shown on a larger screen, equivalent to that 'view' from a vehicle, and an eye tracker device that allows for natural movements. Such a test would not be reliant on press-button defined hazard detection but could simply monitor the patient's natural gaze. A post-hoc analysis of gaze patterns, compared to visually healthy control subjects, as illustrated in this study, could determine if patients 'saw' hazards, road/traffic signs and events that might provide evidence for them being visually 'safe' drivers. Taken alone it is very unlikely that such an idea would solve the difficulty of determining the vision standard for fitness to drive, the skills for which are so multifactorial that it defies one simple standard. Besides, the low task demand of watching a film may give an impression of competent driving performance that may not be maintained if someone is controlling a vehicle. Nevertheless, given the debate about current visual field standards for driving [44,45] such an approach may warrant further investigation.

The films showing, frame by frame, a patient's gaze pattern diverging from those of a number of visually healthy subjects provide a revealing insight into the visual impairment caused by glaucoma. This is particularly striking when the individual binocular visual field defects, made dynamic by aligning them to the moving point of regard, are superimposed on the films. One significant output from this work has been the use of these films in educational/awareness programmes for glaucoma in the UK and the subsequent interest they have generated, including a feature on the BBC (British Broadcasting Corporation) News [46].

In conclusion, this exploratory study provides some new evidence that patients with bilateral glaucoma exhibit different eye movement behaviour compared to visually healthy subjects when viewing a driving scene. We hope these results from this exploratory study will at least stimulate investigations into the novel idea that eye movement studies, perhaps coupled with work on patient's adaption to visual field defects, might provide a new 'window' into understanding the functional deficits of glaucoma. We speculate that understanding such 'real world' visual function deficits in glaucoma is perhaps a first step towards designing appropriate strategies for patient education about the impact of a visual field defect and potential rehabilitation, an overlooked area in this condition as compared, for example, to AMD and RP. Further studies in eye movements and glaucoma are already underway in our laboratory.

Supporting Information

Audio/Video S1 Novel 'Point of Regard' Analysis film. Video example of the BCE 'point of regard' analysis superimposed on a HPT film from figure 2. The centre of the red ellipse represents the mean 'point of regard' of the controls with the spatial extent of the ellipse being one standard deviation from this centre along two principal axes, theoretically affording 'coverage' of approximately 67% of the 'point of regard' locations in a given frame.
Found at: doi:10.1371/journal.pone.0009710.s001 (9.16 MB AVI)

Audio/Video S2 Participants 'point of regard' during HPT film. Video of the HPT film from figure 3 showing the 'point of regard' of all the control subjects. The blue point represents the point of regard for a glaucomatous patient Note that in the UK vehicles are driven on the left hand side of the road.
Found at: doi:10.1371/journal.pone.0009710.s002 (7.17 MB AVI)

Audio/Video S3 Participants 'point of regard' during HPT film showing a patient's 'view'. Video of the HPT film from figure 3 showing the 'point of regard' of the glaucomatous patient in video S2 with their binocular integrated visual field superimposed. The degree of transparency relates to the patients defect in that region, with the least transparent regions being most defective. Note that in the UK vehicles are driven on the left hand side of the road.
Found at: doi:10.1371/journal.pone.0009710.s003 (7.48 MB AVI)

Acknowledgments

We thank Darryl de Cunha and Alister Harlow for interfacing the HPT with eye-movement recordings in the original experiment. We also thank Professor Gary Rubin (Institute of Ophthalmology, University College London) for helpful suggestions about quantifying the eye movements.

Author Contributions

Conceived and designed the experiments: DPC JLB DFE. Performed the experiments: FGR CMC. Analyzed the data: DPC NDS. Contributed reagents/materials/analysis tools: NDS. Wrote the paper: DPC DFE DFGH.

References

1. Haymes SA, LeBlanc RP, Nicolela MT, Chiasson LA, Chauhan BC (2007) Risk of Falls and Motor Vehicle Collisions in Glaucoma. Investigative Ophthalmology & Visual Science 48: 1149–1155.
2. White SC, Atchison KA, Gornbein JA, Nattiv A, Paganini-Hill A, et al. (2006) Risk factors for fractures in older men and women: The Leisure World Cohort Study. Gender Medicine 3: 110–123.
3. Szlyk JPP, Mahler CLMS, Seiple WP, Edward DPMD, Wilensky JTMD (2005) Driving Performance of Glaucoma Patients Correlates With Peripheral Visual Field Loss. Journal of Glaucoma 14: 145–150.
4. Jampel HD, Friedman DS, Quigley H, Miller R (2002) Correlation of the Binocular Visual Field with Patient Assessment of Vision. Invest Ophthalmol Vis Sci 43: 1059–1067.
5. Viswanathan AC, McNaught AI, Poinoosawmy D, Fontana L, Crabb DP, et al. (1999) Severity and Stability of Glaucoma: Patient Perception Compared With Objective Measurement. Arch Ophthalmol 117: 450–454.
6. Friedman DS, Freeman E, Munoz B, Jampel HD, West SK (2007) Glaucoma and Mobility Performance: The Salisbury Eye Evaluation Project. Ophthalmology 114: 2232–2237.e2231.
7. Nelson PP, Aspinall PP, Papasouliotis OP, Worton BP, O'Brien CMDFF (2003) Quality of Life in Glaucoma and Its Relationship with Visual Function. Journal of Glaucoma 12: 139–150.
8. Noe G, Ferraro J, Lamoureux E, Rait J, Keeffe JE (2003) Associations between glaucomatous visual field loss and participation in activities of daily living. Clinical & Experimental Ophthalmology 31: 482–486.
9. Altangerel U, Spaeth GL, Steinmann WC (2006) Assessment of Function Related to Vision (AFREV). Ophthalmic Epidemiology 13: 67–80.
10. Kotecha A, O'Leary N, Melmoth D, Grant S, Crabb DP (2009) The Functional Consequences of Glaucoma for Eye-Hand Coordination. Invest Ophthalmol Vis Sci 50: 203–213.
11. Haymes SA, LeBlanc RP, Nicolela MT, Chiasson LA, Chauhan BC (2008) Glaucoma and On-Road Driving Performance. Invest Ophthalmol Vis Sci 49: 3035–3041.
12. Johnson CA, Keltner JL (1983) Incidence of visual field loss in 20,000 eyes and its relationship to driving performance. Arch Ophthalmol 101: 371–375.
13. McGwin G, Jr., Mays A, Joiner W, DeCarlo DK, McNeal S, et al. (2004) Is Glaucoma Associated with Motor Vehicle Collision Involvement and Driving Avoidance? Investigative Ophthalmology & Visual Science 45: 3934–3939.
14. Ang GS, Eke T (2006) Lifetime visual prognosis for patients with primary open-angle glaucoma. Eye 21: 604–608.
15. Owen VMF, Crabb DP, White ET, Viswanathan AC, Garway-Heath DF, et al. (2008) Glaucoma and Fitness to Drive: Using Binocular Visual Fields to Predict a Milestone to Blindness. Invest Ophthalmol Vis Sci 49: 2449–2455.
16. Bhargava JS, Patel B, Foss AJE, Avery AJ, King AJ (2006) Views of Glaucoma Patients on Aspects of Their Treatment: An Assessment of Patient Preference by Conjoint Analysis. Invest Ophthalmol Vis Sci 47: 2885–2888.
17. Chisholm CM, Rauscher FG, Crabb DP, Davies LN, Dunne MC, et al. (2008) Assessing visual fields for driving in patients with paracentral scotomata. Br J Ophthalmol 92: 225–230.
18. Rauscher F, Chisholm C, Crabb D Central scotomata and driving. Road safety research report 79, compiled for UK Department for Transport.
19. Crabb DP, Fitzke FW, Hitchings RA, Viswanathan AC (2004) A practical approach to measuring the visual field component of fitness to drive. Br J Ophthalmol 88: 1191–1196.
20. Grayson G, Sexton B (2002) Hazard Perception Test. Transport Research Laboratory TRL558.
21. Smith ND, Chisholm CM, Edgar DF, Barbur JL, Garway-Heath DF, et al. (2007) Eye Movement analysis in Glaucoma When Viewing a Driving Hazards Perception Test. ECEM. Potsdam, Germany.
22. Crossland MD, Rubin GS (2002) The use of an infrared eyetracker to measure fixation stability. Optometry and Vision Science 79: 735–739.
23. van der Geest J (2002) Recording eye movements with video-oculography and scleral search coils: a direct comparison of two methods. Journal of Neuroscience Methods 114: 185–195.
24. Hsiao JH, Cottrell G (2008) Two Fixations Suffice in Face Recognition. Psychological Science 19: 998–1006.
25. Stampe DM (1993) Heuristic filtering and reliable calibration methods for video based pupil tracking systems. Behavior Research Methods, Instruments, and Computers 25: 137–142.
26. Bellmann C, Feely M, Crossland MD, Kabanarou SA, Rubin GS (2004) Fixation stability using central and pericentral fixation targets in patients with age-related macular degeneration. Ophthalmology 111: 2265–2270.
27. González E, Teichman J, Lillakas L, Markowitz S, Steinbach M (2006) Fixation stability using radial gratings in patients with age-related macular degeneration. Can J Ophthalmol 41: 333–339.
28. Goldstein RB, Woods RL, Peli E (2007) Where people look when watching movies: Do all viewers look at the same place? Computers in Biology and Medicine 37: 957–964.
29. Altman DG (1978) Plotting Probability Ellipses. Applied Statistics 27: 347–349.
30. Healy HJR (1972) Drawing a Probability Ellipse. Applied Statistics 21: 202–204.
31. Crabb DP, Viswanathan AC (2005) Integrated visual fields: a new approach to measuring the binocular field of view and visual disability. Graefe's Archive for Clinical and Experimental Ophthalmology 243: 210–216.
32. Cornelissen FWP, Bruin KJP, Kooijman ACP (2005) The Influence of Artificial Scotomas on Eye Movements during Visual Search. Optometry & Vision Science 82: 27–35.
33. Henderson JM, McClure KK, Pierce S, Schrock G (1997) Object identification without foveal vision: Evidence from an artificial scotoma paradigm. Perception & Psychophysics 59: 323–346.
34. Vargas-Martin F, Peli E (2006) Eye Movements of Patients with Tunnel Vision While Walking. Invest Ophthalmol Vis Sci 47: 5295–5302.
35. Turano KA, Geruschat DR, Baker FH, Stahl JW, Shapiro MD (2001) Direction of Gaze while Walking a Simple Route: Persons with Normal Vision and Persons with Retinitis Pigmentosa. Optometry and Vision Science 78: 667–675.
36. Crossland MD, Rubin GS (2006) Eye movements and reading in macular disease: further support for the shrinking perceptual span hypothesis. Vision Res 46: 590–597.
37. Cheong AMY, Geruschat DR, Congdon N (2008) Traffic Gap Judgment in People with Significant Peripheral Field Loss. Optometry and Vision Science 85: 26–36.
38. Geruschat DR, Hassan SE, Turano KA, Quigley HA, Congdon NG (2006) Gaze Behavior of the Visually Impaired During Street Crossing. Optometry and Vision Science 83: 550–558.
39. Coeckelbergh TRM, W. Cornelissen F, H. Brouwer W, C. Kooijman A (2002) The effect of visual field defects on eye movements and practical fitness to drive. Vision Research 42: 669–677.
40. Land MF, Lee DN (1994) Where we look when we steer. Nature 369: 742–744.

41. Underwood G, Phelps N, Wright C, Loon E, Galpin A (2005) Eye fixation scanpaths of younger and older drivers in a hazard perception task. Ophthalmic and Physiological Optics 25: 346–356.
42. Underwood G, Chapman P, Bowden K, Crundall D (2002) Visual search while driving: skill and awareness during inspection of the scene. Transportation Research Part F: Traffic Psychology and Behaviour 5: 87–97.
43. Underwood G, Chapman P, Brocklehurst N, Underwood J, Crundall D (2003) Visual attention while driving: sequences of eye fixations made by experienced and novice drivers. Ergonomics 46: 629–646.
44. Kotecha A, Spratt A, Viswanathan A (2008) Visual function and fitness to drive. Br Med Bull 87: 163–174.
45. Westlake W (2000) Another look at visual standards and driving. BMJ 321: 972–973.
46. BBC (2008) Available at: http://news.bbc.co.uk/1/hi/health/7660570.stm. BBC News. UK.

2

Serum and Antibodies of Glaucoma Patients Lead to Changes in the Proteome, Especially Cell Regulatory Proteins, in Retinal Cells

Katharina Bell, Sebastian Funke, Norbert Pfeiffer, Franz H. Grus*

Experimental Ophthalmology, Department of Ophthalmology, Medical Center of the Johannes Gutenberg University, Mainz, Germany

Abstract

Purpose: Previous studies show significantly specifically changed autoantibody reactions against retinal antigens in the serum of glaucoma and ocular hypertension (OHT) patients in comparison to healthy people. As pathogenesis of glaucoma still is unknown the aim of this study was to analyze if the serum and antibodies of glaucoma patients interact with neuroretinal cells.

Methods: R28 cells were incubated with serum of patients suffering from primary open angle glaucoma (POAG), normal tension glaucoma (NTG) or OHT, POAG serum after antibody removal and serum from healthy people for 48 h under a normal or an elevated pressure of 15000 Pa (112 mmHg). RGC5 cells were additionally incubated with POAG antibodies under a normal pressure. Protein profiles of the R28 cells were measured with Seldi-Tof-MS, protein identification was performed with Maldi-TofTof-MS. Protein analysis of the RGC5 cells was performed with ESI-Orbitrap MS. Statistical analysis including multivariate statistics, variance component analysis as well as calculating Mahalanobis distances was performed.

Results: Highly significant changes of the complex protein profiles after incubation with glaucoma and OHT serum in comparison to healthy serum were detected, showing specific changes in the cells (e.g. Protein at 9192 Da ($p<0.001$)). The variance component analysis showed an effect of the serum of 59% on the cells. The pressure had an effect of 11% on the cells. Antibody removal led to significantly changed cell reactions ($p<0.03$). Furthermore, the incubation with POAG serum and its antibodies led to pro-apoptotic changes of proteins in the cells.

Conclusions: These studies show that the serum and the antibodies of glaucoma patients significantly change protein expressions involved in cell regulatory processes in neuroretinal cells. These could lead to a higher vulnerability of retinal cells towards stress factors such as an elevated IOP and eventually could lead to an increased apoptosis of the cells as in glaucoma.

Editor: Demetrios Vavvas, Massachusetts Eye & Ear Infirmary, Harvard Medical School, United States of America

Funding: DOG (Deutsche Ophthalmologische Gesellschaft) funding for innovative scientific work; 2008. The funders had no role in study design, data collection and analysis, decision to publish, or preparation of the manuscript.

Competing Interests: The authors have declared that no competing interests exist.

* E-mail: grus@eye-research.org

Introduction

Glaucoma, a group of diseases leading to loss of retinal ganglion cells (rgc) with still unknown pathogenesis, is a leading cause for blindness worldwide, as the estimated number of affected people counting nearly 7 million shows [1]. The most common form of glaucoma, the primary open angle glaucoma (POAG), is accompanied by an elevated intraocular pressure (IOP). But approximately 30% of the patients don't show an elevated IOP (normal tension glaucoma (NTG)) [2]. Additionally 4–7% of people over the age of 40 have ocular hypertension (OHT) [3] but per year only 1% develop glaucoma [4,5]. Therefore, although still a major risk factor, the presumption that an elevated IOP is the only cause for glaucoma is long out-dated. Glaucoma can be added to the long list of neurodegenerative diseases with mostly unknown pathogenesis, conditions characterized by progressive nervous system dysfunction and often accompanied by the atrophy of the affected central or peripheral nervous system structures [6].

As in other neurodegenerative diseases, such as amyotrophic lateral sclerosis, Alzheimer's and Parkinson disease, glaucoma leads to the apoptotic loss of one specific neuron population, the rgc [7]. An atrophy of central structures such as the lateral geniculate nucleus [8] can also be found. Keeping the number of people affected in mind, glaucoma can be contemplated as one of the most common neurodegenerative diseases [9]. Many possible aspects to the pathway of destruction of the rgc other than an apoptosis [10,11] through elevated IOP are being discussed, most importantly an elevated nitric oxide level [12], a T-cell mediated process [13] or an autoimmune process [14], all including an involvement of intracellular cascades leading to cell death [15,16], which could be possibly caused by a crucial serum factor present in glaucoma patients. Changes in the antibody spectra towards retinal or optic nerve antigens in glaucoma patients (POAG and

NTG) but also OHT patients in comparison to healthy people [17,18] were demonstrated and give a hint to this crucial serum factor. The existence of autoantibodies against retinal or optic nerve head antigens also in healthy people is part of the so called natural autoimmunity [19], which has been demonstrated in many other studies [20].

Considering antibody (Ab) expressions changes and studies showing rgc apoptosis after treatment with an elevated hydrostatic pressure [11], our aim was to determine the effect of serum and Abs from glaucoma patients and different pressure levels on R28 and RGC5 cells, not only by analyzing the viability, but also taking a deeper look at the processes of the cell during different treatments by measuring their protein expression profiles. A cell cultural approach with the established neuroretinal cells R28 [21] [provided as a gift by G M. Seigel; Ross Eye Institute, University of Buffalo] and the established RGC5 cell line [22,23] [provided as a gift by N. Agarwal; Fort Worth, Texas USA] was performed, incubating the cells with serum from POAG, NTG and OHT patients, serum from healthy people and POAG serum after Ab removal under a normal or elevated pressure. Furthermore the cells were treated with the Ab's from POAG patients.

We hypothesize that the serum of glaucoma patients can lead to changes in cell regulatory processes of the cells which make the cells more vulnerable to stress factors and eventually can lead to apoptosis of the cells. Furthermore we believe that the antibodies in the serum of glaucoma patients play a major role in this effect.

Materials and Methods

Ethics Statement

The studies were performed in accordance with the Declaration of Helsinki on medical research involving human subjects. Informed consent from all participants giving serum in for this study was obtained in a written form. The ethics committee of the Landesärztekammer Rheinland-Pfalz approved this study, approval number: No: 817.219.07(5754).

Cell culture

The neuroretinal cell line R28 [provided as a gift by G M. Seigel; Ross Eye Institute, University of Buffalo] and RGC5 cells [provided as a gift by N. Agarwal; Fort Worth, Texas USA] were used. The R28 cells were cultured in Dulbecco's modified Eagles Medium (DMEM) containing 10% Fetal Bovine Serum (FBS; Cambrex Bioscience, Verviers, Belgien), 5 mg/ml Gentamicine-Glutamine Solution (Sigma-Aldrich GmbH, Steinheim), 10% MEM Vitamins (100× (Invitrogen)) and 10% MEM non essential amino acids (100× (Invitrogen)). RGC5 cells were cultured in DMEM containing 10% FBS, 1% Penicillin/Streptomycin (Sigma-Aldrich GmbH) and 4% L-Alanyl-L-Glutamine (Biochrom). Both were grown in a humidified atmosphere of 95% air and 5% CO_2 at 37°C.

Experimental setup

R28 cells were incubated with 10% non heat inactivated serum from POAG, NTG or OHT patients or healthy people for 48 h. One experiment was conducted using POAG and healthy serum (n each group = 9). In a further experiment additionally NTG and OHT serum was used (n each group = 12). An experiment using POAG, healthy and POAG serum after Ab removal with protein G beads was conducted (n each group = 4). The cells were incubated at a normal pressure or an elevated pressure of 15000 Pa in culture dishes with an 82.7 mm inner diameter. 250 000 cells were used. After 48 h, cell lysis was performed (Buffer: Urea 9.5 M, Chaps 2%, DTT 1%+proteinase inhibitor mix (P 1860 (Sigma-Aldrich)) with an ultrasonic pulse echo instrument (Labsonic®M (Sartorius). Protein concentration was determined with the method of Lowry [24].

A titration curve using different concentrations of healthy or POAG serum was performed. R28 cells were incubated under an elevated and normal pressure with different serum concentrations (2.5, 5, 7.5 and 10%; n in each group = 4).

Protein profiles were measured with Seldi-TOF MS. Protein identification was performed with Maldi-TOFTOF-MS.

Additionally, RGC5 cells were incubated with 5% FBS+ 5% healthy or 5% POAG serum or+the ABs of 5% POAG serum. After cell lysis, a SDS gel was performed with the pooled samples. The lanes were divided into 15 pieces and digested with trypsin, to measure the peptide profile with capillary LC-ESI-MSMS.

The viability of R28 cells after treatment with different serum types (POAG, healthy, bovine) and under different pressure conditions was measured with WST-1 test (Roche, Mannheim). The cells were grown in 96 well plates and treated as described above (n of each group = 20). After 48 h WST-1 reagent was added and the cells were measured using an Elisa plate reader at 450 nm.

Serum samples

The serum was collected from patients suffering from POAG, NTG or OHT according to the classification of the guidelines of the European glaucoma society as well as from healthy volunteers after given informed consent. Furthermore patients suffering from autoimmune diseases or other neurodegenerative diseases were excluded from the study. In general no systemic diseases were dominantly represented in one of the experimental groups and therefore a correlation between the measured effects and a systemic disease can be excluded.

Protein profiling with Seldi- TOF-MS

An acetone precipitation of 150 µg protein was undertaken. 8 times the amount of −80°C acetone was added and incubated on ice (30 min). The samples were centrifuged (14000 rpm, 4°C, 30 min). 2 µl of the sample was spotted on the protein chips for Seldi-Tof-MS using weak cationic exchanger (CM10) or reversed-phase surface (H50) chips. A surface-enhanced laser desorption/ionisation time-of-flight mass spectrometer (PBS-II SELDI-TOF (Ciphergen Biosystems Inc., Fremont) was used. The samples were covered with sinapic acid matrix (20 mg Sinapic acid, 750 µl acetonitrile (ACN), 750 µl H_2O-HPLC, 15 µl Trifluoroacetic acid (TFA)). Measurements were performed according to the manufacturer's protocol.

Protein identification with Maldi-TOFTOF-MS

Matrix-**A**ssisted-**L**aser-**D**esorption/**I**onization based **mass-s**pectrometry (Ultraflex MALDI TOF/TOF (Bruker Daltonik GmbH, Bremen)) was used to identify the significantly changed proteins. After protein separation via SDS-Page (Invitrogen), a tryptic digestion of the bands including the significantly changed proteins was performed. In order to detect whether the specific protein was included in the protein band of the gel, an elution of the proteins was performed and measured with Seldi-TOF-MS. Only after detecting the wanted protein in the measurement, the tryptic digestion was performed. 1 µl of the digested proteins was loaded onto a Maldi anchor target using 2×0.5 µl cinnamic-acid matrix (17 mg α-Cyano-4-hydroxycinnamic acid, 4.8 mL HPLC H_2O, 5 mL ACN, 200 µl TFA). Measurements were performed according to the manufacturer's protocol. Protein identification was performed using the mascot search engine using SwissProt database.

Protein profiling with capillary LC-ESI-MSMS

RGC5 cells were analyzed with capillary LC-ESI-MSMS using a C-18 pre-column (30 mm×0.5 mm) and a C18 analytical column (150 mm×0.5 mm, both Thermo Scientific,). A Rheos Allegro HPLC Pump (Thermo Scientific) was the solvent delivery system. The pump flow rate was 200 µl/min, and reduced to a column flow of 10 µl/min (M-472 graduated microsplit valve (Upchurch, Scientific, USA)). With two running buffers (A(98%H_2O, 1.94% ACN, 0,06% methanol, 0.05% TFA)+B(95% ACN, 3% methanol, 2% H_2O, 0.05% TFA) a linear gradient of 80 min was performed (0–47 min: 0–100%B, 47–49 min: 100% B, 49–58: 100% -0% B, 58–80 min: 0%B). Mass spectra were obtained using an LTQ OrbitrapXL.

Statistical analysis

A list of peak clusters measured with Seldi-TOF MS was generated and exported to a statistical analysis program (Statistica, ver. 8.0; Statsoft, Tulsa, OK). Multivariate discriminant analysis based on combinations of multiple protein peaks was calculated. A variance component and mixed model ANOVA was calculated to determine the influence of the dependent (serum, pressure) and independent variables on the protein profiles. The Mahalanobis distances were calculated to show changes after Ab removal.

The data from the capillary LC-ESI-MSMS analysis was used for quantification of the identified proteins in the different samples, after normalizing the intensity of the proteins using the total ion current (TIC). A comparison to the cells incubated with healthy serum was performed.

Antibody depletion

The Ab's for the first study were removed using magnetic protein G beads (Dynabeads®Protein G; Dynal Biotech). 20 µl beads were used to purify 35 µl serum. They were washed (2×600 µl NaAc, pH5 2 min, 1×5 min), added to the POAG serum and incubated at 12°C on an orbital shaker for 6 h. The beads with Abs were discarded and the remaining serum was used for cell incubation. The antibodies were washed from the beads and measured with Seldi-Tof-MS to prove the removal from the serum or at least a large amount of Ab depletion (see Figure S1 for Seldi-spectrum).

For the following study with Ab depletion, the Abs were removed with the Nab Protein G Spin Kit (Thermo scientific), which removes IgG from samples, e.g. serum. The Abs can be released from the columns. Ab removal from the serum was confirmed by measuring the Abs in a SDS gel (see Figure S2) showing Ab bands and their fractions [25].

Results

Glaucoma serum changes cell proteins

The very complex protein and peptide profiles of the R28 cells showed approximately 400 different protein clusters ranging from 3078 Dalton (Da) to 180 kDa. Some sample measurements can be seen in Figure 1 showing Seldi-TOF MS measurements from cells of different experimental groups. The analysis of discriminance showed several highly significantly different regulated proteins, when comparing cells incubated with POAG serum to cells incubated with healthy serum, The significantly changed proteins are listed in Table S1. The table shows the molecular weight of the proteins as well as the calculated p- values. Some of the differently expressed proteins of R28 cells incubated with POAG serum could successfully be identified using Maldi-TofTof-MS e.g. the protein at 9192 Da (Histone4) and the protein at 12390 Da (Profilin) (also listed in Table S1).

Figure 2 A and B shows several of the significantly differently regulated proteins. The proteins at 9192 Da ($p = 0.000058$) and at12390 Da ($p = 0.000086$) are shown. To also detect overall changes in the protein profiles of the cells, the Mahalanobis distances were calculated, showing not only significant changes of single proteins but also of the protein profiles in general. We were able to detect the largest Mahalanobis distance between the cells incubated with POAG serum and an elevated pressure in comparison to control cells incubated with healthy serum (28.1, p-value<0.01). The Mahalanobis distance between cells incubated with POAG serum to healthy controls was 6.5 and between cells incubated with healthy serum+pressure and control cells 4.6 (p-values<0.01). The Mahalanobis distances show the overall changes between experimental groups in comparison to one known/control group.. The larger the distance, the larger the difference between the protein profiles in the experimental groups.

In the second experiment the analysis showed significant differences between cells incubated with OHT serum and healthy or POAG serum, as well as cells incubated with NTG serum and healthy or POAG serum. Significant differences between protein profiles of cells incubated with NTG or OHT serum were detected. Figure S3 of the supplementary information shows an overview of measured protein profiles of cells incubated with NTG serum in comparison to POAG or healthy serum showing different expression levels of proteins depending on the treatment group. Cells incubated with POAG or healthy serum in comparison to OHT serum also showed significant differences in their protein profiles. Canonical roots were calculated showing a clear differentiation between cells incubated either with POAG, OHT or healthy serum (Figure 3).

Serum influence's cells most significantly

We detected a 60% loss of viability after stress through an elevated pressure after 48 h (T-test, $p<0.01$; Table S2). When comparing the viability of the cells incubated either with glaucoma or healthy serum no differences between the experimental groups were detected (T-test, $p = 0.94$, see Table S3). The calculated variance component analysis demonstrated that the serum had the largest effect on the protein profiles of the cells (59%, Table 1). The pressure only had an 11.6% influence, but had an additional effect of 14% on the serum influence. The large influence of the serum also was detected for the significantly changed proteins, e.g. on the protein at 9192 Da (55.2%, Table 1).

Antibodies cause part of effect

After Ab removal the variance component analysis (Table 2) showed an influence of the Abs on the protein profiles of 50.5%. The calculated Mahalanobis distances showed that the overall protein expression profiles of these cells changed significantly when removing the antibodies from the POAG serum ($p<0.03$; Table 3).

To detect whether cells reacted similar to incubation with POAG serum and the Abs of POAG patients, RGC5 cells were incubated with healthy serum, POAG serum and the Abs of POAG patients. A protein profiles analysis was performed. We identified 3124 proteins. 198 Proteins were significantly differently regulated (<-4 or >4 fold different expression) in cells incubated with POAG serum in comparison to cells incubated with healthy serum (The significantly differently regulated proteins are listed in Table S4). 82 Proteins were significantly up- or down- regulated (<-4 or >4 fold different expression) in those cells incubated with the POAG Abs (list of proteins: see Table S5). 56% of the significantly changed proteins in cells incubated with POAG Abs were concordantly regulated in cells incubated with POAG serum.

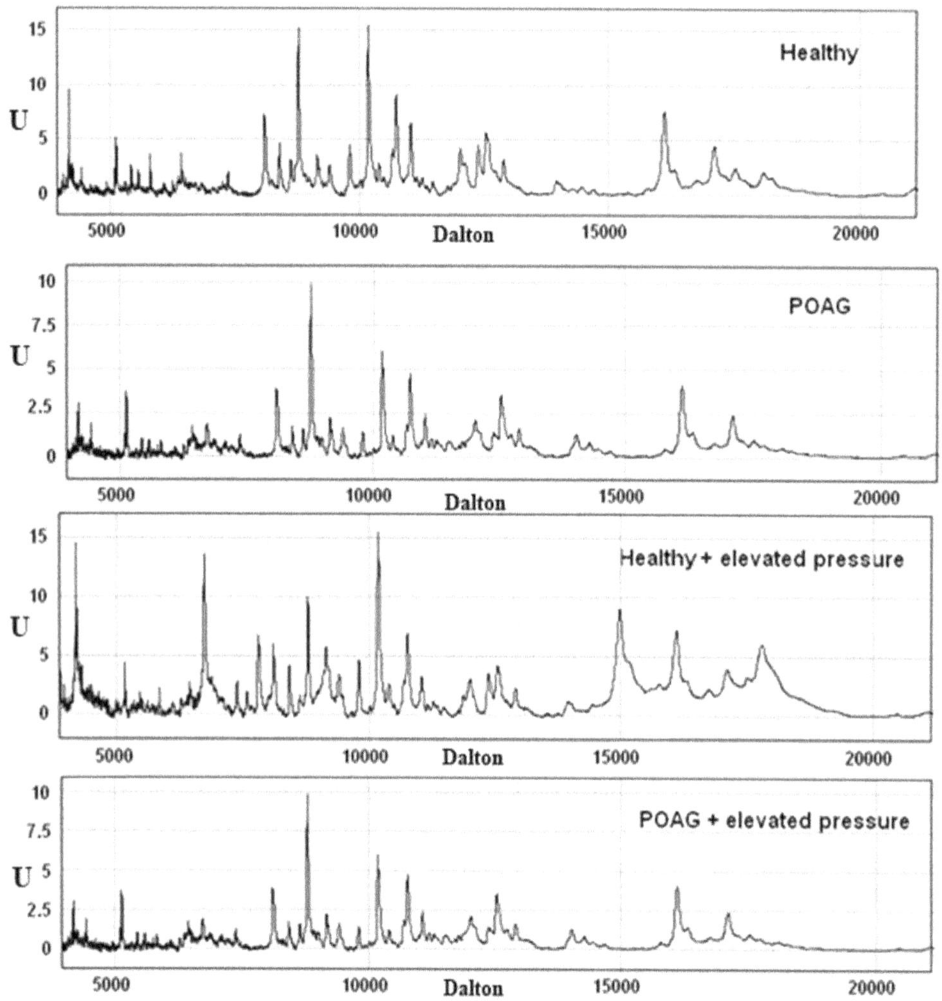

Figure 1. Complex protein profiles in every experimental group. Figure 1 shows examples of protein profiles measured with Seldi-TOF MS. Protein profiles from different experimental groups are shown. The X axis shows the molecular weight in Dalton and the Y axis the intensity of the protein in the sample. Differences between the experimental groups can be seen.

34% of the proteins significantly changed in cells incubated with POAG Abs showed the same tendency of regulation in cells incubated with POAG serum without being significant in both groups. Only 5% of the significantly changed proteins in cells incubated with POAG Abs showed significant changes in the opposite direction in cells incubated with POAG serum.

The analysis of the changed proteins showed that they mostly were associated with cell regulatory functions (see Table S6). Using Ingenuity pathway analysis (Ingenuity® Systems, Redwood City, California, USA) we found, that many of the significantly changed proteins were associated with cell death pathways, cell growth and proliferation pathways or RNA- posttranscriptional modification pathways.

Some of the significantly changed proteins were regulated in a pro-apoptotic manner. One of the pathways affected by incubation with POAG serum was a mitochondrial pathway. We found an up-regulation of BAK and BAX both involved in the mitochondrial apoptosis pathway [26] as well as an up-regulation of Gas2 which leads to cell shrinkage and cell blebbing [27]. Furthermore we were able to detect a down-regulation of the anti-apoptotic protein PARP which has a DNA-repair function. The connection between the different proteins is shown in Figure 4. Proteins indicated in a red colour are up-regulated whereas proteins indicated with green are down-regulated.

Proteins differently regulated in the cells incubated with POAG Abs were mostly associated with pathways regulating cellular development and cell cycle. A list of proteins involved in apoptosis and significantly differently regulated in cells incubated with POAG Abs is shown in Table S6.

Serum effect seems to be dependent on serum concentration

We detected that some of the proteins showed a concentration dependent behavior e.g. the significantly up-regulated protein at 4432 Da (Fig. 5A). When looking at other proteins, we detected many showing a concentration dependent behavior, e.g. the protein at 11572 Da (Fig. 5B).

Discrimination between glaucoma and non-glaucoma possible

Based on the protein profiles of R28 cells incubated with POAG, NTG or healthy serum, artificial networks were calculated to detect the discrimination potential between glaucoma and non-glaucoma. A receiver operating characteristic (ROC) curve was

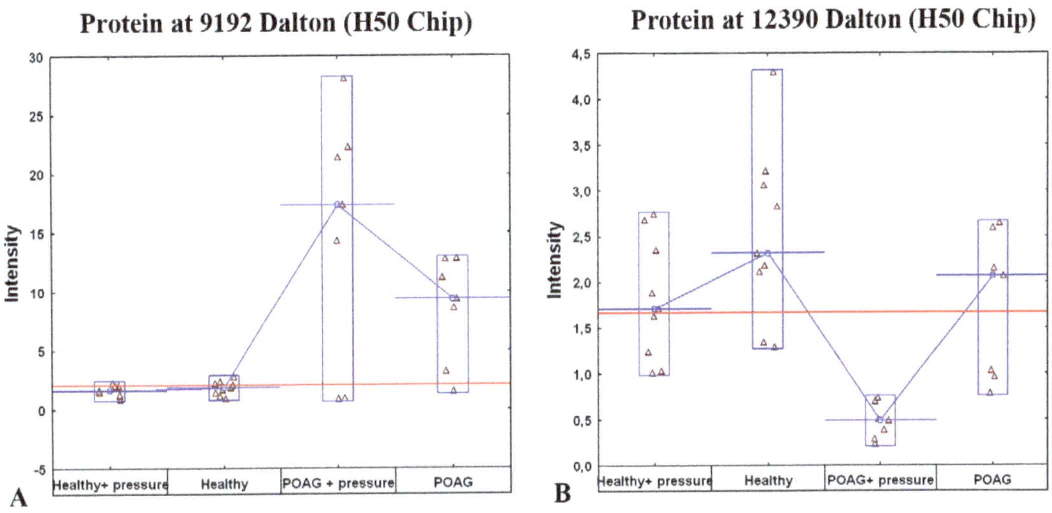

Figure 2. Significantly differently regulated proteins in cells incubated with glaucoma serum. Figure 2A and 2B show several variability plots of the calculated significantly changed proteins with the molecular weights of 9192 and 12390 Dalton. The X axis represents the different experimental groups and the Y axis shows the intensity of the protein measured by Seldi-Tof-MS. Each triangle in a plot represents one sample of the specific group. The protein at 9192 Da is up-regulated in those cells incubated with POAG serum as well as the cells incubated with POAG serum and an elevated pressure, whereas the protein at 12390 Da is down-regulated in those cells incubated with POAG and an elevated pressure.

calculated showing, that discrimination between glaucoma and non-glaucoma serum is possible with a sensitivity of 88% and a specificity of 90%. The area under the curve is 0.92.

Discussion

The first experiments demonstrated in this manuscript focused on the effect of elevated pressure on the cells as well as the effect the serum had on the protein profiles of the cells. We were able to detect a significant loss of viability (60%) of cells incubated with an elevated pressure, correlating with already published data showing a loss of viability of neuronal cells [28] and rgc in vitro under elevated pressure [11]. However, we did not detect significant changes in the viability of cells incubated with glaucoma in comparison to healthy serum. As glaucoma is a slow proceeding disease we believe that significant changes of viability of cells after a short incubation time with patient's serum seems unlikely.

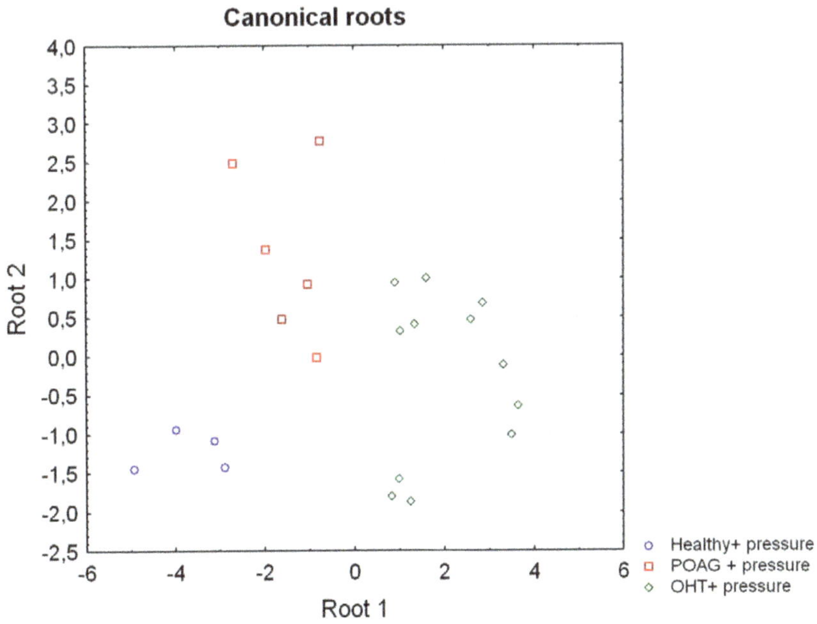

Figure 3. OHT serum also provokes different cell reactions. The graph shows the calculated canonical roots based on the analysis of discriminance of the cells incubated with serum from healthy people, patients suffering from POAG as well as OHT patients. A clear discrimination between the cells on the different experimental groups can be found showing that there are significant differences between the protein profiles and therefore the cell reactions in the different experimental groups.

Table 1. Variance component analysis.

Relative Variance components (in percent)		
Variable	**Influence on general protein profile**	**Influence on protein 9192 Dalton**
Serum type	59.1%	55.2%
Pressure	11.6%	
Combination serum type and pressure	14.0%	9.7%
Other influences	15.3%	35.1%

Table 1 shows the calculated relative variance components analysis in percent for both the overall protein profiles of the cells as well as the influence of the different components on one of the significantly differently regulated proteins (9192 Da). The serum type has a large influence on both the overall protein profiles as well as on the single protein. Furthermore an additional effect of serum type and elevated pressure can be detected in both groups.

However we were able to detect that the serum of glaucoma patients had a very large (59%) and significant influence on the protein profiles of the cells. This influence was potentiated through an elevated pressure (Fig. 2C and 4A). This analysis underlines the hypothesis that the serum of glaucoma patients, by influencing the proteins in the cells, leads to imbalance of proteins in cell regulatory processes and eventually can lead a higher vulnerability of the cells against stress factors such as an elevated pressure.

Specific changes in the protein profiles depending on serum type

We detected highly complex protein and peptide profiles in all experimental groups, showing significant differences not only in the expression of single proteins, but also in the overall protein profiles of the cells. This effect was demonstrated not only for POAG serum but also in cells incubated with NTG serum or OHT serum. In comparison to serum from healthy people, POAG and NTG serum showed significantly different effects. But also when analyzing the protein expression levels between cells incubated with POAG serum or NTG serum we were able to find significant differences. Cells incubated with OHT serum reacted significantly different than cells incubated with either POAG or healthy serum.

Studies show changes of several antibodies in the serum from glaucoma patients that are significantly correlated to different forms of glaucoma. These include specific antibodies against small heat shock proteins e.g. Hsp 27 or α-crystallins [29], α-fodrin [30], antiphosphatidylserine [31] or γ-enolase [32], but also complex changes in the autoantibody profiles against retinal or other ocular antigens [17]. POAG patients show many autoantibodies against retinal antigens, whereas NTG patients show the largest differences in the autoantibodies against optic nerve antigens [17,33].

Table 2. Variance components analysis after antibody removal.

Relative Variance components after antibody removal (in percent)	
Variable	**Influence on general protein profile**
Antibodies	50.5%
Serum type	13.4%
Other influences	36.1%

Table 2 shows the calculated relative variance components after antibody removal. We were able to calculate that the antibody removal had a 50% effect on the protein profiles of the cells.

Changes between OHT and POAG patients or healthy people were also observed in other studies [18]. Combining this information with the results shown in this manuscript underlines the theory that the antibodies in the serum of glaucoma patients have a significant influence in the pathogenesis of the disease glaucoma and could be the serum factor leading to changes in cell regulatory processes.

Significantly changed proteins have regulatory functions

In the first study shown in this manuscript several of the significantly changed proteins were identified. Using the Seldi-TOF-MS approach limits the amount of protein identifications. Using Seldi-TOF MS in combination with the statistical analysis we gained information about the molecular weight of the significantly changed proteins. In order to identify the proteins a SDS-Page had to be performed and the proteins of the bands possibly containing the proteins of interest had to be eluted. These then were measured with Seldi-Tof-MS in order to detect whether the protein of interest was enriched in the fraction. This was the first limiting step of the procedure. If the protein was in the eluted fraction a tryptic digestion was performed and the peptide measured with Maldi-TOF-MS in order to identify the wanted protein. Even after this step the identification of the protein was only secure if the score received from the database was high enough and the measured peptide additionally was a known fragment of the protein. This is a very well-known limitation of top-down Seldi-Tof analysis, which also has been discussed in the literature before [34]. Nevertheless, even those proteins not identified and only known by their molecular weight, can add

Table 3. Mahalanobis distances in comparison to control cells.

Mahalanobis distances to control cells	
Experimental group	**Distance**
POAG – Antibodies	19,6
POAG	56,1

Table 3 shows the calculated Mahalanobis distances for the cells incubated with POAG serum or POAG serum after antibody removal in comparison to the control cells. The Mahalanaobis distances are a measure to show the similarity or the difference between experimental groups to one defined group, in this case the cells incubated with control serum. The largest Mahalanobis distance can be seen for the protein profiles of the cells incubated with POAG serum. A significant change can be seen for the cells incubated with POAG serum after antibody removal.

apoptosispathway example for POAG serum

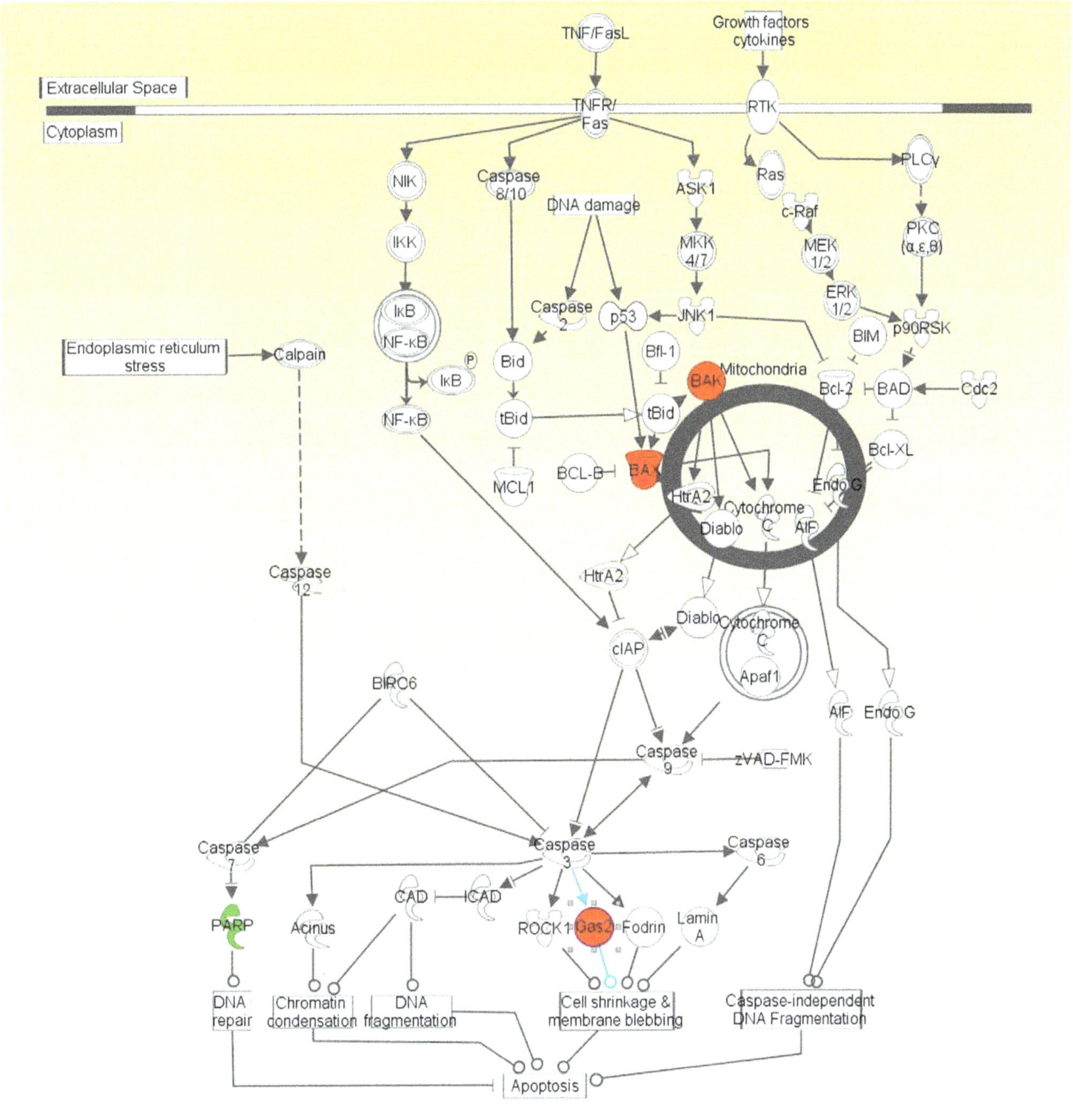

Figure 4. Cell regulatory pathways changed through glaucoma serum. Figure 4 shows changes of proteins belonging to apoptosis pathways in the cells incubated with POAG serum. Red highlighting shows a significant up-regulation of the protein in the cells whereas green highlighting demonstrates a significant down-regulation, both in a pro-apoptotic manner. The pro-apoptotic proteins BAK, BAX and GAS2 were up-regulated whereas the anti-apoptotic protein PARP was significantly down-regulated in the cells incubated with POAG serum. The pathway was built using the Ingenuity pathway analysis software.

important knowledge as shown in many proteome publications [35,36]. Therefore, in our set-up, only a few of the significantly changed proteins were identified. Those proteins securely identified are known to be part of cellular regulatory processes.

We detected changes in the expression level of histone 4 and profilin in cells incubated with POAG serum in comparison to healthy serum. Histones are core proteins of eukaryotic cells and responsible for the spooling of the DNA and the regulation of genes. Histones, can be post-translationally modified e.g. by acetylation or methylation. Changes in the modifications and location of histones have been found in several other neurodegenerative diseases e.g. Alzheimer disease [37,38], but also

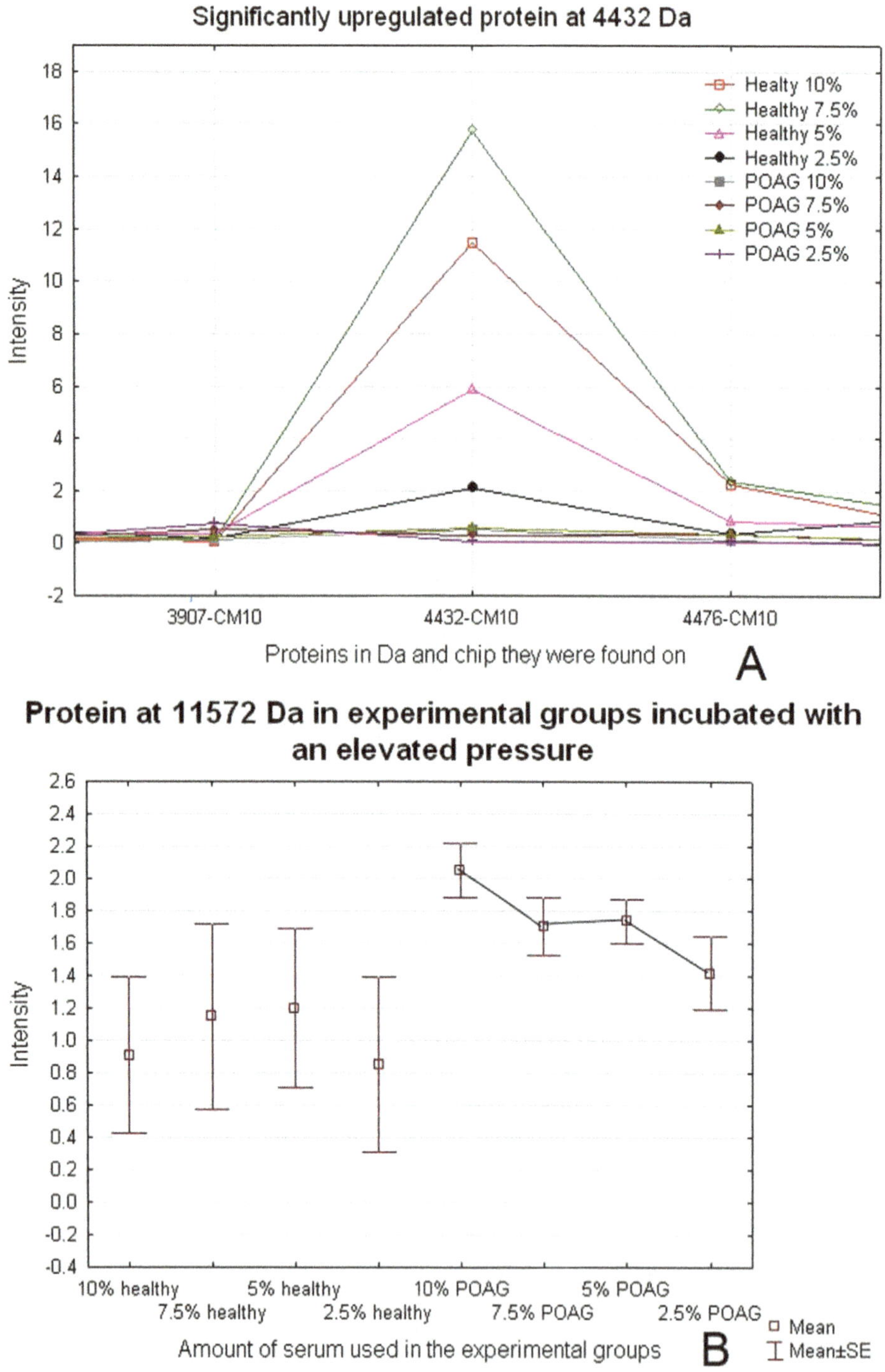

Figure 5. Serum effect is concentration dependant. Figure 5A shows one of the significantly changed proteins in the cells incubated with healthy serum. A concentration dependant behaviour is shown. The cells incbuated with the highest serum levels show the highest protein expression, whereas the cells incubated with the lowest serum concentration show the lowest protein expression. Figure 5B shows a not significantly changed protein either in the cells incubated with POAG or healthy serum. A concentration dependant expression level can be detected in the cells incubated with POAG serum.

changes of the histones of Parkinson disease patients have been detected [39]. Diseases, such as Alzheimer, show overall similarities in terms of apoptosis of neurons [40] as well as autoimmune components [41,42], but also more specific similarities such as changed beta amyloid and Tau protein levels either in the cerebral fluid of Alzheimer patients [43] or the vitreous of glaucoma patients [44]. Profilin, down-regulated in those cells incubated with POAG serum and an elevated pressure, is an actin binding protein and plays a role in membrane trafficking [45]. Studies show a correlation of Profilin with glaucoma and were able to show a hypotensive effect, when applying Profilin topically [46]. Profilin was shown to be up-regulated in the substantia nigra of

Parkinson patients [47]. In contrast we were able to show a down-regulation of Profilin in the cells incubated with glaucoma serum in combination with an elevated pressure. Profilin also has a function in neuronal excitability and plays a role in actin dynamics [45,48]. Changes in the expression level of Profilin in cells therefore can lead to changes in cell dysfunction as shown in other studies [49]. These results emphasize the hypothesis that the serum, respectively a serum component, of glaucoma patients has an influence on cell regulatory processes possibly leading to a higher vulnerability of the cells towards stress factors. Additionally, as discussed above, the different cell reactions towards the different serum types could be correlated with the different autoantibody levels in the serum depending on the type of glaucoma the patient was suffering from. Therefore further experiments were performed in order to analyze the antibody effect on the cells.

Antibodies play a role in the serum effect on the cells

After removal of the antibodies from the POAG serum we were able to detect a large influence (50%; Fig. 5A and B) of the Ab removal on the protein profiles of the cells. By removing the antibodies from the serum we could demonstrate that the antibodies seem to be involved in the serum effect of POAG serum on the cells. Using this approach we were not able to show which changes the Abs themselves provoke in the cells. Therefore further experiments were performed incubating the cells also with POAG Abs after their removal from the serum. By performing a capillary LC-ESI-MSMS rather than a Seldi-TOF-MS measurement we also were able to directly identify the proteins. When comparing the significantly changed proteins of cells incubated either with POAG serum or just with POAG Abs we found that only 5% of the proteins were significantly differently regulated, meaning an up-regulation in one group and a down-regulation on the other group in comparison to cells incubated with healthy serum.

In the cells incubated with POAG serum we found, that several of the proteins involved in the apoptosis of cells, e.g. BAX (5 fold up-regulated), BAK1 (22.9 fold up-regulated), PARP1 (8.8 fold down-regulated) and GAS2 (7.8 fold up-regulated), were significantly differently regulated in a pro-apoptotic manner. BAX belongs to the Bcl-2 family and is involved in the intrinsic apoptosis pathway as a pro-apoptotic protein [50].BAK1 also is a pro-apoptotic member of the Bcl-2 family [51]. Up-regulation of these factors can lead to apoptosis of cells. Furthermore the up-regulation of GAS2, a pro-apoptotic protein [27], as well as the down-regulation of PARP1, an enzyme involved in the repair of the DNA [52], can lead to increase of apoptosis of the cells. In previous studies BAX was correlated with neurodegeneration in glaucoma [53].

When analyzing the proteins changed in the cells incubated with just the POAG Abs we were also detect many changes in proteins involved in apoptosis pathways of the cells. Many of the proteins were regulated in a pro-apoptotic manner, e.g. GAS2, which was also found to be regulated in a pro-apoptotic manner in the cells incubated with POAG serum, but we also found proteins regulated in an anti-apoptotic manner. 11 of the significantly differently regulated proteins involved in the apoptosis of cells were changed in a pro-apoptotic manner whereas 8 proteins were changed in an anti-apoptotic manner.BAK1 was found to be down-regulated in the cells incubated with POAG Abs, whereas it was up-regulated in the cells incubated with POAG serum. Looking at the complexity of cell cycle processes it would be surprising to find a concordant regulation of all of the significantly changed proteins involved in cell cycle/apoptosis processes in the different experimental groups.

But we believe that these results underline our first hypothesis that the serum of glaucoma patients can lead to changes in cell regulatory processes. The balance between proteins in charge of cell survival and cell death, e.g. apoptosis, gets disturbed and long-term, possibly in combination with a further stress factor can lead to a predominance of the pro-apoptotic proteins. The anti-apoptotic counterpart proteins eventually can no longer countersteer and cell apoptosis is induced. Furthermore our second hypothesis is underlined by the fact that many of the proteins significantly differently regulated in the cells incubated with POAG serum are found to be regulated in the same way in in cells incubated with POAG Abs. Additionally these cells also show many changes in proteins concerning apoptotic processes.

Are the protein expression changes specific for rgcs in glaucoma?

When analyzing the cells incubated with POAG or healthy serum we were able to show that the discrimination between glaucoma or non-glaucoma serum was possible with a sensitivity of 88% and a specificity of 90%. In order to answer the question whether these changes are specific for retinal ganglion cells in glaucoma further experiments are needed, as the cells used in these studies (R28 cells or RGC5 cells) both are not pure rgc cultures. R28 cells are known to have properties of other cells such as photoreceptors or glial cells and have to be looked at as neuroretinal cells or retinal precursor cells. [54,55]. Furthermore the RGC5 cells show properties at least also of neuronal cells and therefore also should be used as neuroretinal cells rather than rgc. Furthermore not all of the RGC5 cells show the rgc specific marker Thy1.2 [23]. In the past these cells have been used in many studies to explore the pathogenesis of glaucoma.

In summary, this study shows significant and specific changes in the way the neuroretinal cells react to serum of glaucoma patients. Significantly differently expressed proteins were detected, that play crucial roles in cellular signaling pathways not only in cells incubated with POAG serum but also in cells only incubated with the Abs of POAG patients. We were able to underline both our hypothesis that the serum of glaucoma patients can lead to changes of protein profiles of retinal cells, which then can lead to a higher vulnerability of the cells toward stress factors, as well as the assumption that the antibodies in the serum of glaucoma patients could be the serum factor in charge of the seen serum effects.

Supporting Information

Figure S1 Confirmation of the AB removal after treatment of the POAG serum with Protein G beads. The antibodies of the POAG serum were removed with Protein G Beads. The AB fraction was eluted from the beads and measured with Seldi-TOF MS. Only if we were able to detect an AB peak in the Seldi-TOF-MS measurements the serum was used as AB free serum. The beads were used in abundance to the serum.

Figure S2 Confirmation of the AB removal after treatment of the POAG serum with Protein G beads. Ab removal from POAG serum was performed using Nab Protein G Spin Kit (Thermo scientific). The Ab removal was performed according to the manufacturer's protocol for the amount of 5% (500 µl) serum for each experiment. The Ab's then were used in order to incubate the cells. Beforehand the Kit was performed several times to assure that we were able to show reproducible Ab removal. The bands show different proteolytic components fof serum IgG. The lanes A, B and C show Ab fractions, the 4th lane shows SeeBluePlus marker.

Figure S3 Significantly changed protein profiles in cells incubated with NTG serum. Figure S3 shows a pullout of the measured protein profiles including cells incubated with NTG serum. Again complex protein profiles are shown. Changes in the proteins profiles between the experimental groups can be seen. The cells incubated with NTG serum react differently than cells incubated either with POAG serum or healthy serum.

Table S1 Significantly changed proteins with their p-value and identification. Table S1 shows the proteins significantly differently regulated in R28 after incubation with healthy or POAG serum und a normal or an elevated pressure of 15000 Pa (112 mmHg). The first column shows the molecular weight of the protein with information of the Seldi chip the protein was measured on. The second column shows the p- Value of the significantly changed protein. In the third column the identified proteins are named.

Table S2 Loss of cell viability after incubation with elevated pressure. The cells were incubated with bovine serum under a normal or an elevated pressure of 112 mmHg. We were able to detect that the cells incubated with bovine serum and an elevated pressure showed a loss of viability of nearly 60%.

Table S3 No difference in viability when incubating cells either with POAG or healthy serum. The viability of the cells incubated either with POAG or healthy serum under a normal or elevated pressure was measured and compared. We were not able to detect a significant difference between the viability of the cells incubated with POAG serum and an elevated pressure or the cells incubated with healthy serum and an elevated pressure. Both groups showed a loss of viability after incubation with an elevated pressure of nearly 62%. The table shows the values measured in the WST-1 test.

Table S4 Significantly changed proteins in RGC5 cells after incubation with POAG serum. We identified 3124 proteins in RGC 5 cells incubated with healthy serum, POAG serum or POAG antibodies. 198 Proteins were significantly differently regulated (<−4 or >4 fold expression) in cells incubated with POAG serum in comparison to cells incubated with healthy serum. The first column shows the short name of the protein and the second column shows the fold change of the protein in the cells incubated wit POAG serum in comparison to healthy serum.

Table S5 Significantly changed proteins in cells incubated with POAG Abs in comparison to healthy serum. We identified 3124 proteins in RGC 5 cells incubated with healthy serum, POAG serum or POAG antibodies. 82 Proteins were significantly up- or down- regulated in those cells incubated with the POAG Abs.

Table S6 Significantly changed proteins involved in apoptosis in cells incubated with POAG Abs. RGC5 cell were incubated with healthy serum, POAG serum or POAG antibodies. Proteins involved in apoptosis regulation were found to be significantly differently regulated in those cells incubated with either POAG serum or POAG Abs. The proteins differently regulated in the cells incubated with POAG Abs are shown in this table. The ID of the protein as well as the Gene information is given. Furthermore in column 3 the prediction whether the protein is regulated in a pro-apoptotic manner (increased) or an anti-apoptotic manner (decreased) is shown. Column 4 shows the fold change of the protein in the cells and the last column shows whether in general the protein is pro-apoptotic (increased) or anti-apoptotic (decreased).

Acknowledgments

We thank Dr. Gail Seigel for the R28 retinal cell line.

Author Contributions

Conceived and designed the experiments: KB FHG SF. Performed the experiments: KB. Analyzed the data: KB FHG. Contributed reagents/materials/analysis tools: FHG NP. Wrote the paper: KB.

References

1. Quigley HA (1996) Number of people with glaucoma worldwide. Br J Ophthalmol 80: 389–393.
2. Gutteridge IF (2000) Normal tension glaucoma: diagnostic features and comparisons with primary open angle glaucoma. Clin Exp Optom 83: 161–172.
3. Sommer A (2010) Treatment of ocular hypertension: Hamlet's Lament revisited. Arch Ophthalmol 128: 363–364.
4. Pfeiffer N (2005) [Results of the "Ocular hypertension treatment study"]. Ophthalmologe 102: 230–234.
5. Gordon MO, Beiser JA, Brandt JD, Heuer DK, Higginbotham EJ, et al. (2002) The Ocular Hypertension Treatment Study: baseline factors that predict the onset of primary open-angle glaucoma. Arch Ophthalmol 120: 714–720; discussion 829–730.
6. Przedborski S, Vila M, Jackson-Lewis V (2003) Neurodegeneration: what is it and where are we? J Clin Invest 111: 3–10.
7. Quigley HA (1999) Neuronal death in glaucoma. Prog Retin Eye Res 18: 39–57.
8. Weber AJ, Chen H, Hubbard WC, Kaufman PL (2000) Experimental glaucoma and cell size, density, and number in the primate lateral geniculate nucleus. Invest Ophthalmol Vis Sci 41: 1370–1379.
9. Gupta N, Yucel YH (2007) Glaucoma as a neurodegenerative disease. Curr Opin Ophthalmol 18: 110–114.
10. Okisaka S, Murakami A, Mizukawa A, Ito J (1997) Apoptosis in retinal ganglion cell decrease in human glaucomatous eyes. Jpn J Ophthalmol 41: 84–88.
11. Agar A, Li S, Agarwal N, Coroneo MT, Hill MA (2006) Retinal ganglion cell line apoptosis induced by hydrostatic pressure. Brain Res 1086: 191–200.
12. Neufeld AH (1999) Nitric oxide: a potential mediator of retinal ganglion cell damage in glaucoma. Surv Ophthalmol 43 Suppl 1: S129–135.
13. Schwartz M (2007) Modulating the immune system: a vaccine for glaucoma? Can J Ophthalmol 42: 439–441.
14. Wax MB (2000) Is there a role for the immune system in glaucomatous optic neuropathy? Curr Opin Ophthalmol 11: 145–150.
15. Sukharev SA, Pleshakova OV, Sadovnikov VB (1997) Role of proteases in activation of apoptosis. Cell Death Differ 4: 457–462.
16. Yun HY, Dawson VL, Dawson TM (1996) Neurobiology of nitric oxide. Crit Rev Neurobiol 10: 291–316.
17. Joachim SC, Pfeiffer N, Grus FH (2005) Autoantibodies in patients with glaucoma: a comparison of IgG serum antibodies against retinal, optic nerve, and optic nerve head antigens. Graefes Arch Clin Exp Ophthalmol 243: 817–823.
18. Reichelt J, Joachim SC, Pfeiffer N, Grus FH (2008) Analysis of autoantibodies against human retinal antigens in sera of patients with glaucoma and ocular hypertension. Curr Eye Res 33: 253–261.
19. Lacroix-Desmazes S, Kaveri SV, Mouthon L, Ayouba A, Malanchere E, et al. (1998) Self-reactive antibodies (natural autoantibodies) in healthy individuals. J Immunol Methods 216: 117–137.
20. Poletaev AB (2002) The immunological homunculus (immunculus) in normal state and pathology. Biochemistry (Mosc) 67: 600–608.
21. Sun W, Seigel GM, Salvi RJ (2002) Retinal precursor cells express functional ionotropic glutamate and GABA receptors. Neuroreport 13: 2421–2424.
22. Krishnamoorthy RR, Agarwal P, Prasanna G, Vopat K, Lambert W, et al. (2001) Characterization of a transformed rat retinal ganglion cell line. Brain Res Mol Brain Res 86: 1–12.

23. Van Bergen NJ, Wood JP, Chidlow G, Trounce IA, Casson RJ, et al. (2009) Recharacterization of the RGC-5 retinal ganglion cell line. Invest Ophthalmol Vis Sci 50: 4267–4272.
24. Lowry OH, Rosebrough NJ, Farr AL, Randall RJ (1951) Protein measurement with the Folin phenol reagent. J Biol Chem 193: 265–275.
25. Li L, Kalaga R, Paul S (2000) Proteolytic components of serum IgG preparations. Clin Exp Immunol 120: 261–266.
26. Pang X, Moussa SH, Targy NM, Bose JL, George NM, et al. (2011) Active Bax and Bak are functional holins. Genes Dev 25: 2278–2290.
27. Benetti R, Del Sal G, Monte M, Paroni G, Brancolini C, et al. (2001) The death substrate Gas2 binds m-calpain and increases susceptibility to p53-dependent apoptosis. Embo J 20: 2702–2714.
28. Agar A, Yip SS, Hill MA, Coroneo MT (2000) Pressure related apoptosis in neuronal cell lines. J Neurosci Res 60: 495–503.
29. Tezel G, Seigel GM, Wax MB (1998) Autoantibodies to small heat shock proteins in glaucoma. Invest Ophthalmol Vis Sci 39: 2277–2287.
30. Grus FH, Joachim SC, Bruns K, Lackner KJ, Pfeiffer N, et al. (2006) Serum autoantibodies to alpha-fodrin are present in glaucoma patients from Germany and the United States. Invest Ophthalmol Vis Sci 47: 968–976.
31. Kremmer S, Kreuzfelder E, Klein R, Bontke N, Henneberg-Quester KB, et al. (2001) Antiphosphatidylserine antibodies are elevated in normal tension glaucoma. Clin Exp Immunol 125: 211–215.
32. Maruyama I, Ohguro H, Ikeda Y (2000) Retinal ganglion cells recognized by serum autoantibody against gamma-enolase found in glaucoma patients. Invest Ophthalmol Vis Sci 41: 1657–1665.
33. Grus FH, Joachim SC, Hoffmann EM, Pfeiffer N (2004) Complex autoantibody repertoires in patients with glaucoma. Mol Vis 10: 132–137.
34. Huang F, Clifton J, Yang X, Rosenquist T, Hixson D, et al. (2009) SELDI-TOF as a method for biomarker discovery in the urine of aristolochic-acid-treated mice. Electrophoresis 30: 1168–1174.
35. Lin Q, Peng Q, Yao F, Pan XF, Xiong LW, et al. (2012) A Classification Method Based on Principal Components of SELDI Spectra to Diagnose of Lung Adenocarcinoma. PLoS One 7: e34457.
36. Lee SM, Park JS, Norwitz ER, Kim SM, Kim BJ, et al. (2011) Characterization of discriminatory urinary proteomic biomarkers for severe preeclampsia using SELDI-TOF mass spectrometry. J Perinat Med 39: 391–396.
37. Ogawa O, Zhu X, Lee HG, Raina A, Obrenovich ME, et al. (2003) Ectopic localization of phosphorylated histone H3 in Alzheimer's disease: a mitotic catastrophe? Acta Neuropathol (Berl) 105: 524–528.
38. Duce JA, Smith DP, Blake RE, Crouch PJ, Li QX, et al. (2006) Linker histone H1 binds to disease associated amyloid-like fibrils. J Mol Biol 361: 493–505.
39. Kontopoulos E, Parvin JD, Feany MB (2006) Alpha-synuclein acts in the nucleus to inhibit histone acetylation and promote neurotoxicity. Hum Mol Genet 15: 3012–3023.
40. Cotman CW, Su JH (1996) Mechanisms of neuronal death in Alzheimer's disease. Brain Pathol 6: 493–506.
41. D'Andrea MR (2005) Add Alzheimer's disease to the list of autoimmune diseases. Med Hypotheses 64: 458–463.
42. Mruthinti S, Buccafusco JJ, Hill WD, Waller JL, Jackson TW, et al. (2004) Autoimmunity in Alzheimer's disease: increased levels of circulating IgGs binding Abeta and RAGE peptides. Neurobiol Aging 25: 1023–1032.
43. Grundke-Iqbal I, Rolkova G, Konstekova E, Iqbal K (2006) Biological markers in Alzheimer's disease. Bratisl Lek Listy 107: 359–365.
44. Yoneda S, Hara H, Hirata A, Fukushima M, Inomata Y, et al. (2005) Vitreous fluid levels of beta-amyloid((1–42)) and tau in patients with retinal diseases. Jpn J Ophthalmol 49: 106–108.
45. Pilo Boyl P, Di Nardo A, Mulle C, Sassoe-Pognetto M, Panzanelli P, et al. (2007) Profilin2 contributes to synaptic vesicle exocytosis, neuronal excitability, and novelty-seeking behavior. Embo J 26: 2991–3002.
46. Morales M, Gomez-Cabrero A, Peral A, Gasull X, Pintor J (2007) Hypotensive effect of profilin on rabbit intraocular pressure. Eur J Pharmacol 567: 145–148.
47. Basso M, Giraudo S, Corpillo D, Bergamasco B, Lopiano L, et al. (2004) Proteome analysis of human substantia nigra in Parkinson's disease. Proteomics 4: 3943–3952.
48. Witke W, Podtelejnikov AV, Di Nardo A, Sutherland JD, Gurniak CB, et al. (1998) In mouse brain profilin I and profilin II associate with regulators of the endocytic pathway and actin assembly. Embo J 17: 967–976.
49. Bae YH, Ding Z, Zou L, Wells A, Gertler F, et al. (2009) Loss of profilin-1 expression enhances breast cancer cell motility by Ena/VASP proteins. J Cell Physiol 219: 354–364.
50. Kumarswamy R, Chandna S (2009) Putative partners in Bax mediated cytochrome-c release: ANT, CypD, VDAC or none of them? Mitochondrion 9: 1–8.
51. Gelinas C, White E (2005) BH3-only proteins in control: specificity regulates MCL-1 and BAK-mediated apoptosis. Genes Dev 19: 1263–1268.
52. Bacalini MG, Tavolaro S, Peragine N, Marinelli M, Santangelo S, et al. (2011) A subset of chronic lymphocytic leukemia patients display reduced levels of PARP1 expression coupled with a defective irradiation-induced apoptosis. Exp Hematol.
53. Libby RT, Li Y, Savinova OV, Barter J, Smith RS, et al. (2005) Susceptibility to neurodegeneration in a glaucoma is modified by Bax gene dosage. PLoS Genet 1: 17–26.
54. Seigel GM, Mutchler AL, Adamus G, Imperato-Kalmar EL (1997) Recoverin expression in the R28 retinal precursor cell line. In Vitro Cell Dev Biol Anim 33: 499–502.
55. Seigel GM, Mutchler AL, Imperato EL (1996) Expression of glial markers in a retinal precursor cell line. Mol Vis 2: 2.

3

Cholesterol-Lowering Drugs and Incident Open-Angle Glaucoma

Michael W. Marcus[1], Rogier P. H. M. Müskens[1], Wishal D. Ramdas[2,3], Roger C. W. Wolfs[2,3], Paulus T. V. M. De Jong[4,5], Johannes R. Vingerling[2,3], Albert Hofman[2], Bruno H. Stricker[2,6,7]*, Nomdo M. Jansonius[1,2]

1 Department of Ophthalmology, University Medical Center Groningen, University of Groningen, Groningen, The Netherlands, **2** Department of Epidemiology, Erasmus Medical Center, Rotterdam, The Netherlands, **3** Department of Ophthalmology, Erasmus Medical Center, Rotterdam, The Netherlands, **4** Department of Ophthalmogenetics, Netherlands Institute for Neuroscience, Amsterdam, The Netherlands, **5** Department of Ophthalmology, Academic Medical Center, Amsterdam, The Netherlands, **6** Department of Internal Medicine, Erasmus Medical Center, Rotterdam, The Netherlands, **7** Department of Medical Informatics, Erasmus Medical Center, Rotterdam, The Netherlands

Abstract

Background: Open-angle glaucoma (OAG) is a progressive neurodegenerative disease that may lead to blindness. An elevated intraocular pressure (IOP) is its major risk factor. OAG treatment is currently exclusively directed towards the lowering of the IOP. IOP lowering does not prevent disease progression in all patients and thus other treatment modalities are needed. Earlier studies reported cholesterol-lowering drugs to have neuroprotective properties. The aim of this study was to determine the associations between the use of cholesterol-lowering drugs and incident OAG.

Methodology/Principal Findings: Participants in a prospective population-based cohort study underwent ophthalmic examinations, including IOP measurements and perimetry, at baseline and follow-up. The use of statins and non-statin cholesterol-lowering drugs was monitored continuously during the study. Associations between the use of cholesterol-lowering drugs and incident OAG were analyzed with Cox regression; associations between cholesterol-lowering drugs and IOP at follow-up were analyzed with multiple linear regression. During a mean follow-up of 9.8 years, 108 of 3939 eligible participants (2.7%) developed OAG. The hazard ratio for statin use was 0.54 (95% confidence interval 0.31–0.96; P = 0.034) and for non-statin cholesterol-lowering drugs 2.07 (0.81–5.33; P = 0.13). The effect of statins was more pronounced with prolonged use (hazard ratio 0.89 [0.41–1.94; P = 0.77] for use two years or less; 0.46 [0.23–0.94; P = 0.033] for use more than two years; P-value for trend 0.10). The analyzes were adjusted for age and gender, baseline IOP and IOP-lowering treatment, the family history of glaucoma, and myopia. There was no effect of statins on the IOP.

Conclusions/Significance: Long-term use of statins appears to be associated with a reduced risk of OAG. The observed effect was independent of the IOP. These findings are in line with the idea that statins have neuroprotective properties and may open a way to a new OAG treatment modality.

Editor: Pablo Villoslada, Institute Biomedical Research August Pi Sunyer (IDIBAPS) - Hospital Clinic of Barcelona, Spain

Funding: Stichting Lijf en Leven, Krimpen aan de Lek; MD Fonds, Utrecht; Rotterdamse Vereniging Blindenbelangen, Rotterdam; Stichting Oogfonds Nederland, Utrecht; Blindenpenning, Amsterdam; Blindenhulp, The Hague; Algemene Nederlandse Vereniging ter Voorkoming van Blindheid (ANVVB), Doorn; Landelijke Stichting voor Blinden en Slechtzienden, Utrecht; Swart van Essen, Rotterdam; Stichting Winckel-Sweep, Utrecht; Henkes Stichting, Rotterdam; Professor Mulder Stichting, Groningen; Stichting Nederlands Oogheelkundig Onderzoek, Rotterdam; Laméris Ootech BV, Nieuwegein; Medical Workshop, de Meern; Topcon Europe BV, Capelle aan de IJssel, all in the Netherlands and Heidelberg Engineering, Dossenheim, Germany. The funders had no role in study design, data collection and analysis, decision to publish, or preparation of the manuscript.

Competing Interests: This study was partly funded by the following companies: Laméris Ootech BV, Medical Workshop, Topcon Europe BV and Heidelberg Engineering. The funding was unrestricted and did not, in any way, interfere with the conception and/or design and/or outcome and/or publication of the study. There are no patents, products in development or marketed products to declare. This does not alter the authors' adherence to all the PLoS ONE policies on sharing data and materials.

* E-mail: b.stricker@erasmusmc.nl

Introduction

Open-angle glaucoma (OAG) is a progressive neurodegenerative disease that leads to glaucomatous optic neuropathy and eventually, through glaucomatous visual field loss, to loss of sight. Together with age-related maculopathy it is the most common cause of irreversible blindness. An elevated intraocular pressure (IOP) is the major risk factor of OAG, and OAG treatment is currently exclusively directed towards the lowering of the IOP. However, OAG progression often continues despite an apparently sufficient reduction of the IOP. For that reason, the search for other OAG treatment modalities is a very active field of research.

Statins are selective inhibitors of 3-hydroxyl-3-methylglutaryl coenzyme A reductase (HMG-CoA) [1]. Currently, they are the most important lipid lowering medications for the treatment of hypercholesterolemia [2–4]. Previous studies have reported beneficial effects of statins on a variety of eye diseases, including age-related maculopathy, cataract and diabetic retinopathy [5–11]. Several observational studies addressed the effects of statins on OAG. Some reported a protective effect [12–14] whereas others did not [15,16]. Studies including animal models as well as clinical trials have reported neuroprotective properties of statins [17–22]. Since OAG is characterized by the loss of neuronal cells, the use of statins, and possibly non-statin cholesterol-lowering drugs (NSCLDs) as well, might modify the risk of OAG through neuroprotection. With the current recommendations of lower primary prevention thresholds [23,24], the use of statins and NSCLDs has increased markedly over the years [25]. For these reasons, it is expedient to clarify the associations between these drugs and OAG.

The aim of the present study was to determine the associations between the use of cholesterol-lowering drugs and incident OAG in a large prospective population-based cohort study.

Methods

Ethics statement

All measurements were conducted after the Medical Ethics Committee of the Erasmus University Rotterdam had approved the study protocol and all participants had given written informed consent in accordance with the declaration of Helsinki.

Study population

The present study was performed as part of the Rotterdam Study, a prospective population-based cohort study investigating age-related disorders. The study population consisted of 7983 individuals aged 55 years and older living in the Ommoord district of Rotterdam, the Netherlands [26]. For this study, data from 3939 participants who did not have OAG (see below) at baseline and who completed at least one follow-up examination were used. The baseline examination took place from 1991 to 1993; follow-up examinations were performed from 1997 to 1999 and from 2002 to 2006.

Ophthalmic assessment

Participants underwent similar eye examinations at baseline and at the two follow-up rounds [27]. These examinations included refraction, measurement of the best-corrected visual acuity, Goldmann applanation tonometry (Haag-Streit AG, Bern, Switzerland), fundoscopy, fundus photography of the posterior pole, simultaneous stereoscopic fundus photography of the optic disc, and visual field testing.

At each visit, three IOP measurements were taken on each eye and the median value of these three measurements was recorded [28]; the higher median of both eyes was used in the analysis. The visual field of each eye was screened using a 52-point supra-threshold test that covered the central visual field with a radius of 24° (Humphrey Field Analyzer [HFA]; Carl Zeiss, Oberkochen, Germany) [27,29]. Visual field loss was defined as non-response to a light stimulus of 6 dB above a threshold-related estimate of the hill of vision in at least three contiguous test points, or four including the blind spot. In participants with reproducible abnormalities on supra-threshold testing, Goldmann perimetry (Haag-Streit AG, Bern, Switzerland; baseline and first follow-up) or full-threshold HFA 24-2 testing (second follow-up) was performed on both eyes. Visual field loss was considered to be glaucomatous visual field loss only if reproducible and after excluding all other possible causes [29,30].

Incident open-angle glaucoma

We defined incident OAG as no glaucomatous visual field loss in both eyes at baseline and glaucomatous visual field loss in at least one eye at follow-up [30]. All identified cases were examined by an experienced ophthalmologist (PTVMdJ and RCWW) who performed gonioscopy and a dilated ophthalmic exam. Cases with a history or signs of angle closure or secondary glaucoma were excluded.

Medication data

Data on cholesterol-lowering drugs prescriptions for all participants were obtained from seven fully automated pharmacies using a centralized computer network in the study district, from January 1, 1991, onward. This included the product name, Anatomical Therapeutic Chemical (ATC) code, duration of use, and the date of first prescription. Cholesterol-lowering drugs were classified as statins (C10AA; simvastatin, pravastatin, fluvastatin, atorvastatin, cerivastatin, rosuvastatin) or NSCLDs (C10AB, C10AC, C10AD, C10A; fibrates, bile acid-binding resins or nicotinic acid and derivatives). The use of cholesterol-lowering drugs was recorded as the number of days with use during follow-up. Usage before baseline was not taken into account.

Other covariates

Other covariates included age, gender, smoking, diabetes mellitus, cardiovascular diseases, the use of antihypertensive drugs, body mass index, total cholesterol, IOP, IOP-lowering treatment, and family history of glaucoma. All these covariates were measured at baseline. Smoking status was self reported and categorized as ever or never smoker. Data on diabetes mellitus and cardiovascular disorders such as angina pectoris, atrial fibrillation, myocardial infarction, heart failure, hypertension, and stroke were obtained from the participants through interviews, electrocardiogram readings, and non-fasting and fasting serum blood glucose levels. Diabetes was defined as the use of antidiabetic medication or by a non-fasting or post-load plasma glucose level above 200 mg/dl (11.1 mmol/l). Hypertension was defined as the use of antihypertensive medication for the indication of hypertension or as a systolic blood pressure of 140 mmHg or more, or a diastolic pressure of 90 mmHg or more. Body mass and height were measured at the research center. Total serum cholesterol was measured in non-fasting blood. IOP-lowering treatment was defined as the use of IOP-lowering medication or a history of glaucoma surgery or laser trabeculoplasty. The family history of glaucoma was determined by interviews and was considered positive if the participant reported a history of glaucoma in parents, siblings or offspring. Myopia was defined as a spherical equivalent refractive error of −4 D and more myopia [30]. Eyes with a cataract extraction before baseline were excluded from this analysis. In cases with one eye with incident OAG, the refraction of that eye was used. In participants without OAG or OAG in both eyes, the refraction of a random eye was used.

Statistical analysis

Differences in baseline characteristics between participants with and without incident OAG and differences in baseline characteristics between cholesterol-lowering drug users and non-users were evaluated using chi-square tests for categorical variables and t-tests for normally distributed continuous variables. To determine the associations between the use of cholesterol-lowering drugs and incident OAG, the use of statins or NSCLDs was initially defined as any use during follow-up and the associations were initially analyzed with chi-square tests. Subsequently, a Cox proportional hazards model was used to calculate hazard ratios (HR) and corresponding 95% confidence intervals (CI) for the associations between the use of statins or NSCLDs and incident OAG. Follow-up duration was used as the time axis in the model. For participants without incident OAG, the follow-up duration was counted from the baseline visit to the last visit with reliable perimetry. For incident OAG cases, the follow-up ended at the first visit in which glaucomatous visual field loss was detected. The cholesterol-lowering drugs, age and gender, and other covariates with P<0.20 in the univariate comparisons were included in the multivariate analysis. Subsequently, the cholesterol-lowering drugs, age and gender, and other covariates with P<0.05 in the initial multivariate model were included in the final model. The use of cholesterol-lowering drugs was entered in the model as any use during follow-up. To allow for the evaluation of a possible dose-response relationship, we also performed analysis after making three nominal categories based on the duration of medication use, being no use, cumulative use during two years or less, and cumulative use during more than two years (see Discussion section). The dose-response relationship was evaluated with a trend test. To explore the influence of cholesterol-lowering drugs on the IOP, we conducted a multiple linear regression analysis with IOP at follow-up as the dependent variable. This analysis was adjusted for IOP-lowering treatment at follow-up and for the same covariates as the final Cox model except for baseline IOP and IOP-lowering treatment at baseline. All analyzes were performed using SAS 9.2 (SAS Institute Inc., Cary, NC). A *P*-value of 0.05 or less was considered statistically significant.

Results

During a mean follow-up of 9.8 years, 108 of 3939 eligible participants (2.7%) developed OAG. Table 1A depicts the baseline characteristics of the study population for participants with and without incident OAG. Participants with incident OAG were older, more often male, more often had a positive family history of glaucoma, and more often had myopia. They also had a higher IOP and more frequently received IOP-lowering treatment. There was no difference between the groups regarding total serum cholesterol levels. Table 1B shows the baseline characteristics for cholesterol-lowering drug users and non-users. Participants using cholesterol-lowering drugs were younger, smoked less frequently and more often had diabetes mellitus, a myocardial infarction or hypertension. They also used more often antihypertensive drugs and had a higher total serum cholesterol level and a slightly higher IOP.

Table 2 presents the results of the univariable analyses for the use of statins and NSCLDs at any time during follow-up. These univariable comparisons revealed no significant differences between participants with and without incident OAG. Amongst the 811 participants using statins at any time during follow-up, the median duration of use was 1424 days, with a range from 8 to 4114 days; amongst the 113 participants using NSCLDs, the median duration of use was 298 days, with a range from 7 to 3544 days.

Table 3 presents the final multivariate model, adjusting for age and gender, baseline IOP and IOP-lowering treatment, the family history of glaucoma, and myopia. Participants using statins had a significant risk reduction (HR 0.54; 95% CI 0.31 to 0.96; P = 0.034). The use of NSCLDs was not significantly associated with incident OAG (HR 2.07; 95% CI 0.81 to 5.33; P = 0.13). There was a trend towards a reduced risk of incident OAG with prolonged statin use. The HR was 0.89 (95% CI 0.41 to 1.94, P = 0.77) for use during two years or less and 0.46 (95% CI 0.23 to 0.94, P = 0.033) for use during more than two years. The overall P-value for trend was 0.10.

The protective effect of statins could be either caused by an IOP-lowering effect of statins or by a direct protective effect of statins on the neural tissue. To differentiate between these two possibilities, we conducted a multiple linear regression analysis with IOP at follow-up as the dependent variable. Table 4 shows the results. As can be seen in this table, there was no significant IOP-lowering effect of statins.

Discussion

In this large prospective population-based study, the use of statins was associated with a reduced risk of OAG. This effect was independent of the IOP. The risk reduction tended to increase with the duration of cumulative use, which supports the observed association, but this trend did not reach statistical significance. The use of NSCLDs was not associated with the development of OAG.

The association between the use of statins and OAG we found is consistent with the results of McGwin et al. (odds ratio 0.60; 95% CI 0.39 to 0.92) [12]. They performed a nested case-control study in a clinical administrative database. In contrast, Owen et al. found no evidence for a protective effect of statins (odds ratio 0.97; 95% CI 0.88 to 1.06) [15]. They employed a case-control study design in a primary care database. Similarly, Iskedjidan et al. did not find a significant association between the use of statins and OAG [16]. They performed a retrospective population-based evaluation in an administrative prescription claims database. The designs of the latter two studies might have complicated the classification of OAG, and the resulting misclassification might have biased the effect estimate. The trend of the effect seen in our study is consistent with previously published studies. McGwin et al. reported a significant reduction in the risk of OAG in patients using statins for more than 23 months [12]. De Castro et al. reported that the use of statins was associated with a slower progression of glaucomatous optic nerve atrophy [14]. In their clinical retrospective cohort study, patients using statins for two years showed less optic nerve head changes than patients not using statins. Nagaoka, et al studied the effect of statins on the retinal circulation and the IOP [31]. They found an IOP decrease after the administration of statins. At first sight, this seems to corroborate with our findings. However, our data suggested the protective effect of statins to be IOP independent. A possible explanation for this discrepancy might be that they studied the effects of statins up to one week after the initial administration whereas we found the most pronounced effect in those OAG cases that used statins for more than two years. Leung et al. reported that the use of simvastatin was associated with visual field stabilization in patients with normal tension glaucoma (relative risk 0.36; 95% CI 0.14 to 0.91; P = 0.030) [13]. In their prospective cohort study, 256 patients with normal tension glaucoma of whom thirty-one were taking simvastatin and 225 were not taking simvastatin were followed-up for 36 months.

The use of NSCLDs was not associated with incident OAG in our study. This result contradicts the result of the study by McGwin et al. who found a protective effect among those who used NSCLDs (odds ratio 0.59; 95% CI 0.37 to 0.97) [12]. This discrepancy might be attributed to the low number of users of NSCLDS in our study, as depicted by the wide CIs.

Strengths of our study include its prospective design, the large number of participants, the long follow-up period and the population-based setting, which minimizes selection bias. An inextricable limitation of the population-based design is the limited

Table 1. Baseline characteristics of participants with and without incident open-angle glaucoma (A) and of cholesterol-lowering drug users (either statins or NSCLDs, or both) and non-users (B), with univariable comparisons (mean values with standard deviation between brackets unless stated otherwise).

A	Incident open-angle glaucoma (N = 108)	No incident open-angle glaucoma (N = 3831)	P-value
Age (year)	68.4(7.1)	65.7(6.8)	<0.001
Gender (%female)	49.1	58.7	0.046
Smoking (%)	33.3	33.4	0.98
Diabetes mellitus (%)	8.4	6.9	0.54
Angina pectoris (%)	1.9	3.1	0.46
Atrial fibrillation (%)	2.8	2.1	0.63
Myocardial infarction (%)	13.2	9.7	0.23
Heart failure (%)	0.9	1.2	0.81
Hypertension (%)	52.9	47.1	0.49
Blood pressure lowering drugs (%)	28.0	26.0	0.63
Stroke (%)	2.8	1.2	0.16
Body mass index (kg/m^2)	25.8(2.9)	26.3(3.5)	0.12
Total cholesterol (mmol/l)	6.5(1.1)	6.7(1.2)	0.17
IOP (mmHg)	17.3(4.7)	15.0(3.1)	<0.001
IOP-lowering treatment (%)	15.7	2.3	<0.001
Family history of glaucoma (%)	16.7	8.1	0.002
Myopia	9.5	4.9	0.033
B	**Cholesterol-lowering drug users (N = 848)**	**Non-users (N = 3091)**	
Age	64.3(5.5)	66.1(7.1)	<0.001
Gender (%female)	56.6	58.9	0.23
Smoking (%)	27.5	35.0	<0.001
Diabetes mellitus (%)	10.2	6.1	<0.001
Angina pectoris (%)	3.8	2.8	0.15
Atrial fibrillation (%)	2.4	2.1	0.57
Myocardial infarction (%)	15.3	8.2	<0.001
Heart failure (%)	1.2	1.2	0.97
Hypertension (%)	58.7	47.1	<0.001
Blood pressure lowering drugs (%)	38.3	22.6	<0.001
Stroke (%)	1.4	1.2	0.65
Body mass index (kg/m^2)	26.5(3.5)	26.2(3.5)	0.055
Total cholesterol (mmol/l)	7.4(1.3)	6.5(1.1)	<0.001
IOP (mmHg)	15.3(3.2)	15.0(3.2)	0.044
IOP-lowering treatment (%)	2.0	2.9	0.18
Family history of glaucoma (%)	9.7	8.0	0.13
Myopia	6.3	4.7	0.063

NSCLDs = non-statin cholesterol-lowering drugs; IOP = intraocular pressure.

Table 2. Univariable analyses of the use of cholesterol-lowering medication at any time during follow-up and the development of open-angle glaucoma.

	Incident open-angle glaucoma (N = 108)	No incident open-angle glaucoma (N = 3831)	P-value
Statins (n[%])	16(14.8)	795(20.8)	0.13
NSCLDs (n[%])	5(4.6)	108(2.8)	0.27

NSCLDs = non-statin cholesterol-lowering drugs.

Table 3. Final multivariate model of the risk of developing open-angle glaucoma for cholesterol-lowering medication.

	Hazard ratio	95% confidence interval	P-value
Statins	0.54	0.31–0.96	0.034
NSCLDs	2.07	0.81–5.33	0.13
Age (per year)	1.07	1.04–1.10	<0.001
Gender (female)	0.56	0.38–0.83	0.004
IOP (per mmHg)	1.12	1.08–1.18	<0.001
IOP treatment	3.39	1.82–6.32	<0.001
Family history of glaucoma	1.85	1.08–3.15	0.024
Myopia	2.30	1.19–4.43	0.013

NSCLDs = non-statin cholesterol-lowering drugs; IOP = intraocular pressure.

number of OAG cases – due to the low prevalence of OAG - and the limited number of participants using NSCLDs. Information bias was prevented by prospectively collected and completely automated pharmacy records of all prescriptions. Although this approach guarantees accurate prescription data, it cannot be guaranteed that all participants actually took their medication. Such exposure misclassification is usually similar in cases and controls and leads to conservative risk estimates. Hence, it may have contributed to the lack of effect of NSCLDs, but not to the protective effect of statins.

Several other factors have been reported to be a risk factor for the incidence of OAG, including myopia [32], pseudoexfoliation [33], central corneal thickness [34], and age [30]. Of these factors, only pseudoexfoliation and age may be associated with statin use and may thus be confounding factors in our analysis [35–37]. Pseudoexfoliation is relatively rare in the Netherlands and in our study population (which might or might not be due to underreporting) – hampering a meaningful adjustment for pseudoexfoliation in our analysis. However, the absence of adjustment should have resulted in an increased risk whereas we found a protective effect. Age is associated with statin use but we adjusted our models for that. Age as a linear covariable – as we did – might result in under-adjustment, but in that case an increased risk should have been the result, not a protective effect. We included only participants aged 55 years and older. This is not a limitation for this specific study question, as both statin use at younger age is relatively rare and the prevalence of OAG below 55 years of age is very low (0.1–0.2%; to be compared to 1–2% above 55 years of age [27]. Finally, myopia appeared to occur – presumably by chance – slightly more frequent amongst cholesterol-lowering drug users compared to non-users (P = 0.063; Table 1B) and was included in the final model.

A possible limitation of this study is potential misclassification of exposure. However, such misclassification will be random because the outcome is – inextricably - gathered irrespective of exposure status. To appreciate this approach, it is important to realize that glaucoma development often takes more than a decade and cannot be detected in the earliest stages. Some factors slow down or accelerate the disease development, and thus make it less likely or more likely that the disease can be detected at a certain point in time (being our follow-up examination). Cumulative exposure stratified into biologically plausible nominal categories as we used in our analyses is the best proxy for studying the overall influence of the use of medication on the rate of glaucoma development during follow-up. Details of this technique were published earlier [38]. Because the exposure misclassification is random, it will tend to bias the results towards the null hypothesis. This might mean that the significant protection we found is an underestimation of the true effect.

Our finding of a protective effect of statins may offer potential therapeutic possibilities for OAG or its prevention. We showed the effect to be independent of the IOP. Hence, the protective effect of statins could be caused by lowering serum cholesterol or by (other) neuroprotective properties of statins on neuronal cells, as mentioned in the Introduction section [17–22]. Our incident OAG cases did not have an elevated serum cholesterol level at baseline (Table 1), but that observation does not exclude a beneficial effect of a further lowering of this level - cardiovascular trials have shown beneficial effects of further lowering cholesterol levels even if initially already within normal limits [39,40]. Studies with serum cholesterol level monitoring during follow-up should enable the uncovering of more details of the mechanism underlying the protective effect of statins. Given the current level of evidence and the fact that statins are widely available and thoroughly investigated drugs, a neuroprotective OAG treatment could become reality and a randomised clinical trial seems to be a viable next step.

In conclusion, we confirmed that statins appear to have a protective effect on OAG. Due to our study design, we were able to add that this protective effect is IOP independent. Hence, statins should be further explored as a new class of medications for the treatment of OAG, especially for those patients in whom disease progression continues despite an apparently sufficient IOP reduction.

Table 4. Multiple linear regression analysis with intraocular pressure at follow-up as the dependent variable.

	beta	95% confidence interval	P-value
Statins	−0.006	−0.262–0.249	0.96
Age (year)	−0.011	−0.026–0.005	0.18
Gender (female)	−0.269	−0.479–−0.060	0.012
IOP-lowering treatment at follow-up	1.761	1.340–2.181	<0.001
Family history of glaucoma	0.378	0.001–0.755	0.050
Myopia	0.597	0.124–1.069	0.013

IOP = intraocular pressure.

Author Contributions

Conceived and designed the experiments: NMJ RPHMM JRV AH PTVMdJ BHS. Performed the experiments: WDR RCWW JRV. Analyzed the data: MWM WDR. Wrote the paper: MWM RPHMM WDR RCWW PTVMdJ JRV AH BHS NMJ.

References

1. Endo A (1992) The discovery and development of HMG-CoA reductase inhibitors. J Lipid Res 33: 1569–1582.
2. Corsini A, Bellosta S, Baetta R, Fumagalli R, Paoletti R, et al. (1999) New insights into the pharmacodynamic and pharmacokinetic properties of statins. Pharmacol Ther 84: 413–428.
3. Schachter M (2005) Chemical, pharmacokinetic and pharmacodynamic properties of statins: An update. Fundam Clin Pharmacol 19: 117–125.
4. Grundy SM (1988) HMG-CoA reductase inhibitors for treatment of hypercholesterolemia. N Engl J Med 319: 24–33.
5. Van Leeuwen R, Vingerling J, Hofman A, de Jong P, Stricker B (2003) Cholesterol lowering drugs and risk of age related maculopathy: Prospective cohort study with cumulative exposure measurement. BMJ 326: 255–256.
6. McGwin G, Owsley C, Curcio C, Crain R (2003) The association between statin use and age related maculopathy. Br J Ophthalmol 87: 1121–1125.
7. Tan JS, Mitchell P, Rochtchina E, Wang JJ (2007) Statin use and the long-term risk of incident cataract: The blue mountains eye study. Am J Ophthalmol 143: 687–689.
8. Chodick G, Heymann AD, Flash S, Kokia E, Shalev V (2010) Persistence with statins and incident cataract: A population-based historical cohort study. Ann Epidemiol 20: 136–142.
9. Li J, Wang JJ, Chen D, Mott R, Yu Q, et al. (2009) Systemic administration of HMG-CoA reductase inhibitor protects the blood-retinal barrier and ameliorates retinal inflammation in type 2 diabetes. Exp Eye Res 89: 71–78.
10. Sen K, Misra A, Kumar A, Pandey RM (2002) Simvastatin retards progression of retinopathy in diabetic patients with hypercholesterolemia. Diabetes Res Clin Pract 56: 1–11.
11. Klein BE, Klein R, Lee KE, Grady LM (2006) Statin use and incident nuclear cataract. JAMA: The Journal of the American Medical Association 295: 2752–2758.
12. McGwin G, Jr., McNeal S, Owsley C, Girkin C, Epstein D, et al. (2004) Statins and other cholesterol-lowering medications and the presence of glaucoma. Arch Ophthalmol 122: 822–826.
13. Leung DY, Li FC, Kwong YY, Tham CC, Chi SC, et al. (2010) Simvastatin and disease stabilization in normal tension glaucoma: A cohort study. Ophthalmology 117: 471–476.
14. De Castro DK, Punjabi OS, Bostrom AG, Stamper RL, Lietman TM, et al. (2007) Effect of statin drugs and aspirin on progression in open-angle glaucoma suspects using confocal scanning laser ophthalmoscopy. Clin Experiment Ophthalmol 35: 506–513.
15. Owen CG, Carey IM, Shah S, de Wilde S, Wormald R, et al. (2010) Hypotensive medication, statins, and the risk of glaucoma. Invest Ophthalmol Vis Sci 51: 3524–3530.
16. Iskedjian M, Walker J, Desjardins O, Robin A, Covert D, et al. (2009) Effect of selected antihypertensives, antidiabetics, statins and diuretics on adjunctive medical treatment of glaucoma: A population based study. Curr Med Res Opin 25: 1879–1888.
17. Vaughan CJ, Delanty N (1999) Neuroprotective properties of statins in cerebral ischemia and stroke. Stroke 30: 1969–1973.
18. Stepien K, Tomaszewski M, Czuczwar SJ (2005) Neuroprotective properties of statins. Pharmacol Rep 57: 561–569.
19. Wood WG, Eckert GP, Igbavboa U, Muller WE (2010) Statins and neuroprotection: A prescription to move the field forward. Ann N Y Acad Sci 1199: 69–76.
20. van der Most PJ, Dolga AM, Nijholt IM, Luiten PG, Eisel UL (2009) Statins: Mechanisms of neuroprotection. Prog Neurobiol 88: 64–75.
21. Sierra S, Ramos MC, Molina P, Esteo C, Vazquez JA, et al. (2011) Statins as neuroprotectants: A comparative in vitro study of lipophilicity, blood-brain-barrier penetration, lowering of brain cholesterol, and decrease of neuron cell death. J Alzheimers Dis 23: 307–318.
22. McGuinness B, O'Hare J, Craig D, Bullock R, Malouf R, Passmore P (2010) Statins for the treatment of dementia. Cochrane Database Syst Rev 4: CD007514.
23. De Backer G, Ambrosioni E, Borch-Johnsen K, Brotons C, Cifkova R, et al. (2004) European guidelines on cardiovascular disease prevention in clinical practice. third joint task force of european and other societies on cardiovascular disease prevention in clinical practice (constituted by representatives of eight societies and by invited experts). Atherosclerosis 173: 381–391.
24. Expert Panel on Detection, Evaluation, and Treatment of High Blood Cholesterol in Adults (2001) Executive summary of the third report of the national cholesterol education program (NCEP) expert panel on detection, evaluation, and treatment of high blood cholesterol in adults (adult treatment panel III). JAMA 285: 2486–2497.
25. Walley T, Folino-Gallo P, Schwabe U, van Ganse E, EuroMedStat group (2004) Variations and increase in use of statins across europe: Data from administrative databases. BMJ 328: 385–386.
26. Hofman A, Breteler MM, Van Duijn CM, Janssen HL, Krestin GP, et al. (2009) The Rotterdam Study: 2010 objectives and design update. Eur J Epidemiol 24: 553–572.
27. Wolfs RC, Borger PH, Ramrattan RS, Klaver CC, Hulsman CA, et al. (2000) Changing views on open-angle glaucoma: Definitions and prevalences-the Rotterdam Study. Invest Ophthalmol Vis Sci 41: 3309–3321.
28. Dielemans I, Vingerling JR, Hofman A, Grobbee DE, Jong PT (1994) Reliability of intraocular pressure measurement with the Goldmann applanation tonometer in epidemiological studies. Graefe's Archive for Clinical and Experimental Ophthalmology 232: 141–144.
29. Skenduli-Bala E, de Voogd S, Wolfs RC, et al. (2005) Causes of incident visual field loss in a general elderly population: the Rotterdam study. Arch Ophthalmol 123: 233–238.
30. Czudowska MA, Ramdas WD, Wolfs RC, Hofman A, De Jong PT, et al. (2010) Incidence of glaucomatous visual field loss: A ten-year follow-up from the Rotterdam Study. Ophthalmology 117: 1705–1712.
31. Nagaoka T, Takahashi A, Sato E, Izumi N, Hein TW, et al. (2006) Effect of systemic administration of simvastatin on retinal circulation. Arch Ophthalmol 124: 665–670.
32. Marcus MW, de vries MM, Montolio FG, Jansonius NM (2011) Myopia as a risk factor for open-angle glaucoma: a systematic review and meta-analysis. Ophthalmology;In press.
33. Ekström C (2010) Risk factors for incident open-angle glaucoma: a population-based 20-years follow-up study. Acta Ophthalmol;DOI: 10.1111/j.1755-3768.2010.01943.x.
34. Gordon MO, Beiser JA, Brandt JD, Heuer DK, Higginbotham EJ, et al. (2002) The Ocular Hypertension Treatment Study: baseline factors that predict the onset of primary open-angle glaucoma. Arch Ophthalmol 120: 714–720.
35. Mitchell P, Wang JJ, Smith W (1997) Association of pseudoexfoliation syndrome with increased vascular risk. Am J Ophthalmol 124: 685–687.
36. Citirik M, Acaroglu G, Batman C, Yildiran L, Zilelioglu O (2007) A possible link between the pseudoexfoliation syndrome and coronary artery disease. Eye 21: 11–15.
37. Andrikopoulos GK, Mela EK, Georgakopoulos CD, Papadopoulos GE, Damelou AN, Alexopoulos DK, Gartaganis SP (2009) Pseudoexfoliation syndrome prevalence in Greek patients with cataract and its association to glaucoma and coronary artery disease. Eye 23: 442–447.
38. Stricker BH, Stijnen T (2010) Analysis of individual drug use as a time-varying determinant of exposure in prospective population-based cohort studies. Eur J Epidemiol 25: 245–251.
39. Colhoun HM, Betteridge DJ, Durrington PN, Hitman GA (2004) Primary prevention of cardiovascular disease with atorvastatin in type 2 diabetes in the collaborative atorvastatin diabetes study (CARDS): Multicentre randomised placebo-controlled trial. The Lancet 364: 685–696.
40. Collins R, Armitage J, Parish S, Sleigh P, Peto R, et al. (2003) MRC/BHF heart protection study of cholesterol-lowering with simvastatin in 5963 people with diabetes: A randomised placebo-controlled trial. Lancet 361: 2005–2016.

4

Prevention of Ocular Scarring Post Glaucoma Filtration Surgery Using the Inflammatory Cell and Platelet Binding Modulator Saratin in a Rabbit Model

Jeff Min[1], Zachary L. Lukowski[1], Monica A. Levine[1], Craig A. Meyers[1], Ashley R. Beattie[1], Gregory S. Schultz[2], Don A. Samuelson[3], Mark B. Sherwood[1]*

1 Department of Ophthalmology, College of Medicine, University of Florida, Gainesville, Florida, United States of America, **2** Department of Ob/Gyn and Institute of Wound Healing, College of Medicine, University of Florida, Gainesville, Florida, United States of America, **3** College of Veterinary Medicine, University of Florida, Gainesville, Florida, United States of America

Abstract

Clinical Relevance: Late complications can occur with use of current antimetabolites to prevent scarring following glaucoma filtration surgery (GFS). Safer, more targeted, anti-fibrosis agents are sought.

Objectives: The protein saratin has been shown to exhibit anti-fibrotic and anti-thrombotic properties in response to injury, but had not been used for glaucoma surgery. The goal of this study was to compare the efficacy of saratin with that of the widely accepted mitomycin-C (MMC) in prolonging bleb survival following GFS in the rabbit model. Two saratin delivery routes were compared; a single intraoperative topical application versus a combination of intraoperative topical application with two additional postoperative injections.

Methods: Twenty-four New Zealand White rabbits underwent GFS and received either intraoperative topical saratin, intraoperative topical saratin plus two injections on post-operative days 4 and 8, balanced saline solution (BSS), or MMC. The bleb tissues and their elevation durations were compared based on clinical and histological findings.

Results: Rabbits receiving topical+injections of saratin had a mean bleb survival of 33.6±8.5 days, significantly higher than the negative BSS controls, which averaged 17.4±6.0 days ($p = 0.018$). No improvement over BSS was seen for rabbits receiving topical saratin only (15.5±4.8 days, $p = 0.749$). Rabbits receiving saratin did not develop bleb avascularity and thinning associated with MMC treatment and there were no apparent clinical signs of toxicity.

Conclusions: Treatment with a single intraoperative topical application plus two additional postoperative injections significantly prolonged bleb elevation comparable to MMC, but without toxicity; however, topical application alone was ineffective.

Editor: Demetrios Vavvas, Massachusetts Eye & Ear Infirmary, Harvard Medical School, United States of America

Funding: Biovasc Incorporated supplied the protein Saratin used in the study as well as funding for the research with Award # 00067832 (http://www.biovascularinc.com/saratin.html). Research to Prevent Blindness also provided grant support for the study on project # 00068545 (www.rpbusa.org/). The funders had no role in study design, data collection and analysis, decision to publish, or preparation of the manuscript.

Competing Interests: Biovasc Incorporated supplied the protein Saratin used in the study as well as funding for the research with Award # 00067832(http://www.biovascularinc.com/saratin.html). This does not alter the authors' adherence to all the PLoS ONE policies on sharing data and materials.

* E-mail: Sherwood@ufl.edu

Introduction

Glaucoma filtration surgery (GFS) remains the gold standard for the management of intraocular pressure (IOP) when medication and laser surgery have proven insufficient [1,2]. However, scar tissue due increased fibroblast proliferation and activation can form between the conjunctiva/Tenon's capsule and the sclera at the surgical site often months or years after surgery, obstructing aqueous flow and causing the filter to fail [3,4].

The antimetabolites mitomycin-C (MMC) and 5-fluorouracil (5-FU) are used in current clinical practice to help limit post-operative ocular scar tissue formation. While these agents have been shown to improve the IOP outcome of GFS, they do so in a non-selective manner [5]. As a result, antimetabolite treatment is associated with a significant side-effect profile, including hypotony, blebitis, endophthalmitis, bleb leakage, and vision loss in a few [2,3,5–8]. Recent studies into alternative methods of preventing tissue fibrosis have focused on the inhibition of Tenon's capsule fibroblasts through the regulation of various growth factors [9–11]. Some success in reducing scar formation after GFS by inhibiting vascular endothelial growth factor (VEGF) and transforming growth factor-β (TGF-β) has been reported in recent literature [5,12,13].

The focus of this investigation is to examine the ability of saratin to limit ocular scarring following GFS. Saratin is a 12 kD protein which was originally isolated from the saliva of the leech *Hirudo medicinalis*. It has been shown to interfere with platelet integrin $\alpha_2\beta_1$-collagen and von Willebrand factor-collagen binding, preventing platelet aggregation in response to injury [14–17]. To date, saratin has been shown to be effective in preventing platelet adhesion and intimal hyperplasia in both animal and human models [18,19]. Recent studies in human models have shown that the protein has potent antithrombotic properties, making it useful in the treatment of atherosclerotic lesions [20].

Evidence also suggests that saratin can potentially reduce inflammation by limiting the immune response at the site of tissue injury. Primarily, it is thought that the protein interferes with the binding of inflammatory cells to extracellular matrix proteins, a necessary step for cell migration toward wound sites [21]. *In vitro* Boyden chamber assays indicated that saratin inhibits the chemotaxis of human monocytes and T-lymphocytes toward the chemokines MCP-1 and MIP-1α, respectively [22]. Secondarily, by interfering with platelet aggregation at the wound site, saratin limits the release of platelet-derived growth factor (PDGF), TGF-β, insulin-like growth factor (IGF), and epidermal growth factor (EGF) [23]. These growth factors have been shown to contribute toward accelerated ocular wound healing by stimulating proliferation, migration, and collagen production in Tenon's capsule fibroblasts [10,11,24,25].

The rabbit model is well-established as a standard animal model for the investigation of wound healing and scarring following GFS [25–28]. Our experiment investigates the ability of saratin to reduce fibrotic activity at the site of GFS. To our knowledge, this is the first reported ocular use of the saratin protein. The primary goals of this study were to evaluate potential methods of delivering saratin, as well as to compare the overall efficacy of saratin versus a BSS negative control and a MMC positive control. An additional aim for this project was to identify potential side effects of treatment using saratin.

Methods and Materials

Twenty four New Zealand White rabbits weighting between 2 kg and 4 kg were used for this study. All animal experiments performed adhered to the ARVO Statement for the Use of Animals in Ophthalmic and Vision Research and were approved by the University of Florida's Institutional Animal Care and Use Committee.

Study Design

The rabbits were randomized to one of 4 different treatment groups of six rabbits each. All 24 rabbits underwent glaucoma filtering operation in their left eyes with one surgeon (MBS) performing the procedures; the right eyes were not operated on and served as controls.

Rabbits in the first experimental group received a single topical application of saratin at 5 mg/ml applied intraoperatively using a standardized 5 mm×5 mm partial-thickness Weck cell (Alcon Surgical, Fort Worth, TX), immediately following the fashioning of a fornix-based conjunctival flap.

Rabbits in the second experimental group also received a topical application with the partial-thickness Weck cell sponge at the time of surgery. In addition, two 0.1 ml subconjunctival injections of saratin at 5 mg/ml were administered on postoperative days (POD) 4 and 8. The protein saratin used in both experimental groups one and two was supplied by BioVascular, Inc., is now made by recombinant expression in yeast (*Hansenula polymorpha*) and purified to greater than 95% purity.

To provide a more accurate comparison to the experimental groups, all rabbits in the negative control group received an intraoperative topical application of BSS. Three (half) of the rabbits in this group also received 0.1 ml subconjunctival injections of BSS on POD 4 and 8 to match group 2 rabbits and three did not in order to mimic group 1 rabbits and MMC positive controls. All postoperative subconjunctival injections were given following bleb examination by the masked observer, and the injection material remained unknown to both the observer and the clinician giving the injection.

Finally, rabbits in the positive control group received a topical application of 0.4 mg/ml mitomycin-C at the time of surgery and were not given any post-operative injections.

Glaucoma Filtering Operation

The rabbits were anesthetized with an intramuscular injection of a combination of 50 mg/kg ketamine ("Ketaject", Phoenix, Mo) and 10 mg/kg xylazine ("Xyla-ject", Phoenix, Mo). A topical anesthetic, 0.1% proparacaine eye drop (Bausch & Lomb, Tampa, FL), was also administered. The surgical technique for the glaucoma filtration operations was similar to the procedures described in previous publications [25]. In brief, an eyelid speculum retracted the eyelids. A partial-thickness, corneal traction suture made in the superior cornea rotated the eye inferiorly. In the superior lateral quadrant of the eye at the limbus, a measured standard sized 5 mm fornix-based conjunctival flap was created. Blunt dissection helped undermine the conjunctiva and Tenon's capsule. At this point, a 5 mm×5 mm partial-thickness Weck cell (Alcon Surgical, Fort Worth, TX) soaked in 5 mg/ml saratin, 0.4 mg/ml mitomycin-C, or BSS depending on the treatment group was placed locally between the conjunctiva/Tenon's capsule and the sclera. After 5 minutes, the sponge was removed and the area was washed with 30 ml of saline. Next, a clear corneal paracentesis tract was fashioned in the superonasal quadrant using a # 75 Beaver™ blade (Becton Dickinson & Co., Franklin Lakes, NJ). A viscoelastic material (Healon® 10mg/ml, Pharmacia & Upjohn) was injected to maintain the anterior chamber.

A 25-gauge needle was then used to create a beveled, full-thickness tract through the sclera into the anterior chamber about 1 mm posterior to the limbus. This was followed by insertion of a 22-gauge, IV cannula (Insyte® Becton Dickinson Vascular Access, Sandy, UT) along this tract into the anterior chamber. The cannula needle was pulled out, and the cannula was positioned beyond the pupillary margin to prevent the tube from being occluded by iris. The cannula was trimmed at its scleral end so it would not protrude more than approximately 1 mm from the point of insertion. A 10–0 nylon suture (Ethicon Inc., Somerville, NJ) was used to anchor the tube to the sclera.

A running suture of 8–0 absorbable suture material (*Vicryl®*, Ethicon Inc., Somerville, NJ) was used to close the conjunctiva/Tenon's capsule at the limbus in a watertight fashion. At the end of the procedure, saline was injected into the anterior chamber via the paracentesis tract to elevate the bleb and a Seidel test performed to ensure that there was no bleb leak. An ointment of neomycin and dexamethasone was applied topically immediately following the surgery.

Post-Operative Injections and Clinical Evaluations

Following the operation, the eyes were examined three times per week by an examiner masked to the treatment group. The examiner looked for the presence of bleb elevation as well as for any complications that may have resulted from the surgeries or various treatments, including conjunctival injection, edema, anterior chamber shallowing, tube mal-positioning, hyphema or sub-conjunctival hemorrhage, bleb leaks, and corneal or lens opacification. Bleb failure was declared after the masked observer deemed the bleb to be flat in two consecutive examinations. The first of the two dates was recorded as the endpoint. When applicable, rabbits in the saratin and BSS treatment groups were also given injections of 0.1 ml saratin or 0.1 ml BSS respectively on POD 4 and 8.

The rabbits were anesthetized with isoflurane during their post-operative examinations, and a topical 0.1% proparacaine anesthetic eye drop was administered for those that required a post-op injection. A speculum was used to retract the eyelids. Non-toothed Bishop-Harmon forceps were used to tent the conjunctiva, and the 0.1 ml injections were given near the bleb using a 30-gauge needle on a 1 ml syringe on POD 4 and 8.

Histology

Eyes were obtained from one rabbit in each of the four groups on post-operative day (POD) 12 so bleb tissues could be examined at a uniform time. Eyes were obtained from all other rabbits after the bleb was observed to be flat in two consecutive clinical evaluations.

The tissues were fixed for 24 hours in a 10% neutral buffered formalin solution. The globes were placed in tissue cassettes, and then processed through graded ethanol and xylene using a Sakura Tissue-Tek VIP 5 tissue processor (Torrance, CA). The tissues were infiltrated with paraffin (Richard-Allan Scientific, Kalamazoo, MI) and embedded on a Tissue Tek III embedding center. Sagittal serial sections of the globes were taken. Once deparaffinized, the sections were stained using either standard Harris hematoxylin and eosin or Masson's trichrome. The slides were examined under light microscopy by an observer masked to the treatment groups and representative sections were photographed using a Canon EOS T1i digital camera attached to an Olympus Vanox microscope. The slides were qualitatively graded based upon collagen and fibroblast densities and vascularity in the tissues around the end of the cannula, plus preservation of the conjunctival tissue morphology including goblet cell numbers.

Statistical Analysis

Analysis of Variance (ANOVA) testing was used to determine any significant difference in bleb survival duration among the treatment groups. Tukey's Honestly Significantly Different (HSD) post hoc test was then used to determine significance between pairs of relevant groups.

Results

Bleb Survival

Rabbits receiving a single 5 minute topical application of saratin had an average time to bleb failure of 15.5+/− 4.8 days. Rabbits receiving two additional injections of saratin on POD 4 and 8 had an average time of 33.6+/− 8.5 days. The average time to bleb failure for rabbits receiving BSS injections/topical application was 17.4+/− 6.0 days. Rabbits receiving MMC treatments had bleb elevation durations averaging 41.6+/− 13.0 days. The rabbits from each treatment group sacrificed on POD 12 for histologic comparison were omitted from these data calculations. These results are represented in a Kaplan-Meier survival plot (Fig. 1) and summarized using a box-and-whisker plot (Fig. 2).

Analysis of variance (ANOVA) testing revealed a significant difference among the treatment groups ($p = 0.001$) at a 95% confidence interval. Post-hoc testing with Tukey's Honestly Significant Different (HSD) showed that the MMC rabbit group had a significantly longer bleb survival duration than the BSS group at a 95% confidence interval. In addition, there was a significant difference in bleb survival duration between the topical+injection saratin group and the BSS group at a 90% confidence interval. No significant improvements over BSS were found for the topical-only saratin group at a 90 or 95% confidence interval. Finally, there was no statistically significant difference between the MMC group and the topical+injection saratin treatment group at a 90% or 95% confidence interval.

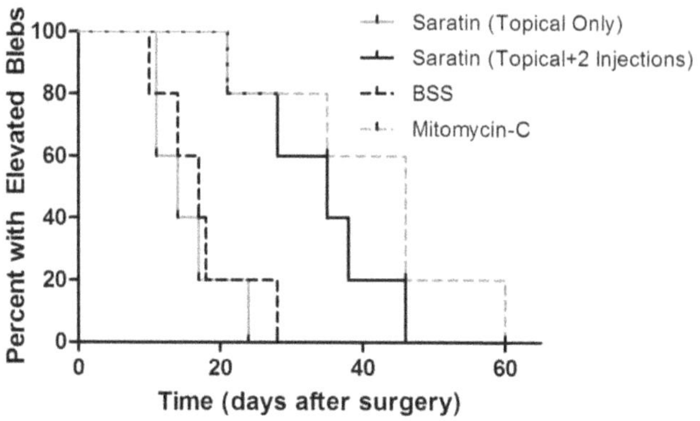

Figure 1. Kaplan-Meier bleb survival plot of eyes in each treatment group. For each rabbit, bleb failure was declared after the bleb appeared flat in two consecutive masked clinical examinations. The first of the two dates was recorded as the endpoint.

Clinical Evaluation

Blebs treated with MMC developed avascularity that was not observed in either saratin or BSS groups. There were no clinical signs of obvious toxicity to saratin treatments.

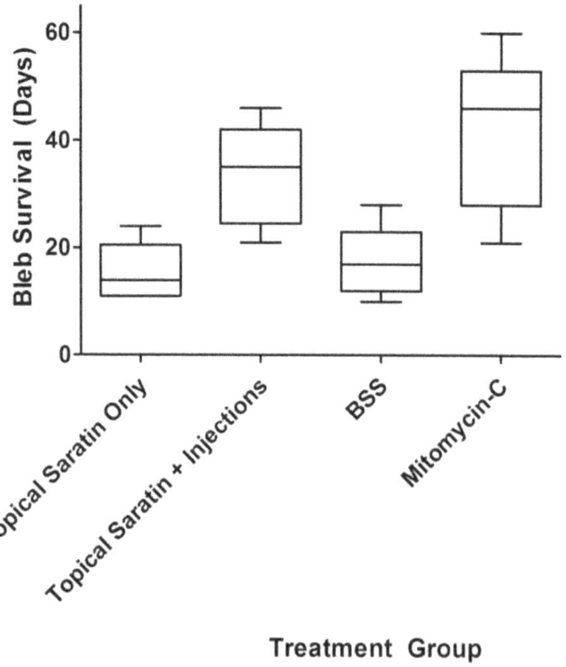

Figure 2. Box-and-whisker plot of bleb survival for each treatment group. First and third quartiles are delineated by boxes. Whiskers represent maxima and minima.

Histology

Histological examination focused on samples taken on post-operative day 12 to provide a common time-point of comparison (Fig. 3 & 4). Among all treatment groups, a zone of fibroblast proliferation with associated intracellular collagen was observed bordering the site of the implant. A variable infiltration of plasma cells and polymorphonuclear leukocytes (PMNLs) was evident within this area. The rabbits that received saratin by either topical application or injections had a mild collagen density and a moderate fibroblast proliferation. The group that received BSS showed a mild to moderate fibroblast density and a collagen density similar to the animals in the saratin group. The MMC group showed slightly less fibrosis, with minimal to mild collagen and fibroblast density highlighted by a large region of acellular fibrosis and necrosis (Fig. 4, right). The conjunctiva of rabbits treated with saratin did not exhibit avascularity, tissue thinning, and change in epithelial morphology from pseudostratified columnar to stratified squamous with a loss of mucin-producing (goblet) cells typical of MMC treatment (Fig. 5).

Discussion

In this study we examined the antifibrotic effects of saratin, a protein which has been previously investigated as an antithrombotic agent. Because the application of saratin in GFS was a novel use for the protein, we tested two methods of delivering the drug. The first experimental group received only an intraoperative topical application similar to the method in which MMC is currently administered. A second experimental group received a combined treatment of topical saratin with additional subconjunctival injections on POD 4 and 8. Because the amount of saratin retained in ocular tissues is unknown, the injections in the latter treatment modality ensured high amounts of the protein over an extended duration.

Statistical analysis showed that intraoperative topical saratin alone did not improve bleb survival compared to BSS negative controls. The Kaplan-Meier survival plot (Fig. 1) and box-and-whisker plot (Fig. 2) show that rabbits in the topical saratin group performed similarly to those in the BSS group. However, the group which received postoperative injections of saratin in addition to topical application had a significant improvement over BSS negative controls and was comparable to the MMC positive control group. While the mean for the topical+injection saratin group was slightly less than that of the MMC group ($33.6^{+}/-$ 8.5 days vs. 41.6+/− 13.0 days), the difference was not statistically significant.

When applied topically for a brief period of 1–5 minutes, MMC has an immediate effect on local tissues by alkylating and crosslinking DNA, as well as inhibiting DNA synthesis, transcription, and translation [29]. Topical saratin, when administered in a similar manner for 5 minutes did not improve bleb survival beyond that of the BSS control. When two post-operative subconjunctival injections were given in addition, there was a significant improvement over BSS control and the bleb survival was not significantly different from the MMC positive control. The ineffectiveness of topical saratin when administered at surgery using a partial-thickness Weck cell sponge suggests three possibilities; either a lack of local uptake of the saratin from the sponge, or that contact with the tissues was not long enough to produce an effect, or that peroperative application is not the most effective time to deliver saratin compared to early post-operative treatment. The optimal delivery route, number of applications, and the half-life of saratin in the ocular tissues warrant further study.

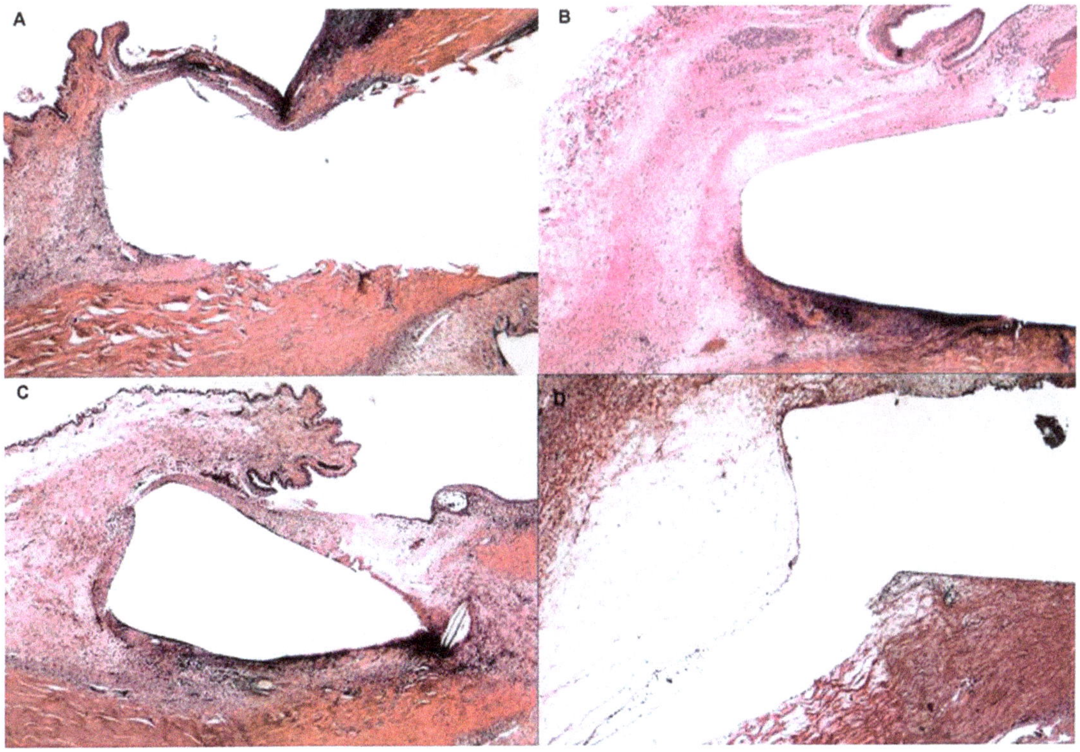

Figure 3. Representative sections of the implant site taken on POD 12, H&E 20x; (A) Topical saratin; (B) Topical+2 injections of saratin; (C) Balanced saline solution; (D) Mitomycin-C.

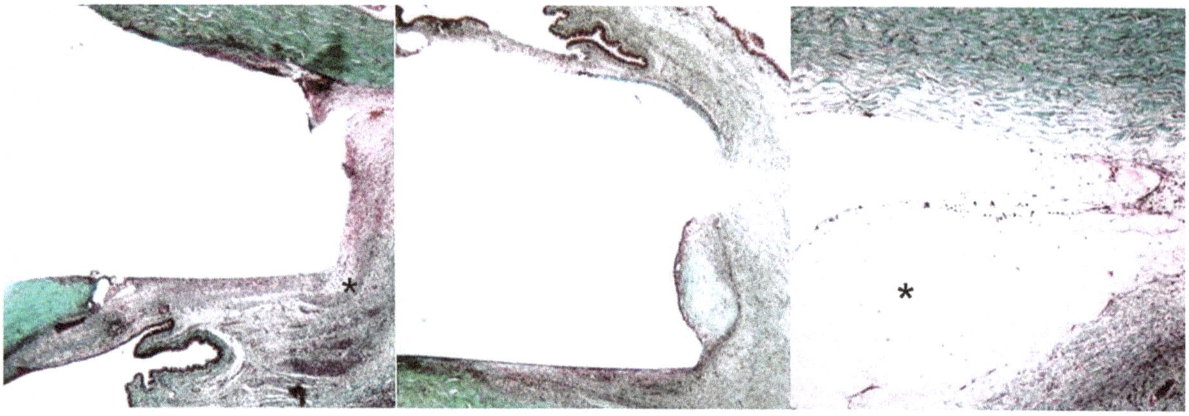

Figure 4. Representative sections of the implant site taken on POD 12, Masson's Trichrome 20x; Left: Topical+2 injections of saratin; *asterisk*, mild collagen density and moderate fibroblast proliferation Middle: Balanced saline solution; Right: Mitomycin-C; *asterisk*, acellular fibrosis and necrosis.

Clinically and histologically, saratin did not appear to cause bleb avascularity and tissue thinning, including alteration in epithelial structure, commonly associated with MMC treatment. While the topical+injection group did not outperform MMC, the effects of MMC have been extensively studied and the dosage optimized [2,3,5–8,29]. Further studies on saratin may be necessary to improve the dosing regimen and to provide additional information regarding potential side-effects.

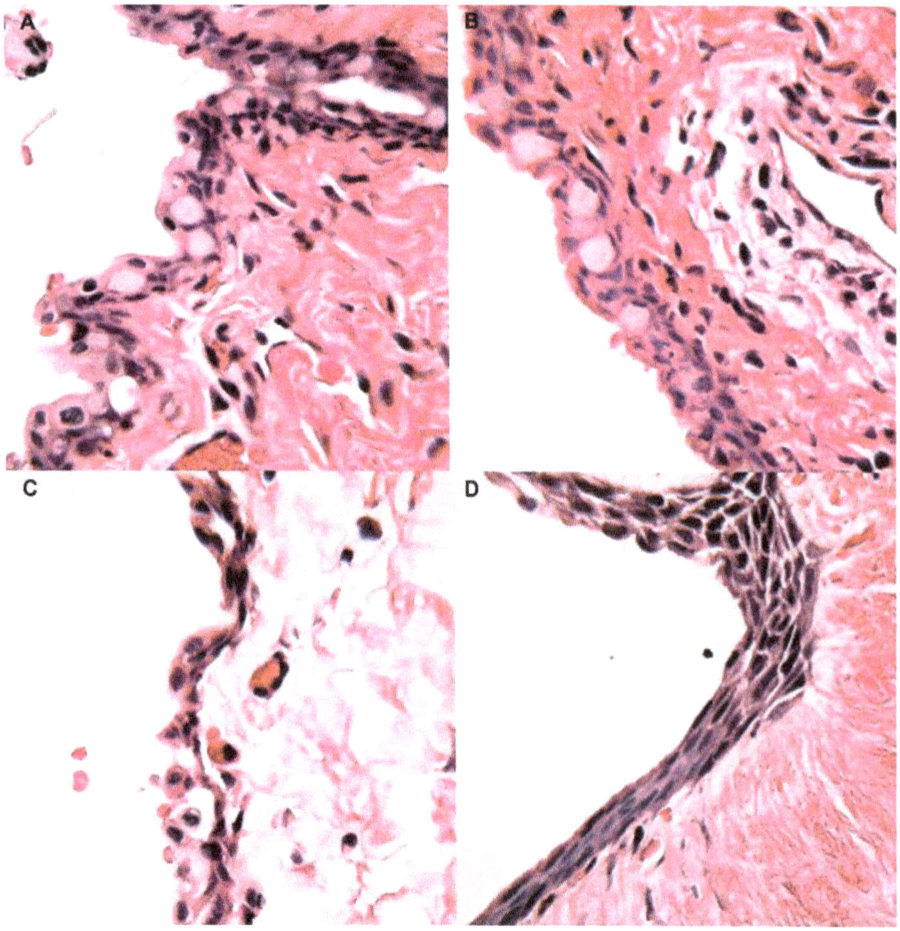

Figure 5. Representative sections of the bleb conjunctiva taken on POD 12, H&E 250x; (A) Topical saratin; (B) Topical+2 injections of saratin; (C) Balanced saline solution; (D) Mitomycin-C.

Acknowledgments

The authors would like to thank BioVasc Incorporated for supplying the protein saratin used in the study as well as funding for the research. We also extend thanks to the Research to Prevent Blindness for their generous grant.

Author Contributions

Conceived and designed the experiments: ZLL JM MBS. Performed the experiments: ZLL JM MAL CAM ARB MBS. Analyzed the data: JM MAL ZLL. Contributed reagents/materials/analysis tools: GSS DAS. Wrote the paper: MAL JM ZLL MBS.

References

1. Burr J, Azuara-Blanco A, Avenell A (2005) Medical versus surgical interventions for open angle glaucoma. Cochrane Database Syst Rev 18: CD004399.
2. DeBry PW, Perkins TW, Heatley G, et al. (2002) Incidence of late-onset bleb-related complications following trabeculectomy with mitomycin. Arch Ophthalmol 120: 297–300.
3. Muckley ED, Lehrer RA (2004) Late-onset blebitis/endophthalmitis: incidence and outcomes with mitomycin C. Optom Vis Sci 81: 499–504.
4. Francis BA, Du LT, Najafi K, Murthy R, Kurumety U, et al. (2005) Histopathologic features of conjunctival filtering blebs. Arch Ophthalmol 123: 166–70.
5. Li Z, Van Bergen T, Van de Veire S, Van de Vel I, Moreau H, et al. (2009) Inhibition of vascular endothelial growth factor reduces scar formation after glaucoma filtration surgery. Invest Ophthal Vis Sci 50: 5217–5225.
6. Bindlish R, Condon GP, Schlosser JD, D'Antonio J, Lauer KB, et al. (2002) Efficacy and safety of mitomycin-C in primary trabeculectomy: five year follow-up. Ophthalmology 109: 1336–1341.
7. Anand N, Arora S, Clowes M (2006) Mitomycin C augmented glaucoma surgery: evolution of filtering bleb avascularity, transconjunctival oozing, and leaks. Br J Ophthalmol. 90: 175–180.
8. Beckers HJ, Kinders KC, Webers CA (2003) Five-year results of trabeculectomy with mitomycin C. Graefes Arch Clin Exp Opthalmol 241: 106–10.
9. Denk PO, Hoppe J, Hoppe V, Knorr M (2003) Effect of growth factors on the activation of human Tenon's capsule fibroblasts. Curr Eye Res 27: 35–44.
10. Schultz G, Khaw PT, Oxford K, MaCauley S, Van Setten G, et al. (1994) Growth factors and ocular wound healing. Eye 8: 184–187.
11. Khaw PT, Occleston NL, Schultz G, Grierson I, Sherwood MB, et al. (1994) Activation and suppression of fibroblast function. Eye 8: 188–195.
12. Meyer-ter-Vehn T, Katzenberger B, Han H, Grehn F, Schlunck G (2008) Lovastatin inhibits TGF-β-induced myofibroblast transdifferentiation in human tenon fibroblasts. Invest Ophthal Vis Sci 49: 3955–3960.
13. Xiao YQ, Liu K, Shen JF, Xu G, Ye W (2009) SB-431542 inhibition of scar formation after filtration surgery and its potential mechanism. Invest Ophthal Vis Sci 50: 1698–1706.
14. Barnes CS, Krafft B, Frech M, Hofmann UR, Papendieck A (2001) Production and characterization of saratin, an inhibitor of von Willebrand factor-dependent platelet adhesion to collagen. Semin Thromb Hemost 24: 337–348.
15. Bonnefoy A, Romijn RA, Vandervoort PA, VAN Rompaey I, Vermylen J, et al. (2006) Von Willebrand factor A1 domain can adequately substitute for A3 domain in recruitment of flowing platelets to collagen. J Thromb Taemost 4: 2151–61.
16. White TC, Berny MA, Robinson DK, Yin H, DeGrado WF, et al. (2007) The leech product saratin is a potent inhibitor of platelet integrin alpha2beta1 and von Willebrand factor binding to collagen. FEBS J 274: 1481–1491.
17. Gronwald W, Bomke J, Maurer T, Domogalla B, Huber F, et al. (2008) Structure of the leech protein saratin and characterization of its binding to collagen. J Mol Biol 381: 913–927.
18. Smith TP, Alshafie TA, Cruz CP, Fan CY, Brown AT, et al. (2003) Saratin, an inhibitor of collagen-platelet interaction, decreases venous anastomotic intimal hyperplasia in a canine dialysis access model. Vasc Endovascular Surg 37: 259–69.
19. Davis JA, Brown AT, Alshafie T, Poirier LA, Cruz CP, et al. (2004) Saratin (an inhibitor of platelet-collagen interaction) decreases platelet aggregation and homocysteine-mediated postcarotid endarterectomy intimal hyperplasia in a dose-dependent manner. Am J Surg 188: 778–785.
20. Vilahur G, Duran X, Juan-Babot O, Casani L, Badimon L (2004) Antithrombotic effects of saratin on human atherosclerotic plaques. Thromb Haemost 95: 191–200.
21. Dugrillon A, Eichler H, Kern S, Kluter H (2002) Autologous concentrated platelet-rich plasma (cPRP) for local application in bone regeneration. Int J Oral Maxillofac Surg 31: 615–9.
22. Glidden PF (2010) Methods and compositions for blocking platelet and cell adhesion, cell migration and inflammation. Patent No. US7691839B2 p.
23. Gehring S, Hoerauf H, Laqua H, Kirchner H, Kluter H (1999) Preparation of autologous platelets for the ophthalmic treatment of macular holes. Transfusion 39: 144–148.
24. Knorr M, Volker M, Denk PO, Wunderlich K, Thiel HJ (1997) Proliferative response of cultured human Tenon's capsule fibroblasts to platelet-derived growth factor isoforms. Graefe's Arch Clin Exp Ophthalmol 235: 667–671.
25. Cordeiro MF, Constable PH, Alexander RA, Bhattacharya SS, Khaw PT (1997) Effect of varying the mitomycin-C treatment area in glaucoma filtration surgery in the rabbit. Invest Ophthalmol Vis Sci 38: 1639–1646.
26. Sherwood MB, Esson DW, Neelakantan A, Samuelson DA (2004) A new model of glaucoma filtering surgery in the rat. J Glaucoma 13: 407–12.
27. Doyle JW, Sherwood MB, Khaw PT, McGrory S, Smith MF (1993) Intraoperative 5-fluorouracil for filtration surgery in the rabbit. Invest Ophthalmol Vis Sci 34: 3313–3319.
28. Connon CJ, Meek KM (2003) Organization of corneal collagen fibrils during the healing of trephined wounds in rabbits. Wound Repair Regen 11: 71–78.
29. Khaw PT, Doyle JW, Sherwood MB, Smith MF, McGorray S (1993) Effects of intraoperative 5-fluorouracil or mitomycin C on glaucoma filtration surgery in the rabbit. Ophthalmology100: 367–72.

5

Autotaxin-Lysophosphatidic Acid Axis Is a Novel Molecular Target for Lowering Intraocular Pressure

Padma Iyer[1], Robert Lalane III[1], Corey Morris[1], Pratap Challa[1], Robin Vann[1], Ponugoti Vasantha Rao[1,2]*

1 Department of Ophthalmology, Duke University School of Medicine, Durham, North Carolina, United States of America, **2** Department of Pharmacology and Cancer Biology, Duke University School of Medicine, Durham, North Carolina, United States of America

Abstract

Primary open-angle glaucoma is the second leading cause of blindness in the United States and is commonly associated with elevated intraocular pressure (IOP) resulting from diminished aqueous humor (AH) drainage through the trabecular pathway. Developing effective therapies for increased IOP in glaucoma patients requires identification and characterization of molecular mechanisms that regulate IOP and AH outflow. This study describes the identification and role of autotaxin (ATX), a secretory protein and a major source for extracellular lysophosphatidic acid (LPA), in regulation of IOP in a rabbit model. Quantitative proteomics analysis identified ATX as an abundant protein in both human AH derived from non-glaucoma subjects and in AH from different animal species. The lysophospholipase D (LysoPLD) activity of ATX was found to be significantly elevated (by ~1.8 fold; $n = 20$) in AH derived from human primary open angle glaucoma patients as compared to AH derived from age-matched cataract control patients. Immunoblotting analysis of conditioned media derived from primary cultures of human trabecular meshwork (HTM) cells has confirmed secretion of ATX and the ability of cyclic mechanical stretch of TM cells to increase the levels of secreted ATX. Topical application of a small molecular chemical inhibitor of ATX (S32826), which inhibited AH LysoPLD activity *in vitro* (by >90%), led to a dose-dependent and significant decrease of IOP in Dutch-Belted rabbits. Single intracameral injection of S32826 (~2 µM) led to significant reduction of IOP in rabbits, with the ocular hypotensive response lasting for more than 48 hrs. Suppression of ATX expression in HTM cells using small-interfering RNA (siRNA) caused a decrease in actin stress fibers and myosin light chain phosphorylation. Collectively, these observations indicate that the ATX-LPA axis represents a potential therapeutic target for lowering IOP in glaucoma patients.

Editor: Asad U. Khan, Aligarh Muslim University, India

Funding: This work was supported by the National Eye Institute, National Institutes of Health grants RO1 EY18950 and EY18950 ARRA stimulus supplement to PVR. The funding agencies had no role in study design, data collection and analysis, decision to publish, or preparation of the manuscript.

Competing Interests: The authors have declared that no competing interests exist.

* E-mail: rao00011@mc.duke.edu

Introduction

Glaucoma, a leading cause of blindness characterized by optic nerve degeneration and progressive visual field loss, is commonly associated with elevated intraocular pressure (IOP) [1]. Ocular hypertension (OH) or elevated IOP is a definite and primary risk factor for primary open angle glaucoma (POAG) [1,2,3]. The risk of developing glaucoma decreases significantly when a 20% reduction in IOP is achieved in patients with OH, and ocular hypotensive therapy remains the mainstay of glaucoma treatment [4,5]. However, while there are several classes of ocular hypotensive drugs available for treatment of glaucoma, there remains a significant unmet medical need for novel, more efficacious and targeted therapy [5,6]. This need requires that we address the gap which currently exists in our understanding of regulation of IOP and AH outflow and identification of physiological and pathological factors that influence IOP and AH outflow in both normal and glaucoma patients.

The conventional or trabecular AH outflow pathway is composed of the trabecular meshwork (TM), juxtacanalicular connective tissue (JCT) and Schlemm's canal (SC). In humans, this pathway represents a predominant route of AH drainage [3]. AH is secreted by non-pigmented epithelial cells that line the ciliary body and flows into the anterior chamber, which then drains through the TM into Schlemm's canal and the episcleral veins on a continuous basis. While there is a general agreement that decreased AH outflow through the trabecular pathway is the primary cause for increased IOP in glaucoma patients, little is known about the molecular basis for increased resistance to AH outflow through the trabecular pathway [3,7]. Various extracellular factors including TGF-beta, bioactive lipids (lysophosphatidic acid and Sphingosine-1 phosphate), endothelin-1, myocilin, interleukins, prostaglandins, steroids, CD44, matrix metalloproteinases and extracellular matrix proteins have been reported to influence AH outflow and IOP [3,8,9,10,11,12,13,14,15,16,17,18]. Importantly, the levels of some of these factors have been shown to be elevated in the AH of human glaucoma patients [2,13,19,20,21].

In our previous work, we demonstrated that TM and SC cells express different G-protein coupled receptors specific for both lysophosphatidic acid (LPA) and sphingosin-1-phosphate (S1P), and perfusion of enucleated eyes with these lipids was noted to influence AH outflow concomitant with changes in TM cell contractile properties, Rho GTPase activation and expression of extracellular matrix proteins [15,22]. These initial observations were subsequently confirmed by independent investigators and collectively supported the importance of bioactive lipids in regulation of AH outflow and potentially IOP [15,17,23]. Although these observations implied the significance of LPA and SIP in the regulation of AH outflow, we currently know very little about how the levels of these bioactive lipids are regulated in AH, and the different molecular mechanisms involved in the generation of these lipids in the AH. To explore these questions, we recently performed quantitative proteomic analysis of human AH derived from cataract surgery patients with normal IOP. This initial analysis revealed that ATX [24], which is a well characterized secretory protein with lysophospholipase D (LysoPLD) activity, was one of the abundant proteins in human AH. Since this protein has been considered a major source for extracellular LPA [25,26], and LPA has in turn been demonstrated to influence AH outflow facility [15], in this study we investigated the role of ATX in IOP using a small molecular weight chemical inhibitor of this protein. This study reports that inhibition of ATX LysoPLD activity by topical and intracameral delivery of a chemical inhibitor significantly decreases IOP, suggesting that ATX is a potential therapeutic target for lowering IOP in glaucoma patients.

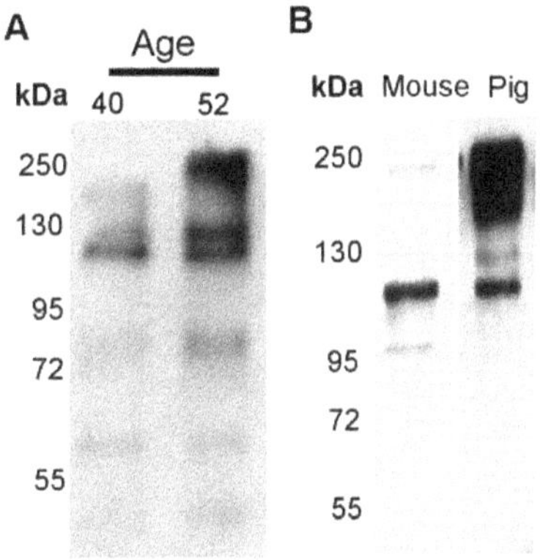

Figure 1. Detection of ATX in the AH from human and other species. A. Immunoblot analysis of AH (10 µg protein) derived from two different human donors (aged 40 and 52 years) revealed multiple immunopositive bands with molecular mass ranging between 65 to 250 kDa. B. Detection of ATX by immunoblot analysis of mouse and porcine AH (10 µg protein). Similar to human AH, both mouse and porcine exhibit ATX immunopositive bands with molecular mass ranging from 95 to 250 kDa.

Results

ATX is an abundant protein of human aqueous humor

Towards our objective to identifying extracellular factors regulating AH outflow and IOP, an LC-MS (liquid chromatography- mass spectrometry) proteomic analysis was performed to identify abundant proteins of human AH, using one µg of pooled AH total protein derived from 8 individual donors who underwent cataract surgery. This analysis identified eighty nine non-redundant proteins with high confidence based on 2 or more matching peptides. Individual proteins were quantified by comparison of signal intensity, using an internal standard of yeast alcohol dehydrogenase (label free). Table S1 lists AH proteins identified by proteomic analysis, together with their respective Swiss-Prot protein accession number, protein common name and relative concentration (fmol/1 µg total protein). Of the different easily detectable proteins present in the human AH sample, ATX, also known as Ectonucleotide pyrophosphatase/phosphodiesterase (ENNP2), was found to be one of 25 most abundant proteins (Table S1).

To independently confirm the presence of ATX in AH by an alternative means, we performed immunoblotting analysis of AH using a rabbit polyclonal anti-ATX antibody. Immunoblotting analysis of 10 µg of human AH total protein derived from two independent donors (aged 40 and 52 years) identified multiple immunopositive bands with molecular mass ranging from 65 to 250 kDa, confirming the presence of ATX isoforms in different proteolytically and postranslationally processed forms (Fig. 1A). Protein blots of the AH sample were also probed with primary antibody which was pre-blocked with antigen specific peptide or secondary antibody alone, to confirm specificity of the primary antibody used for immunoblotting, and confirmed lack of non-specific reactions in the observed results. We also confirmed the presence of ATX in mouse and porcine AH by immunoblot analysis (Fig. 1B) and comparative analysis revealed interesting differences and similarities in the profiles of ATX isoforms between the human, mouse and porcine species.

Elevated levels of LysoPLD activity in the AH of POAG patients

To measure LysoPLD activity in human AH, we utilized a modified fluorogenic enzyme-coupled assay protocol [27] using a commercially available Amplex Red PLD Assay kit. Human AH samples derived from 20 different cataract and POAG patients were tested for LysoPLD activity. While age and sex were matched between the cataract and glaucoma groups, race demography was found to be significantly ($p<0.05$) different between the two groups based on both Fisher's exact and Chi-Square tests. As shown in Figure 2A, the racial composition of the POAG sample group consisted of 75% African American, 15% Caucasian/white and 5% Hispanic patients. On the other hand, the cataract control group comprised of 85% Caucasian/white and 15% African American patients. LysoPLD activity measured in these specimens was expressed as micromoles of H_2O_2 generated per milligram of AH protein, with the activity measured for POAG patients being significantly elevated (by 1.8 fold, $n = 20$), as compared to the cataract control specimen values, based on the Wilcoxon Rank Sum test of differences in medians with one-way Chi-Square approximation (Fig. 2B and 2C). Figure 2C provides Box-and-whisker plots of the AH LysoPLD activity of glaucoma and cataract controls, with the box showing median and interquartile ranges.

ATX is expressed and secreted by TM cells

Since ATX was easily detectable in human AH samples, we hypothesized that this protein is expressed and secreted by cells of the AH outflow pathway. RT-PCR analysis confirmed expression of all three isoforms of ATX (α, β and γ, Fig. 3A) [28] in primary cultures of HTM cells derived from three different donors (aged 33, 54 and 75 years; representative data from a single TM cell strain (donor) is shown). Examination of the cellular distribution profiles of ATX in primary cultures of HTM cells by immunofluorescence analysis using a polyclonal antibody specific for ATX (Fig. 3B) reveals a distinct vesicular/punctate distribution pattern, which is a characteristic feature of secretory proteins. Immunoblotting analysis of ATX protein profiles in cell lysates (20 µg protein) derived from primary cultures of HTM and porcine TM cells (Fig. 3C and 3D, respectively) revealed multiple immunopositive bands with molecular mass ranging from 55 to 250 kDa. On the other hand, the HTM cell conditioned media (10 µg protein) exhibited a single immunopositive band with a molecular mass of ~95 kDa (Fig. 3C). Compared to the HTM cells, the PTM cell conditioned media (10 µg) showed the 95 kDa protein similar to

A

	Cataract	POAG
Age	47-85	25-86
Males	30%	30%
Females	70%	70%
Race - White	85%	15%
- Black	15%	70%
- Hispanic	0%	5%

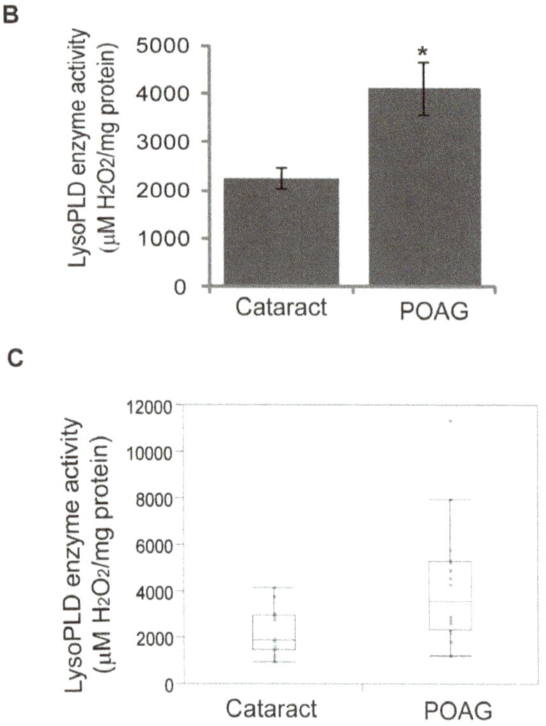

Figure 2. Elevated levels of LysoPLD activity in AH derived from primary open angle glaucoma human patients. A. Details of the demographics for the Cataract control and POAG patients. B. LysoPLD activity (expressed per unit of AH total protein) in the AH of POAG patients (n = 20) revealed a significant (* $p <= 0.005$) increase relative to age-matched cataract control specimens based on the Wilcoxon Rank Sum test. C. Box-and-whisker plot of the AH LysoPLD activity of glaucoma and cataract controls with box showing median and interquartile range.

the HTM cells and an additional immunopositive band at around ~65 kDa (Fig. 3D).

In vitro inhibition of AH ATX activity by S32826

For this experiment, the water soluble chemical inhibitor-S32826 [4-(Tetradecanoylamino) benzyl phosphonic acid disodium salt] which inhibits ATX in the nanomolar range [29], was used to assess inhibition of LysoPLD activity in AH derived from the rabbits *in vitro*. Ten microgram aliquots of rabbit AH total protein were incubated with different concentrations (5–25 µM) of S32826 at 37°C for 20 minutes prior to determining LysoPLD activity using Amplex Red reagent [27]. While S32826 is reported to have an IC_{50} in the nanomolar range (9 nM) for purified ATX, and a low IC_{50} for the phosphodiesterase activity of ATX, the IC_{50} for inhibition of LPA release from adipocytes is much higher (200 nM) [29]. Therefore, we used µM range drug concentrations

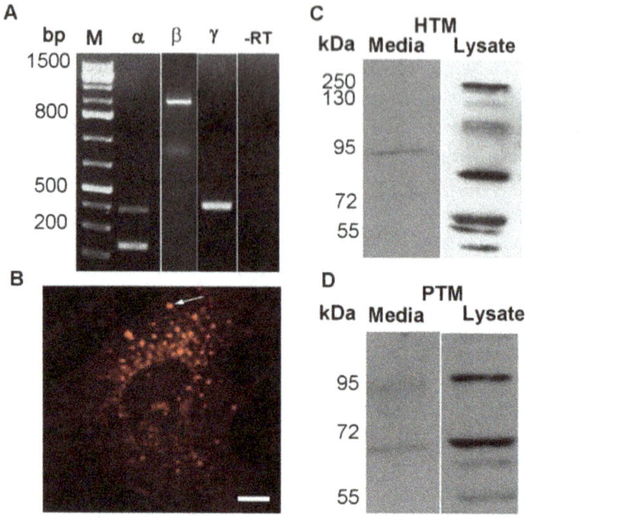

Figure 3. Expression and secretion of ATX by primary cultures of trabecular meshwork cells derived from human and porcine eyes. A. RT-PCR based amplification of total RNA derived from human TM cells confirmed expression of the α, β and γ variants of ATX. PCR products were sequenced to confirm identity. Similar observations were noted in TM cells from three different human donors. -RT represents negative controls run without reverse transcriptase. B. Immunofluorescence localization of ATX in primary cultures of human TM cells reveals a vesicular/punctate distribution, characteristic of a secretory protein. C and D. Human (C) and porcine (D) TM cell lysates (20 µg protein) and conditioned media from TM cells (10 µg protein) show the presence of various isoforms of ATX by immunoblot analysis. Bar: 10 µm.

to assess the effect of S32828 in AH samples to account for possible matrix effects of a heterogeneous biological sample. Incubation of rabbit AH with 10 µM S32826 inhibited LysoPLD enzyme activity by 90% (n = 4; $p<0.01$; based on Student's t-test, Fig. 4).

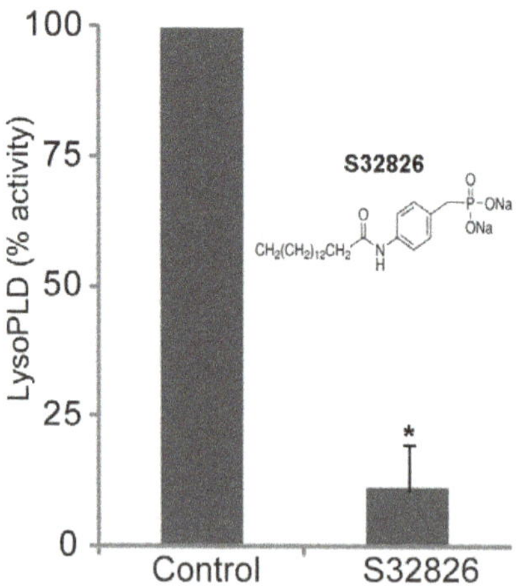

Figure 4. *In vitro* inhibition of rabbit AH LysoPLD activity by S32826. To confirm that S32826 inhibits LysoPLD activity of AH, 10 µg of AH protein derived from rabbits was pre-treated with S32826 *in vitro* for 20 minutes prior to analysis of LysoPLD activity using Amplex Red reagent and fluorimetric detection as described in methods. Rabbit AH LysoPLD activity was inhibited by more than 90% by 10 µM S32826 based on 4 independent observations. The chemical structure of S32826 is shown in the figure inset [29].

Effects of topically administered S32826 on IOP in rabbits

Nine Dutch-Belted normal male rabbits were used in two different experiments (4 and 5 in the first and second experiment, respectively). Prior to drug treatment, IOP was monitored for several days using a pneumotonometer to confirm steady baseline values. Of the three different concentrations (2, 5, and 10 mM) of drug tested topically, the highest dose (10 mM) caused a significant drop in IOP starting 2 hrs and continuing for at least for 24 hrs post-application in all nine rabbits evaluated. IOP values decreased by 10–17% from basal IOPs in the drug treated eyes, and by 15–22% between drug-treated and control eyes ($p<0.005$, $n=9$). Further, this response to drug treatment was consistently observed in three different experiments (twice with the first set of rabbits, and for the third time with a second set of rabbits). Figure 5A shows IOP changes with time, and 5B depicts the net change in IOP values in drug-treated eyes as compared to control eyes. We noted a steady increase or shift in basal IOPs to higher levels in these experiments, although the differences were not significant from the basal value in the control eyes, perhaps due to alkaline sham treatment. Daily topical administration of a 5 mM dose (mornings only) for 5 days also caused a significant, but smaller net decrease in IOP (by ~3 mm Hg between drug and control groups; $n=4$) as compared to sham treated controls (Fig. 5C). In contrast, while topical treatment with the 2 mM (daily morning dose for 5 days) concentration of drug did not yield a steady significant drop in IOP between drug treated and control eyes, IOP values in the drug treated rabbits were consistently lower than in control animals by 1.5 to 2 mm Hg (Fig. 5D). Throughout these experiments, topical application of all three doses of drug dissolved in aqueous medium was associated with drug precipitation on the corneal surface as a fine thin film. Further, topical application of the 10 mM dose of drug was observed to cause conjunctival hyperaemia within the first 2 hrs of drug application, which disappeared within 24 hrs, at which time we still noted a significant decrease in IOP in the drug treated animals compared to the controls (Fig. 6A). Based on slit lamp microscopic examination performed on these animals by a board certified glaucoma specialist, drug treated eyes did not exhibit any noticeable inflammation. Further, post-mortem histology analysis of the cornea (Fig. 6B) and iridocorneal angle (not shown) of rabbit eyes treated with 5 mM drug for 5 days revealed no obvious or toxicological changes relative to control eyes.

Effects of intracameral administration of S32826 on IOP of rabbits

Since topical drug application was observed to result in drug precipitating on the cornea and causing conjunctival hyperaemia, we decided to change the route of administration. The effects of intracameral injections (delivering the drug directly into the anterior chamber of the eye) were assessed by administering S32826 dissolved in phosphate buffered saline (pH 7.4) at a much lower concentration (μM) than the topical dose (mM). Four Dutch-Belted normal rabbits were used for this experiment. Drug was dissolved initially in dimethyl sulfoxide (DMSO) and subsequently diluted with PBS containing 2% DMSO. In each rabbit one eye was injected with 5 μl of 100 μM drug dissolved in PBS with 2% DMSO, while the other eye served as a non-injected control. The effect of vehicle alone was tested by administering 5 μl of PBS containing 2% DMSO into the contralateral eyes of the same rabbits used for evaluating the effect of active drug. Vehicle administration was performed after waiting at least for one week following completion of the drug treatment experiments, and after ensuring that IOP values were confirmed to be similar to basal values. Intracameral delivery of drug did not result in precipitation as evaluated using a slit lamp microscope. Drug-injected eyes exhibited a significant decrease in IOP (33% ($p<0.0036$) at 24 hrs, 31.5% ($p<0.001$) at 48 hrs and 18% ($p<0.001$) at 72 hrs post drug injection) compared to contralateral non-injected eyes (Fig. 7). Similarly, in comparison to the vehicle injected control eyes, IOP was observed to decrease by 18% ($p<0.007$) at 24 hrs and 30% ($p<0.007$) at 48 hrs after drug injection in S32826 treated eyes. Further, IOP values of drug treated eyes were significantly lower relative to basal IOP values (prior to drug injection) measured in the same animals (Fig. 7). At the 96 hr time point post drug injection, we missed recording IOP in two of the animals used in the experiment, resulting in an $n=2$ observations for this time point, as indicated in Figure 7. There were no notable ocular abnormalities in any group of animals used in this experiment, either during or after completion of the tests described.

Effects of siRNA-based suppression of ATX expression in TM cells

To explore the role of ATX in TM cell morphological and contractile properties, we suppressed the expression of this protein in HTM cells using the small interfering RNA (siRNA) approach. As shown in Figure 8A, treatment of HTM cells with ATX specific siRNA resulted in significant decreases in the intracellular levels of ATX protein relative to cells treated with scrambled FITC-conjugated siRNA and untreated control cells ($n=4$). As can be seen from the figure, ATX siRNA treatment affected the levels of different isoforms of ATX. Based on densitometric analysis using β-tubulin as internal standard, the protein levels of a predominant isoforms of ATX (125 kDa) was reduced by 70% in ATX siRNA treated HTM cells (Fig. 8B), while some isoforms (~100 kDa) were decreased to undetectable levels in HTM cells treated with ATX siRNA (Fig. 8A), relative to control cells treated with scrambled FITC-siRNA. Although the ATX siRNA treated HTM cells did not reveal any obvious changes in cell morphology, F-actin staining by TRITC-phalloidin revealed decreased levels of actin stress fibers compared to the scrambled FITC-siRNA treated controls (Fig. 8C). Additionally, we observed a significant ($p<0.03$; $n=4$) decrease in the levels of phosphorylated myosin light chain, a regulatory subunit of myosin II activity, in HTM cells treated with ATX siRNA, based on immunoblotting analysis (Fig. 8D) and semi-quantitative measurement using densitometric scanning (Fig. 8E).

Effects of S32826 on cultured TM cells

To determine the effects of S32826 on cultured TM cells, confluent cultures of HTM cells (derived from two different donors) maintained under serum free conditions or in the presence of 0.5% fetal bovine serum (FBS) were treated with 5 or 10 μM S32826 for 24 hrs along with respective sham treated controls. Time dependent observations based on phase contrast microscopy revealed presence of large floating membranous clumps in drug-treated cell culture dishes starting as early as 30 minutes from the time of drug addition, and relative to sham treated cells (Fig. 9A. 10 μM drug; arrows). However, drug treatment did not cause changes in cell morphology or cytotoxic response, as assessed by propidium iodide and fluorescein diacetate in live cell labeling (data not shown), [15] or changes in actin stress fiber distribution (data not shown). However, since floating membranous material was consistently noted in drug treated cell cultures in three independent experiments, the material was collected by centrifugation, rinsed with PBS, dissolved in Laemmli sample buffer, and separated by SDS-PAGE. Predominant protein bands were then gel extracted and subjected to mass spectrometry-based identification (Fig. 9B) [30]. Intriguingly, the majority of the proteins

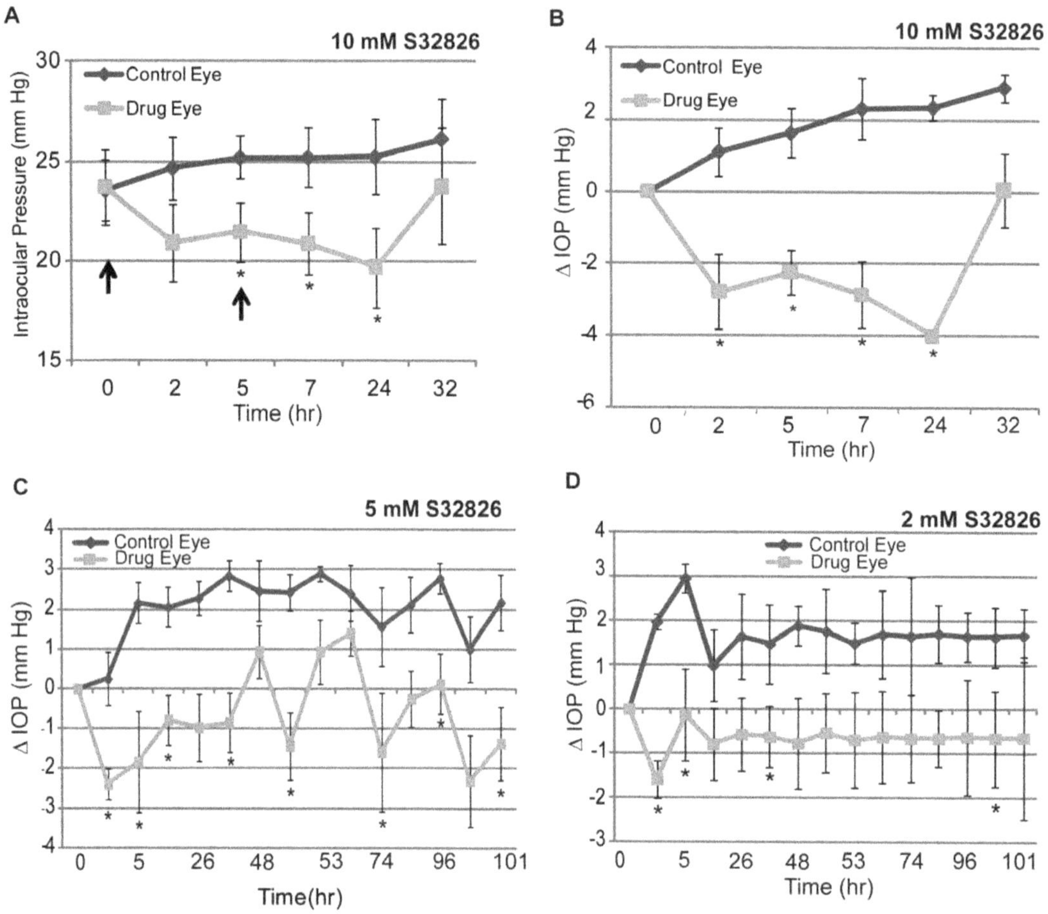

Figure 5. Topical application of ATX inhibitor (S32826) decreases IOP in rabbits. Topical application of S32826 (dissolved in water, pH~8–9) decreased IOP in a dose- and time- dependent manner in Dutch-Belted adult male rabbits, as determined using pneumotonometer under waking conditions. A. 10 mM S32826 exhibited the maximum and statistically significant effect in lowering IOP (by 5–6 mm Hg; n = 9) with drug application at 0 and 5 hrs (indicated with arrows, 35 μl×2) relative to sham controls receiving pH adjusted water. The IOP-lowering effect of drug lasted for a minimum of 24 hrs, after which, the changes in IOP began to normalize and were similar to control values by 48 hrs after initial drug application. B. The effects of S32826 (10 mM) on net change in IOP from basal values in the same animals. Net IOP values were significantly reduced from basal values, and between 2 to 24 hours following drug administration, based on a paired t-test. Further, IOP in the drug treated eyes was significantly reduced as compared to IOP in the control eyes based on the Wilcoxon Rank Sum test of differences in median's (n = 9). C and D. Effects of 5 and 2 mM S32826 on IOP with a daily (single morning dose, 35 μl×2; n = 4) dose of drug application, respectively. Relative to the 2 mM concentration of drug, administration of 5 mM drug resulted in a significant drop in IOP starting from 2 hrs post drug injection as compared the control values, with the IOP lowering effect lasting till the end of the study (5 days later). While eyes treated with 2 mM S32826 exhibited IOP values that were significantly reduced relative to control values throughout the 5-day study period, based on the Wilcoxon Rank Sum test of differences in medians, significance was not consistent across all time points as shown in the figure. In all these experiments, sham treatment alone increased IOP; the difference was not significant relative to the basal IOP values in any of the experiments. *$P<0.05$.

found in the floating membranous material shed from drug treated cells belonged to the class of proteins involved in membrane trafficking, exocytosis and membrane repair mechanisms, and included Annexin-2, 5 and 1, myosin-9 and 10, filamin A, radixin, actin, lysozyme C, cathepsin G, α2-macroglobulin, various ECM molecules, heat shock proteins-60, 70 and 90, myoferlin, 14-3-3 adaptor protein zeta/delta, protein S100-09/08, serotransferin, peptidyl-prolyl cis-trans-isomerase, cystatin-A, protein disulfide isomerise and vimentin. The protein profile of membranous material derived from drug treated HTM cells was similar regardless of whether cells had been maintained under serum starved conditions or in medium containing 0.5% FBS.

Influence of Cyclic Mechanical Stretch on ATX Expression and Secretion in TM cells

TM cells are mechano-sensitive and fluctuations in IOP are thought to influence paracrine and autocrine activity of these cells and thereby influence the homeostatic mechanisms involved in maintenance of normal AH outflow and IOP [8]. To explore the possible involvement of ATX in the effects of cyclic mechanical stretch, serum starved confluent cultures of porcine TM cells (passage 4) were subjected to 17 hrs of cyclic mechanical stretch with one cycle/second with 10% final stretch. In this experiment we used porcine TM cells due to limited availability of HTM cells. Cells exposed to these conditions exhibited significantly elevated levels of ATX both in the conditioned media (Fig. 10A and 10B) and in cell lysates (Fig. 10C and 10D), relative to unstretched control cells as determined by immunoblotting analysis. Figure 10A and 10C show the cyclic stretch-induced changes in ATX protein

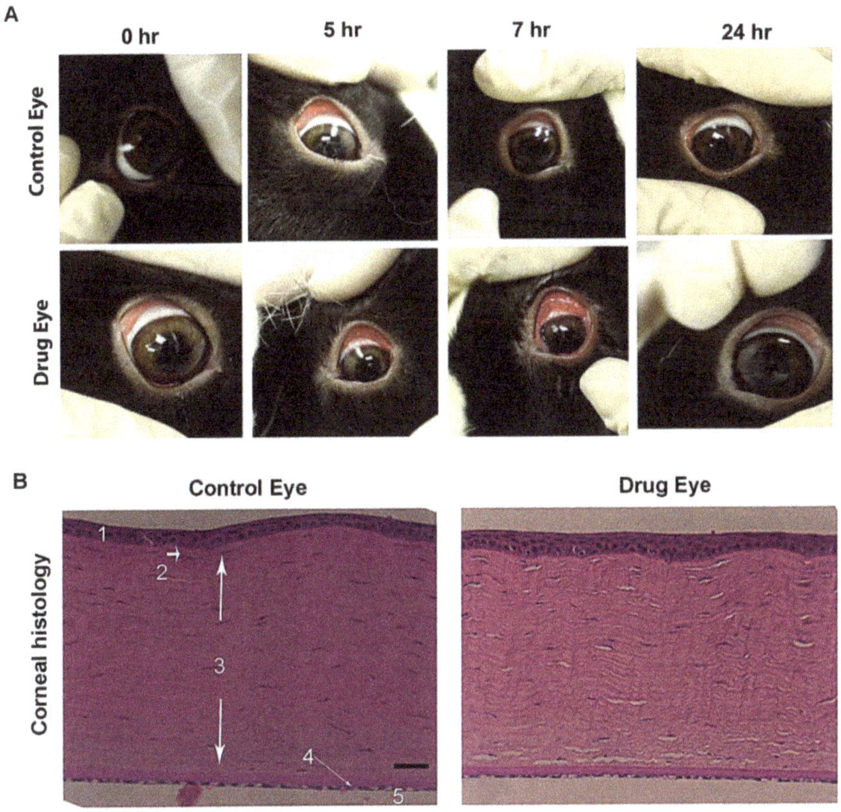

Figure 6. Effects of topical application of S32826 on the rabbit cornea. A. Topical application of 10 mM S32826 (twice daily, 35 µl aliquots) in Dutch-Belted adult male rabbits caused conjunctival hyperemia within the first 2 hrs after drug application, in association with drug precipitation on the cornea and conjunctival tissue as a fine thin film. However, hyperemia and all evidence of drug precipitation disappeared within 24 hrs following drug application. B. Topical effects of S32826 on rabbit corneal histology. Rabbits treated with a topical dose of 5 mM S32826 for 5 days (single daily dose) and which showed a decrease in IOP were enucleated and examined for corneal histological changes relative to sham treated specimens. As shown in the figure, drug application did not cause any apparent change on the integrity of corneal epithelium, endothelium, Bowman's layer, Stroma or Descemet's membrane (based on hematoxylin and eosin staining) relative to the control cornea. Bar: 10 µm. Labels: 1. Corneal Epithelium; 2. Bowman's layer; 3. Corneal Stroma; 4. Descemet's membrane; 5. Corneal Endothelium.

levels in media and cell lysates, respectively. Densitometric scanning of immunoblots from 4 independent experiments showed a significant ($p<0.005$) increase in secretory (Fig. 10B) and intracellular (Fig. 10D) ATX protein levels in stretched cells as compared to unstretched control cells.

Discussion

Increased IOP is a well recognized risk factor for development of POAG, which is a blinding disease [3]. Although lowering IOP is the primary treatment available for different types of glaucoma at present and different classes of ocular hypotensive drugs are used in clinical management of IOP in POAG patients, we lack a mechanism-based and targeted therapy for elevated IOP in glaucoma patients [5,6]. As part of our ongoing research to identify and characterize molecular mechanisms that lead to ocular hypertension and regulate AH outflow, we have in this study identified ATX/LysoPLD, which is a major source for extracellular LPA, as an abundant protein of human AH and found that AH LysoPLD activity is abnormally elevated in POAG patients. Significantly, topical or intracameral delivery of a small molecular weight chemical inhibitor of ATX (S32826) results in lowering IOP in normal rabbits. Collectively, these observations reveal the importance of the ATX-LPA axis in homeostasis of IOP and its potential as a therapeutic target for development of novel ocular hypotensive agents to treat glaucoma patients. To our knowledge, this is the first report on the possible therapeutic importance of the ATX-LPA axis in treatment of ocular hypertension in glaucoma patients.

The AH contains various extracellular factors of both protein and non-protein makeup which influence trabecular meshwork cell physiology, phagocytic function, contractile responses, autocrine activity and extracellular matrix turnover, several of which have been found to influence AH outflow and IOP [3,8,18,31]. Further, there is convincing experimental and clinical evidence in support of the contention that changes in levels of certain physiologically relevant factors present in the AH might be linked to increased resistance to AH outflow and elevated IOP [11,18,19,32]. To identify such AH factors, we and other investigators have begun to analyze the protein composition of AH derived from the human subjects using recent technical advancements in proteomics capabilities. In our previous studies we demonstrated a role for bioactive lipids (LPA and SIP) and lipid metabolizing enzymes (iPLA2) in regulating AH outflow through the trabecular meshwork [15,33]. Therefore, we were particularly interested in understanding the role played by AH lipid metabolizing enzymes and exploring the relevance of changes in the levels of these proteins in normal and glaucoma patients.

While it is known that ATX is present in human AH, [34,35] our quantitative proteomics analysis, revealed that this protein is

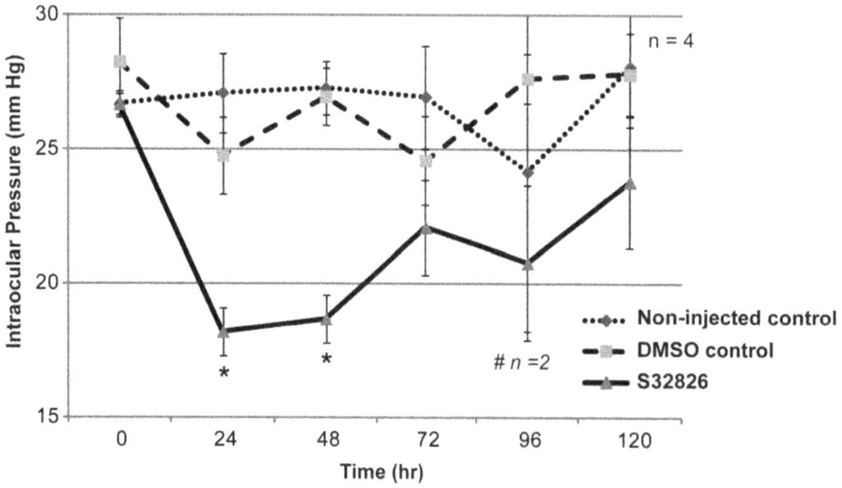

Figure 7. Intracameral injections of ATX inhibitor decreases IOP in rabbits. To determine the effects of intracameral delivery of S32826 on IOP, Dutch belted adult male rabbits (one eye from each animal, n = 4) were intracamerally injected with 5 µl of 100 µM drug. IOP was monitored in drug treated and contralateral (untreated) control eyes using a pneumotonometer. Drug treated eyes showed a significant decrease in IOP from the baseline (by 6–7 mm Hg) at 24 and 48 hrs based on paired t-test. This IOP lowering effect continued for more than 96 hrs, with IOP gradually returning to basal value by120 hrs post- injection. Further, IOP in drug treated eyes was significantly reduced as compared to IOP of the contralateral untreated eyes and eyes treated with sham control (PBS containing 2%DMSO) based on the Wilcoxon Rank Sum test of differences in medians. For the sham treatment, we used the contralateral eyes of the same animals in which we tested the effects of drug, with the sham treatment being performed 2 weeks after completion of the drug treatments (n = 4 for drug treated, sham treated and untreated controls). However, at the 96 hr time point, IOP was recorded in only two of the four rabbits from the drug treated and untreated control groups. $^{*}P<0.05$.

present in abundant amounts in human AH. ATX, a secretory protein, which was initially characterized as autocrine factor involved in cell motility, proliferation, differentiation and survival, has been identified as an extracellular LysoPLD which generates LPA and to a lesser extent S1P [24,25,26,36,37,38]. LPA is a bioactive lipid that in turn regulates several cellular processes including Rho GTPase regulated cell adhesion, contraction and migration by acting through different G-protein coupled receptors [39]. Importantly, abnormal regulation of the ATX-LPA axis has been shown to be associated with various pathological conditions including cancer and fibrosis [24,37]. Our analysis of AH samples derived from POAG and control (cataract) patients revealed significantly elevated levels of LysoPLD activity (expressed per unit of total protein) in POAG patients.

Although there was a significant difference in racial demography between the glaucoma and control specimens tested in this study, it is unlikely that the 1.8 fold elevation in the LysoPLD activity that we noted in POAG patients relative to age-matched cataract control samples is solely related to differences in the racial demography. Further, there is no known currently available information on racial differences in gene expression profiles of TM or other ocular tissues of the anterior segment of the eye. However, it is important to note that POAG is more prevalent in African Americans and Hispanics relative to Caucasians [40,41]. While it would have been ideal to determine and confirm whether the observed elevated levels of LysoPLD activity in the AH of POAG patients is associated with elevated levels of LPA, the product of ATX, we could not however, establish this association due to inadequate amounts of AH obtained from each patient.

Based on abundant levels of ATX in AH, and elevated LysoPLD activity in the AH of POAG patients, we hypothesized that inhibition of ATX in the eye would likely impact AH outflow through the trabecular meshwork, and thereby IOP as well. To set the stage for addressing this hypothesis, we first performed *in vitro* studies using a relevant cell type, confirming that TM cells derived from humans and other species express and secrete ATX. Additionally, both secretion and expression of ATX by TM cells was found to be responsive to cyclic mechanical stretch, further supporting the mechanosensitive nature of TM cells and the impact of mechanotransducing stimuli on TM cell physiology [8,14]. To test whether inhibition of ATX in the AH influences IOP, we evaluated the effects of a well characterized small molecular weight water soluble pharmacological inhibitor of ATX (S32826) [29] on IOP using topical and intracameral drug delivery in rabbits. Both routes of S32826 administration were found to cause significant reductions in IOP in these animals. Since the topical route of administration requires use of millimolar concentrations of S32826, we could not use DMSO to dissolve the drug. Dissolution of drug in sterile filtered water resulted in a solution with an alkaline pH of ~8–9. Since the drug precipitates out of solution at neutral pH, we used pH adjusted water as sham control in our experiments. S32826 treatment resulted in a dose - dependent ocular hypotensive effect on IOP in rabbits relative to control (sham-treated) eyes. This decrease in IOP was also significant relative to basal IOP in the same animal, and lasted for a minimum of 24 hrs post-treatment in rabbits treated twice a day with 10 mM S32826. It was noted that topical application of alkaline water (sham control) per se caused an upward shift in IOP values by ~2 to 2.5 mm Hg. The reason for this effect of the sham treatment is not clear. Topical drug application, especially at the 10 mM concentration, was found to cause a transient conjunctival hyperaemia, a response which appears to be associated with drug precipitation on the cornea and conjunctival tissue. However, the decrease in IOP in drug treated eyes was not related to conjunctival hyperaemia since IOP was found to be significantly less in the drug treated animals even after 24 hrs after drug application, by which time there was no evidence of hyperaemia or drug precipitation.

To substantiate the ocular hypotensive effects of S32826 and to circumvent both drug precipitation and resulting conjunctival hyperaemia noted with topical drug delivery in rabbit eyes, S32826 was delivered into the eye anterior chamber by

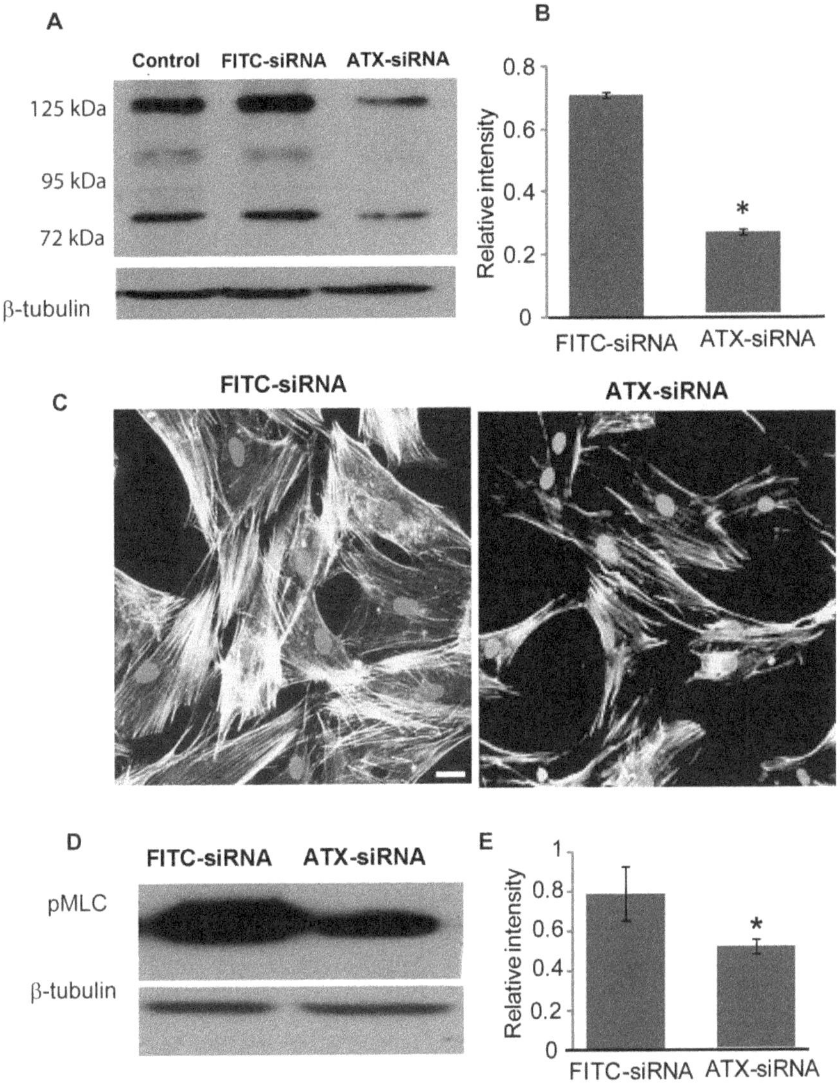

Figure 8. Suppression of ATX expression in human TM cells induces changes in actin cytoskeletal organization and myosin II phosphorylation. A. Primary cultures of human TM cells treated with ATX-specific siRNA revealed significant suppression of ATX expression (different isoforms) relative to cells treated with FITC-conjugated scrambled siRNA control. β-tubulin was used as a loading control. B. Protein levels of one of the variants (~125 kDa) of ATX were significantly reduced (by >75%) in ATX siRNA treated HTM cells based on densitometric semi-quantification. C. The ATX siRNA treated human TM cells (after 72 hrs) maintained under serum starved conditions for 24 hrs revealed a marked decrease in actin stress fibers (labelled using rhodamine-phalloidin) relative to cells treated with scrambled siRNA (FITC-siRNA). D. ATX siRNA treated human TM cells (for 72 hrs) maintained under serum starved conditions for 24 hrs showed a significant decrease in the levels of phosphorylated myosin light chain (pMLC), a regulatory subunit of myosin II, as compared to cells treated with scrambled siRNA (FITC-siRNA). β-tubulin was blotted as a loading control. E. Changes in the levels of phospho-MLC in the ATX siRNA treated cells compared to the scrambled siRNA treated control, based on densitometric semi-quantitative analysis.

intracameral injections. Importantly, in this case, drug was dissolved initially in DMSO and subsequently diluted in phosphate buffered saline, pH 7.4. Using this method, there was no evidence for drug precipitation or ocular hyperaemia, and IOP was found to be significantly decreased in drug treated eyes by more than 5 mm Hg, with the ocular hypotensive response lasting for more than 48 hrs in response to a single injection of 5 µl of 100 µM S32826. The final concentration of drug in the AH was estimated be in the range of 2 to 2.5 µM based on the volume of AH (approximately 200 to 250 µl) in the adult rabbit eye. Although this experiment provided convincing evidence for the ocular hypotensive effect of S32826, and the ability of S32826 to inhibit LysoPLD activity in rabbit AH was confirmed using an *in vitro* assay, we could not validate that the ocular hypotensive response of S32826 was indeed associated with decreased levels of LPA. Our preliminary attempts to determine levels of LPA in the limited amounts of AH obtained from rabbit eyes by mass spectrometric analysis were not successful. Further work is needed to establish protocols for determining LPA levels in AH. However, S32826 has been shown to decrease LPA levels produced by adipocytes [29].

Finally, siRNA-mediated suppression of ATX expression in TM cells resulted in a decrease in actin stress fibers and myosin light chain phosphorylation, indicating a role for ATX in cell contractile properties, cell tension and cell adhesive properties of TM cells. Consistent with these observations, our previous studies demonstrated that LPA, which is a direct product of ATX activity,

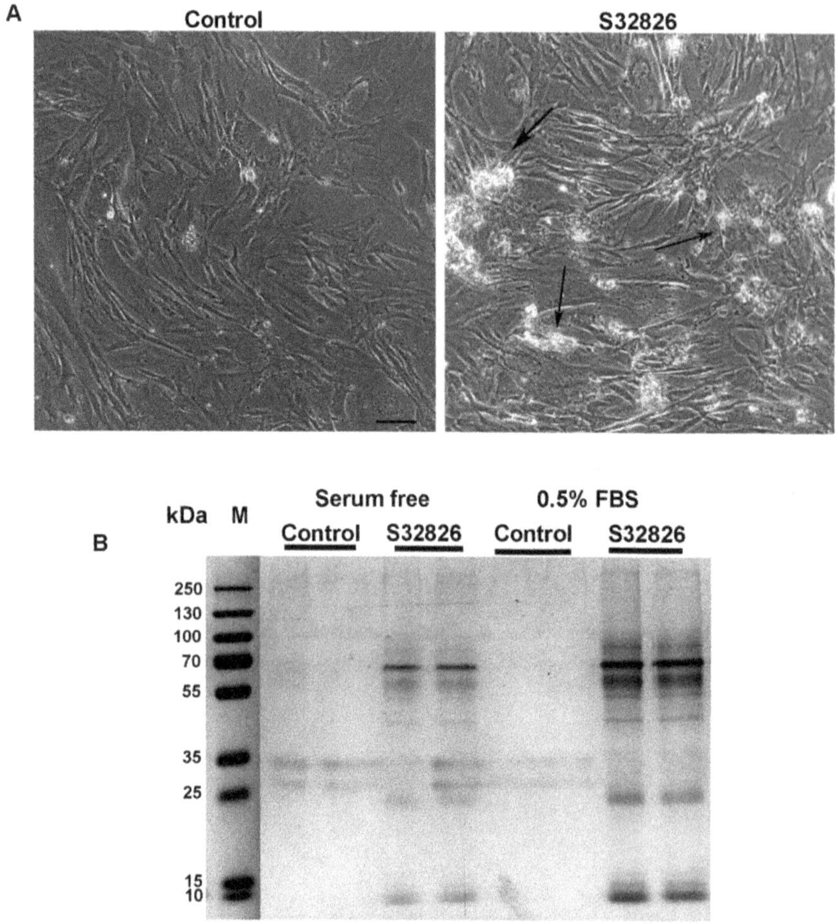

Figure 9. ATX inhibitor-S32826 induced changes in cultured human TM cells. A. Primary cultures of human TM cells cultured either on gelatin-coated glass coverslips or in plastic petridishes were treated with S32826 (10 μM) in the absence of serum or in the presence of 0.5% fetal bovine serum for 24 hrs. Based on phase contrast microscopic examination, treatment of TM cells cultures with drug caused the appearance of membranous floating clumps (arrows) in culture medium, without any noticeable changes in cell morphology and cell adhesion relative to control cells treated with DMSO vehicle. This response appeared to increase progressively with time. B. The membranous floating material generated from drug (S32826) treated cells (A) was extracted from the cell culture media by centrifugation, rinsed with PBS, dissolved in Laemmli sample buffer, separated by SDS-PAGE and stained with gelcode blue as shown in the figure (two independent samples are shown from each treatment). Subsequently, the predominant protein bands were gel extracted and subjected to mass spectrometry-based identification. This analysis revealed presence of proteins involved in lysosomal exocytosis, trafficking and membrane repair as discussed in the results section.

induces formation of actin stress fibers, focal adhesions and myosin light chain phosphorylation and Rho GTPase activation in TM cells [15]. Further, in contrast to the ocular hypotensive effects of the ATX inhibitor S32826 noted in this study, perfusion of LPA has been demonstrated to decrease AH outflow facility, leading to increased IOP [15]. Intriguingly, S32826 showed no detectable effects either on cell morphology or actin cytoskeletal reorganization of TM cells maintained in serum free media. Instead, drug treated TM cell cultures maintained either under serum-starved conditions or with 0.5%FBS were observed to generate cell-derived membranous floating material with no evidence of a cytotoxic response. The analysis of protein composition of this material by mass spectrometry analysis confirmed presence of proteins involved in membrane trafficking, repair and exocytosis. It is not clear whether inhibition of autotaxin, which is known to act locally at cell surface by interacting with integrins and to produce LPA close to the cell surface receptors, influences membrane recycling properties in TM cells [42,43,44].

In conclusion, this initial study reports the ocular hypotensive effect of an ATX inhibitor in live rabbits, suggesting potential significance of ATX as a therapeutic target for lowering IOP in glaucoma patients. Further studies are necessary to delineate the molecular mechanisms by which inhibition of ATX mediates decrease of IOP.

Methods

Ethics Statement

Animals. This study was carried out in strict accordance with the recommendations in the Guide for the Care and Use of Laboratory Animals of the National Institutes of Health and Association for Research in Vision and Ophthalmology. The protocol was approved by the Committee on the Ethics of Animal Experiments of the Duke University School of Medicine (Protocol Number: A094-10-04). Intracameral injections were performed under ketamine/xylazine anesthesia, and all efforts were made to minimize pain and suffering during experiments.

Human Subjects. All research involving collection of human aqueous humor samples has been approved by the Duke University School of Medicine's institutional review board (IRB).

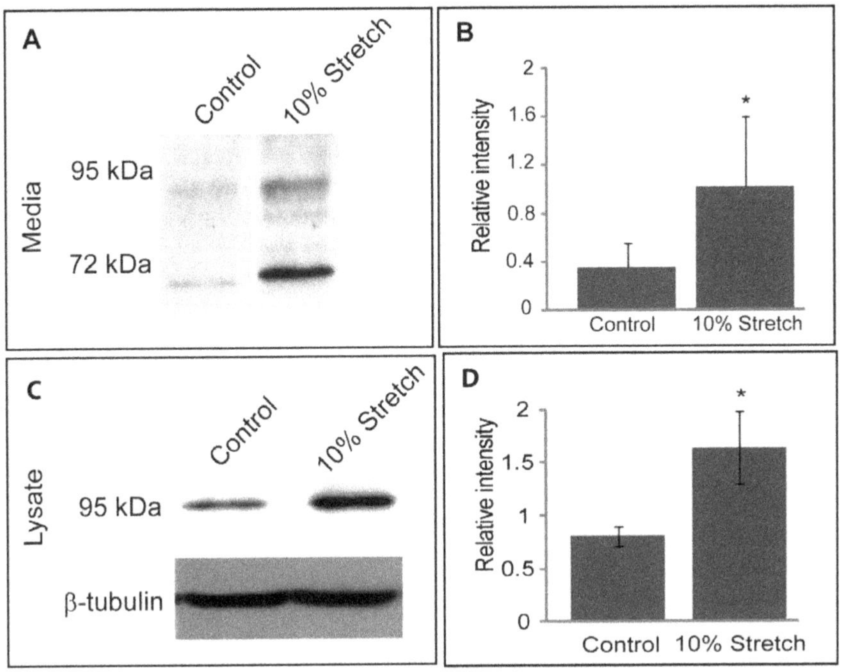

Figure 10. Cyclic mechanical stretch of TM cells induces ATX extracelluar and intracellular protein. A. Confluent cultures of primary porcine TM cells maintained under serum free condition and subjected to 10% cyclical mechanical stretch (one cycle/second) for 17 hrs revealed increased levels of ATX protein levels in the conditioned media as compared to the media derived from the un-stretched control cells based on immunoblot analysis with equal amount (10 µg) of total protein. For a loading control, SDS-PAGE separated proteins were stained with Coomassie blue and the staining intensity was compared (not shown). B. Densitometric semi-quantitative analysis of the immunoblots shown in panel A. $^*P<0.05$, $n=4$. C. Cell lysates derived from TM cells subjected to the cyclic mechanical stretch revealed increased levels of ATX protein compared to the samples of unstretched controls based on immunoblot analysis of equal amounts of protein (20 µg). β-tubulin was immunoblotted as a loading control. D. Densitometric semi-quantitative analysis of ATX immunoblots of cell lysates shown in panel C. * $P<0.05$, $n=4$.

Informed written patient consent was obtained prior to sample collection and the principles expressed in the Declaration of Helsinki were followed. This study does not involve minors or children.

Reagents

RNeasy Mini kit (Qiagen, Valencia, CA), Advantage RT for PCR kit and Advantage cDNA PCR kit (BD Biosciences Clontech, Palo Alto, CA) were procured from the respective commercial sources. Mouse monoclonal anti-tubulin antibodies and Tetramethyl rhodamine isothiocyanate (TRITC)–conjugated phalloidin were from Sigma-Aldrich (St. Louis, MO). Polyclonal phospho-MLC antibody (C.No. 36745) was from Cell Signalling Technology (Danvers, MA). L-α-Lysophosphatidylcholine (C.No. 830071P) was from Avanti Polar Lipids, Inc. (Alabaster, AL). ATX polyclonal antibody (C. No. 10005375) and its blocking peptide (C. No. 10007193) were obtained from Cayman Chemicals (Ann Arbor, MI), and S32826 (ATX inhibitor) were from Cayman Chemicals (C. No. 13664) and Sigma-Aldrich (C. No. S1825). Amplex Red PLD Assay Kit (C.No. A12219) was from Molecular Probes/Invitrogen (Grand Island, NY). Fetal Bovine Serum (FBS) and Dulbecco's Modified Eagle's Medium (DMEM) with low glucose were obtained from Gibco-BRL (Gaithersburg, MD). Bio-Rad protein assay reagent (C. No. 500-0006) was purchased from Bio-Rad. FITC (Fluorescein isothiocyanate) conjugated scrambled siRNA (C. No. sc-36869) and human ATX siRNA (C. No. sc-44906) were from Santa Cruz Biotechnology (Santa Cruz, CA).

Collection of Aqueous Humor

Humans. Aqueous humor was collected from patients undergoing elective cataract surgery or surgery for glaucoma at the Duke Eye Center by the glaucoma and comprehensive clinical service clinicians. A cannula attached to a tuberculin syringe was inserted into the anterior chamber through a paracentesis tract at the start of surgery and AH was slowly aspirated until shallowing of the anterior chamber. The sample was transferred from the syringe to a microcentrifuge tube and was centrifuged at 3000 rpm for 10 min at 4°C. The supernatant was collected and stored at −80°C until further use.

Animals. Mouse AH was collected from 1 year old male C57BL/6 mice. The mice were first sacrificed using sodium phenobarbital intraperitoneally and a 25 µl Hamilton syringe (22 s/2″/2) was carefully inserted into the anterior chamber of the eye to withdraw the AH. Porcine eye AH was collected using a sterile insulin syringe (29G) from freshly enucleated eyes obtained from a local slaughterhouse. AH from anaesthetized (using ketamine/xylazine) New Zealand white rabbits was collected using an insulin syringe (29G). AH derived from these different species was centrifuged at 3000 rpm, 4°C for 10 minutes and the supernatant was collected and stored at −80°C till further use.

Quantitative Proteomics of human AH

Briefly, human AH samples were collected from 8 patients during cataract surgery, centrifuged at 3000 RPM, 4°C for 10 minutes and equal volumes of supernatant from individual specimens were pooled. Protein content of the pooled specimen was determined using a Bio-Rad dye protein assay reagent with bovine serum albumin as the standard. The AH sample was reduced with 10 mM dithiothreitol, alkylated with 20 mM iodoacetamide and digested with trypsin in the presence of 0.1% w/v RapiGest SF surfactant (Waters). The sample was spiked with 50 fmol of yeast alcohol dehydrogenase digest (Waters Mass Prep) per μg of total AH protein. One μg of protein from the digested AH was injected onto a nanoAcquity LC system, coupled to a Synapt HDMS mass spectrometer. The sample was analyzed in triplicate using MS^E (data-independent acquisition) for quantitative/qualitative analysis, followed by a single data-dependent analysis (DDA) for supplementary identifications. Data were searched against the Swissprot Human (v57.5) database, with 20 ppm precursor and 0.04 Da product ion mass accuracy and trypsin specificity, with either PLGS 2.4/IdentityE (MSE) or Mascot v2.2 (DDA) search engine. Data was loaded into Scaffold 2 Proteome Software version 2.06 to generate a list of the most abundant proteins detected by mass spectrometry. Raw data alignment, feature detection, and label-free quantitation were performed within Rosetta Elucidator v3.3 software. The fmol quantity of each protein (per μg injected) was performed according to the method of Silva et al. [45] for the 89 proteins detected based on 2 or more peptides using yeast alcohol dehydrogenase as an internal standard. These analyses were performed at the Duke Proteomics Core Facility.

TM cell cultures

Human primary TM cells were cultured from fresh corneal rings donated by the Duke Ophthalmology Clinical Service after they were used for corneal transplantation as described previously [22]. Porcine primary TM cells were isolated and cultured using collagen IV digestion as described earlier by us [46]. Cell passages between 4 and 6 were used in this study.

LysoPLD assay

LysoPLD enzyme activity was assayed by measuring hydrolysis of lysophosphatidylcholine to choline and lysophosphatidic acid as described by Gijsbers et al. [27]. Briefly, choline derived from the hydrolysis of lysophosphatidylcholine was coupled with choline oxidase to oxidize choline into betaine and H_2O_2. Subsequently, the H_2O_2 generated reacts with Amplex Red reagent in the presence of horseradish peroxidase to generate resorufin, which is measured using a fluorescence spectrometer with excitation and emission filters at 530 nm and 590 nm, respectively. The original PLD assay was modified for lysoPLD by replacing the substrate phosphatidylcholine with lysophosphatidylcholine. The enzyme reactions were performed in duplicate in a final volume of 200 μl at 37°C for 30 minutes using a 96 well microtiter plates and Molecular Probe Spectramax M3. H_2O_2 standards, heat inactivated AH control and enzyme assays lacking lysophosphatidylcholine substrate were run simultaneously. Enzyme activity was expressed as μM H_2O_2 generated per mg of total AH protein.

Immunofluorescence

TM cells were plated on glass coverslips coated with 2% gelatin and grown till they were 80% confluent. After treatments in serum-free media, they were washed twice with 1× phosphate buffered saline (PBS) and fixed in 4% paraformaldehyde for 15 min at room temperature. Cells were permeabilized in 0.5% Triton-X 100 for 15 minutes, and blocked in serum buffer containing 10% FBS. Following this, cells were incubated with respective primary and Alexa fluor-conjugated secondary antibodies as we described earlier [22]. Finally, coverslips were washed and mounted onto glass slides with Aqua Mount (Lerner Laboratories, Pittsburg, PA) and observed under a Nikon confocal system (C1 Digital Eclipse).

Immunoblotting

Total cell lysates were prepared from confluent serum-starved TM cells. Briefly, cells were washed twice with cold PBS, and collected into lysis buffer containing 10 mM Tris, pH 7.4, 0.2 mM $MgCl_2$, 5 mM N-ethylmaleimide, 0.4 mM iodoacetamide and 60 μM PMSF and protease inhibitor (cocktail tablets complete, Mini, EDTA-free, Roche, Basel, Switzerland), and phosphatase inhibitors (Phosphostop, Basel, Switzerland), sonicated on ice (probe sonicator, followed by bath sonicator for 30 min) and centrifuged at 800 g, 4°C for 15 min. The supernatant was collected and protein was measured as described below. Media was collected and centrifuged at 3000 rpm for 10 min at 4°C to remove cellular debris. The supernatant was concentrated using Millipore Centrifugal Filter Units with <30 kDa cutoff. The filters were centrifuged at 2500 rpm at 4°C. Bio-Rad dye protein assay reagent was used to estimate the protein concentrations in both cell lysate and media samples using the Bradford method. Equal amounts of protein were dissolved in Laemmli buffer, boiled for 5 minutes, and separated by SDS-PAGE using 8% acrylamide gels. Proteins were transferred to nitrocellulose membrane, which were then incubated with LysoPLD polyclonal antibody (diluted 1:250 in TBST) overnight at 4°C. Immunoblots were developed using appropriate HRP (horse radish peroxidase)-conjugated secondary antibody and enhanced chemiluminescence, as we described earlier [22]. Densitometry of scanned films was performed using Adobe Photoshop CS3 Software, and results expressed relative to the loading control (β-tubulin).

Myosin Light Chain (MLC) Phosphorylation

Changes in TM cell myosin light chain phosphorylation status were determined by immunoblot analysis using a phospho-MLC specific antibody and urea-glycerol gel electrophoresis as we described earlier [15]. Densitometry of scanned films was performed using Adobe Photoshop CS3 Software, and results expressed relative to the loading control (β-tubulin).

RT-PCR

Total RNA was extracted using RNeasy Micro kit (Qiagen, Valencia, CA) per the user manual from P4 confluent cultures of HTM cells derived from human donors aged 33, 54 and 75 years. 2 μg of total RNA was used for first-strand synthesis using Superscript first-strand synthesis system for RT-PCR (Life Technologies, Carlsbad, CA). The resultant cDNA was used to amplify DNA specific to ATX isoforms in a total volume of 50 μl with 1.5 mM $MgCl_2$, 0.2 mM dNTPs, 2 U *Taq* polymerase (Life Technologies), and 0.5 μM sense and antisense primers for the α, β, and γ variants of ATX. GAPDH primers were used as positive control. The primer sequences (forward/reverse) used to amplify the different isoforms of ATX are listed below:

1. α – ATGGATTACAGCCACCAAGC/TCTTCCATTCCATGGTCTCC
2. β - TCGGCCCTGAGATGACAAATC/GAGGTGTCTCTCTTCTGTAG
3. γ – ATGTCCGTGTTTCTCCGAGT/ATTGCAGCTCTCCTCGTTGT
4. GAPDH – TGCACCACCAACTGCTTAGC/GGCATGGACTGTGGTCATGAG.

The amplification was carried out using GeneAmp Amplification System (Applied Biosciences) with a denaturation step at 94°C for 4 min, followed by 94°C for 1 min, annealing at 57°C for 60 s, and extension at 72°C for 60 s. This cycle was repeated 30 times with a final step at 72°C for 7 min. The resulting products were separated by 1% agarose gel electrophoresis and visualized by ethidium bromide staining and using a Fotodyne Trans-illuminator (Fotodyne Inc., Wisconsin). Control reactions containing no reverse transcriptase were run simultaneously.

Cyclic Mechanical Stretch

Porcine TM cells between passages 4 and 5 were plated onto BioFlex six-well plates pre-coated with collagen (Flexcell International, Hillsborough, NC). Once they reached confluence, cells were serum starved for 24 hrs and then stretched using the FlexCell FX-4000 system (Flexcell International, Hillsborough, NC). A cyclic stretch of 1 cycle/second was applied to the experimental plates for 17 hrs at 37°C as we described earlier [47]. Control plates were incorporated into the same system, but did not undergo stretch. Experimental plates were exposed to a total stretch of 10% as compared to control plates. After stretch treatment, media were collected, centrifuged (3000 rpm, 4°C for 10 minutes) and supernatants were used for detection of ATX by immunoblotting. The cells were scraped and lysates were prepared for Western blotting analysis as previously described.

siRNA Treatment

HTM cells (passaged between 3 to 5 cycles; derived from donors aged 16, 18 and 74 years) were cultured in 100 cm plates in DMEM with 10% FBS, until they reached about 80% confluency. Medium (containing 10% FBS) was changed a day before and on the day of transfection. Cells were trypsinized and counted prior to transfection, and 5×10^5 cells were used for each nucleofector transfection. Two different controls: untransfected control, and FITC-conjugated scrambled siRNA control were set up for these experiments. The Amaxa Nucleofector (program T023) and Basic Endothelial Cell Nucleofector Kit (C. No. VP1-1001) were used and the kit specifications were strictly adhered to. Post transfection, cells were plated in 6-well plates and coverslips coated with 2% gelatin for immunostaining. Cells were changed into fresh medium on the day following transfection. FITC fluorescence was detected after 24–36 hours of transfection. Prior to cell lysate preparation for Western blot analysis, cells were changed into serum-free media overnight and the standard procedure was followed for cell lysate preparation. Coverslips were fixed for actin filament staining using TRITC-phalloidin as described earlier.

Animal experimentation

Topical drug effects. In the first set of experiments, we used four Dutch-Belted adult male rabbits. One eye was treated with drug while the other (contralateral) eye was used as control (sham treatment). Basal IOPs were measured using a pneumotonometer (Model 30, Medtronic) for a week before beginning the experiments to monitor for any irregularities in IOP. The ATX inhibitor (S32826; Sigma) was dissolved in sterile autoclave distilled water (resulting in an alkaline pH~8) to obtain a desired concentration (2–10 mM) for the topical dosing. pH adjusted (pH~8) distilled water served as a control for the contralateral eye. Before administering drug or sham control vehicle, the eyes were treated with a drop of topical anesthetic (0.5% proparacaine HCl). The animals were awake during the IOP measurements. Basal IOPs were measured prior to drug treatments. 35 µl of the drug or sham control vehicle were applied to the respective eyes. This volume was found to be appropriate, covered the entire cornea and did not spill over from the eye. During drug application, the rabbit eyes were kept open physically to prevent blinking for a minute before applying a second aliquot of 35 µl drug solution. In the first set of rabbits, 3 different concentrations of the drug (10, 2 and 5 mM) were tested in separate experiments (sequentially). Only for the 10 mM concentration, a second dose of drug was administered 5–6 hrs (typically at ~4 PM) after the first dose (typically at ~10 AM). The effects of 10 mM drug were repeated in a second set of rabbits under identical conditions as the first experiment, using 5 additional rabbits. IOPs were measured at 2, 5, 7, 24, 32 and 50 hrs after the first dose of drug application. An average of four readings was used to plot the IOP data for each time point. For the lower concentrations of drug (5 mM and 2 mM), only one morning dose was applied every day (~10/11 AM) for 5 days, and IOPs were monitored twice a day. For the concentration response experiments, animals received sufficient recovery time after each concentration experiment was completed, and the next concentration experiment was tested only after IOP returned to the basal or normal level. The rabbits from the first set of experiments were sacrificed after they received the 5 mM drug for 5 days, after which AH was collected and enucleated eyes fixed for histological analysis.

Intracameral drug effects. Due to drug precipitation on the corneal surface and conjunctival hyperaemia associated with topical drug delivery, an intracameral injection experiment was designed using a new batch of four rabbits (same strain as the previous experiments). The volume of AH in adult rabbits was estimated to be ~200–250 µl based on our previous observations. For this study, the drug stock was prepared initially in DMSO and subsequently diluted in PBS, such that the final DMSO concentration in the aqueous humour would be ~0.05%. Prior to intracameral injections, basal IOPs were measured in awake rabbits as described above. The rabbits were anesthetized using intramuscular injections of ketamine and xylazine cocktail, followed by a topical drop of 0.5% proparacaine HCl. An operating microscope was positioned over the eye undergoing surgery and the anterior chamber was entered in the superotemporal quadrant using a 0.3 cc insulin syringe positioned at an angle and 5 µl of drug (100 µM stock in PBS with 2% DMSO) was injected into the eye anterior chamber. The injections and follow-up ocular changes were performed by a board certified glaucoma specialist. The contralateral eye served as the non-injected control. IOP values in both eyes were measured at 24, 48, 72, 96, and 120 hrs post drug injections, until the pressures in the injected eyes returned to normal. During this time, the eyes were monitored for ocular changes using a slit lamp. Once these rabbits recovered from drug injections after 2 weeks, the contralateral eye was injected with 5 µl of PBS containing 2% DMSO and served as the DMSO-injected sham control. IOPs were measured in both eyes at 24, 48, 72, 96, and 120 hrs post injection.

Histology

Rabbit eyes from the topical drug experiment (5 mM drug) were enucleated, rinsed in 1× PBS and fixed in 4% paraformaldehyde (PFA) for 1 hr at room temperature. After this, the lens was carefully removed and the anterior segment was cut into two halves, one half being processed for assessment of corneal toxicity. Briefly, tissue was immersed in 10% buffered formalin at room temperature and sent for pathological analysis, where it was processed and stained with haematoxylin and eosin (H&E). The other half was processed for histological changes at the AH outflow angle. The tissue was immersed in 2.5% glutaraldehyde, 50 mM cacodylate buffer (pH 7.2) containing 4% sucrose and 2 mM $CaCl_2$ for 2 hrs, then transferred to 10% buffered formalin for 48 hrs. The specimens were then embedded in methyl methacrylate, and 2 µm sections were cut and stained with hematoxylin and eosin stain using conventional methods. Micrographs were captured using a Zeiss light microscope.

Statistical analysis

In figures, all data are presented as mean ± SEM. The Wilcoxon Rank Sum test of differences in medians was performed to compare the ATX enzyme activity between glaucoma and cataract controls with one-way Chi-square approximation. IOP changes between drug treated and sham treated rabbits were assessed for significance using the Wilcoxon Rank Sum test. IOP changes within the same group before and after drug treatment was tested using the paired t-test. Racial difference between glaucoma and cataract groups was tested by the Fisher's exact test. Student's t-test was used for evaluating significance in biochemical studies performed with cultured cells. A p-value<0.05 was considered significant. A box-and-whisker plot was used to represent the AH LysoPLD activity in glaucoma and cataract control subjects.

Supporting Information

Table S1 Quantitative proteome of aqueous humor from control (cataract) eyes with proteins listed in order of abundance. Values represent mean ± standard deviation (SD).

Acknowledgments

We are grateful to J. Will Thompson, Ph.D., and Nikolai Skiba, Ph.D., for their help with the proteomics analysis and Sandra Stinnett, D.P.H., for her help with statistical analysis. We thank David Epstein, M.D., for his helpful comments and suggestions during the conduction of these studies and manuscript preparation, and Padmanabhan Pattabiraman, Ph.D., for his help in the cell culture studies.

Author Contributions

Conceived and designed the experiments: PVR. Performed the experiments: PI RL CM PC RV. Analyzed the data: PI PVR. Wrote the paper: PI PVR.

References

1. Quigley HA, Broman AT (2006) The number of people with glaucoma worldwide in 2010 and 2020. Br J Ophthalmol 90: 262–267.
2. Weinreb RN, Khaw PT (2004) Primary open-angle glaucoma. Lancet 363: 1711–1720.
3. Gabelt BT, Kaufman PL (2005) Changes in aqueous humor dynamics with age and glaucoma.Prog Retin Eye Res 24: 612–637.
4. The AGIS Investigators (2000) The advanced glaucoma intervention study, 6: effect of cataract on visual field and visual acuity. Arch Ophthalmol 118: 1639–1652.
5. Lee AJ, Goldberg I (2011) Emerging drugs for ocular hypertension. Expert Opin Emerg Drugs 16: 137–161.
6. Toris CB (2010) Pharmacotherapies for glaucoma. Curr Mol Med 10: 824–840.
7. Tamm ER, Fuchshofer R (2007) What increases outflow resistance in primary open-angle glaucoma? Surv Ophthalmol 52 Suppl 2: S101–104.
8. Acott TS, Kelley MJ (2008) Extracellular matrix in the trabecular meshwork. Exp Eye Res 86: 543–561.
9. Clark AF, Wordinger RJ (2009) The role of steroids in outflow resistance. Exp Eye Res 88: 752–759.
10. Fautsch MP, Bahler CK, Vrabel AM, Howell KG, Loewen N, et al. (2006) Perfusion of his-tagged eukaryotic myocilin increases outflow resistance in human anterior segments in the presence of aqueous humor. Invest Ophthalmol Vis Sci 47: 213–221.
11. Gottanka J, Chan D, Eichhorn M, Lutjen-Drecoll E, Ethier CR (2004) Effects of TGF-beta2 in perfused human eyes. Invest Ophthalmol Vis Sci 45: 153–158.
12. Keller KE, Aga M, Bradley JM, Kelley MJ, Acott TS (2009) Extracellular matrix turnover and outflow resistance. Exp Eye Res 88: 676–682.
13. Knepper PA, Mayanil CS, Goossens W, Wertz RD, Holgren C, et al. (2002) Aqueous humor in primary open-angle glaucoma contains an increased level of CD44S. Invest Ophthalmol Vis Sci 43: 133–139.
14. Liton PB, Luna C, Bodman M, Hong A, Epstein DL, et al. (2005) Induction of IL-6 expression by mechanical stress in the trabecular meshwork. Biochem Biophys Res Commun 337: 1229–1236.
15. Mettu PS, Deng PF, Misra UK, Gawdi G, Epstein DL, et al. (2004) Role of lysophospholipid growth factors in the modulation of aqueous humor outflow facility. Invest Ophthalmol Vis Sci 45: 2263–2271.
16. Shepard AR, Millar JC, Pang IH, Jacobson N, Wang WH, et al. (2010) Adenoviral gene transfer of active human transforming growth factor-{beta}2 elevates intraocular pressure and reduces outflow facility in rodent eyes. Invest Ophthalmol Vis Sci 51: 2067–2076.
17. Stamer WD, Read AT, Sumida GM, Ethier CR (2009) Sphingosine-1-phosphate effects on the inner wall of Schlemm's canal and outflow facility in perfused human eyes. Exp Eye Res 89: 980–988.
18. Wiederholt M, Thieme H, Stumpff F (2000) The regulation of trabecular meshwork and ciliary muscle contractility. Prog Retin Eye Res 19: 271–295.
19. Tripathi RC, Li J, Chan WF, Tripathi BJ (1994) Aqueous humor in glaucomatous eyes contains an increased level of TGF-beta 2. Exp Eye Res 59: 723–727.
20. Mackay EO, Kallberg ME, Gelatt KN (2008) Aqueous humor myocilin protein levels in normal, genetic carriers, and glaucoma Beagles. Vet Ophthalmol 11: 177–185.
21. Howell KG, Vrabel AM, Chowdhury UR, Stamer WD, Fautsch MP (2010) Myocilin levels in primary open-angle glaucoma and pseudoexfoliation glaucoma human aqueous humor. J Glaucoma 19: 569–575.
22. Pattabiraman PP, Rao PV (2010) Mechanistic basis of Rho GTPase-induced extracellular matrix synthesis in trabecular meshwork cells. Am J Physiol Cell Physiol 298: C749–763.
23. Kumar J, Epstein DL (2011) Rho GTPase-mediated cytoskeletal organization in Schlemm's canal cells play a critical role in the regulation of aqueous humor outflow facility. J Cell Biochem 112: 600–606.
24. Moolenaar WH, Perrakis A (2011) Insights into autotaxin: how to produce and present a lipid mediator. Nat Rev Mol Cell Biol 12: 674–679.
25. Umezu-Goto M, Kishi Y, Taira A, Hama K, Dohmae N, et al. (2002) Autotaxin has lysophospholipase D activity leading to tumor cell growth and motility by lysophosphatidic acid production. J Cell Biol 158: 227–233.
26. Tokumura A, Majima E, Kariya Y, Tominaga K, Kogure K, et al. (2002) Identification of human plasma lysophospholipase D, a lysophosphatidic acid-producing enzyme, as autotaxin, a multifunctional phosphodiesterase. J Biol Chem 277: 39436–39442.
27. Gijsbers R, Aoki J, Arai H, Bollen M (2003) The hydrolysis of lysophospholipids and nucleotides by autotaxin (NPP2) involves a single catalytic site. FEBS Lett 538: 60–64.
28. Giganti A, Rodriguez M, Fould B, Moulharat N, Coge F, et al. (2008) Murine and human autotaxin alpha, beta, and gamma isoforms: gene organization, tissue distribution, and biochemical characterization. J Biol Chem 283: 7776–7789.
29. Ferry G, Moulharat N, Pradere JP, Desos P, Try A, et al. (2008) S32826, a nanomolar inhibitor of autotaxin: discovery, synthesis and applications as a pharmacological tool. J Pharmacol Exp Ther 327: 809–819.
30. Maddala R, Skiba NP, Lalane R III, Sherman DL, Brophy PJ, et al. (2011) Periaxin is required for hexagonal geometry and membrane organization of mature lens fibers. Dev Biol 357: 179–190.
31. Lutjen-Drecoll E (1999) Functional morphology of the trabecular meshwork in primate eyes. Prog Retin Eye Res 18: 91–119.
32. Fleenor DL, Shepard AR, Hellberg PE, Jacobson N, Pang IH, et al. (2006) TGFbeta2-induced changes in human trabecular meshwork: implications for intraocular pressure. Invest Ophthalmol Vis Sci 47: 226–234.
33. Pattabiraman PP, Lih FB, Tomer KB, Rao PV (2012) The role of calcium-independent phospholipase A2gamma in modulation of aqueous humor drainage and Ca2+ sensitization of trabecular meshwork contraction. Am J Physiol Cell Physiol 302: C979–991.
34. Chowdhury UR, Madden BJ, Charlesworth MC, Fautsch MP (2010) Proteome analysis of human aqueous humor. Invest Ophthalmol Vis Sci 51: 4921–4931.
35. Bennett KL, Funk M, Tschernutter M, Breitwieser FP, Planyavsky M, et al. (2011) Proteomic analysis of human cataract aqueous humour: Comparison of one-dimensional gel LCMS with two-dimensional LCMS of unlabelled and iTRAQ(R)-labelled specimens. J Proteomics 74: 151–166.
36. Stracke ML, Krutzsch HC, Unsworth EJ, Arestad A, Cioce V, et al. (1992) Identification, purification, and partial sequence analysis of autotaxin, a novel motility-stimulating protein. J Biol Chem 267: 2524–2529.
37. Nakanaga K, Hama K, Aoki J (2010) Autotaxin–an LPA producing enzyme with diverse functions. J Biochem 148: 13–24.
38. Clair T, Aoki J, Koh E, Bandle RW, Nam SW, et al. (2003) Autotaxin hydrolyzes sphingosylphosphorylcholine to produce the regulator of migration, sphingosine-1-phosphate. Cancer Res 63: 5446–5453.
39. Moolenaar WH, van Meeteren LA, Giepmans BN (2004) The ins and outs of lysophosphatidic acid signaling. Bioessays 26: 870–881.

40. Tielsch JM, Sommer A, Katz J, Royall RM, Quigley HA, et al. (1991) Racial variations in the prevalence of primary open-angle glaucoma. The Baltimore Eye Survey. JAMA 266: 369–374.
41. Sample PA, Girkin CA, Zangwill LM, Jain S, Racette L, et al. (2009) The African Descent and Glaucoma Evaluation Study (ADAGES): design and baseline data. Arch Ophthalmol 127: 1136–1145.
42. Fulkerson Z, Wu T, Sunkara M, Kooi CV, Morris AJ, et al. (2011) Binding of autotaxin to integrins localizes lysophosphatidic acid production to platelets and mammalian cells. J Biol Chem 286: 34654–34663.
43. Hausmann J, Kamtekar S, Christodoulou E, Day JE, Wu T, et al. (2011) Structural basis of substrate discrimination and integrin binding by autotaxin. Nat Struct Mol Biol 18: 198–204.
44. Nishimasu H, Okudaira S, Hama K, Mihara E, Dohmae N, et al. (2011) Crystal structure of autotaxin and insight into GPCR activation by lipid mediators. Nat Struct Mol Biol 18: 205–212.
45. Silva JC, Gorenstein MV, Li GZ, Vissers JP, Geromanos SJ (2006) Absolute quantification of proteins by LCMSE: a virtue of parallel MS acquisition. Mol Cell Proteomics 5: 144–156.
46. Rao PV, Deng PF, Kumar J, Epstein DL (2001) Modulation of aqueous humor outflow facility by the Rho kinase-specific inhibitor Y-27632. Invest Ophthalmol Vis Sci 42: 1029–1037.
47. Chudgar SM, Deng P, Maddala R, Epstein DL, Rao PV (2006) Regulation of connective tissue growth factor expression in the aqueous humor outflow pathway. Mol Vis 12: 1117–1126.

6

Biophysical Characterization of the Olfactomedin Domain of Myocilin, an Extracellular Matrix Protein Implicated in Inherited Forms of Glaucoma

Susan D. Orwig, Raquel L. Lieberman*

School of Chemistry and Biochemistry, Georgia Institute of Technology, Atlanta, Georgia, United States of America

Abstract

Myocilin is an eye protein found in the trabecular extracellular matrix (TEM), within the anatomic region that controls fluid flow. Variants of myocilin, localized to its olfactomedin (OLF) domain, have been linked to inherited forms of glaucoma, a disease associated with elevated intraocular pressure. OLF domains have also been implicated in psychiatric diseases and cancers by their involvement in signaling, neuronal growth, and development. However, molecular characterization of OLFs has been hampered by challenges in recombinant expression, a hurdle we have recently overcome for the myocilin OLF domain (myoc-OLF). Here, we report the first detailed solution biophysical characterization of myoc-OLF to gain insight into its structure and function. Myoc-OLF is stable in the presence of glycosaminoglycans, as well as in a wide pH range in buffers with functional groups reminiscent of such glycosaminoglycans. Circular dichroism (CD) reveals significant β-sheet and β-turn secondary structure. Unexpectedly, the CD signature is reminiscent of α-chymotrypsin as well as another ocular protein family, the βγ-crystallins. At neutral pH, intrinsic tryptophan fluorescence and CD melts indicate a highly cooperative transition with a melting temperature of ~55°C. Limited proteolysis combined with mass spectrometry reveals that the compact core structural domain of OLF consists of approximately residues 238-461, which retains the single disulfide bond and is as stable as the full myoc-OLF construct. The data presented here inform new testable hypotheses for interactions with specific TEM components, and will assist in design of therapeutic agents for myocilin glaucoma.

Editor: Anna Delprato, Institut Européen de Chimie et Biologie, France

Funding: This work was supported by grants to R.L.L. from the Glaucoma Research Foundation and American Health Assistance Foundation. S.D.O. was supported in part by a United States Department of Education Graduate Assistance in Areas of National Need program P200A060188. The funders had no role in study design, data collection and analysis, decision to publish, or preparation of the manuscript.

Competing Interests: The authors have declared that no competing interests exist.

* E-mail: raquel.lieberman@chemistry.gatech.edu

Introduction

Myocilin, the protein most closely associated with inherited forms of open angle glaucoma (OAG) through genetic linkage studies, is a ~57 kDa glycoprotein composed of a secretion signal sequence, coiled-coil region, and a ~30 kDa olfactomedin (OLF) domain (Figure 1), which harbors 90% of all reported pathogenic lesions [1]. The molecular mechanisms that lead to glaucoma are not well established but are of significant biomedical interest given that glaucoma is a leading cause of blindness worldwide, and early-onset myocilin glaucoma accounts for ~4% of glaucoma cases, primarily afflicting children [1].

Wild-type (WT) myocilin is secreted from human trabecular meshwork (HTM) cells to the trabecular meshwork extracellular matrix (TEM) [2,3,4], the anatomical region believed to regulate intraocular pressure [4,5]. By contrast, mutant myocilins aggregate in the endoplasmic reticulum (ER), leading to cell death and a malfunctioning matrix. The net result is an increase in intraocular pressure and retina degeneration, a hallmark of glaucoma [6]. A gain-of-toxic-function is thought to underlie the pathophysiology of myocilin glaucoma [7,8]. Temperature-sensitive secretion of some myocilin variants [9,10] indicates that when protein production is slowed, some mutant proteins appear native-like and competent for trafficking out of the cell and to the TEM. In cell culture, the toxicity of mutant myocilins can be reduced by the addition of certain chemical chaperones [11,12], and in vitro, the compromised stability of mutant myoc-OLFs can be restored with some of the same compounds [13].

In spite of the importance of myocilin in inherited glaucoma pathogenesis, little is known about its normal biological function in the TEM, especially the OLF (myoc-OLF) domain. Full-length myocilin has been shown to bind to TEM proteins such as laminin and the Hep II domain of fibronectin [14,15], as well as the glycosaminoglycan (GAG) heparan sulfate, but these interactions are localized to the coiled-coil region of myocilin, and not myoc-OLF [16]. The normal biological roles of myocilin are further complicated by reports of myocilin localized to the mitochondria of HTM cells [2,17], calpain-II dependent cleavage prior to secretion [18], as well as its expression in other ocular tissues including sclera, ciliary body, iris, retina and optic nerve head [19]. Moreover, beyond the eye, OLF domains are found in numerous multicellular organisms, and more than half of reported OLF domains are found in neural tissues. OLF domains are proposed to play roles in neurogensis, neural crest formation, dorsal ventral patterning, cell-cell adhesion, cell-cycle regulation, cell-cell signaling, tumorigenesis, and have been implicated in psychiatric disorders [20]. The explicit roles of myocilin in any of these tissues and processes, however, are not clear due to a lack of functional assays.

```
Mutations                                                                        * *
gi_3065674         1 M---RFFCARCCSFGPEMPAVQLLLLACLVWDVGARTAQLRK------------ANDQSGRCQYTFSVAS  55
gi_62632725        1 M---WF-------------LAVLWISSLLMGSQVQSSANLRR------------ANAGNGRCQYTFMVDS  42
gi_74356501        1 -----------------MPAVQLLLLACLLGGVGARTAQFQK------------ANDRSGRCQYTFSVAS  41
gi_47522798        1 -----------------MPAVQLLLLACLVWSAGARTAQLWK------------ANDRSGQCQYTFKVAS  41
gi_15077142        1 -----------------MPALHLLFLACLVWGMGARTAQFRK------------ANDRSGRCQYTFTVAS  41
gi_3845607         1 ----MPSCARCCSCGPKMPALQLLFLACLVWGMGARTAQFRK------------ANDRSGRCQYTFTVAS  54
gi_28453877        1 MKYPTFFAPF---------RALMTAVIICLFVETSKCQEATPLGPAYMRTTSGVVETSSGRCQCETAFPP  61
Consensus_ss:            hh hhh         hhhhhhhhhhhhhhhh                       eeeeeeee

Mutations                                                *       *
gi_3065674        56 PNESSCPE---------QSQAMSVIHNLQRDSSTQRLDLEATKARLSSLESLLHQLTLDQAARPQETQEG 116
gi_62632725       43 PTEASCP---------------------SPGSTPEMEALMSRLGLLEALVARLVGGEAMPESSQSSG  88
gi_74356501       42 PSESSCPE---------QGQAMLAIQELQRDSSEQRATLESTKARLSSLEALLHRLTSGQPAGPLETHQG 102
gi_47522798       42 PNESSCPE---------QGQTMSALQDLQRDSSEQRAALESTKARLSSLEALLHRLILGQATGPWEAQEG 102
gi_15077142       42 PNESSCPR---------EDQAMSAIQDLQRDSSIQHADLESTKARVRSLESLLHQMTLGRVTGTQEAQEG 102
gi_3845607        55 PSESSCPR---------EDQAMSAIQDLQRDSSIQHADLESTKARVRSLESLLHQMTSGGVTGTQEVQEG 115
gi_28453877       62 L--VTCQDYVETGYPERLEAAEREIALLGHQLEEYNHTVIRLHIDLELADSQLNVTMMTLEGVLDGTVVV 129
Consensus_ss:                              hhhhhhhhhhhhhhhhh  hhhhhhhhhhhhhhhhhhhhhhh       h

Mutations                       *                              *
gi_3065674       117 LQRELGTLRRERDQLETQTRELETAYSNLLRDKSVLEEEKKRLRQENENLARR--LESSSQEVARLR--- 181
gi_62632725       89 S----GLQDSYNQVMGENAQLKREKQRLDRQVQDLQQRMEELRQEAERLRSRPCMQQTSSRVPQKDNSF 153
gi_74356501      103 LQRELEALRREREQLETQTQELESAYSNLVRDKSALEEEKRRLQAENEDLARR--LESSSQEVASLR--- 167
gi_47522798      103 LEKELGTLRREREQLETQNRELETTYNNLTRDKSALEEEKRQLETENEDLARR--LESSSQELAKL---- 166
gi_15077142      103 LQGQLGALRRERDQLETQTRDLEAAYNNLLRDKSALEEEKRQLEQENEDLARR--LESSSEEVTRLR--- 167
gi_3845607       116 LQGQLGALRRERDQLETQTRDLEVAYNNLLRDKSALEEEKRQLEQENKDLARR--LEGSSQEVARLR--- 180
gi_28453877      130 TVAELELVKEELKEMSLLLERIEEVASEI--------PEVQQLREELNNFTEL--IKQLEVTRPT----- 184
Consensus_ss:              hhhhhhhhhhhhhhhhhhhhhhhhhhhhhh hhhhhhhhhhhhh hhhh  hhhhh

Mutations                                                     *
gi_3065674       182 RGQCPQTRDTARAV------PPGSREVSTWNLDTLAFQELKSELTEVPASRILKES-PSGYLRSGEGDTG 244
gi_62632725      154 RPGSGHVPSNLASRPGNPQEDKSSLRDPAWQYSNPGYQELTAVVTEVTAPN----------QDGPADISG 213
gi_74356501      168 RGQCPQAHSSSQDV------PSGSREVAKWNLENMDFQELKSELTEVPASQILKES-PSGHPRNEEGGTG 230
gi_47522798      167 KVQCPQAHSMSQDV------PLGSREVSKWNVENLDFQELKSELTEVPAARILKES-VSGHSGSEEGGSG 229
gi_15077142      168 RGQCPSTQYPSQDM------LPGSREVSQWNLDTLAFQELKSELTEVPASQILKEN-PSGRPRSKEGDKG 230
gi_3845607       181 RGQCPSTHHPSQDM------LPGSREVSQWNLDTLAFQELKSELTEVPASQILKN--QSGHPRSKEGDKG 242
gi_28453877      185 ---------------------------EVRVLQRKIDDLKSKLAECERYTRTEDESLFQPWSDFPSQDS 226
Consensus_ss:                                            hhhhhhhhh

Mutations                   **        *         *           **      *      *
gi_3065674       245 CGELVWVGEPLTLRTAETITGKYGVWMRDPKPTYPYTQETTWRIDTVGTDVRQVFEYDLISQFMQGYP-- 312
gi_62632725      214 CGDLVWVENPEVHRKADSIAGKYGVWMQDPEAKEPYGPDMVWRIDSVGSEVRQLFGYENMDQLTRGFP-- 281
gi_74356501      231 CGELVWVGEPITLRTAETITGKYGVWMRDPQATFPYTGETTWRIDTVGTDIRQVFEYDHIRQFTQGYP-- 298
gi_47522798      230 CGELVWVGEPVTLRTAETITGKYGVWMRDPKATYPYTQETTWRIDTVGTDIRQVFEYDRISQFAQGYP-- 297
gi_15077142      231 CGALVWVGEPVTLRTAETIAGKYGVWMRDPKPTHPYTQESTWRIDTVGTEIRQVFEYSQISQFEQGYP-- 298
gi_3845607       243 CGVLMWVGEPVTLRTAETITGKYGVWMRDPKPTHPYTQETTWRIDTVGTGIRQVFEYSQISQFEQGYP-- 310
gi_28453877      227 CRDIIHVSEPFTVRGVG---NKIGAWFRDPLQDYI---KVYYAPFHNPRLTYQVDRFAHVADFRGGTEYE 290
Consensus_ss:            eeeee   eeeeee        eee         eeee        eeeeee  hhhhhh

Mutations                        *            *    *        **      ** **  **  *     *  *
gi_3065674       313 -SKVHILPRPLESTGAVVYSGSLYFQGAESRTVIRYELNTETVKAEKEIPGAGYHGQFPYSWGGYTDIDL 381
gi_62632725      282 -TKVLLLPESVESTGATMYKGSLYYQRRLSRTLIRYDLHAESIAARRDLPHAGFHGQFPYSWGGYTDIDL 350
gi_74356501      299 -SKVHVLPRPLESTGAVVYRGSLYFQAAESRTVLRYDLRTETLKAEKEIPGAGYHGQFPYSWGGYTDIDL 367
gi_47522798      298 -SKVHVLPRRLESTGAVVYQGSLYFQGASSRTVIRYELSTETLKAEKEIPGAGYHGQFPYSWGGYTDIDL 366
gi_15077142      299 -SKVHVLPRALESTGAVVYAGSLYFQGAESRTVVRYELDTETVKAEKEIPGAGYHGHFPYAWGGYTDIDL 367
gi_3845607       311 -SKVHVLPQALESTGAVVYAGSLYFQGAESRTVLRYELNTETVKAEKEIPGAGYHGQFPYAWGGYTDIDL 379
gi_28453877      291 HRYMLPTNLPAQGPGMVAYNGSLYYHAFQSRQIVRYDLENHTVVTTGEISDADI-----NIRGSPSAIDL 355
Consensus_ss:           eeeee        eeee  eeeee      eeeee    eeeeeee                 eee

Mutations                        *     *                      * **     **  *      *    *
gi_3065674       382 AVDEAGLWVIYSTDEAKGAIVLSKLNPENLELEQTWETNIRKQSVANAFIICGTLYTVSSYTSADATVNF 451
gi_62632725      351 AIDENGLWAIYSTNKAKGAIVISQLDPHNLEVKGTWETKIRKTSVANAFMICGKLYTVASYTSPNTTVNY 420
gi_74356501      368 AVDEIGLWVIYSTEAAKGAIVLSKLNPETLELEQTWETNIRKQSVANAFIICGTLYTVSSYSSPDATVNF 437
gi_47522798      367 AVDETGLWVIYSTEAAKGAIVLSKLNPENLELERTWETNIRKQSVANAFIICGTLYTVSSYSSPEATINF 436
gi_15077142      368 AVDESGLWVIYSTEEAKGAIVLSKLNPANLELERTWETNIRKQSVANAFVLCGILYTVSSYSSAHATVNF 437
gi_3845607       380 AVDESGLWVIYSTEETRGAIVLSKLNPENLELESTWETNIRKQSVANAFVICGILYTVSSYSSVHATINF 449
gi_28453877      356 AVDELGLWAIYASVSDQTNTMISRLDPETLDVIETWVAPFPKYQAGSCFMVCGRLYCLSSFFSTDSTVEL 425
Consensus_ss:          eee   eeeeee     eeeeeee     eeeeeee      hhheeeeeeeeeeee      eeee

Mutations                          *    **    *  ** *              *
gi_3065674       452 AYDTGTGISKTLTIPFKNRYKYSSMIDYNPLEKKLFAWDNLNMVTYDIKLSKM----------------- 504
gi_62632725      421 MFDTATSQGKAISVPFKNRYRYNSMVDYNSAKRKLYAWDNYYMVSYSVRLGKQE---------------- 474
gi_74356501      438 AYDTGTGSSKALTVPFKNRYKYSSMIDYNPLERKLFAWDNFNMVSYDIKLSRL----------------- 490
gi_47522798      437 AYDTSTGSSKALTIPFKNRYEYSSMIDYNPLEKKLFAWDNFNMVTYDIRLSRM----------------- 489
gi_15077142      438 AYDTKTGTSKTLTIPFTNRYKYSSMIDYNPLERKLFAWDNFNMVTYDIKLLEM----------------- 490
gi_3845607       450 AYDTNTGISKTLTIPFKNRYKYSSMVDYNPLERKLFAWDNFNMVTYDIKLSEM----------------- 502
gi_28453877      426 VYETSSNVFRVIDVLFDIRFGEMMSLKYNPRDQKLYGWDNGHQVVYDLTFDPPARSQLLPTDTNIPLNLQ 495
Consensus_ss:          eee    eeee           eee   hhh eeeeee eeeeeeeee
```

Figure 1. Multiple sequence alignment for myocilin and non-ocular ortholog amassin. Alignment includes myocilin from *H. sapiens* (gi 3065674), *D. rerio* (gi 62632725), *B. taurus* (gi 74356501), *S. scrofa* (gi 47522798), *M. musculus* (gi 15077142), *R. norvegicus* (gi 3845607), and amassin from *S. purpuratus* (gi 28453877). The region shaded in grey contains the N-terminal signal sequence and coiled-coil region, whereas the OLF domain remains unshaded. The consensus predicted secondary structures are shown in the last line (h, alpha-helix; e, beta-strand). Blue, similar residues; red, conserved residues; asterisk, reported disease-causing mutation in human myocilin [49]. The alignment and predicted secondary structure were generated using PROMALS [53]. Solid black boxes enclose peptides identified in both core-OLF and myoc-OLF by mass spectrometry; whereas dashed boxes enclose peptides identified only in myoc-OLF (see text).

The objective of this study is to probe the molecular properties of myoc-OLF to gain insight into its function and structure. The study was enabled by our recent development of a preparative in vitro expression system in which myoc-OLF is closely fused to a cleavable maltose binding protein (MBP) [13]. Our current work places the OLF domain for the first time in the context of other known proteins. The analysis of myoc-OLF described herein also provides a biophysical basis for the development of a new therapeutic avenue for glaucoma in the context of a protein conformational disorder.

Results

pH stability profile of myoc-OLF

We investigated the pH stability profile of myoc-OLF to elucidate any preferences of this domain as well as to gain insight into its resilience under different pH environments, such as low pH, that might be encountered under a known age-related TEM stressor, oxidative stress [21]. For the broad 96-well pH screen (Table S1), we used the MBP-OLF fusion protein and adapted the differential scanning fluorimetry (DSF) technique used originally to assess thermal stability differences between WT and glaucoma-causing myoc-OLF variants [13]. The melting of MBP is deconvoluted from the melting of OLF by the addition of 50 mM maltose. The melting curves of MBP and OLF are readily distinguished in the stability assay throughout the pH range tested. MBP is stable from pH 4-10.5 [22], OLF is not affected by the presence of maltose [13], and Sypro Orange is not pH sensitive in the range 4-10 (not shown).

To cross-validate the results obtained using the MBP-OLF fusion protein, we subsequently tested cleaved myoc-OLF in a subset of stabilizing and destabilizing buffers (Table S1). There was no difference in melting temperature (T_m) between the MBP-OLF and cleaved myoc-OLF among the pHs tested (Table S1), reinforcing the independence of the domains in the fusion protein. Interestingly, myoc-OLF is stable in 100 mM buffers corresponding to a range in pH of 4.6 to 7.4, but specifically in sodium lactate, acetate, MES, phosphate and Hepes (Table 1, Table S1). Bicine at pH 7.0 and glycine at pH 8.2 were also stabilizing buffers, albeit within a more limited pH range (Table 1, Table S1). By contrast, OLF was destabilized in pH 4.0–4.6, as well as the full pH range tested of Bis-Tris, Imidazole, Tris, and CHES buffers (Table 1, Table S1).

The concentration dependence of buffer stabilization or destabilization was further investigated using acetate buffer pH 4.6 or Tris buffer pH 7.5 as examples, respectively (Table S1). Myoc-OLF is more stable in 10 mM Tris pH 7.5 compared to 100 mM Tris pH 7.5. For Tris buffer, increasing the ionic strength by the addition of NaCl partially restores stability, suggesting that counterions may play a role in this buffer system. Conversely, for acetate buffer pH 4.6, a further increase of 2°C in the T_m value for myoc-OLF is observed when 100 mM acetate buffer pH 4.6 is used compared to 10 mM (Table S1), with no additional effects due to the presence of NaCl (not shown).

Stability analysis in the presence of GAGs

Interestingly, the preferred buffers for myoc-OLF contain sulfate and acetate functional groups that are reminiscent of GAGs, whereas those that are destabilizing in an overlapping pH range harbor aliphatic amines (Table 1). Thus, we sought to evaluate the stability of myoc-OLF in the presence of individual GAGs found in the TEM [23] at physiologically relevant concentrations [24] (Table 2). Indeed, a modest ($\Delta T_m = 4.5°C$) stabilizing effect was observed for myoc-OLF in the presence of a relatively low concentration (0.75 mg/ml) of heparan sulfate, whereas a similar increase in stability for chondroitin sulfate and hyaluronic acid were observed only at higher concentrations of 10 mg/ml, at the outer limit of the physiological range, suggesting a weaker effect. The addition of dermatan sulfate did not change the T_m value of myoc-OLF in the full range tested.

Conformational analysis of myoc-OLF at pH 4.6, 5.8, and 7.2

In order to detect structural changes across the stable pH regime, we next compared the secondary structure of myoc-OLF by conducting CD melts in stabilizing buffers of varying pH. We measured the CD spectrum in 10 mM acetate buffer pH 4.6, below the calculated [25] pI = ~5 of myoc-OLF, at the lower end of the stable range, as well as in 10 mM phosphate buffer pH 5.8 where OLF was the most stable in our assay (Table 1, Table S1), and at the physiological pH 7.2 expected in the TEM under normal conditions.

Table 1. Summary of stabilization of myoc-OLF by buffers of varying pH.

Buffer	pH range	Stabilizing Buffer[a]
Sodium Lactate/HCl	4.0–4.4	No
Sodium Lactate/HCl	**4.8–5.2**	**Yes**
Sodium Acetate/Acetic Acid	4.2	No
Sodium Acetate/Acetic Acid	**4.6–6.2**	**Yes**
MES/NaOH	**5.0–7.4**	**Yes**
Bis-Tris/HCl	5.2–8.0	No
Imidazole/HCl	5.4–8.2	No
K_2HPO_4/NaH_2PO_4	**5.8–7.4**	**Yes**
K_2HPO_4/NaH_2PO_4	7.8–8.6	No
Hepes/NaOH	**6.0–7.2**	**Yes**
Hepes/NaOH	7.6–8.4	No
Tris/HCl	6.6–8.6	No
Bicine/NaOH	**7.0**	**Yes**
Bicine/NaOH	7.2–8.6	No
CHES/NaOH*	8.0–8.8	No
Glycine/NaOH	**8.2**	**Yes**
Glycine/NaOH	8.6	No

[a]No: T_m<51.7°C; Yes: T_m>51.7°C. The lower limit cutoff is 1°C less than the originally reported T_m of myoc-OLF in phosphate buffer, using DSF [13]. Full data are presented in Table S1.

Table 2. Stabilization of myoc-OLF by GAGs.

	T_m (°C)	ΔT_m (°C)
None	52.4±0.1	0
Chondroitin Sulfate	57.7±0.0	5.3
Dermatan Sulfate	52.7±0.0	0.3
Heparan Sulfate [a]	57.2±0.0	4.8
Hyaluronic Acid	55.4±0.1	3.0

[a]For these experiments, heparan sulfate concentration was 0.75 mg/ml, whereas all other GAGs were present at 10 mg/ml.

No major changes are observed among the three CD spectra at different pH values. The 200–210 nm range is more positive at pH 4.6 than the others, suggestive of non-native features of OLF in this buffer environment, but otherwise there are only slight differences in the intensity of the two major minima at ~217 and ~230 nm (Figure 2A). Component spectra, identified using singular value decomposition (SVD) analysis, reveal three significant spectral contributions. By far the most predominant component is one that contains both minima, followed by two minor contributions from spectra that resemble random coils (Figure 2B). Notably, there is no significant contribution from features at 208 nm and/or another at 222 nm; thus, there is no evidence of α-helices in myoc-OLF. The broad ~217 nm minimum, which is characteristic of antiparallel β-sheets, resembles the CD spectrum of a smaller OLF construct expressed in *P. pastoris* [26], but the prominent shoulder near 230 nm has not been seen previously. The lack of this latter feature in the *P. pastoris* OLF construct may have been a result of its N-terminal truncation or the use of Tris pH 8.0 [26], a destabilizing buffer (Table 1, Table S1).

Consistent with the aggregation propensity observed in mutants that lead to myocilin glaucoma, the unfolding transitions of myoc-OLF are irreversible. Sample precipitation was seen under all experimental conditions tested, including all concentrations, pH and temperature ranges. Nevertheless, there is substantial evidence for a highly cooperative transition [27]. First, at all three pH values, a sharp transition and similar isodichroic point near 238 nm are observed for myoc-OLF (Figure 3). Second, the differences in T_m for the melting curves monitored at the two local minima are consistently within 1°C of each other, and within error of the fit to the T_m obtained from the Boltzmann sigmoid equation, which assumes a two-state model (Table S2). Third, there is no obvious scan rate dependence of denaturation (not shown), suggesting that the melting transition is under thermodynamic, rather than kinetic control. Nevertheless, because we were not able to find experimental conditions of reversibility for myoc-OLF, the extent of the validity of thermodynamic parameters obtained using a two-state model cannot be assessed. We note, however, that thermodynamic parameters we obtained using this assumption with excellent error statistics (Text S1, Figure S1, Table S2) are similar to those of α-chymotrypsin [28], a protein that exhibits both similar mass and CD spectrum as myoc-OLF (see Discussion).

The transition to the denatured state for myoc-OLF at pH 4.6 occurs between 40–50°C (Figure 3A). Upon denaturation, the ellipticity is reduced by 50% and there is a shift in minimum at 216 nm in the folded state to 220 nm in the denatured state. SVD deconvolution (not shown) reveals a significant reduction in the β-sheet component and an increase in the random coil component, suggesting the precipitated sample is likely a molten globule with local secondary structure. By comparison, for both unfolding experiments conducted at pH 5.8 (Figure 3B) and pH 7.2 (Figure 3C), the transition occurs between 50 and 60°C with a fourfold reduction in signal intensity between folded and unfolded states of myoc-OLF. Less residual secondary structure remaining in these higher pH experiments may be attributed to the difference in net charge per residue. In conditions far from the pI of myoc-OLF, such as at pH 7.2, secondary structure would be expected to be disrupted due to the high net charge per residue. By contrast, at pH 4.6, myoc-OLF is closest to its pI where it may experience less repulsion and therefore retain secondary structure in the denatured state [29].

The T_m of myoc-OLF at pH 4.6 is nearly 10°C lower than the T_m at pH 5.8 or 7.2, and ~3°C lower than that measured by DSF using the same ionic strength buffer (Table 1). Using a two-state assumption (see caveats above), comparison of the free energy of unfolding, as well as both enthalpy and entropy components, also indicate a lower barrier to unfolding (Table S2). Nevertheless, even the values at pH 4.6 are well within parameters obtained from numerous other folded proteins [28]. The thermodynamic values fit for myoc-OLF above its pI indicate a larger energy barrier and more stable protein, consistent with the measured increase in T_m. Finally, the unfolding transition at neutral pH was further corroborated by a thermal melt in which intrinsic tryptophan fluorescence was monitored at pH 7.2 (Figure 3D). Indeed, the intrinsic T_m measured by both CD and Trp fluorescence melts is close to the $T_m = 52.7$°C we previously reported using the more

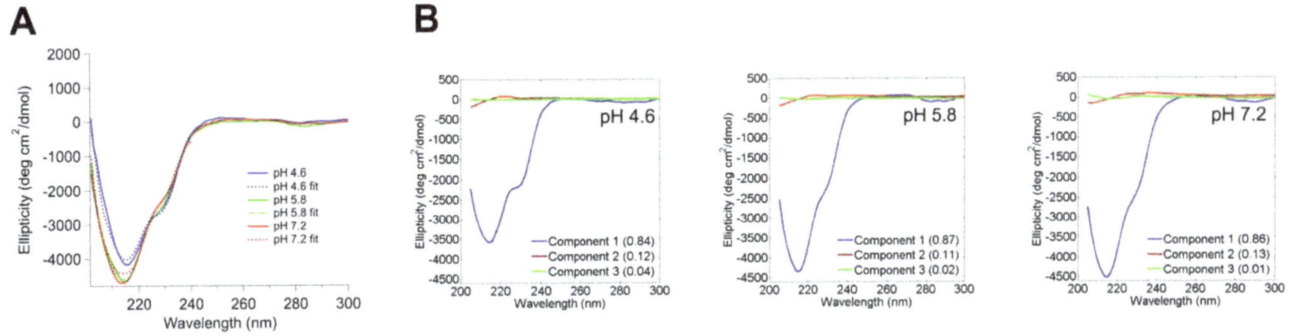

Figure 2. CD signatures of myoc-OLF domain at varying pH. (A) Prominent minima are observed at ~217 nm and ~230 nm for both experimental spectra (solid) and reconstructed spectral fit from SVD analysis (dashed). (B) Top component spectra from SVD analysis. Inset: relative contribution.

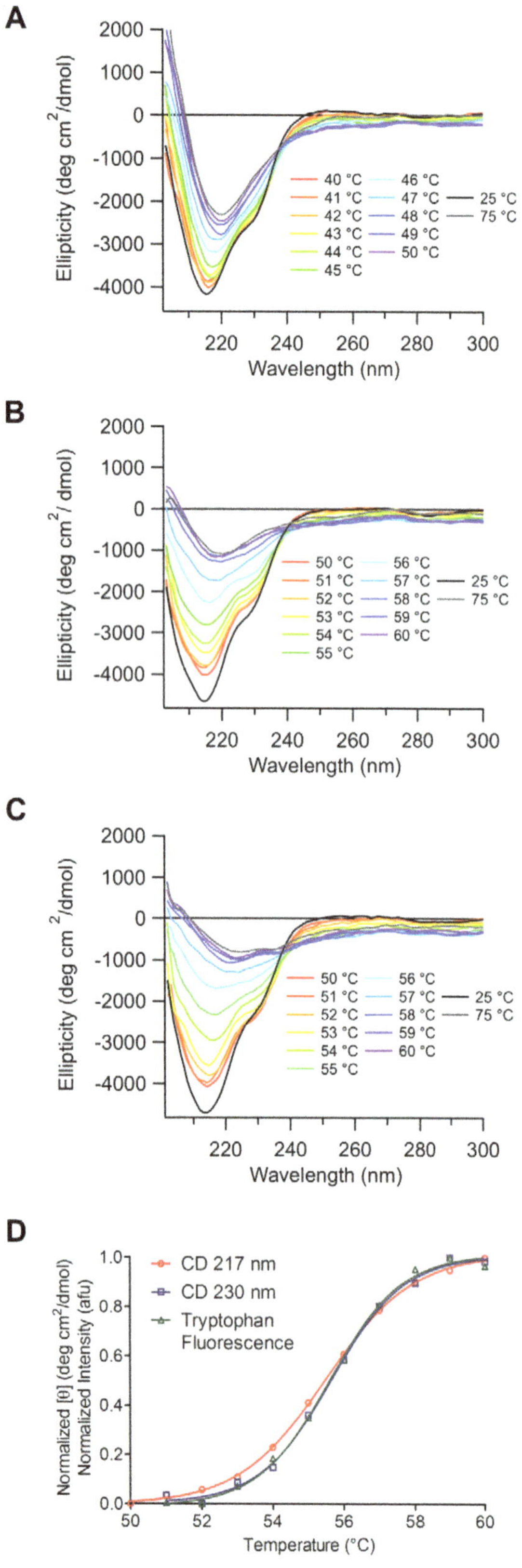

Figure 3. Thermal unfolding of myoc-OLF monitored by CD spectropolarimetry. Melts were conducted at (A) pH 4.6 (B) pH 5.8 and (C) pH 7.2. For each, 11 spectra are overlayed in the region of melting as well as two additional extrema. (D) Comparison of tryptophan fluorescence melt with CD melts from above. Each curve is normalized to the range of its respective signal.

facile, if indirect, DSF technique [13]. The melting thermogram overlays particularly well with the curve obtained monitoring ~230 nm by CD, suggesting tryptophan residues contribute to this CD signal (see Discussion).

Limits of the myoc-OLF core domain

We subjected myoc-OLF to limited proteolysis to identify its three dimensional core structure(s). In most constructs of myoc-OLF studied in the laboratory, a disulfide bond is formed between the only two available cysteine residues (Cys 245 and Cys 433) [13,26], which are 189 residues apart. Yet, protein domains are typically composed of ~150 amino acids [30]. It is possible that the two cysteine residues, far apart in sequence, are nevertheless topologically close. This could lead to either two or more smaller structural domains or one larger than average single domain.

Overall, myoc-OLF is resistant to cleavage by proteases at room temperature, including trypsin, α-chymotrypsin, pepsin, and V_8 protease (not shown) suggesting that our construct consisting of residues 228–504 of myocilin, comprises a well folded, ~30 kDa protein. However, incubation with subtilisin A, a non-specific protease that cleaves after large uncharged residues, generated a smaller domain of ~25 kDa (Figure 4A). Similar results were obtained with the likewise promiscuous protease papain (not shown). The CD spectrum of core-OLF is similar to that of myoc-OLF with some minor exceptions, a 202 nm shoulder characteristic of a type I β-turn [31], and a more pronounced 230 nm shoulder (Figure 4B). As seen previously with myoc-OLF [13], the disulfide bond remains intact in core-OLF. Observed using the thiol-sensitive fluorogenic reagent, ThioGlo (see Materials and Methods), fluorescence increases only in samples in which the disulfide bond in core-OLF has been reduced with tris(2-carboxyethyl)phosphine (TCEP) (Table 3). Finally, the T_m is unchanged, 53.4±0.2°C measured by DSF.

Peptide mass fingerprinting reveals that the N- and C-termini of core-OLF are truncated compared to myoc-OLF (Figure 1, Table 4). For core-OLF, the most N-terminal fragment observed in the spectrum encompasses residues 238–258, the extreme C-terminal peptide observed for core-OLF comprises residues 408–422 (Table 4), whereas the peptides TLTIPFK (residues 462–468, Figure 4C, Table 4) and YSSMIDYNPLEK (residues 473–484, Figure 4D, Table 4) are absent. The truncated C-terminal 44 residues may form a structural element not detected by SDS-PAGE due to its small size, or it may be largely unordered. In sum, consistent with the ~25 kDa fragment size, and digest analysis, the main structural domain of myoc-OLF harbors a disulfide bond and is likely inclusive of residues Ser 238 and Lys 461.

Discussion

Functional significance

The human TEM, a microenvironment in the eye consisting of fibrillar and curly collagens, elastic fibrils, basement membrane and amorphous basement membrane-like materials, as well as other specific proteins, proteoglycans and GAGs, is the anatomical region that controls outflow of aqueous humor in the eye [23]. The structural and functional details of this interconnected matrix, its receptor-mediated interactions with HTM cells, and mechanisms leading to phenotypes observed in the diseased state, are poorly understood [1]. The proper functioning of this complex tissue involves adaptation to a host of cellular and environmental stressors over time, and cumulative long-term detrimental effects of oxidative stress have been implicated in decreased aqueous humor outflow. Eventually, poor flow control leads to an impaired ability to regulate eye pressure, and subsequently, glaucoma [21]. Changes in GAG

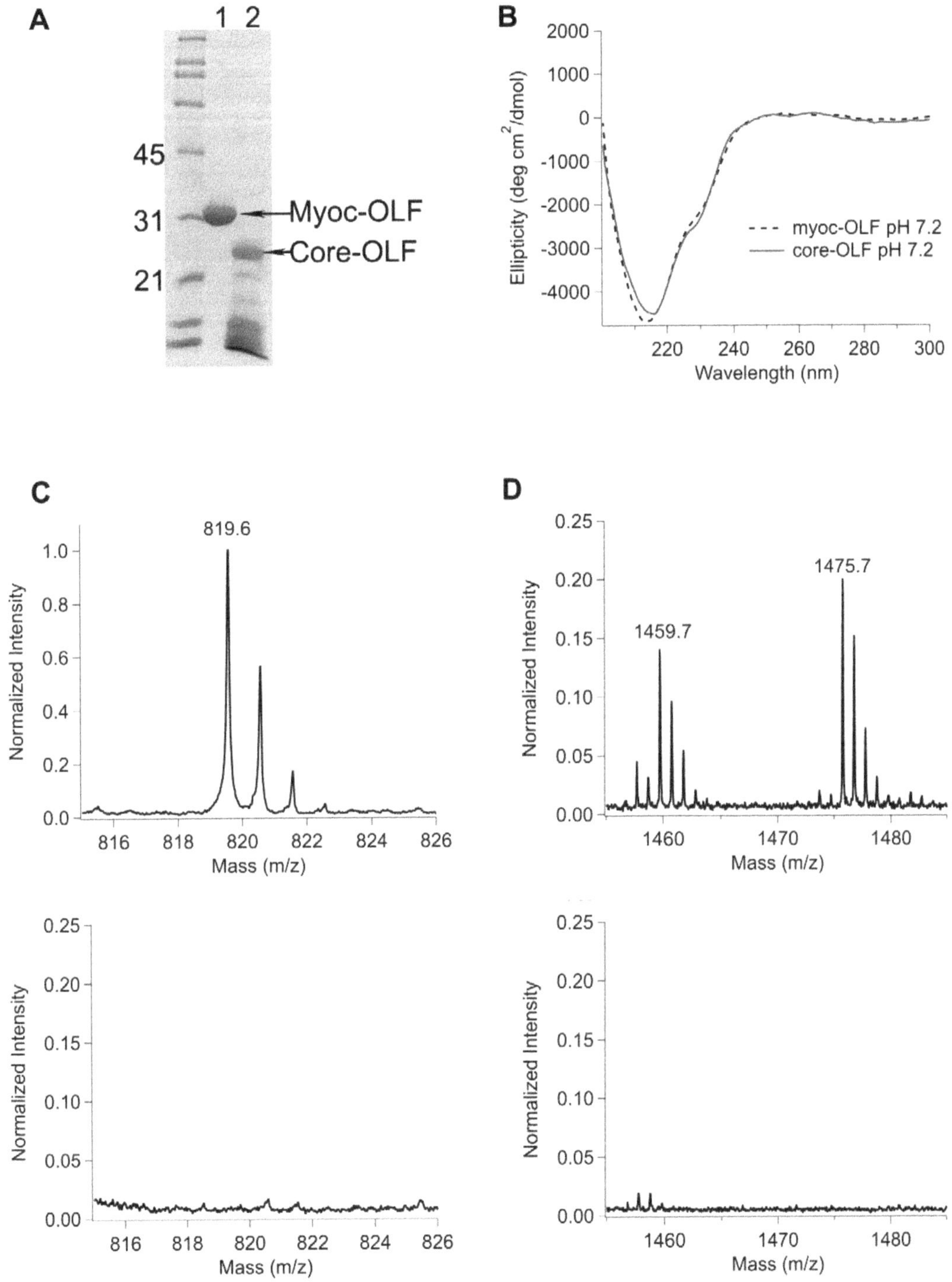

Figure 4. Analysis of core OLF domain. (A) SDS-PAGE analysis of myoc-OLF before and after limited proteolysis by subtilisin A. Lane 1, myoc-OLF, Lane 2, core-OLF. Molecular mass markers denoted in kDa. (B) Overlay of core-OLF and myoc-OLF CD spectra at pH 7.2. (C, D) Comparison of trypsin digest/MALDI TOF/TOF mass spectra of myoc-OLF (top) and core OLF domain (bottom) in two key regions (see text, Table 4).

Table 3. Characterization of disulfide bond in core-OLF.

Sample	Fluorescence Intensity (513 nm)
core-OLF (6 μM)	0.7
core-OLF (6 μM), TCEP (5 mM)	184.4

composition have also been observed in glaucoma-patient derived samples [32,33], but the mechanisms that bring about these changes are unknown. In addition, the roles played by myocilin in the TEM, either normal or pathogenic, are not clear. In this study, we have unraveled some of the molecular characteristics of the myoc-OLF domain in the context of its TEM microenvironment, which will aid future functional characterization.

Several lines of evidence support the notion that GAGs provide a favorable environment for myoc-OLF to function, even though

Table 4. Observed and calculated mass spectrum peaks for myoc-OLF and core-OLF.

	Residue Range	Calculated Mass	Observed Mass	ΔMass	MS/MS	Sequence
Core-OLF	267–272	827.3868	827.3786	−0.0082		YGVWM[a]R
	288–296	975.5105	975.5100	−0.0005	yes	IDTVGTDVR
	347–355	1096.5521	1096.5477	−0.0044	yes	YELNTETVK
	273–287	1882.8970	1882.8944	−0.0026		DPKPTYPYTQETTWR
	406–422	2099.0403	2099.0400	−0.0003	yes	LNPENLELEQTWETNIR
	238–258	2232.0601	2232.0674	0.0073	yes	SGEGDTGC[b]GELVWVGEPLTLR
Myoc-OLF	462–468	819.4974	819.5486	0.0512		TLTIPFK
	267–272	843.3817	843.3954	0.0137		YGVWM[c]R
	288–296	975.5105	975.5311	0.0206		IDTVGTDVR
	347–355	1096.5521	1096.5712	0.0191		YELNTETVK
	473–484	1459.6672	1459.6852	0.0180		YSSMIDYNPLEK
	273–287	1882.8970	1882.9452	0.0482		DPKPTYPYTQETTWR
	406–422	2099.0403	2099.0972	0.0569		LNPENLELEQTWETNIR
	297–314	2180.0369	2180.0801	0.0432		QVFEYDLISQFMQGYPSK

[a]A indicates oxidation of methionine,
[b]B designates carbamidomethyl cysteine,
[c]C indicates methionine sulphone.

to date, no experiments have identified specific GAGs binders in the myoc-OLF region from any organism. Four GAG attachment sites to the myoc-OLF domain are predicted by the ELM database [34] within residues 232–235, 237–240, 330–333 and 443–446, suggesting that direct linkages are possible. The microenvironment of myoc-OLF in the TEM is also replete with GAGs at a total concentration of 1–2 mg/ml [35], with the approximate composition of 20–25% hyaluronic acid or hyaluronan, 40–60% chondroitin and dermatan sulfates, 5–10% karatan sulfate, and 15–20% heparan sulfate [23]. Our experiments reveal a modest increase in stability for myoc-OLF in the presence of heparan sulfate, chondroitin sulfate, and hyaluronic acid. Although no change in T_m was observed in the presence of dermatan sulfate, no GAGs tested destabilized myoc-OLF. Interestingly, whereas direct binding of chondroitin sulfate to another OLF-containing protein, mouse photomedin, has been shown [36], the presence of chondroitin sulfate only weakly influences thermal properties of myoc-OLF. This result suggests that chondroitin sulfate may have different functional significance for related OLF-containing proteins.

By contrast, a more pronounced effect on myoc-OLF stability was observed under physiologically relevant concentrations of heparan sulfate. Even though direct binding to the OLF domain has been ruled out by a previous study demonstrating binding via the N-terminal coiled-coil domain of myocilin [16], the knowledge that heparan sulfate binds to myocilin indicates that this GAG is in the local milieu of myoc-OLF. The observation that heparan sulfate thermally stabilizes myoc-OLF should prompt experiments to further clarify the nature of the mechanism of stabilization.

In addition, although heparan sulfate appears to exert a modest stabilizing effect on myoc-OLF in the absence of other analytes, it seems plausible that cations might enhance the favorable specific interactions between the negatively charged GAGs and the negatively charged OLF domain under physiological conditions. For example, detailed functional studies of amassin, a related, but non-ocular, OLF-containing protein (Figure 1) from the invertebrate animal sea urchin, demonstrates the requirement of the amassin OLF domain for cell-cell adhesion in coelomocytes. This process also requires the presence of Ca^{2+}, and higher multimeric states of the amassin OLF domain [37]. To date, however, no canonical Ca^{2+}-binding sites have been identified in myoc-OLF, and to the best of our knowledge, Ca^{2+} has not been included in any assays. In our hands, myoc-OLF does not bind Tb^{3+}, a Ca^{2+} mimic [38] (not shown), and has only been isolated as a monomer by gel filtration [13]. Although it is possible that these two related proteins have unique modes of interactions and binding partners, based on our study we raise the possibility that certain key components, such as GAGs and/or metal ions, may be missing from functional assays of myocilin attempted to date.

Lastly, the importance of elucidating the mechanism by which GAGs stabilize myoc-OLF is underscored by the finding that the concentrations of GAGs in glaucomatous eyes deviate from those of healthy eyes [32,33]. Specifically, concentrations of sulfated GAGs, such as chondroitin sulfate, are higher in samples derived from early-onset glaucoma patients than from controls [33], and the concentration of hyaluronan decreases in adult-onset OAG patient-derived specimens compared to controls [32]. Given the connection between myocilin and early-onset glaucoma [39], an understanding of the nuances of different GAG interactions with myoc-OLF may pave the way to a better comprehension of myocilin glaucoma pathogenesis.

Structural significance

Although predominantly β-sheet-containing proteins, such as the immunoglobulins [40], exhibit a trough at ~217 nm that is characteristic of antiparallel β-sheets [31], of particular interest is the prominent ~230 nm shoulder that had not been observed previously. One possibility is that a β-turn [41] is present, a hypothesis supported by prediction of β-turns in myoc-OLF by bioinformatics [42]. Alternatively, or in addition, the 230 nm feature may arise from aromatic residues, as observed in certain serine proteases. For example, a notable 230 nm band in α-chymotrypsin has been attributed to a tryptophan residue whose conformation is sensitive to changes in its environment upon activation of α-chymotrypsinogen to α-chymotrypsin [43]. In support of this assignment, the Trp fluorescence melt curve overlays closely with that from 230 nm observed in CD (Figure 3D). Of the seven Trp residues in myoc-OLF, two, Trp 270 and Trp 286, are in and near, respectively, a proline-rich region. Alternatively, Trp 373 is within a region with significant disorder probability as predicted by GlobPlot [44]. Future studies involving systematic mutagenesis of each Trp residue may shed more light on the properties of this unusual feature of the CD spectrum.

Intriguingly, the CD spectrum of core-OLF is similar to that of the βγ-crystallin superfamily. Crystallins are cytoplasmic lens cell proteins associated with genetic forms of cataract, a condition in which the crystallins precipitate. Regardless of their quaternary structure, which often exhibits functionally significant polydisperse, domain-swapped oligomers [45], CD spectra of crystallins include the same features at ~202 nm, ~217 nm, and ~230 nm as seen with core-OLF [46], albeit with different relative intensities. Myoc-OLF exhibits no significant sequence homology with crystallins, is ~10 kDa larger, is not known to oligomerize, nor observed to harbor two structural domains [47]. Nevertheless, OLF likely shares structural features such as similar length or twist of its β-strands, and/or the unusually strained torsion angles in a β-hairpin. Further characterization of the three-dimensional structure of an OLF domain will help elucidate the extent of similarity of features with the crystallins, including repeat structures in myoc-OLF that may be important for myocilin self assembly and/or function in the TEM, or plausible molecular mechanisms for the severe aggregation properties observed upon thermal unfolding.

Implications for new therapeutic directions

The details of the unfolding mechanisms of WT and disease-causing myoc-OLF domains variants, particularly at physiological pH, are informative for a pharmacological chaperone therapeutic effort [48] for myocilin glaucoma. In this approach, the binding of small molecules will enhance the stability of the mutant myocilins to WT levels so that after folding in the ER, mutant myocilins will meet quality control requirements and be competent for secretion to the TEM.

Both thermodynamics and kinetics may be important in chaperone therapy for myocilin glaucoma. The therapeutic small molecule might bind to a folded mutant protein to restore its stability to that of WT, and/or bind to a non-native conformation and accelerate folding to the native state. From this study we know that the ~31 kDa WT myoc-OLF domain is a stable entity that appears to unfold under thermodynamic control in a highly cooperative transition. We can now move forward to compare unfolding pathways of the numerous missense mutants of OLF. If mutant OLFs unfold in similarly cooperative transitions, thermal stabilization of the fully folded protein may be sufficient for preventing aggregation and improving secretion, and screening for candidate chaperone molecules would be based on thermal stability alone. However, a more likely scenario is that deviations from two-state unfolding exist for at least some of the reported mutants [49]. In this case, a pharmacological chaperone may need to be tailored in such a way that it alters the folding pathway back to a fully cooperative mechanism observed in WT myoc-OLF. Future studies will examine to what extent such unfolding intermediates exist for specific glaucoma-causing myoc-OLF mutants.

Materials and Methods

Expression and purification of myoc-OLF

The myoc-OLF gene was introduced into the MBP fusion vector, pMAL-c4x, as described previously [13]. Expression and purification of MBP-OLF followed previously described procedures, as did generation of cleaved myoc-OLF by incubation with Factor Xa and further purification [13]. SDS-PAGE analysis was conducted as described [50].

Thermal stability assay for buffer and pH analysis

Our fluorescence thermal stability assay [13] utilizing DSF [51] was adapted to identify buffer and pH preferences for myoc-OLF. Reactions of 30 μL were prepared at room temperature and delivered to 96-well optical plates (Applied Biosystems) before sealing with optical film (Applied Biosystems). The reaction mixture consisted of 1 μM myoc-OLF or MBP-OLF in 10 mM sodium phosphate dibasic/potassium phosphate monobasic, 200 mM NaCl pH 7.2 (Buffer A) and 5X Sypro Orange (Invitrogen). Buffers from pH 4 to pH 9 were obtained from the pHat™ Buffer screen (Emerald Biosciences) and added to each reaction at a final concentration of 100 mM, with the exception of N-Cyclohexyl-2-aminoethanesulfonic acid (CHES), which had a final concentration of 50 mM. Only for the initial screen was MBP-OLF used and 50 mM maltose added to the reaction mixture. Selected DSF measurements were repeated with cleaved myoc-OLF in acetate, MES, phosphate, Tris, bicine, and glycine buffers. Fluorescence data were acquired on an Applied Biosciences Step-One Plus RT-PCR instrument equipped with a fixed excitation wavelength (480 nm) and a ROX emission filter (610 nm). Melts were conducted from 25–95°C with a 1°C per min increase. Collected data were baseline subtracted, trimmed to include both the boundaries and the transition of interest, and subjected to Boltzmann sigmoid analysis (see below).

Thermal stability assay in the presence of GAGs

The thermal stability assay described above was employed to test for increased myoc-OLF stability in the presence of GAGs including chondroitin sulfate (shark cartilage, Sigma), dermatan sulfate (TCI America), heparan sulfate (bovine kidney, Sigma), and hyaluronic acid (rooster comb, Sigma) at concentrations ranging from 0 mg/ml to 10 mg/ml. Samples were prepared in 10 mM Tris, pH 7.5 and 200 mM NaCl, diluted from a 5x stock solution. GAGs were added from 20 mg/ml stock solutions in water, keeping protein and Sypro Orange concentration the same as above. Data analysis was performed as described above.

Circular dichroism (CD) spectropolarimetry

CD was performed on a Jasco J-810 spectropolarimeter with purified myoc-OLF (8–10 μM) prepared in Buffer A, Buffer A adjusted to pH 5.8, as well as in 10 mM sodium acetate/acetic acid and 200 mM NaCl, pH 4.6. Melts were performed in triplicate on each of the samples by raising the temperature from 5 to 90°C in 1°C /min increments using a Neslab RTE-111 (Thermo Scientific) circulating water bath and monitoring the profiles between 200 and 300 nm in a 0.1 cm cuvette. Ten spectra, scanned from 300 to 200 nm at rate of 500 nm•min^{-1}, were then averaged at the designated temperature. Our attempts to acquire reliable data below 200 nm were not successful due to voltage limits of the instrument and available nitrogen flow rate. Temperature increase and spectra acquisition lasted about five minutes per degree Celsius, and no differences in melting transitions were observed when the scan rate was reduced to 0.5°C /min (data not shown). In all cases, samples precipitated after melting, including reversibility tests in which the temperature was raised just to the T_m and then cooled (not shown).

Each averaged spectrum was background-corrected and converted to mean residue ellipticity

$$[\Theta] = \frac{M_{res} \times \Theta_{obs}}{10 \times d \times c}$$

where $M_{res} = 112.9$ is the mean residue mass calculated from the protein sequence; θ_{obs} is the observed ellipticity (degrees) at wavelength λ; d is the pathlength (cm); and c is the protein concentration (g/ml). CD melt data from 205 – 300 nm were deconvoluted into component spectra using the singular value decomposition procedure in Matlab (The Mathworks), and their statistical significance was calculated based on singular values. The top three components comprising ≥95% of the CD signal were then selected for reconstitution for the final fit plotted in Figure 2. Inspection of difference spectra confirmed that additional components consist of noise.

Tryptophan fluorescence spectroscopy

Measurements were carried out in triplicate on a FluoroMax-3 spectrofluorimeter (Horiba Scientific). Intrinsic tryptophan fluorescence of myoc-OLF (2 μM) in Buffer A was excited at 280 nm (slit width 1 nm) and emission recorded in the range 300–400 nm (slit width 5 nm) with a maximum at 340 nm corresponding to tryptophan fluorescence emission. Each sample was heated from 20 to 70°C or 45 to 65°C, with a rate of three minutes per degree Celsius, using a Neslab RTE-7 Digital Plus (Thermo Scientific) circulating water bath.

Boltzmann sigmoid analysis

The baseline-subtracted and trimmed melt curves acquired by the fluorescence thermal stability assay, CD, and intrinsic fluorescence were processed using GraphPad Prism. The reported T_m is the inflection point of the sigmoidal curve, and is calculated using the Boltzmann sigmoid equation

$$Y = \frac{LL + (UL - LL)}{1 + \exp((T_m - X)/Slope)}$$

where UL and LL are the values of minimum and maximum intensities, respectively [51].

Limited proteolysis

Myoc-OLF was pre-screened at room temperature against a variety of proteases including trypsin, α-chymotrypsin, pepsin, papain, V_8 protease and subtilisin A to identify a protease and concentration capable of producing a discrete smaller construct detectable by SDS-PAGE. The optimal reaction condition consisted of a 1:200 dilution of subtilisin A (Sigma Aldrich, 1 mg/ml) in 0.2 mg/ml myoc-OLF in 10 mM Hepes pH 7.5 or 1:200 dilution of papain (Sigma, 1 mg/ml) in 0.2 mg/ml myoc-OLF in 10 mM MES pH 6.2. The reaction was incubated at room temperature for 30 minutes followed by subsequent quenching by either the addition of Complete Protease Inhibitor Cocktail (Roche) or SDS-PAGE sample loading buffer for SDS-PAGE analysis and in-gel digestion for mass spectrometry analysis. The core OLF product was fractionated from smaller digestion products on a Superdex 75 GL column (GE Healthcare) equilibrated with Buffer A. The core-OLF sample was further analyzed by CD as described above. Disulfide bond formation was confirmed with ThioGlo (EMD Biosciences) and the T_m measured as described [13].

In-gel digestion and MALDI-TOF/TOF MS analysis

In-gel digestion of myoc-OLF and core-OLF was carried out as described previously [52]. Digested and dried samples were subjected to peptide mass fingerprinting analysis using the Georgia Institute of Technology Bioanalytical Mass Spectrometry Facility. Spectra were acquired on an Applied Biosystems 4700 Proteomics Analyzer MALDI-TOF/TOF tandem mass spectrometer. Core-OLF was also analyzed by MS/MS. Peaks were analyzed by using MASCOT (GPS Explorer, Applied Biosystems). Only identified peptide fragments with a>3:1 signal-to-noise intensity were included in analysis. Samples were analyzed in duplicate. Due to the nonspecific nature of subtilisin cleavage, N-/C-terminal sequencing was not undertaken.

Supporting Information

Figure S1 Melt data fit to a two-state transition. Melt curves and fitting residuals are presented. (A) pH 4.6, (B) pH 5.8, (C) pH 7.2. See values in Table S2.

Table S1 Melting temperature of myoc-OLF and MBP-OLF in buffer.

Table S2 Thermodynamic data for myoc-OLF unfolding assuming a two-state transition.

Text S1 Supporting methods for two-state (Van't Hoff) thermodynamic analysis.

Acknowledgments

We gratefully acknowledge the Hud (GA Tech), Lyon (GA Tech), Lutz (Emory) laboratories, the Institute for Bioengineering and Biosciences core facility for access to instrumentation and D. Vollrath (Stanford) for helpful discussions. We are also grateful to Chad Bernier and Loren Williams (GA Tech) for use of their two-state folding fitting program and to Tanay Desai for assistance with SVD analysis.

Author Contributions

Conceived and designed the experiments: RLL. Performed the experiments: SDO. Analyzed the data: RLL SDO. Contributed reagents/materials/analysis tools: RLL SDO. Wrote the paper: SDO RLL.

References

1. Resch Z, Fautsch M (2009) Glaucoma-associated myocilin: A better understanding but much more to learn. Exp Eye Res 88: 704–712.
2. Ueda J, Wentz-Hunter K, Yue BY (2002) Distribution of myocilin and extracellular matrix components in the juxtacanalicular tissue of human eyes. Invest Ophthalmol Vis Sci 43: 1068–1076.
3. Tawara A, Okada Y, Kubota T, Suzuki Y, Taniguchi F, et al. (2000) Immunohistochemical localization of MYOC/TIGR protein in the trabecular tissue of normal and glaucomatous eyes. Curr Eye Res 21: 934–943.
4. Filla MS, Liu X, Nguyen TD, Polansky JR, Brandt CR, et al. (2002) In vitro localization of TIGR/MYOC in trabecular meshwork extracellular matrix and binding to fibronectin. Invest Ophthalmol Vis Sci 43: 151–161.
5. Wentz-Hunter K, Kubota R, Shen X, Yue B (2004) Extracellular myocilin affects activity of human trabecular meshwork cells. J Cell Physiol 200: 45–52.
6. Kwon YH, Fingert JH, Kuehn MH, Alward WL (2009) Primary open-angle glaucoma. N Engl J Med 360: 1113–1124.
7. Kim BS, Savinova OV, Reedy MV, Martin J, Lun Y, et al. (2001) Targeted disruption of the myocilin gene (myoc) suggests that human glaucoma-causing mutations are gain of function. Mol Cell Biol 21: 7707–7713.
8. Lam DS, Leung YF, Chua JK, Baum L, Fan DS, et al. (2000) Truncations in the TIGR gene in individuals with and without primary open-angle glaucoma. Invest Ophthalmol Vis Sci 41: 1386–1391.
9. Gobeil S, Letartre L, Raymond V (2006) Functional analysis of the glaucoma-causing TIGR/myocilin protein: integrity of amino-terminal coiled-coil regions

and olfactomedin homology domain is essential for extracellular adhesion and secretion. Exp Eye Res 82: 1017–1029.
10. Vollrath D, Liu Y (2006) Temperature sensitive secretion of mutant myocilins. Exp Eye Res 82: 1030–1036.
11. Yam GH-F, Zuber C, Roth J (2005) A synthetic chaperone corrects the trafficking defect and disease phenotype in a protein misfolding disorder. FASEB J 19: 12–18.
12. Jia L-Y, Gong B, Pang C-P, Huang Y, Lam DS-C, et al. (2009) Correction of the disease phenotype of myocilin-causing glaucoma by a natural osmolyte. Invest Ophthalmol Vis Sci 50: 3743–3749.
13. Burns JN, Orwig SD, Harris JL, Watkins JD, Vollrath D, et al. (2010) Rescue of glaucoma-causing mutant myocilin thermal stability by chemical chaperones. ACS Chem Biol 5: 477–487.
14. Fautsch MP, Vrabel AM, Johnson DH (2006) The identification of myocilin-associated proteins in the human trabecular meshwork. Exp Eye Res 82: 1046–1052.
15. Peters DM, Herbert K, Biddick B, Peterson JA (2005) Myocilin binding to Hep II domain of fibronectin inhibits cell spreading and incorporation of paxillin into focal adhesions. Exp Cell Res 303: 218–228.
16. Goldwich A, Scholz M, Tamm ER (2009) Myocilin promotes substrate adhesion, spreading and formation of focal contacts in podocytes and mesangial cells. Histochem Cell Biol 131: 167–180.
17. Mertts M, Garfield S, Tanemoto K, Tomarev SI (1999) Identification of the region in the N-terminal domain responsible for the cytoplasmic localization of Myoc/Tigr and its association with microtubules. Lab Invest 79: 1237–1245.
18. Sanchez-Sanchez F, Martinez-Redondo F, Aroca-Aguilar JD, Coca-Prados M, Escribano J (2007) Characterization of the intracellular proteolytic cleavage of myocilin and identification of calpain II as a myocilin-processing protease. J Biol Chem 282: 27810–27824.
19. Tamm ER (2002) Myocilin and glaucoma: facts and ideas. Prog Retin Eye Res 21: 395–428.
20. Tomarev SI, Nakaya N (2009) Olfactomedin domain-containing proteins: possible mechanisms of action and functions in normal development and pathology. Mol Neurobiol 40: 122–138.
21. Liton PB, Gonzalez P, Epstein DL (2009) The role of proteolytic cellular systems in trabecular meshwork homeostasis. Exp Eye Res 88: 724–728.
22. Ganesh C, Shah AN, Swaminathan CP, Surolia A, Varadarajan R (1997) Thermodynamic characterization of the reversible, two-state unfolding of maltose binding protein, a large two-domain protein. Biochemistry 36: 5020–5028.
23. Acott TS, Kelley MJ (2008) Extracellular matrix in the trabecular meshwork. Exp Eye Res 86: 543–561.
24. Knepper PA, Fadel JR, Miller AM, Goossens W, Choi J, et al. (2005) Reconstitution of trabecular meshwork GAGs: influence of hyaluronic acid and chondroitin sulfate on flow rates. J Glaucoma 14: 230–238.
25. Gasteiger E, Hoogland C, Gattiker A, Duvaud S, Wilkins MR, et al. (2005) Protein identification and analysis tools on the ExPASy Server. In: Walker JM, ed. The proteomics Protocol Handbook. Totowa, NJ: Humana Press. pp 571–607.
26. Nagy I, Trexler M, Patthy L (2003) Expression and characterization of the olfactomedin domain of human myocilin. Biochem Biophys Res Commun 302: 554–561.
27. Greenfield NJ (2004) Analysis of circular dichroism data. Methods Enzymol 383: 282–317.
28. Robertson AD, Murphy KP (1997) Protein structure and the energetics of protein stability. Chem Rev 97: 1251–1268.
29. Pace CN, Huyghues-Despointes BMP, Fu HL, Takano K, Scholtz JM, et al. (2010) Urea denatured state ensembles contain extensive secondary structure that is increased in hydrophobic proteins. Protein Sci 19: 929–943.
30. Xu D, Nussinov R (1998) Favorable domain size in proteins. Fold Des 3: 11–17.
31. Wu J, Yang JT, Wu CS (1992) Beta-II conformation of all-beta proteins can be distinguished from unordered form by circular dichroism. Anal Biochem 200: 359–364.
32. Knepper PA, Goossens W, Hvizd M, Palmberg PF (1996) Glycosaminoglycans of the human trabecular meshwork in primary open-angle glaucoma. Invest Ophthalmol Vis Sci 37: 1360–1367.
33. Kuleshova ON, Zaidman AM, Korel AV (2007) Glycosaminoglycans of the trabecular meshwork of the eye in primary juvenile glaucoma. Bull Exp Biol Med 143: 381–384.
34. Gould CM, Diella F, Via A, Puntervoll P, Gemund C, et al. (2010) ELM: the status of the 2010 eukaryotic linear motif resource. Nucleic Acids Res 38: D167–180.
35. Knepper PA, Miller AM, Choi J, Wertz RD, Nolan MJ, et al. (2005) Hypophosphorylation of aqueous humor sCD44 and primary open-angle glaucoma. Invest Ophthalmol Vis Sci 46: 2829–2837.
36. Furutani Y, Manabe R, Tsutsui K, Yamada T, Sugimoto N, et al. (2005) Identification and characterization of photomedins: novel olfactomedin-domain-containing proteins with chondroitin sulphate-E-binding activity. Biochem J 389: 675–684.
37. Hillier BJ, Vacquier VD (2007) Structural features and functional domains of amassin-1, a cell-binding olfactomedin protein. Biochem Cell Biol 85: 552–562.
38. Rajini B, Graham C, Wistow G, Sharma Y (2003) Stability, homodimerization, and calcium-binding properties of a single, variant betagamma-crystallin domain of the protein absent in melanoma 1 (AIM1). Biochemistry 42: 4552–4559.
39. Stone EM, Fingert JH, Alward WL, Nguyen TD, Polansky JR, et al. (1997) Identification of a gene that causes primary open angle glaucoma. Science 275: 668–670.
40. Johnson PM, Scopes PM, Tracey BM, Watkins J (1974) A comparison of the circular dichroism spectra of the subclasses of human immunoglobulin G. Immunology 27: 27–31.
41. Brahms S, Brahms J (1980) Determination of protein secondary structure in solution by vacuum ultraviolet circular dichroism. J Mol Biol 138: 149–178.
42. Fuchs PF, Alix AJ (2005) High accuracy prediction of beta-turns and their types using propensities and multiple alignments. Proteins 59: 828–839.
43. Morrisett JD, Broomfield CA (1971) Active site spin-labeled alpha-chymotrypsin. Guanidine hydrochloride denaturation studies using electron paramagnetic resonance and circular dichroism. J Am Chem Soc 93: 7297–7304.
44. Linding R, Russell RB, Neduva V, Gibson TJ (2003) GlobPlot: Exploring protein sequences for globularity and disorder. Nucleic Acids Res 31: 3701–3708.
45. Bloemendal H, de Jong W, Jaenicke R, Lubsen NH, Slingsby C, et al. (2004) Ageing and vision: structure, stability and function of lens crystallins. Prog Biophys Mol Biol 86: 407–485.
46. Evans P, Bateman OA, Slingsby C, Wallace BA (2007) A reference dataset for circular dichroism spectroscopy tailored for the betagamma-crystallin lens proteins. Exp Eye Res 84: 1001–1008.
47. Mandal K, Chakrabarti B, Thomson J, Siezen RJ (1987) Structure and stability of gamma-crystallins. Denaturation and proteolysis behavior. J Biol Chem 262: 8096–8102.
48. Chaudhuri TK, Paul S (2006) Protein-misfolding diseases and chaperone-based therapeutic approaches. FEBS J 273: 1331–1349.
49. Gong G, Kosoko-Lasaki O, Haynatzki GR, Wilson MR (2004) Genetic dissection of myocilin glaucoma. Hum Mol Genet 13 Spec No 1: R91–102.
50. Sambrook J, Russell DW (2001) Molecular cloning: a laboratory manual. Cold Spring Harbor, N.Y.: Cold Spring Harbor Laboratory Press. 3 v. p.
51. Niesen FH, Berglund H, Vedadi M (2007) The use of differential scanning fluorimetry to detect ligand interactions that promote protein stability. Nat Protoc 2: 2212–2221.
52. Shevchenko A, Wilm M, Vorm O, Mann M (1996) Mass spectrometric sequencing of proteins from silver stained polyacrylamide gels. Analytical Chemistry 68: 850–858.
53. Pei J, Grishin NV (2007) PROMALS: towards accurate multiple sequence alignments of distantly related proteins. Bioinformatics 23: 802–808.

7

Status of Systemic Oxidative Stresses in Patients with Primary Open-Angle Glaucoma and Pseudoexfoliation Syndrome

Masaki Tanito*, Sachiko Kaidzu, Yasuyuki Takai, Akihiro Ohira

Department of Ophthalmology, Shimane University Faculty of Medicine, Izumo, Shimane, Japan

Abstract

Background: The involvement of local and systemic oxidative stress in intraocular pressure (IOP) elevation and optic nerve damage has been hypothesized in the pathogenesis of glaucoma. To test this, we measured the systemic levels of prooxidants and antioxidants by analyzing the blood biochemistry in patients with glaucoma.

Methods: Peripheral blood samples were collected from Japanese patients with primary open-angle glaucoma (PG) (n = 206), exfoliation syndrome (EX) (n = 199), and controls (n = 126). Plasma levels of lipid peroxides, ferric-reducing activity, and thiol antioxidant activity were measured by diacron reactive oxygen metabolites (dROM), biological antioxidant potential (BAP), and sulfhydryl (SH) tests, respectively, using a free radical analyzer.

Results: In the PG, EX, and control groups, the mean ± standard deviation values were 355±63, 357±69, and 348±56 (U. Carr), respectively, for dROM; 1,951±282, 1,969±252, and 2,033±252 (μmol/L), respectively, for BAP (μmol/L); and 614±98, 584±91, and 617±99 (μmol/L), respectively, for SH. The differences in the BAP values were significant between the PG and control groups (p = 0.0062), for SH between the EX and control groups (p = 0.0017), and for SH between the PG and EX groups (p = 0.0026). After adjustment for differences in age and sex among groups using multiple regression analysis, lower BAP values were correlated significantly with PG (p = 0.0155) and EX (p = 0.0049). Higher dROM values with and without glaucoma were correlated with female gender, and lower SH values with older age. There were no significant differences between the higher (≥21 mmHg) and lower (<21 mmHg) baseline IOPs in the PG group or between the presence or absence of glaucoma in the EX group.

Conclusions: Lower systemic antioxidant capacity that measured by ferric-reducing activity is involved in the pathogenesis of PG and EX.

Editor: Karin Jandeleit-Dahm, Baker IDI Heart and Diabetes Institute, Australia

Funding: This study was supported by research grants from the Imai Memorial Glaucoma Research Foundation, the Suda Memorial Glaucoma Research Foundation, and a Grant-in-Aid for Scientific Research (C) from the Japan Society for the Promotion of Science (JSPS). The funders had no role in study design, data collection and analysis, decision to publish, or preparation of the manuscript.

Competing Interests: The authors have declared that no competing interests exist.

* E-mail: tanito-oph@umin.ac.jp

Introduction

Glaucoma, characterized by progressive "glaucomatous" optic neuropathy and corresponding visual field loss, is a leading cause of irreversible blindness worldwide [1,2], including in Japan [3]. Retinal ganglion cell (RGC) death due to apoptosis and loss of RGC axons leads to glaucomatous optic neuropathy, in which elevated intraocular pressure (IOP) is the main risk factor [2]. In open-angle glaucoma (OAG) including primary open-angle glaucoma (PG) and glaucoma secondary to pseudo-exfoliation syndrome (EX), the IOP increases because of reduced aqueous humor outflow at the trabecular meshwork (TM) [4]. The increased aqueous humor outflow resistance results from changes in the amount and quality of the extracellular matrix (ECM) in the TM [5]. In EX, an age-related, complex, generalized disorder of the ECM, the progressive accumulation of intraocular abnormal fibrillar materials in the TM is considered the primary cause of chronic IOP elevation [6,7]. Although the involvement of various genetic and internal and external stress factors, such as immune reactions [8,9], inflammation [10], ischemia [11], and hypoxia [12], have been proposed, the exact mechanisms of the ECM changes in the TM and progressive loss of RGC bodies and axons in OAG is still not well understood. Clinical and experimental studies have shown the possible involvement of oxidative stress in the pathogenesis of glaucoma, including increased aqueous outflow resistance with increased dysfunction of the TM cell viability [13–15] and glaucomatous neurodegeneration in the retina, optic nerve, and brain [16,17]. Thus, oxidative stress seems to explain the wide range of tissue and/or cellular damage in glaucoma.

Oxidative stress generally is induced through formation of multiple reactive oxygen species including superoxide, hydrogen peroxide, and hydroxyl radicals that can initiate and propagate free radicals. The net oxidative burden between prooxidant and antioxidant systems is the oxidative stress that damages cellular and tissue macromolecules such as lipids, proteins, and nucleic acids, and results in cellular and tissue dysfunction and cellular death. After identification of the circulating autoantibodies against antioxidative stress enzymes and chaperone molecules glutathione S-transferase [18] and heat shock proteins [19,20] in the serum of patients with glaucoma, the systemic status of redox (reduction/oxidation) in glaucoma has become a topic of interest. Until now, a number of studies have assessed this topic [21–29]. However, these studies may not be sufficiently comprehensive in that they included relatively small numbers of subjects (mostly only 20–40 subjects in each case and control groups), analyzed only one glaucoma type (either PG or EX) or unclassified mixed types of glaucoma in the case group, and/or analyzed either prooxidant or antioxidant status only.

Therefore, the aim of the current study was to examine the systemic redox status of glaucoma more comprehensively by including more patients with PG and EX in each group and by simultaneously testing the oxidative and antioxidative status.

Subjects and Methods

Subjects

A total of 531 Japanese subjects comprised the PG (n = 206), EX (n = 199), and non-glaucomatous control (n = 126) groups. These subjects were recruited consecutively at Shimane University Hospital and Iinan Hospital, Shimane, Japan. The current study adhered to the tenets of the Declaration of Helsinki. The institutional review boards of both hospitals reviewed and approved the research. All subjects provided written informed consent. All subjects underwent ophthalmologic examinations including measurements of the best-corrected visual acuity (VA) and IOP by Goldmann applanation tonometry and slit-lamp, gonioscopic, and funduscopic examinations under pupillary dilatation. PG was diagnosed based on the presence of an open iridocorneal angle bilaterally, the characteristic appearance of glaucomatous optic neuropathy such as enlargement of the optic disc cup or focal thinning of the neuroretinal rim, and corresponding visual field defects identified using the Humphrey Visual Field Analyzer (Carl Zeiss Meditec, Dublin, CA) in at least one eye, and no evidence of secondary glaucoma bilaterally. In the PG group, 117 subjects with the history of untreated IOP of 21 mmHg or higher in at least one eye were considered to have high-tension glaucoma (HTG), and the other 89 subjects who did not have a history of untreated IOP of 21 mmHg or higher were considered to have normal tension glaucoma (NTG). EX was diagnosed based on the presence of an open iridocorneal angle and characteristic pseudoexfoliation material deposits on the anterior capsule and/or pupillary margin in at least in one eye. In the EX group, 131 subjects with a history of IOP elevations of 21 mmHg or higher or the characteristic appearance of glaucomatous optic neuropathy in at least in one eye were considered to be exfoliation glaucoma (EXG), and the other 68 subjects who did not have a history of IOP elevations and glaucomatous optic neuropathy were considered to be exfoliation syndrome without glaucoma (EXS). The control subjects had a corrected visual acuity (VA) of 0.7 or better measured in both eyes using a decimal VA chart, and no glaucomatous optic neuropathy or history of IOP of 21 mmHg or higher. Except for a cataract and/or glaucoma, no subjects had ocular pathologies such as clinically detectable ocular inflammation, infection, neuropathies, retinopathies, or maculopathies.

Recording Clinical Parameters and Collecting Blood Samples

To avoid the possible confounding effect of systemic diseases [30–32], the subjects were questioned about a history of severe systemic diseases during an interview before entry into the study. These diseases included acute brain infarction and hemorrhage, systemic neurologic diseases, cardiac diseases requiring catheter placement or surgery, cardiac failure and other systemic diseases affecting the subjects' physical activity, lung diseases causing dyspnea, chronic and acute hepatitis requiring interferon therapy, liver cirrhosis, renal failure requiring hemodialysis, autoimmune diseases requiring systemic steroids and other immunosuppressive therapies, severe anemia requiring blood transfusions, major visceral surgery, malignancies, and severe hypertension causing cardiac and kidney failure, severe diabetes requiring insulin therapy. In addition to a history of severe systemic diseases, to adjust for the possible confounding effects of other factors such as differences in nutrition, blood pressure, blood glucose, and smoking habits [33–35], the presence or absence of diabetes, current smoking, the time since the last meal, and the systolic (SBP) and diastolic (DBP) blood pressures and pulse rate were recorded before the blood sample were collected. Venous blood specimens were collected from the antecubital vein into evacuated tubes. Plasma samples obtained by centrifugation of the collected venous blood were stored at 4°C until oxidative stress measurements. During all handling procedures, including transportation from the clinical setting to the laboratory and centrifugation, the temperature was maintained at 4°C.

Oxidative Stress Measurements

All blood analyses were performed using a free radical analyzer system (FREE Carpe Diem, Wimerll Company Ltd., Tokyo, Japan) that included a spectrophotometric device reader and a thermostatically regulated mini-centrifuge, and the measurement kits were optimized to the FREE Carpe Diem System, according to the manufacturer's instructions. Based on the recommendation from the manufacturer, all analyses were performed within 48 hours of venous blood collection to avoid falsely high or low results. To analyze the plasma levels of reactive oxygen metabolites, antioxidant capacity, and thiol-antioxidant capacity, diacron reactive oxygen metabolite (dROM), biological antioxidant potential (BAP), and sulfhydryl (SH) tests were performed, respectively.

The dROM test reflects the amount of organic hydroperoxides that is related to the free radicals from which they are formed. When the samples are dissolved in an acidic buffer, the hydroperoxides react with the transition metal (mainly iron) ions liberated from the proteins in the acidic medium and are converted to alkoxy and peroxy radicals. These newly formed radicals oxidize an additive aromatic amine (*N,N*-diethyl-*para*-phenylen-diamine) and cause formation of a relatively stable colored cation radical that is spectrophotometrically detectable at 505 nm [33,36]. The results are expressed in arbitrary units (U. Carr), one unit of which corresponds to 0.8 mg/L of hydrogen peroxide [33,36].

The BAP test provides an estimate of the global antioxidant capacity of blood plasma, measured as its reducing potential against ferric ions. When the sample is added to the colored solution obtained by mixing a ferric chloride solution with a thiocyanate derivative solution, decoloration results. The intensity of the decoloration is spectrophotometrically detectable at 505 nm and is proportional to the ability of plasma to reduce ferric ions [34,37]. The results are expressed in μmol/L of the reduced ferric ions.

Table 1. Demographic subject data.

	Control	PG			EX			p value
		Total	NTG	HTG	Total	EXS	EXG	
N	**126**	**206**	**89**	**117**	**199**	**68**	**131**	
Age (yrs)								
Mean ± SD	70.6±10.8	70.5±11.3	72.6±10.7	68.9±11.5	78.2±7.8	78.6±7.3	78.0±8.1	<0.0001[a]**
range	23-93	24-89	25-89	24-88	50-96	61-96	50-94	
p value, v.s. CT [c]		0.9677	0.1694	0.2534	<0.0001##	<0.0001##	<0.0001##	
p value, v.s. PG [c]		-	-	-	<0.0001##	-	-	
p value, v.s. NTG [c]		-	-	0.0196	-	-	-	
p value, v.s. EXS [c]		-	-	-	-	-	0.5852	
Sex								
Men, n (%)	40 (31.7)	95 (46.1)	36 (40.4)	59 (50.4)	96 (48.2)	19 (27.9)	77 (58.8)	0.0079[b]**
Women, n (%)	86 (68.3)	111 (53.9)	53 (59.6)	58 (49.6)	103 (51.8)	49 (72.1)	54 (41.2)	
p value, v.s. CT [d]		0.0113#	0.1960	0.0040#	0.0039#	0.6265	<0.0001##	
p value, v.s. PG [d]		-	-	-	0.6912	-	-	
p value, v.s. NTG [d]		-	-	0.1616	-	-	-	
p value, v.s. EXS [d]		-	-	-	-	-	<0.0001##	
SBP (mmHg)								
Mean ± SD	136.2±19.4	139.8±20.0	139.7±19.4	139.9±20.5	141.1±21.1	139.2±21.1	142.1±21.1	0.0964[a]
range	94-223	89-211	90-182	89-211	85-203	85-203	85-191	
p value, v.s. CT [c]		0.1146	0.1951	0.1462	0.0326	0.3156	0.0197	
p value, v.s. PG [c]		-	-	-	0.5124	-	-	
p value, v.s. NTG [c]		-	-	0.9829	-	-	-	
p value, v.s. EXS [c]		-	-	-	-	-	0.3563	
DBP (mmHg)								
Mean ± SD	74.6±12.0	76.8±12.9	74.2±11.3	78.7±13.7	76.1±13.2	73.2±10.7	77.7±14.2	0.3223[a]
range	45-119	47-133	47-100	51-133	46-123	51-100	46-123	
p value, v.s. CT [c]		0.1349	0.8182	0.0132#	0.2929	0.4167	0.0626	
p value, v.s. PG [c]		-	-	-	0.6189	-	-	
p value, v.s. NTG [c]		-	-	0.0133#	-	-	-	
p value, v.s. EXS [c]		-	-	-	-	-	0.0237	
Pulse rate (/min.)								
Mean ± SD	73.3±12.0	75.3±14.6	73.3±14.2	76.8±14.7	75.5±12.6	73.4±12.2	76.6±12.7	0.2914[a]
range	46-109	42-131	51-114	42-131	48-120	48-120	53-112	
p value, v.s. CT [c]		0.1817	0.9842	0.0425	0.1407	0.9581	0.0315	
p value, v.s. PG [c]		-	-	-	0.8663	-	-	
p value, v.s. NTG [c]		-	-	0.0906	-	-	-	
p value, v.s. EXS [c]		-	-	-	-	-	0.0847	
Duration from last meal (h)								
Mean ± SD	4.0±2.9	3.8±2.0	3.7±1.3	3.9±2.4	3.8±2.0	3.5±1.3	3.9±1.6	0.6024[a]
range	1-18	1-19	1.5-8	1-19	0.5-14	1.5-7.5	0.5-14	
p value, v.s. CT [c]		0.3873	0.3084	0.7525	0.3479	0.1879	0.7586	
p value, v.s. PG [c]		-	-	-	0.9271	-	-	
p value, v.s. NTG [c]		-	-	0.4279	-	-	-	
p value, v.s. EXS [c]		-	-	-	-	-	0.0826	
Diabetes								
Yes, n (%)	18 (14.3)	47 (22.8)	15 (16.9)	32 (27.3)	35 (17.6)	13 (19.1)	22 (16.8)	0.1310[b]
No, n (%)	108 (85.7)	159 (77.2)	74 (83.1)	85 (72.7)	164 (82.4)	55 (80.9)	109 (83.2)	
p value, v.s. CT [d]		0.0644	0.7015	0.0167	0.5379	0.4147	0.6093	
p value, v.s. PG [d]		-	-	-	0.2167	-	-	

Table 1. Cont.

	Control	PG			EX			p value
		Total	NTG	HTG	Total	EXS	EXG	
N	126	206	89	117	199	68	131	
p value, v.s. NTG [d]		-	-	0.0938	-	-	-	
p value, v.s. EXS [d]		-	-	-	-	-	0.6978	
Current smoking habit								
Yes, n (%)	12 (9.5)	25 (12.2)	7 (7.9)	18 (15.5)	11 (5.5)	2 (2.9)	9 (6.9)	0.0573[b]
No, n (%)	114 (90.5)	180 (87.8)	82 (92.1)	98 (84.5)	188 (94.5)	66 (97.1)	122 (93.1)	
p value, v.s. CT [d]		0.4795	0.8089	0.1756	0.1876	0.1440	0.4990	
p value, v.s. PG [d]		-	-	-	0.0226	-	-	
p value, v.s. NTG [d]		-	-	0.1313	-	-	-	
p value, v.s. EXS [d]		-	-	-	-	-	0.3377	

The SH test provides an estimate of the total thiol groups in the biologic samples, using a modified Ellman method [38,39]. When the sample is added to the solution, sulfhydryl groups in the sample react with 5,5-dithiobus-2-nitrobenzoic acid, which is followed by development of a stained complex that is spectrophotometrically detectable at 405 nm and is proportional to their concentration according to the Beer-Lambert law [34,36]. The results are expressed as μmol/L of the sulfhydryl groups.

Statistical Analysis

Data are expressed as the mean ± standard deviation and analyzed using StatView version 5.01 statistical software (SAS Institute, Inc., Cary, NC). For comparisons between the control, PG, and EX groups, the differences in continuous data (age, SBP, DBP, pulse rate, time from the last meal, dROM, BAP, and SH tests) were calculated using one-way analysis of variance followed by post-hoc un-paired t tests, and the differences in categorical data (sex, diabetes, and current smoking) were calculated using the G-test followed by the post-hoc Fisher's exact probability test. To correct for multi-group comparisons, p values of 0.0167 and 0.0033 for the unpaired or Fisher's exact probability test were considered significant with significance levels of 5% and 1%, respectively, based on the Bonferroni's method. The same statistical tests were used for the comparisons among the control, NTG, and HTG groups or among the control, EXS, and EXG groups. To adjust for differences in age and sex distributions among the groups, the values of the dROM, BAP, and SH tests were compared between the PG and control groups or the EX and control groups using multiple regression analysis; p values of 0.0167 and 0.0033 were considered significant with significance levels of 5% and 1%, respectively.

Results

The demographic patient data, including age, sex, SBP, DBP, pulse rate, time from the last meal, diabetes, and smoking status, are summarized in Table 1. The comparisons among the control, PG, and EX groups showed that the patients in the EX group were significantly older (78.2 years) than those in the control (70.6 years, $p<0.0001$) and the PG (70.5 years, $p<0.0001$) groups, and there were significantly fewer women in the PG (53.9%, $p = 0.0113$) and EX (51.8%, $p = 0.0039$) groups than in the control group (68.3%). Other parameters did not differ significantly among the three groups. The subgroup analyses among the controls (68.3%), NTG, and HTG groups showed that significantly fewer women had HTG (49.6%, $p = 0.0040$) compared with the control group, and the DBP was significantly higher in the HTG (78.7 mmHg) group than in the control (74.6 mmHg, $p = 0.0132$) and the NTG (74.2 mmHg, $p = 0.0133$) groups. The subgroup analyses among the control, EXS, and EXG groups showed that significantly fewer women had EXG (41.2%) compared with the control (68.3%, $p<0.0001$) and EXS (72.1%, $p<0.0001$) groups.

The measured levels of oxidative and antioxidative parameters in plasma of subjects are shown in Table 2. The dROM levels, a measure of oxidative status, did not differ significantly in any comparisons. The BAP levels, a measure of antioxidative status, were significantly lower in the PG group (1,951 μmol/L, $p = 0.0062$) than the control group (2,033 μmol/L); although the BAP level was lower in the EX (1,969 μmol/L) group than the control group but did not reach significance ($p = 0.0360$). The subgroup analyses showed that compared to the control group, The BAP level was significantly lower in the HTG group (1,917 μmol/L, $p = 0.0005$). The SH level, a measure of thiol-mediated antioxidative status, was significantly lower in the EX group (584 μmol/L) than in the control (617 μmol/L, $p = 0.0026$) and PG (614 μmol/L, $p = 0.0017$) groups. The subgroup analyses also showed that compared to the control group the SH levels were lower in the EXS (585 μmol/L, $p = 0.0227$) and EXG (584 μmol/L, $p = 0.0066$) groups, but the difference did not reach significance between the two ($p = 0.9615$).

Since the age and sex differed among the control, PG, and EX groups (Table 1), multiple regression analyses were performed to adjust for any possible confounding effects of these two parameters on the measured oxidative and antioxidative status (Table 3). Comparisons between the control and PG groups (Table 3) showed that glaucoma was associated significantly with lower BAP levels ($p = 0.0155$), while glaucoma was unrelated to the results of the dROM ($p = 0.1549$) and SH ($p = 0.8187$) tests. We also found a significant correlation between female gender and higher dROM levels ($p = 0.0056$) and between older age and lower SH levels ($p<0.0001$). Comparisons between the control and EX groups (Table 3) showed that EX was related significantly to lower BAP levels ($p = 0.0049$), while glaucoma was not related to the results of the dROM ($p = 0.1938$) and SH ($p = 0.9488$) tests. We also found a significant correlation between female gender and higher dROM

Table 2. The dROM, BAP, and SH values.

	Control	PG			EX			*p-value*
		Total	NTG	HTG	Total	EXS	EXG	
n	126	206	89	117	199	68	131	
dROMs test (U. CARR)								
Mean ± SD	347.9±56.0	354.9±62.7	350.7±66.1	358.2±60.1	357.2±69.0	353.3±64.2	359.2±71.5	*0.4280[a]*
range	219–511	204–555	204–555	219–522	102–551	201–501	102–551	
p-value, v.s. CT[b]		*0.3307*	*0.7425*	*0.1698*	*0.2001*	*0.5428*	*0.1600*	
p-value, v.s. PG[b]		-	-	-	*0.7177*	-	-	
p-value, v.s. NTG[b]		-	-	*0.3964*	-	-	-	
p-value, v.s. EXS[b]		-	-	-	-	-	*0.5681*	
BAP test (μmol/L)								
Mean ± SD	2032.6±251.5	1950.5±282.2	1994.6±301.3	1916.9±263.2	1969.4±252.3	1978.2±301.6	1964.8±223.6	*0.0206[a]**
range	1218–2813	990–2857	1242–2857	990–2723	413–2560	413–2492	1355–2560	
p-value, v.s. CT[b]		*0.0062#*	*0.3162*	*0.0005##*	*0.0360*	*0.1820*	*0.0231*	
p-value, v.s. PG[b]		-	-	-	*0.4717*	-	-	
p-value, v.s. NTG[b]		-	-	*0.0501*	-	-	-	
p-value, v.s. EXS[b]		-	-	-	-	-	*0.7245*	
SH test (μmol/L)								
Mean ± SD	617.0±99.2	614.2±97.9	611.9±97.9	615.9±98.3	584.1±90.7	584.6±83.1	583.9±94.7	*0.0014[a]***
range	320–830	328–884	331–884	328–847	257–833	395–760	257–833	
p-value, v.s. CT[b]		*0.7915*	*0.7068*	*0.9298*	*0.0026##*	*0.0227*	*0.0066#*	
p-value, v.s. PG[b]		-	-	-	*0.0017##*	-	-	
p-value, v.s. NTG[b]		-	-	*0.7706*	-	-	-	
p-value, v.s. EXS[b]		-	-	-	-	-	*0.9615*	

levels ($p = 0.0007$) and between older age and lower SH levels ($p<0.0001$).

Discussion

Several studies have assessed the systemic status of redox in patients with glaucoma [21–29]. Engin et al. analyzed 160 patients with glaucoma and 31 control subjects in the largest study; however, the study included mixed types of glaucoma in a case group [26]. The various types of glaucoma, i.e., open-angle and angle-closure glaucomas or primary and secondary glaucomas, have different etiologies; thus, separate analyses of each glaucoma type seemed more appropriate. Except for the study by Engin et al. [26], the other studies included up to 40 subjects in the glaucoma groups. The current study of 531 subjects is the largest assessment of the systemic redox status in OAG.

We found that the BAP level, a measure of total antioxidative stress activity, was lower in plasma in the PG and EX groups compared with the control groups after adjustment for age and sex (Table 3). Several studies have reported lower systemic levels of antioxidants or antioxidative stress capacity in glaucoma, that is, a reduced form of the glutathione level was lower in the red blood cells of patients with PG [22], Erel's total antioxidant capacity [40] was lower in the serum of patients with OAG [28,29] or EX [24,29], the vitamin E level was lower in the serum of patients with glaucoma [26], and the level of the reduced form of glutathione and the enzymatic activities of catalase, superoxide dismutase, and glutathione peroxidase were lower in the red blood cells of patients with PG [22,27]. Sorkhabi et al. reported a correlation between a higher aqueous humor 8-hydroxy-2′-deoxyguanosine (8-OHdG) level, an established marker for oxidative stress-induced DNA damage, and a higher 8-OHdG level and lower antioxidant capacity levels in the serum of patients with glaucoma [28]. Thus, the systemic antioxidant capacity could reflect the local ocular redox status. In experimental studies, free-radical scavengers effectively prevented glaucomatous tissue injury such as glutamate- and IOP-induced RGC death [41,42] and tumor necrosis factor α-induced axonal injury [43]. Collectively, decreased levels of

Table 3. Multiple regression analyses for dROM, BAP, and SH values.

	PG vs Control (n = 332)			EX vs Control (n = 325)		
	dROM test (U. CARR)	BAP test (μmol/L)	SH test (μmol/L)	dROM test (U. CARR)	BAP test (μmol/L)	SH test (μmol/L)
R^2	0.026	0.038	0.134	0.044	0.033	0.177
P-value for fitting	0.0317	0.0050	<0.0001	0.0023	0.0131	<0.0001
Age (per yr)						
Slope	−0.02	2.1	−3.3	0.4	3.6	−4.1
p-value	0.9564	0.1135	<0.0001**	0.2992	0.0184	<0.0001**
Sex (men = 0, women = 1)						
Slope	18.9	49.2	4.1	24.6	13.7	7.3
p-value	0.0056*	0.1089	0.6954	0.0007**	0.6331	0.4611
Glaucoma (Control = 0, PG or EX = 1)						
Slope	9.7	−75.0	−2.4	10.3	−88.7	−0.7
p-value	0.1549	0.0155*	0.8178	0.1938	0.0049*	0.9488

systemic antioxidant capacity might be involved in glaucomatous TM and neuronal damage as a result of local inadequate defense against oxidative stress. Since the decrease in BAP was more marked in HTG and EXG than in NTG and EXS, reduced antioxidant capacity is related more closely to the IOP elevation than neuronal damage. Engin et al. [26] has suggested the possible association between lower systemic antioxidants levels and clinical parameters of glaucoma, thus the analyses regarding the correlations between BAP values and severity indices of glaucoma such as visual field, optic disc morphology, and IOP level using the data obtained in this study would be interest, and should be tested in the near future.

We found no significant difference in the levels of dROM between the control and any glaucoma groups. Several previous studies have reported higher systemic levels of oxidation in glaucoma; the lipid peroxidation byproduct malondialdehyde level is higher in plasma from patients with PG [21,29], and Erel's total oxidant status measured by the oxidizing activity of the ferrous ion/*o*-dianisidine complex to ferrous ion [44] is higher in the serum from patients with glaucoma [26], PG [29] or EX [24,29]. In the current study, we included eyes with mild cataract with a VA of 0.7 or better in the control group, while most previous studies have included subjects without cataracts as controls. The presence of a cataract might be related to increased systemic oxidation [45,46]; thus, the difference in the control groups between the current and previous studies might explain the discrepancy. In addition, the relatively small difference (around 5%) in BAP between the glaucoma and control groups in the current study might have increased if we had included only non-cataractous control eyes. Current study included both newly and previously diagnosed glaucoma patients. One may imagine that the patients who previously diagnosed had already changed their lifestyle to reduce the oxidative stress or increase the anti-oxidative defense. Therefore, in the same context, the difference in BAP between the glaucoma and control groups in the current study might have increased if we had included only newly diagnosed glaucoma eyes. Alternatively, if the absence of a difference in the systemic dROM levels between the glaucoma and control groups is real, glaucomatous tissue damage might result from a local increase in oxidative stress due to local compensation for systemic oxidative stress by systemic reduction of antioxidant capacity in each individual.

The results suggested that with or without glaucoma the dROM level was higher in women than in men, and the SH level, a measure of the total amount of thiol, was correlated negatively with age (Table 3). The results corroborated previous observations regarding a gender difference in systemic oxidative stress [47,48]. Thus, the evidence supports the suitability of the measurement protocol and statistical analyses in the current study. The glutathione and thioredoxin systems are thought to be major thiol-mediated redox systems in humans, although the plasma glutathione level is 100 to 1,000 times higher than that of thioredoxin [49,50]. Gherghel et al. reported a negative correlation between age and total glutathione levels in red blood cells with no significant difference in the total glutathione level between the patients with glaucoma and controls [22]. Thus, the SH level in the current study might correspond mainly to the total glutathione level, but that remains to be clarified. Previous studies have reported the possible involvement of thioredoxin system dysregulation in the pathogenesis of glaucoma [41,42,51–53]; thus, measurement of the thioredoxin level separately from the other thiol groups should be done in the future.

Based on the personally provided information from the manufacturer, that keeping the blood samples at 4°C enables us to obtain a stable acquisition of data for up to 48 hours, we decided to perform measurements within 48 hours from the blood collection. It is generally recognized as that pro- and anti-oxidants are sometimes unstable, thus relatively long duration between the blood collection and the measurements might affect the results. Instead of fasting before the blood collection, we decided to record the duration after the last meal in this study. Although the duration was not different among the study groups, this factor might affect the results also. Use of antioxidants and other supplements were not defined as the inclusion/exclusion criteria of this study, thus this is another weak point of this study.

Based on the results of this comprehensive large-scale study, we concluded that patients with glaucoma have low levels of serum antioxidative capacity, suggesting a general compromise of the antioxidant defense.

Acknowledgments

The authors are grateful to Ms. Ryoko Takahashi for her technical help with the dROM, BAP, and SH measurements.

Author Contributions

Conceived and designed the experiments: MT SK YT AO. Performed the experiments: SK. Analyzed the data: MT. Contributed reagents/materials/analysis tools: MT YT. Wrote the paper: MT SK YT AO.

References

1. Foster A, Resnikoff S (2005) The impact of Vision 2020 on global blindness. Eye (Lond) 19: 1133–1135.
2. Weinreb RN, Khaw PT (2004) Primary open-angle glaucoma. Lancet 363: 1711–1720.
3. Iwase A, Araie M, Tomidokoro A, Yamamoto T, Shimizu H, et al. (2006) Prevalence and causes of low vision and blindness in a Japanese adult population: the Tajimi Study. Ophthalmology 113: 1354–1362.
4. Alvarado JA, Murphy CG (1992) Outflow obstruction in pigmentary and primary open angle glaucoma. Arch Ophthalmol 110: 1769–1778.
5. Lutjen-Drecoll E, Shimizu T, Rohrbach M, Rohen JW (1986) Quantitative analysis of 'plaque material' in the inner- and outer wall of Schlemm's canal in normal- and glaucomatous eyes. Exp Eye Res 42: 443–455.
6. Ritch R, Schlotzer-Schrehardt U (2001) Exfoliation syndrome. Surv Ophthalmol 45: 265–315.
7. Schlotzer-Schrehardt U, Naumann GO (2006) Ocular and systemic pseudoexfoliation syndrome. Am J Ophthalmol 141: 921–937.
8. Tezel G (2011) The immune response in glaucoma: a perspective on the roles of oxidative stress. Exp Eye Res 93: 178–186.
9. Takai Y, Tanito M, Ohira A (2012) Multiplex cytokine analysis of aqueous humor in eyes with primary open-angle glaucoma, exfoliation glaucoma, and cataract. Invest Ophthalmol Vis Sci 53: 241–247.
10. Li G, Luna C, Liton PB, Navarro I, Epstein DL, et al. (2007) Sustained stress response after oxidative stress in trabecular meshwork cells. Mol Vis 13: 2282–2288.
11. Nakabayashi M (2004) Review of the ischemia hypothesis for ocular hypertension other than congenital glaucoma and closed-angle glaucoma. Ophthalmologica 218: 344–349.
12. Helbig H, Schlotzer-Schrehardt U, Noske W, Kellner U, Foerster MH, et al. (1994) Anterior-chamber hypoxia and iris vasculopathy in pseudoexfoliation syndrome. Ger J Ophthalmol 3: 148–153.
13. Izzotti A, Bagnis A, Sacca SC (2006) The role of oxidative stress in glaucoma. Mutat Res 612: 105–114.
14. Sacca SC, Izzotti A, Rossi P, Traverso C (2007) Glaucomatous outflow pathway and oxidative stress. Exp Eye Res 84: 389–399.
15. Luna C, Li G, Liton PB, Qiu J, Epstein DL, et al. (2009) Resveratrol prevents the expression of glaucoma markers induced by chronic oxidative stress in trabecular meshwork cells. Food Chem Toxicol 47: 198–204.
16. Kumar DM, Agarwal N (2007) Oxidative stress in glaucoma: a burden of evidence. J Glaucoma 16: 334–343.
17. Tezel G (2006) Oxidative stress in glaucomatous neurodegeneration: mechanisms and consequences. Prog Retin Eye Res 25: 490–513.
18. Yang J, Tezel G, Patil RV, Romano C, Wax MB (2001) Serum autoantibody against glutathione S-transferase in patients with glaucoma. Invest Ophthalmol Vis Sci 42: 1273–1276.
19. Wax MB, Tezel G, Saito I, Gupta RS, Harley JB, et al. (1998) Anti-Ro/SS-A positivity and heat shock protein antibodies in patients with normal-pressure glaucoma. Am J Ophthalmol 125: 145–157.
20. Tezel G, Seigel GM, Wax MB (1998) Autoantibodies to small heat shock proteins in glaucoma. Invest Ophthalmol Vis Sci 39: 2277–2287.
21. Yildirim O, Ates NA, Ercan B, Muslu N, Unlu A, et al. (2005) Role of oxidative stress enzymes in open-angle glaucoma. Eye (Lond) 19: 580–583.
22. Gherghel D, Griffiths HR, Hilton EJ, Cunliffe IA, Hosking SL (2005) Systemic reduction in glutathione levels occurs in patients with primary open-angle glaucoma. Invest Ophthalmol Vis Sci 46: 877–883.
23. Yagci R, Ersoz I, Erdurmus M, Gurel A, Duman S (2008) Protein carbonyl levels in the aqueous humour and serum of patients with pseudoexfoliation syndrome. Eye (Lond) 22: 128–131.
24. Cumurcu T, Gunduz A, Ozyurt H, Nurcin H, Atis O, et al. (2010) Increased oxidative stress in patients with pseudoexfoliation syndrome. Ophthalmic Res 43: 169–172.
25. Yuki K, Murat D, Kimura I, Tsubota K (2010) Increased serum total antioxidant status and decreased urinary 8-hydroxy-2′-deoxyguanosine levels in patients with normal-tension glaucoma. Acta Ophthalmol 88: e259–264.
26. Engin KN, Yemisci B, Yigit U, Agachan A, Coskun C (2010) Variability of serum oxidative stress biomarkers relative to biochemical data and clinical parameters of glaucoma patients. Mol Vis 16: 1260–1271.
27. Majsterek I, Malinowska K, Stanczyk M, Kowalski M, Blaszczyk J, et al. (2011) Evaluation of oxidative stress markers in pathogenesis of primary open-angle glaucoma. Exp Mol Pathol 90: 231–237.
28. Sorkhabi R, Ghorbanihaghjo A, Javadzadeh A, Rashtchizadeh N, Moharrery M (2011) Oxidative DNA damage and total antioxidant status in glaucoma patients. Mol Vis 17: 41–46.
29. Erdurmus M, Yagci R, Atis O, Karadag R, Akbas A, et al. (2011) Antioxidant status and oxidative stress in primary open angle glaucoma and pseudoexfoliative glaucoma. Curr Eye Res 36: 713–718.
30. Vassalle C, Pratali L, Boni C, Mercuri A, Ndreu R (2008) An oxidative stress score as a combined measure of the pro-oxidant and anti-oxidant counterparts in patients with coronary artery disease. Clin Biochem 41: 1162–1167.
31. Nakayama K, Terawaki H, Nakayama M, Iwabuchi M, Sato T, et al. (2007) Reduction of serum antioxidative capacity during hemodialysis. Clin Exp Nephrol 11: 218–224.
32. Shimano M, Shibata R, Inden Y, Yoshida N, Uchikawa T, et al. (2009) Reactive oxidative metabolites are associated with atrial conduction disturbance in patients with atrial fibrillation. Heart Rhythm 6: 935–940.
33. Cornelli U, Terranova R, Luca S, Cornelli M, Alberti A (2001) Bioavailability and antioxidant activity of some food supplements in men and women using the D-Roms test as a marker of oxidative stress. J Nutr 131: 3208–3211.
34. Martinovic J, Dopsaj V, Dopsaj MJ, Kotur-Stevuljevic J, Vujovic A, et al. (2009) Long-term effects of oxidative stress in volleyball players. Int J Sports Med 30: 851–856.
35. Kotani K, Koibuchi H, Miyamoto M, Yamada T, Taniguchi N (2010) Relationship between reactive oxygen metabolites and carotid intima-media thickness in subjects with hypercholesterolemia. Med Princ Pract 19: 496–498.
36. Carratelli M, Porcaro L, Ruscica M, De Simone E, Bertelli AA, et al. (2001) Reactive oxygen metabolites and prooxidant status in children with Down's syndrome. Int J Clin Pharmacol Res 21: 79–84.
37. Pasquini A, Luchetti E, Marchetti V, Cardini G, Iorio EL (2008) Analytical performances of d-ROMs test and BAP test in canine plasma. Definition of the normal range in healthy Labrador dogs. Vet Res Commun 32: 137–143.
38. Ellman GL (1959) Tissue sulfhydryl groups. Arch Biochem Biophys 82: 70–77.
39. Sedlak J, Lindsay RH (1968) Estimation of total, protein-bound, and nonprotein sulfhydryl groups in tissue with Ellman's reagent. Anal Biochem 25: 192–205.
40. Erel O (2004) A novel automated direct measurement method for total antioxidant capacity using a new generation, more stable ABTS radical cation. Clin Biochem 37: 277–285.
41. Inomata Y, Nakamura H, Tanito M, Teratani A, Kawaji T, et al. (2006) Thioredoxin inhibits NMDA-induced neurotoxicity in the rat retina. J Neurochem 98: 372–385.
42. Munemasa Y, Ahn JH, Kwong JM, Caprioli J, Piri N (2009) Redox proteins thioredoxin 1 and thioredoxin 2 support retinal ganglion cell survival in experimental glaucoma. Gene Ther 16: 17–25.
43. Kitaoka Y, Munemasa Y, Hayashi Y, Kuribayashi J, Koseki N, et al. (2011) Axonal protection by 17beta-estradiol through thioredoxin-1 in tumor necrosis factor-induced optic neuropathy. Endocrinology 152: 2775–2785.
44. Erel O (2005) A new automated colorimetric method for measuring total oxidant status. Clin Biochem 38: 1103–1111.
45. Li L, Duker JS, Yoshida Y, Niki E, Rasmussen H, et al. (2009) Oxidative stress and antioxidant status in older adults with early cataract. Eye (Lond) 23: 1464–1468.
46. Virgolici B, Stoian I, Muscurel C, Maracine M, Moraru C, et al. (2007) Plasma redox status and premature onset of senile cataract. Rom J Intern Med 45: 59–65.
47. Marra G, Cotroneo P, Pitocco D, Manto A, Di Leo MA, et al. (2002) Early increase of oxidative stress and reduced antioxidant defenses in patients with uncomplicated type 1 diabetes: a case for gender difference. Diabetes Care 25: 370–375.
48. Vassalle C, Novembrino C, Maffei S, Sciarrino R, De Giuseppe R, et al. (2011) Determinants of oxidative stress related to gender: relevance of age and smoking habit. Clin Chem Lab Med 49: 1509–1513.
49. Nakamura H, De Rosa SC, Yodoi J, Holmgren A, Ghezzi P, et al. (2001) Chronic elevation of plasma thioredoxin: inhibition of chemotaxis and curtailment of life expectancy in AIDS. Proc Natl Acad Sci U S A 98: 2688–2693.
50. Michelet F, Gueguen R, Leroy P, Wellman M, Nicolas A, et al. (1995) Blood and plasma glutathione measured in healthy subjects by HPLC: relation to sex, aging, biological variables, and life habits. Clin Chem 41: 1509–1517.
51. Lamoke F, Ripandelli G, Webster S, Montemari A, Maraschi A, et al. (2012) Loss of thioredoxin function in retinas of mice overexpressing amyloid beta. Free Radic Biol Med.
52. Fatma N, Kubo E, Toris CB, Stamer WD, Camras CB, et al. (2009) PRDX6 attenuates oxidative stress- and TGFbeta-induced abnormalities of human trabecular meshwork cells. Free Radic Res 43: 783–795.
53. Miyamoto N, Izumi H, Miyamoto R, Kondo H, Tawara A, et al. (2011) Quercetin induces the expression of peroxiredoxins 3 and 5 via the Nrf2/NRF1 transcription pathway. Invest Ophthalmol Vis Sci 52: 1055–1063.

8

Association of OPA1 Polymorphisms with NTG and HTG

Yatu Guo[1,2,4], Xia Chen[2], Hongtuan Zhang[3], Ningdong Li[2], Xiong Yang[3], Wenbo Cheng[1,5], Kanxing Zhao[2]*

1 Tianjin Medical University, Tianjin, China, 2 Tianjin Eye Hospital, Tianjin Eye Institute, Tianjin Key Lab of Ophthalmology and Visual Science, Tianjin, China, 3 Second Hospital of Tianjin Medical University, Tianjin, China, 4 Krieger Mind/Brain Institute, Johns Hopkins University, Baltimore, Maryland, United States of America, 5 Department of Ophthalmology, the People's Hospital of Changzhi, Shanxi, China

Abstract

Background: Genetic polymorphisms of the Optic atrophy 1 gene have been implicated in altering the risk of primary open angle glaucoma (POAG), especially the susceptibility to normal tension glaucoma (NTG), but the results remain controversial.

Methods: Multiple electronic databases (up to January 20, 2012) were searched independently by two investigators. A meta-analysis was performed on the association between Optic atrophy 1 polymorphisms (rs 166850 and rs 10451941) and normal tension glaucoma (NTG)/high tension glaucoma (HTG). Summary odds ratios (ORs) and 95% confidence intervals (CI) were estimated.

Results: Seven studies of 713 cases and 964 controls for NTG and five studies of 1200 cases and 971 controls for HTG on IVS8+4C>T (rs 166850) and IVS8+32T>C (rs10451941) were identified. There were significant associations between the OPA1 rs10451941polymorphism and NTG susceptibility for all genetic models(C vs. T OR = 1.26, 95% CI 1.09–1.47, **p = 0.002**; CC vs. TT: OR = 1.52, 95% CI 1.04–2.20, **p = 0.029**; CC vs. CT+TT: OR = 1.64, 95% CI 1.16–2.33, **p = 0.005**; CC+CT vs. TT: OR = 1.21, 95% CI 1.02–1.44, **p = 0.032**). However, no evidence of associations was detected between the OPA1 IVS8+32C>T polymorphism and POAG susceptibility to HTG. Similarly, clear associations between the rs 166850 variant and NTG were observed in allelic and dominant models (T vs. C OR = 1.52, 95% CI 1.16–1.99, **p = 0.002**; TT+TC vs. CC OR = 1.50, 95% CI 1.13–2.01, **p = 0.006**) but not to HTG. In subgroup analyses by ethnicity, we detected an association between both OPA1 polymorphisms and risk for NTG in Caucasians but not in Asians. By contrast, no significant findings were noted between OPA1 variants for HTG, either in Caucasians or in Asians.

Conclusions: Both the IVS8+4C>T and IVS8+32T>C variants may affect individual susceptibility to NTG. Moreover, stratified analyses for NTG detecting the effects of both OPA1 polymorphisms seemed to vary with ethnicity. Further investigations are needed to validate the association.

Editor: Yuk Fai Leung, Purdue University, United States of America

Funding: This work was supported by major And key Programs of the Chinese National Natural Science Foundation (30730099) [http://www.nsfc.gov.cn/Portal0/default152.htm], 'Project 211' -The Innovation Fund For Graduate Students of Tianjin Medical University [http://gs.tmu.cn/xyxw/2010/100128.htm]. The funders had no role in study design, data collection and analysis, decision to publish, or preparation of the manuscript.

Competing Interests: The authors have declared that no competing interests exist.

* E-mail: zhaokanxing@yahoo.com.cn

These authors contributed equally to this work.

Introduction

Glaucoma, the leading cause of irreversible blindness worldwide [1], is characterized by visual field defects, retinal ganglion cell death, and progressive degeneration of the optic nerve [1,2,3,4]. Approximately half of all cases are of the angle closure type, which is prevalent among Asian populations [5,6,7,8]. The remaining cases consist of primary open angle glaucoma (POAG) [9] and affect 70 million individuals worldwide [10,11,12]. POAG is clinically classified into high tension glaucoma (HTG), in which elevated intraocular pressure (IOP) is a major feature, and normal tension glaucoma (NTG), in which IOPs are consistently within the statistically normal population range [13,14,15], accounting for approximately a third of all POAG cases [13]. POAG is considered to be a multi-factorial disorder with a significant heritable component [16,17,18,19,20,21,22,23,24,25]. Three causative genes have been identified thus far: optineurin (OPTN, OMIM 602432) on chromosome 10p14-15 [18,26], myocilin (MYOC, OMIM 610652) on chromosome 1q24-25 [27–28], and WDR36 (OMIM 609669) on chromosome 5q21-22 [29,30], but these account for fewer than 10% of patients with sporadic, adult-onset POAG. Multiple POAG susceptibility loci have been identified in populations from different ethnic backgrounds [31,32,33,34,35,36,37,38,39,40,41].The majority of the findings are conflicting, including those for the OPA1 gene located on chromosome 3.

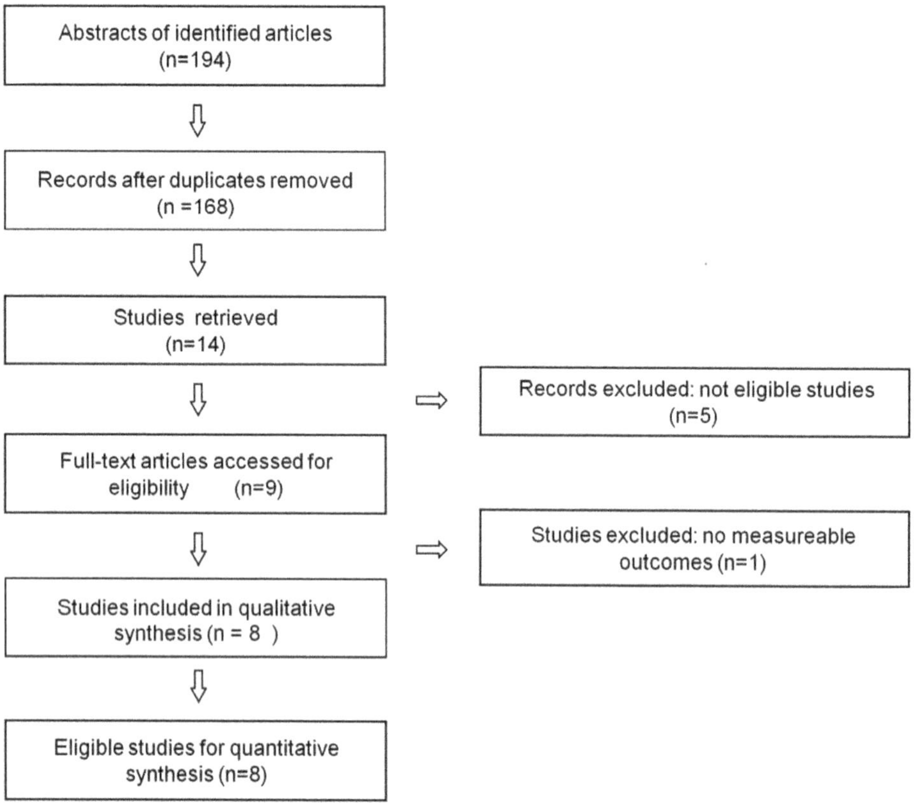

Figure 1. Flow chart of literature search and study selection.

The optic atrophy 1 (OPA1) gene [42] (OMIM 605290, chromosome 3q28) is a nuclear gene encoding a dynamin-related protein. As a family of GTPases, dynamins have been found to be ubiquitous in all human tissues tested and localized to mitochondria, with important functions in mitochondrial biogenesis and membrane integrity [43,44]. Mutations in the OPA1 gene were at first considered to be reasonable candidates for autosomal dominant optic atrophy (ADOA) because the defective The OPA1 gene product may cause a derangement in mitochondrial metabolic function, including respiratory deficiency, which may be involved in the degeneration of retinal ganglion cells and atrophy of the optic nerve [45,46,47].The similarities between the clinical phenotypes and the finding that OPA1 is expressed in the optic nerve made OPA1 an excellent candidate susceptibility gene for POAG, or specifically for NTG [48,49,50].

In recent years, OPA1 polymorphisms have attracted widespread attention. Although several OPA1 polymorphisms have been investigated as risk factors for POAG, two polymorphisms, IVS8+4C>T and IVS8+32T>C, within the OPA1 gene have been the most extensively investigated so far. Aung et al. [48,51] first reported the rs 166850 (IVS8+4C>T) polymorphism to be associated with NTG but not HTG. If so, such a finding would be beneficial for screening those people at risk of developing NTG. On the contrary, Mabuchi and his colleagues [52] reported that this polymorphism influences the phenotypic features in patients with HTG. Their findings, however, could not be replicated in all populations [53,54,55,56]. Whether OPA1 gene polymorphisms may contribute to the pathogenesis of POAG is still vigorously debated.

To date, no meta-analysis has been conducted to validate the association of polymorphisms of OPA1 with normal tension glaucoma (NTG) and high tension glaucoma (HTG). Hence, we performed a meta-analysis of all eligible studies to derive a more precise estimation of the association, to help us better understand its possible influence on POAG.

Methods

Publication Search

MEDLINE, EMBASE, Science Citation Index, the Cochrane Library and the Chinese National Knowledge Infrastructure (CNKI) were searched up to the end of February 2012, using the key terms "OPA1 gene" or "optic atrophy 1 (autosomal dominant)" or "OPA1", "polymorphism" or "SNP" or "single nucleotide polymorphism" or "variation" or "mutation", and "glaucoma" or "primary open-angle glaucoma" or "POAG" or "high tension glaucoma" or "normal tension glaucoma" or "NTG" or "HTG". Relevant publications were examined for references until no further studies were found.

Inclusion Criteria

The following inclusion criteria were used to select literature for the meta-analysis: (1) case-control, nested case-control, or cohort studies; (2) description of the association of OPA1 polymorphisms with POAG; (3) the numbers of cases and controls and the number of different genotypes of IVS8+4C>T, IVS8+32T>C in the cases and controls were provided, or information that could help infer the results in the papers.

Data Extraction

Two observers (YTG, XC) independently abstracted data from all eligible publications onto paper data collection forms. Two

Table 1. Main characteristics of studies included in this meta-analysis.

IVS8+4C>T(rs166850)					Cases			Control		
Author	**Year**	**Ethnicity**	**Location**	**HWE**	**CC**	**CT**	**TT**	**CC**	**CT**	**TT**
HTG										
Yao et al	2006	Barbados	US	0.99	47	1	0	46	2	0
Liu et al	2007	Caucasian	US	1.00	185	84	10	165	57	5
		Black		0.93	179	14	0	90	7	0
		Ghanaian		–	170	0	0	138	0	0
Mabuchi	2007	Asian	Japan	0.99	184	7	0	182	3	0
Fan et al	2010	Asian	HK, China	1.00	217	35	0	173	27	1
Yu-Wai-Man	2010	Caucasian	UK	0.17	49	16	2	59	13	3
NTG										
Aung et al[1]	2002	Caucasian	UK	0.75	57	26	0	86	14	0
Aung et al[2]	2002	Caucasian	UK	0.88	56	24	0	77	9	0
Powwell et al	2003	Caucasian	UK	0.73	41	16	4	111	53	4
Woo et al	2004	Asian	Korea	–	62	3	0	101	0	0
Yao et al	2006	Barbados	US	0.99	58	3	0	46	2	0
Mabuchi	2007	Asian	Japan	0.99	190	4	0	182	3	0
Fan et al	2010	Asian	HK, China	0.99	89	9	1	173	27	1
Yu-Wai-Man	2010	Caucasian	UK	0.17	41	26	3	59	13	3
IVS8+32T>C(rs10451941)					**Cases**			**Control**		
Author	**Year**	**Ethnicity**	**Location**	**HWE**	**TT**	**TC**	**CC**	**TT**	**TC**	**CC**
HTG										
Yao et al	2006	Barbados	US	0.66	20	16	12	16	26	6
Liu et al	2007	Caucasian	US	1.00	95	136	49	79	110	38
		Black		0.99	65	94	34	25	48	24
		Ghanaian		1.00	61	82	27	39	69	30
Mabuchi	2007	Asian	Japan	0.56	137	50	4	146	35	4
Fan et al	2010	Asian	HK, China	0.32	101	125	26	74	104	23
Yu-Wai-Man	2010	Caucasian	UK	1.00	12	36	19	21	37	17
NTG										
Aung et al[1]	2002	Caucasian	UK	0.27	47	36	0	72	28	0
Aung et al[2]	2002	Caucasian	UK	0.13	41	39	0	55	31	0
Powwell et al	2003	Caucasian	UK	**0.003**	17	27	17	43	104	21
Woo et al	2004	Asian	Korea	0.92	40	18	7	68	29	4
Yao et al	2006	Barbados	US	0.66	14	30	17	16	26	6
Mabuchi	2007	Asian	Japan	0.56	125	63	6	146	35	4
Fan et al	2010	Asian	HK, China	0.32	38	49	12	74	104	23
Yu-Wai-Man	2010	Caucasian	UK	1.00	11	37	22	21	37	17

HWE, Hardy-Weinberg equilibrium; HTG, high tension glaucoma; NTG, normal tension glaucoma; Black, African American; –, data not available.

reviewers were blinded to the details (title, author and academic address) of these studies during assessment. Disagreements were resolved by discussion or consensus involving a third reviewer (HTZ) when required. The following items were collected from each study: first author's surname, year of publication, statistical data, ethnicity, total number of cases and controls as well as numbers of cases and controls for each OPA1 genotype.

Statistical Analysis

The Hardy–Weinberg equilibrium (HWE) in controls was recalculated in our meta-analysis. The chi-squared goodness of fit was used to test deviation from HWE (significant at the 0.05 level). The effect measure of choice was pooled OR with its corresponding 95% CI. The assumption of heterogeneity was checked with the Q-test. A P-value less than 0.10 for the Q test indicated a lack of heterogeneity among the studies. Based on the Q-test value, two models of meta-analysis were applied for dichotomous outcomes: A fixed-effects model, using the Mantel-Haenszel (M-H method),

Table 2. Results of meta-analysis for OPA1 polymorphisms and risk of primary open angle glaucoma.

Comparisons	Number of studies	OR	95%CI	P value	Heterogeneity		Effects model	Egger's test
					I^2	P value		P>|t|
IVS8+4								
T vs C								
HTG	5	1.17	0.92–1.49	0.20	0.00%	0.81	Fixed	0.74
Caucasian	2	1.25	0.93–1.68	0.15	0.00%	0.86	Fixed	
Asian	2	1.08	0.67–1.73	0.75	24.7%	0.25	Fixed	
NTG	7	1.52	1.16–1.99	**0.002**	35.9%	0.14	Fixed	0.64
Caucasian	3	1.70	1.25–2.31	**0.001**	42.8%	0.16	Fixed	
Asian	3	1.02	0.57–1.86	0.94	35.80%	0.21	Fixed	
TT vs CC								
HTG	5	1.23	0.52–2.91	0.65	0.00%	0.48	Fixed	–
Caucasian	2	1.43	0.57–3.59	0.45	0.00%	0.48	Fixed	
Asian	2	0.27	0.01–6.61	0.42	0.00%	0.48	Fixed	
NTG	7	1.95	0.71–5.34	0.19	0.00%	0.87	Fixed	0.83
Caucasian	3	1.96	0.66–5.75	0.22	0.00%	0.59	Fixed	
Asian	3	1.93	0.12–31.27	0.64	–	–	Fixed	
TT vs TC+CC								
HTG	5	1.15	0.49–2.71	0.75	0.00%	0.49	Fixed	–
Caucasian	2	1.33	0.53–3.32	0.54	0.00%	0.47	Fixed	
Asian	2	0.27	0.01–6.57	0.42	0.00%	0.49	Fixed	
NTG	7	1.82	0.67–4.94	0.24	0.00%	0.69	Fixed	0.90
Caucasian	3	1.79	0.61–5.22	0.29	0.00%	0.39	Fixed	
Asian	3	2.03	0.13–32.8	0.62	–	–	Fixed	
TT+TC vs CC								
HTG	5	1.17	0.90–1.52	0.23	0.00%	0.86	Fixed	0.85
Caucasian	2	1.24	0.89–1.72	0.20	0.00%	0.96	Fixed	
Asian	2	1.12	0.69–1.83	0.65	16.5%	0.27	Fixed	
NTG	7	1.50	1.13–2.01	**0.006**	35.9%	0.14	Fixed	0.90
Caucasian	3	1.70	1.22–2.38	**0.002**	48.3%	0.12	Fixed	
Asian	3	1.004	0.54–1.87	0.99	38.4%	0.20	Fixed	
IVS8+32								
C vs. T								
HTG	5	0.98	0.87–1.10	0.74	0.00%	0.6	Fixed	0.29
Caucasian	2	1.06	0.87–1.29	0.58	0.00%	0.58	Fixed	
Asian	2	1.03	0.83–1.28	0.80	41.8%	0.19	Fixed	
NTG	7	1.26	1.09–1.47	**0.002**	0.00%	0.56	Fixed	0.08
Caucasian	3	1.27	1.02–1.58	**0.031**	0.00%	0.67	Fixed	
Asian	3	1.24	0.99–1.56	0.06	50.00%	0.14	Fixed	
CC vs. TT								
HTG	5	0.92	0.71–1.19	0.54	0.00%	0.78	Fixed	0.42
Caucasian	2	1.11	0.75–1.72	0.56	0.00%	0.59	Fixed	
Asian	2	0.89	0.51–1.58	0.70	0.00%	0.79	Fixed	
NTG	7	1.52	1.04–2.20	**0.029**	0.00%	0.84	Fixed	0.1
Caucasian	3	1.51	0.87–2.61	0.14	0.00%	0.97	Fixed	
Asian	3	1.40	0.78–2.49	0.26	0.00%	0.42	Fixed	
CC vs. TT+TC								
HTG	5	0.94	0.74–1.20	0.64	0.00%	0.62	Fixed	0.35
Caucasian	2	1.10	0.75–1.63	0.62	0.00%	0.69	Fixed	
Asian	2	0.91	0.53–1.57	0.74	0.00%	0.93	Fixed	

Table 2. Cont.

Comparisons	Number of studies	OR	95%CI	P value	Heterogeneity		Effects model	Egger's test
					I^2	P value		P>|t|
NTG	7	1.64	1.16–2.33	**0.005**	0.00%	0.65	Fixed	0.51
Caucasian	3	1.75	1.06–2.89	**0.030**	0.00%	0.35	Fixed	
Asian	3	1.37	0.78–2.40	0.27	0.00%	0.45	Fixed	
CC+TC vs. TT								
HTG	5	0.99	0.86–1.14	0.9	0.00%	0.83	Fixed	0.63
Caucasian	2	1.05	0.82–1.33	0.72	0.00%	0.70	Fixed	
Asian	2	1.05	0.82–1.35	0.69	34.8%	0.22	Fixed	
NTG	7	1.21	1.02–1.44	**0.032**	0.00%	0.64	Fixed	0.42
Caucasian	3	1.20	0.93–1.55	0.16	0.00%	0.61	Fixed	
Asian	3	1.23	0.95–1.60	0.12	40.50%	0.19	Fixed	

was used to calculate the pooled ORs when the Q-test value ≥0.1. By contrast, a random-effects (DerSimonian and Laird, D+L) model was utilized if the Q-test value < 0.1. First we compared allele frequencies (IVS8+4C>T T vs. C; IVS8+32T>C C vs. T) between cases and controls. We then examined OPA1 genotypes using additive (TT vs. CC; CC vs. TT), recessive (TT vs. CT+CC; CC vs. TT+TC) and dominant (TT+TC vs. CC; CC+TC vs. TT) genetic models for allele T and allele C. Furthermore, subgroup analyses were performed by ethnicity.

One-way sensitivity analyses were performed by iteratively removing one study at a time to assess the stability of the meta-analysis results. Cumulative meta-analysis was performed to evaluate the accumulation of evidence on the association between OPA1 polymorphisms and NTG/HTG. Finally, publication bias was qualitatively assessed by performing Begg's funnel plots, and it was quantitatively evaluated by Egger's test. P<0.05 was considered representative of statistically significant publication bias. All statistical analyses were performed using a commercial statistical softwore package(STATA statistical software Version 11.0; STATA Corporation, College Station, TX,US). Two-sided p-values <0.05 were considered statistically significant.

Results

Literature Search and Characteristics

The initial search yielded 194 articles. Based on the title, the content of the abstract and key words, 185 studies were excluded. Nine articles were reviewed in their entirety. One arm had to be excluded because of no data available [57]. Three studies for NTG [48,53,54], one study for HTG [56] and four studies for both NTG and HTG [52,55,58,59] that met our inclusion criteria were included in this review. The flow chart of the literature search is shown in Figure 1. Seven studies [48,52,53,54,55,58,59] of 713 cases and 964 controls for NTG, and five studies [52,55,56,58,59] of 1200 cases and 971 controls for HTG were included in the meta-analysis of the OPA1 IVS8+4 C>T genotype. Similarly, seven studies (713 cases, 964 controls) for NTG and five studies (1200 cases, 971 controls) for HTG were included in the meta-analysis of the IVS8+32T>C genotype, of which, in one study [53], the distribution of the genotypes in the control group were not in Hardy-Weinberg equilibrium (HWE, Fisher's exact test, P<0.05). Two independent cohort studies were reported in a paper by Aung and his colleagues [48]. For the meta-analysis of OPA1 polymorphisms for NTG, there were three studies on Caucasians [48,53] [59], three studies on Asians [52,54,58], and one study on Barbadians [55]. Meanwhile, for the meta-analysis of OPA1 polymorphisms for HTG, two studies on Asians, one study on Caucasians, one study on Barbadians and one study of three different populations - Ghanaian, African American and Caucasian [56] - were included. Detailed study characteristics are summarized in Table 1.

Meta-analysis Results

The overall analyses suggested significant associations between the IVS8+32T>C polymorphism and normal tension glaucoma (NTG) susceptibility in all genetic models(C vs. T: OR = 1.26, 95% CI 1.09–1.47, P = 0.002; CC vs. TT: OR = 1.52, 95% CI 1.04–2.20, P = 0.029; CC vs. CT+TT: OR = 1.64, 95% CI 1.16–2.33, P = 0.005; CC+CT vs. TT: OR = 1.21, 95% CI 1.02–1.44, P = 0.032), and clear evidence of associations was found between the IVS8+4C>T variant and risk of NTG in allelic or dominant models (T vs. C OR = 1.52, 95% CI 1.16–1.99, P = 0.002; TT+TC vs. CC OR = 1.50, 95% CI 1.13–2.01, P = 0.006). However, no evidence of associations was detected between the two OPA1 polymorphisms and high tension glaucoma (HTG) susceptibility. Because a Q-test of heterogeneity among studies was nonsignificant in all genetic models, a fixed-effects model was used. (Data shown in Table 2 and Figures 2, 3).

To better understand the exact consequence of the relationship between OPA1 polymorphisms and normal tension glaucoma susceptibility, we investigated the effects of the OPA1 IVS8+4C>T and IVS8+32T>C genotypes on the occurrence of NTG by ethnicity. Overall, no evidence of association was observed in any genetic model between the OPA1 IVS8+4C>T or IVS8+32C>T variants and risk of normal tension glaucoma (NTG) in Asians. In contrast to the results for NTG risk in Asians, the analyses showed significant associations between both OPA1 polymorphisms and susceptibility to NTG in Caucasians (rs 166850 T vs. C OR = 1.70, 95% CI 1.25–2.31, P = 0.001; TT+TC vs. CC OR = 1.70, 95% CI 1.22–2.38, P = 0.002; rs 10451941 C vs. T OR = 1.27, 95% CI 1.02–1.58, P = 0.031; CC vs. TT+TC OR = 1.75, 95% CI 1.06–2.89, P = 0.03; Figure 4). In addition, stratified analyses by ethnicity were performed between the OPA1 polymorphisms and high tension glaucoma (HTG) risk. However, no significant finding was noted between either OPA1

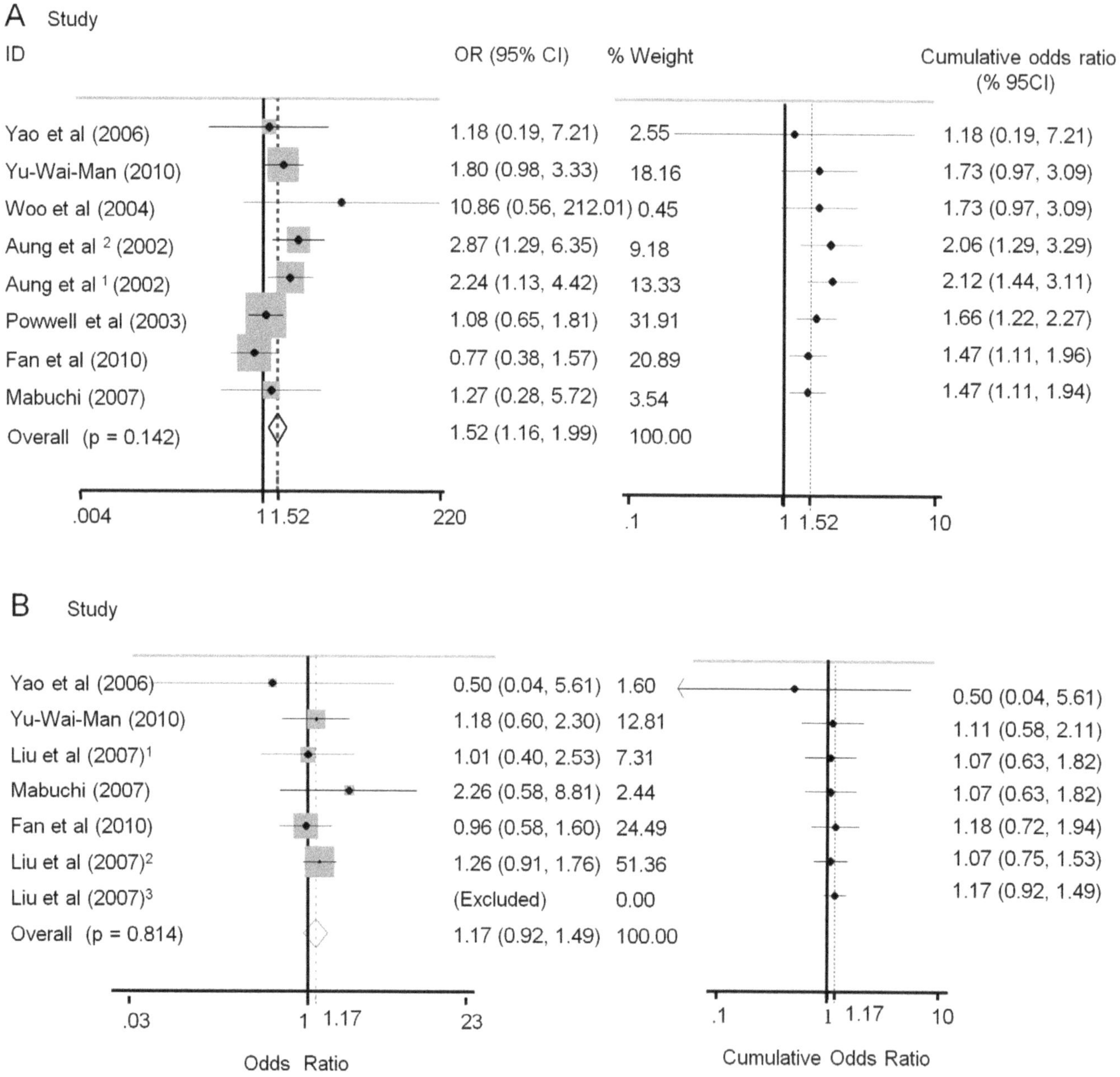

Figure 2. Forest plots describing overall meta-analysis (left) and cumulative meta-analysis (right) of the associations between IVS+4 T>C polymorphism and POAG risk. Odds ratios shown for individual studies for allelic model genotype contrasts (C vs. T). Cumulative odds ratios shown for each additional information step obtained by stepwise inclusion of every new study into pooled estimate. A. meta-analysis of association between IVS+4 T>C variant and NTG in order of sample size; B. meta-analysis of association between IVS+4 T>C variant and HTG in order of sample size.

polymorphism and risk of HTG, either in Asians or in Caucasians (Table 2 and Figure 5).

Sensitivity Analysis and Cumulative Meta-analysis

To evaluate the robustness of the association results, a meta-analysis was performed repeatedly with each study removed. The results indicated that the fixed-effect estimates before or after the deletion of any single study were generally similar, suggesting a high stability of the meta-analysis results (data not shown). Cumulative meta-analysis of both OPA1 polymorphisms and NTG risk revealed that the summary ORs was larger than 1, and the 95% CI was reduced with accumulated sample size. By contrast, the pooled ORs of cumulative meta-analysis for HTG remained centered on 1 with increasing sample size, indicating that rs 166850 and rs 10451941 were unlikely risk variants for HTG, as shown in Figures 2 and 3.

Publication Bias

Publication bars were qualitatively assessed by Begg's funnel plot and quantitatively assessed by Egger's test. Neither Begg's funnel plot nor Egger's test detected obvious evidence of publication bias in the overall and subgroup analyses for all genetic models (Figure 6; data available in Table 2).

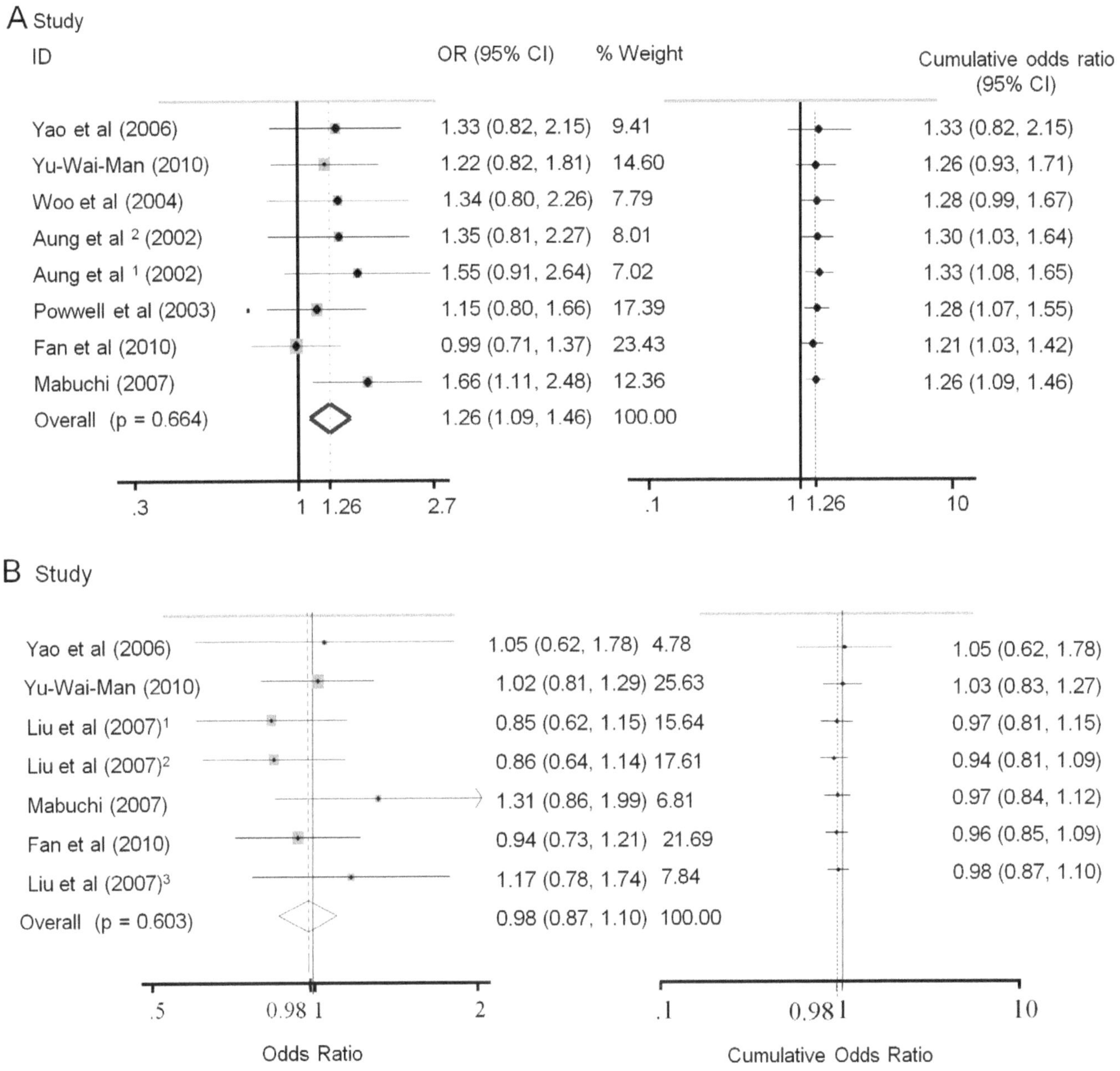

Figure 3. Forest plots describing overall meta-analysis (left) and cumulative meta-analysis (right) of the associations between IVS+32 C>T polymorphism and POAG risk. Odds ratios shown for individual studies for allelic model genotype contrasts (T vs. C). Cumulative odds ratios shown for each additional information step obtained by stepwise inclusion of every new study into pooled estimate. A. meta-analysis of association between IVS+32 C>T variant and NTG in order of sample size. B. meta-analysis of association between IVS+32 C>T variant and HTG in order of sample size.

Discussion

Primary open-angle glaucoma is considered to be a complex trait with a strong genetic component [12,60]. OPA1, the gene responsible for autosomal dominant optic atrophy (ADOA) [61], represents a good candidate genetic risk factor for POAG [49], as the clinical phenotypes between ADOA and POAG are similar, and OPA1 is expressed in the retinal ganglion cells and optic nerve [62]. The OPA1 gene is related to mitochondrial biogenesis and respiration through its product of dynamin-related GTPase. The dysfunction of mitochondria caused by mutations in the OPA1 gene in ADOA is thought to be associated with apoptosis of retinal ganglion cells leading to optic neuropathy [50]. Since the identification of OPA1 polymorphisms, a number of studies have investigated the genetic effects of OPA1 polymorphisms on POAG susceptibility with conflicting results. Meta-analysis, as a powerful statistical method, can provide a quantitative approach to pooling variant results on the same topic to estimate and explain their diversity [63,64]. This advantage stimulated us to conduct this meta-analysis of eight published case-control or cohort studies, which may help elucidate these phenomena and explore a more robust estimate of the effects of these polymorphisms on primary angle glaucoma.

In this meta-analysis, we found that the effect of the OPA1 polymorphisms on POAG risk may vary by subtype of POAG

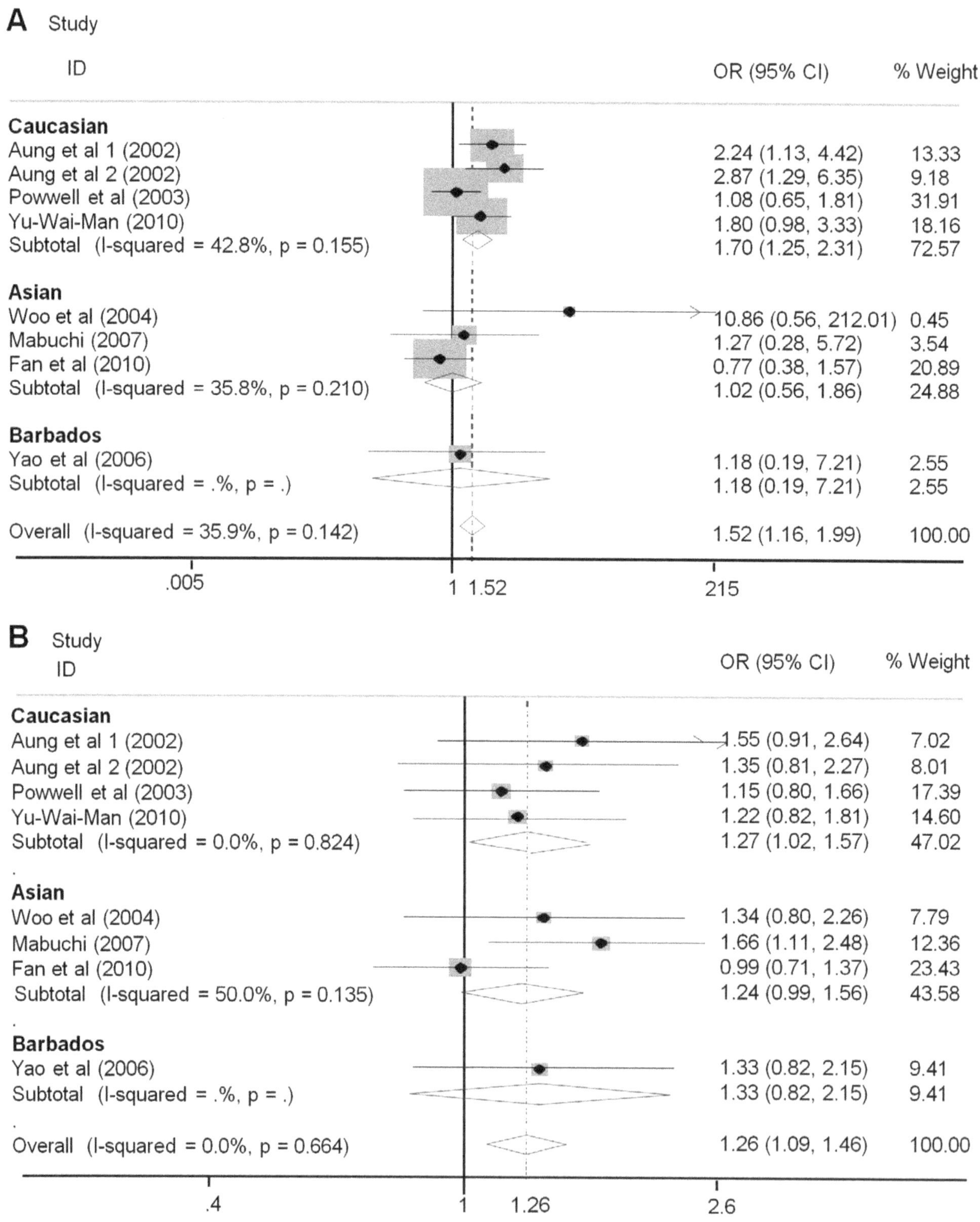

Figure 4. Forest plots describing subgroup analyses of the association between OPA1 polymorphisms and risk for NTG. The size of the square indicate the relative weight of each study.Bars,95% confidence interval(95% CI) A. subgroup analysis of IVS8+4 C>T stratified by ethnicity in order of publication year; B subgroup analysis of IVS8+32 T>C stratified by ethnicity in order of publication year.

[49,56] and ethnicity [54,55,56]. Studies by Aung et al. [48],Yao et al. [55] and Liu et al. [56] revealed that the association of OPA1 variants with POAG may be limited to patients with normal tension glaucoma, suggesting that a genetic mechanism favoring OPA1 would have a greater role in the pathophysiology of NTG than HTG. By contrast, Mabuchi and his colleagues [52]

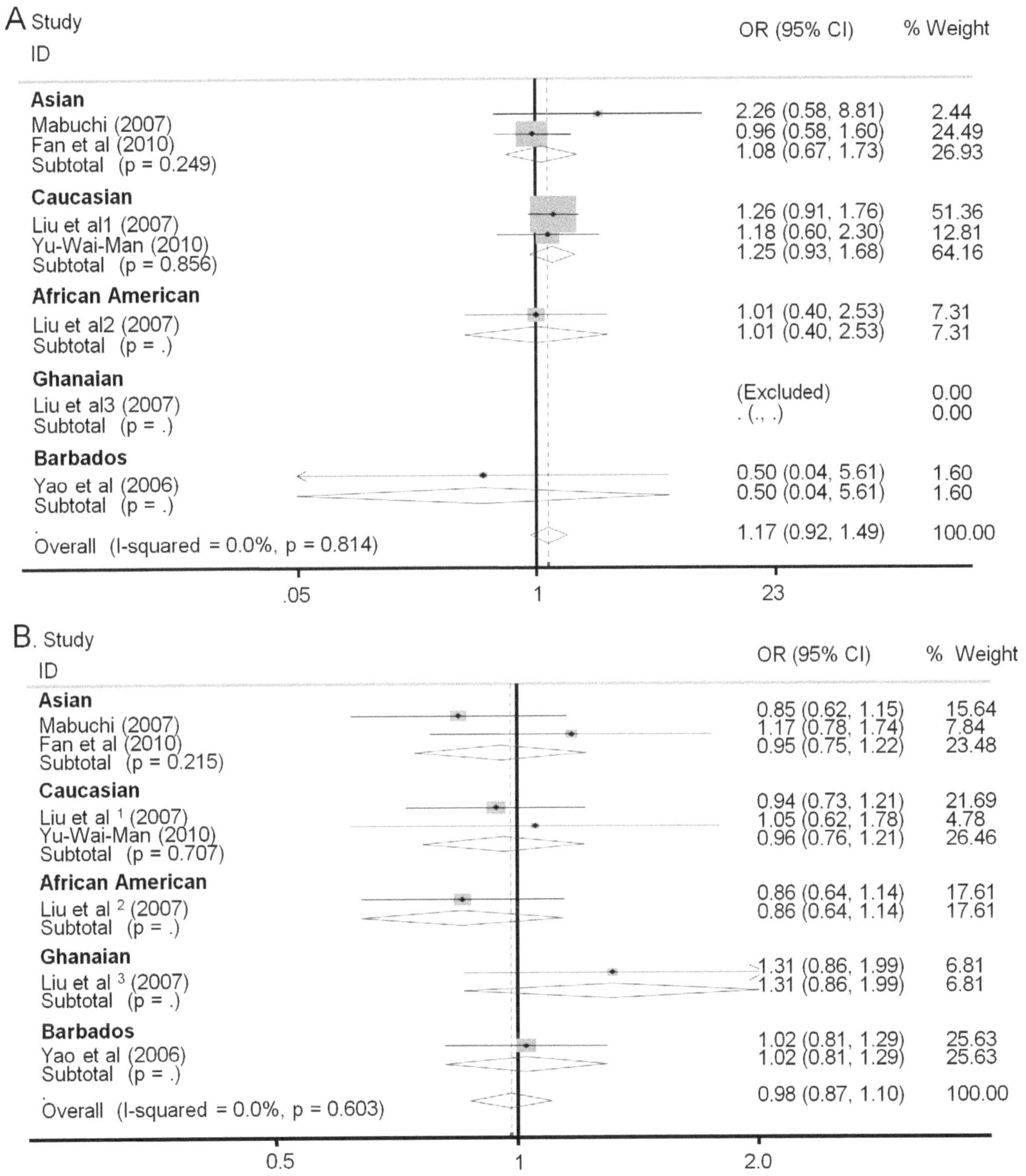

Figure 5. Forest plots describing subgroup analyses of the association between OPA1 polymorphisms and risk for HTG. The size of the square indicate the relative weight of each study.Bars,95% confidence interval(95% CI) A. subgroup analysis of IVS8+4 C>T stratified by ethnicity in order of publication year;B subgroup analysis of IVS8+32 T>C stratified by ethnicity in order of publication year.

presented data that this polymorphism also influences the HTG phenotype and should therefore be considered a genetic risk factor not only for NTG but also for HTG in the Japanese population. Therefore, overall analyses were conducted on normal tension glaucoma (NTG) and high tension glaucoma (HTG). Strong evidence was found that the associations with NTG were significant for the IVS8+4C>T(rs 166850) and IVS8+32T>C (rs 10451941) polymorphisms. There was, however, no clear association between either OPA1 polymorphism and HTG, which is consistent with the findings of the largest cohort study,

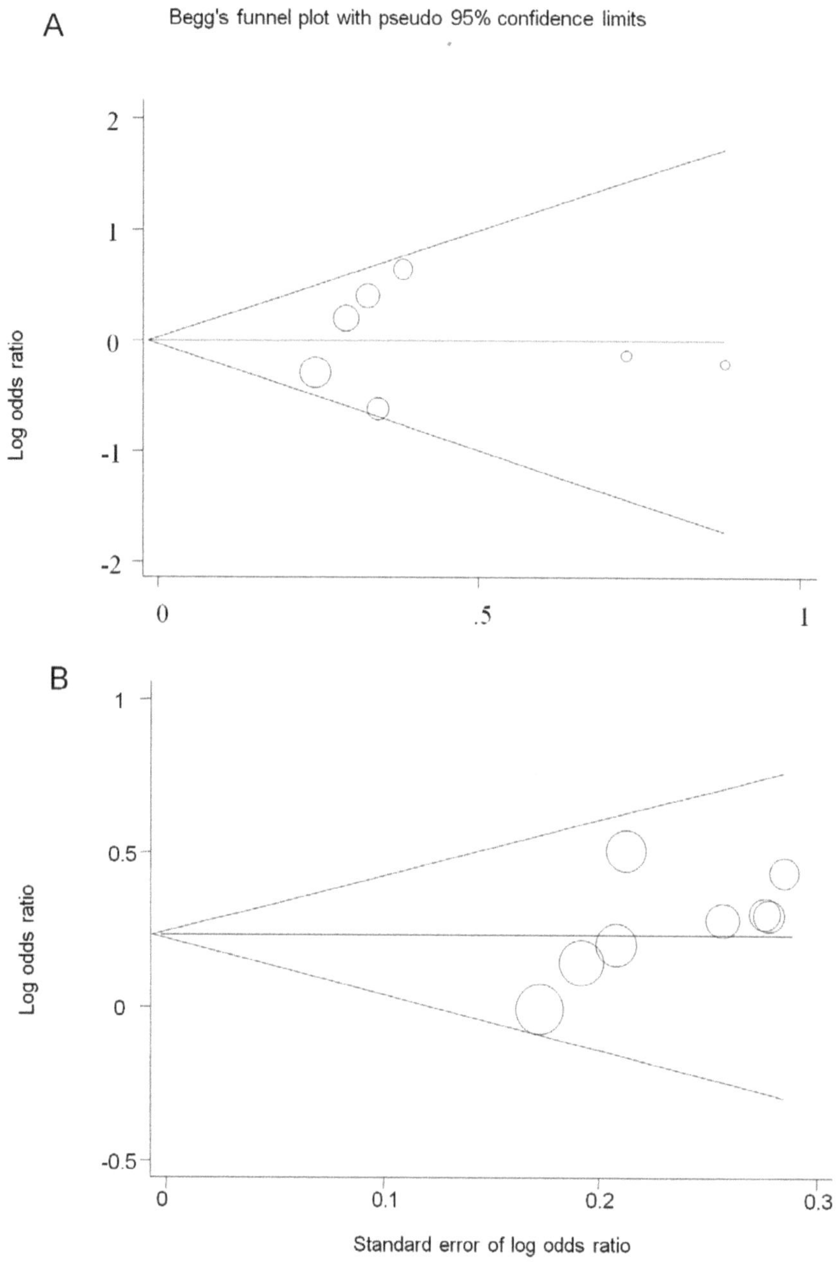

Figure 6. Begg's funnel plot of OPA1 polymorphisms and NTG for allelic model. A: IVS8+4 T vs C; B:IVS8+32 C vs T. Each circle represents a separate study for the indicated association, and its size is proportional to the sample size of each study.

performed by Liu and his colleagues [56]. It is worth noting that the association between the presence of the C allele and the occurrence of HTG presented by Mabuchi is marginal [52]. The explanation for this discrepancy may be that the small sample size reduced its power to detect the association; alternatively, this discrepancy may result from different ethnicities. Thus, it is necessary to confirm the HTG risk in OPA1 variant carriers in other ethnic populations with large numbers of patients and well-defined diagnostic criteria. Meanwhile, reports on the associations of these two polymorphisms with NTG often conflict in different studies. Aung et al. [48] showed that the IVS8+4 C>T genotype was associated with NTG susceptibility, whereas Powell's data [53] only supported an association of the IVS8+32T>C genotype with NTG, for which no independent association was seen by the Aung group. Our data showed that both the IVS8+4C>T and IVS8+32T>C polymorphisms are associated with risk of NTG. It should be noted that the distribution of the control group for IVS8+32T>C(rs 10451941) in Powell's report [53] deviated from Hardy-Weinberg equilibrium, which may have been due to genotyping errors or selection bias in the control and/or population stratification. Therefore, as recommended by Attia [65],we conducted the meta-analysis again with this study removed. The results indicated that the estimates before or after deletion of the study were similar, suggesting a high stability of the meta-analysis results with little effect of this particular study.

As mentioned above, the results of many studies have represented that ethnic differences may affect genetic predisposition to NTG and HTG [52,54]. For this reason, subgroup analyses on different ethnicities were performed. The results showed that OPA1 polymorphisms were significantly associated with NTG from studies of Caucasian individuals, but not in Asian individuals. In contrast to the results with NTG, no difference was found in the associations between OPA1 polymorphisms and HTG in Asians or Caucasians. The discrepancy may have arisen because studies with small sample sizes may be underpowered to detect a slight effect or may have generated a variable risk estimate. More large-scale cohort or case-control studies with sufficient power are needed to study HTG risk in carriers of OPA1 variants in different populations.

If the effect observed in this meta-analysis was truly without bias, several possibilities may explain why such an effect was detected in Caucasians but not in Asians. On the one hand, the possible role of ethnic differences in genetic background is suggested. On the other, the relevant environmental exposure in Asia may differ from that in Western countries. Furthermore, the genetic pathogenesis of NTG may be different between the two ethnic groups. Further studies involving different racial groups from the same geographic areas may help answer this question.

Some limitations in our study should be addressed, and the results should be interpreted with caution. First, controls were not uniformly defined. This study is a meta-analysis of case-control studies, most of which were hospital-based. Thus, some inevitable selection bias might exist in the results, and they may not be representative of the general population. Second, only published studies were included in this meta-analysis. Unpublished data, ongoing studies and articles published in languages other than English and Chinese were not sought, especially those with negative findings, which may have biased our results, although no obvious publication bias was apparent. Third, this meta-analysis was limited by the number of cases and controls as well as small sample sizes, especially in the subgroup analysis by ethnicity. Only a single study was conducted in Barbadian, Ghanaian, and African-American populations. Thus, additional studies are needed to evaluate the effect of these functional polymorphisms on POAG in different races. Fourth, our results were based on unadjusted estimates; a more precise analysis of the various groups should be conducted according to other factors, such as age and sex. Fifth, the genotyping methods used were different among these studies, which might have affected the results. This discrepancy between genotyping methods highlights the need for implementing rigorous quality control procedures in future studies. Finally, the existing literature lacks information about potential gene-gene or gene-environment interactions. Given that the role of several environmental factors in the pathogenesis of open angle glaucoma is established, further research should be performed in this direction.

In conclusion, the results of this meta-analysis suggest that two OPA1 polymorphisms [IVS8+4C>T (rs166850) and IVS8+32T>C (rs10451941)] are associated with an increased risk for normal tension glaucoma. It is also worthwhile to note that OPA1 polymorphisms may be involved in the pathogenesis of NTG in Caucasians but not in Asians. Due to the limitations discussed above, well-designed large-scale cohorts or case-control studies are warranted to confirm our findings.

Acknowledgments

We thank Drs. Qing Liu and Xu Fang for providing helpful information.

Author Contributions

Conceived and designed the experiments: KZ YG. Performed the experiments: YG XC. Analyzed the data: YG XC. Contributed reagents/materials/analysis tools: YG HZ WC XY. Wrote the paper: YG. Suggestion for research design: NL.

References

1. Coleman AL, Brigatti L (2001) The glaucomas. Minerva Med 92: 365–379.
2. Cedrone C, Mancino R, Cerulli A, Cesareo M, Nucci C (2008) Epidemiology of primary glaucoma: prevalence, incidence, and blinding effects. Prog Brain Res 173: 3–14.
3. Wen W, Sun XH (2010) Primary glaucoma and psychological characteristics]. Zhonghua Yan Ke Za Zhi 46: 566–571.
4. Kim E, Varma R (2010) Glaucoma in Latinos/Hispanics. Curr Opin Ophthalmol 21: 100–105.
5. Foster PJ (2002) The epidemiology of primary angle closure and associated glaucomatous optic neuropathy. Semin Ophthalmol 17: 50–58.
6. Bourne RR, Sukudom P, Foster PJ, Tantisevi V, Jitapunkul S, et al. (2003) Prevalence of glaucoma in Thailand: a population based survey in Rom Klao District, Bangkok. Br J Ophthalmol 87: 1069–1074.
7. Chen XY, Cai Y (2011) Epidemiology and classification of primary angle-closure glaucoma today. Zhonghua Yan Ke Za Zhi 47: 949–952.
8. Peng PH, Manivanh R, Nguyen N, Weinreb RN, Lin SC (2011) Glaucoma and clinical characteristics in Vietnamese Americans. Curr Eye Res 36: 733–738.
9. Sugiyama K (2011) A review 45. characteristics of and treatment strategy for primary open-angle glaucoma. Nihon Ganka Gakkai Zasshi 115: 79–92.
10. Rouland JF, Berdeaux G, Lafuma A (2005) The economic burden of glaucoma and ocular hypertension: implications for patient management: a review. Drugs Aging 22: 315–321.
11. Quigley HA, Broman AT (2006) The number of people with glaucoma worldwide in 2010 and 2020. Br J Ophthalmol 90: 262–267.
12. Gemenetzi M, Yang Y, Lotery AJ (2012) Current concepts on primary open-angle glaucoma genetics: a contribution to disease pathophysiology and future treatment. Eye (Lond) 26: 355–369.
13. Klein BE, Klein R, Sponsel WE, Franke T, Cantor LB, et al. (1992) Prevalence of glaucoma. The Beaver Dam Eye Study. Ophthalmology 99: 1499–1504.
14. Sowka J (2005) New thoughts on normal tension glaucoma. Optometry 76: 600–608.
15. Anderson DR, Feuer W, Schiffman J (2008) Normal-tension glaucoma. Ophthalmology 115: 590–591; author reply 591–592.
16. Charliat G, Jolly D, Blanchard F (1994) Genetic risk factor in primary open-angle glaucoma: a case-control study. Ophthalmic Epidemiol 1: 131–138.
17. Chihara E, Liu X, Dong J, Takashima Y, Akimoto M, et al. (1997) Severe myopia as a risk factor for progressive visual field loss in primary open-angle glaucoma. Ophthalmologica 211: 66–71.
18. Bergen AA, Leschot NJ, Hulsman CA, De Smet MD, De Jong PT (2004) [From gene to disease; primary open-angle glaucoma and three known genes: MYOC, CYP1B1 and OPTN]. Ned Tijdschr Geneeskd 148: 1343–1344.
19. Fan BJ, Leung YF, Wang N, Lam SC, Liu Y, et al. (2004) Genetic and environmental risk factors for primary open- angle glaucoma. Chin Med J (Engl) 117: 706–710.
20. Libby RT, Gould DB, Anderson MG, John SW (2005) Complex genetics of glaucoma susceptibility. Annu Rev Genomics Hum Genet 6: 15–44.
21. Ozcura F, Aydin S (2007) Is diabetes mellitus a risk factor or a protector for primary open angle glaucoma? Med Hypotheses 69: 233–234.
22. Bron A, Chaine G, Villain M, Colin J, Nordmann JP, et al. (2008) Risk factors for primary open-angle glaucoma. J Fr Ophtalmol 31: 435–444.
23. Kountouras J, Zavos C, Grigoriadis N, Deretzi G, Katsinelos P, et al. (2008) Helicobacter pylori infection as an environmental familial clustering risk factor for primary open-angle glaucoma. Clin Experiment Ophthalmol 36: 296–297; author reply 297.
24. Yuki K, Dogru M, Imamura Y, Kimura I, Ohtake Y, et al. (2009) Lead accumulation as possible risk factor for primary open-angle glaucoma. Biol Trace Elem Res 132: 1–8.
25. Zanon-Moreno V, Garcia-Medina JJ, Zanon-Viguer V, Moreno-Nadal MA, Pinazo-Duran MD (2009) Smoking, an additional risk factor in elder women with primary open-angle glaucoma. Mol Vis 15: 2953–2959.
26. Rezaie T, Child A, Hitchings R, Brice G, Miller L, et al. (2002) Adult-onset primary open-angle glaucoma caused by mutations in optineurin. Science 295: 1077–1079.
27. Fingert JH, Heon E, Liebmann JM, Yamamoto T, Craig JE, et al. (1999) Analysis of myocilin mutations in 1703 glaucoma patients from five different populations. Hum Mol Genet 8: 899–905.
28. Baird PN, Foote SJ, Mackey DA, Craig J, Speed TP, et al. (2005) Evidence for a novel glaucoma locus at chromosome 3p21–22. Hum Genet 117: 249–257.
29. Pasutto F, Mardin CY, Michels-Rautenstrauss K, Weber BH, Sticht H, et al. (2008) Profiling of WDR36 missense variants in German patients with glaucoma. Invest Ophthalmol Vis Sci 49: 270–274.

30. Blanco-Marchite C, Sanchez-Sanchez F, Lopez-Garrido MP, Inigez-de-Onzono M, Lopez-Martinez F, et al. (2011) WDR36 and P53 gene variants and susceptibility to primary open-angle glaucoma: analysis of gene-gene interactions. Invest Ophthalmol Vis Sci 52: 8467–8478.
31. Stoilova D, Child A, Trifan OC, Crick RP, Coakes RL, et al. (1996) Localization of a locus (GLC1B) for adult-onset primary open angle glaucoma to the 2cen-q13 region. Genomics 36: 142–150.
32. Trifan OC, Traboulsi EI, Stoilova D, Alozie I, Nguyen R, et al. (1998) A third locus (GLC1D) for adult-onset primary open-angle glaucoma maps to the 8q23 region. Am J Ophthalmol 126: 17–28.
33. Sarfarazi M, Child A, Stoilova D, Brice G, Desai T, et al. (1998) Localization of the fourth locus (GLC1E) for adult-onset primary open-angle glaucoma to the 10p15-p14 region. Am J Hum Genet 62: 641–652.
34. Wirtz MK, Samples JR, Rust K, Lie J, Nordling L, et al. (1999) GLC1F, a new primary open-angle glaucoma locus, maps to 7q35-q36. Arch Ophthalmol 117: 237–241.
35. Juronen E, Tasa G, Veromann S, Parts L, Tiidla A, et al. (2000) Polymorphic glutathione S-transferase M1 is a risk factor of primary open-angle glaucoma among Estonians. Exp Eye Res 71: 447–452.
36. Monemi S, Spaeth G, DaSilva A, Popinchalk S, Ilitchev E, et al. (2005) Identification of a novel adult-onset primary open-angle glaucoma (POAG) gene on 5q22.1. Hum Mol Genet 14: 725–733.
37. Junemann AG, von Ahsen N, Reulbach U, Roedl J, Bonsch D, et al. (2005) C677T variant in the methylentetrahydrofolate reductase gene is a genetic risk factor for primary open-angle glaucoma. Am J Ophthalmol 139: 721–723.
38. Suriyapperuma SP, Child A, Desai T, Brice G, Kerr A, et al. (2007) A new locus (GLC1H) for adult-onset primary open-angle glaucoma maps to the 2p15-p16 region. Arch Ophthalmol 125: 86–92.
39. Rocha AV, Talbot T, Magalhaes da Silva T, Almeida MC, Menezes CA, et al. (2011) Is the GSTM1 null polymorphism a risk factor in primary open angle glaucoma? Mol Vis 17: 1679–1686.
40. Fernandez-Martinez L, Letteboer S, Mardin CY, Weisschuh N, Gramer E, et al. (2011) Evidence for RPGRIP1 gene as risk factor for primary open angle glaucoma. Eur J Hum Genet 19: 445–451.
41. Burdon KP, Macgregor S, Hewitt AW, Sharma S, Chidlow G, et al. (2011) Genome-wide association study identifies susceptibility loci for open angle glaucoma at TMCO1 and CDKN2B-AS1. Nat Genet 43: 574–578.
42. Votruba M, Moore AT, Bhattacharya SS (1998) Demonstration of a founder effect and fine mapping of dominant optic atrophy locus on 3q28-qter by linkage disequilibrium method: a study of 38 British Isles pedigrees. Hum Genet 102: 79–86.
43. Olichon A, Guillou E, Delettre C, Landes T, Arnauné-Pelloquin L, et al. (2006) Mitochondrial dynamics and disease, OPA1. Biochimica et Biophysica Acta (BBA) - Molecular Cell Research 1763: 500–509.
44. Pawlikowska P, Orzechowski A (2007) Role of transmembrane GTPases in mitochondrial morphology and activity. Postepy Biochem 53: 53–59.
45. Van Bergen NJ, Crowston JG, Kearns LS, Staffieri SE, Hewitt AW, et al. (2011) Mitochondrial oxidative phosphorylation compensation may preserve vision in patients with OPA1-linked autosomal dominant optic atrophy. PLoS One 6: e21347.
46. Delettre C, Lenaers G, Griffoin J-M, Gigarel N, Lorenzo C, et al. (2000) Nuclear gene OPA1, encoding a mitochondrial dynamin-related protein, is mutated in dominant optic atrophy. Nat Genet 26: 207–210.
47. Alexander C, Votruba M, Pesch UE, Thiselton DL, Mayer S, et al. (2000) OPA1, encoding a dynamin-related GTPase, is mutated in autosomal dominant optic atrophy linked to chromosome 3q28. Nat Genet 26: 211–215.
48. Aung T, Ocaka L, Ebenezer ND, Morris AG, Krawczak M, et al. (2002) A major marker for normal tension glaucoma: association with polymorphisms in the OPA1 gene. Hum Genet 110: 52–56.
49. Turkoski BB (2012) Glaucoma and glaucoma medications. Orthop Nurs 31: 37–41.
50. Buono LM, Foroozan R, Sergott RC, Savino PJ (2002) Is normal tension glaucoma actually an unrecognized hereditary optic neuropathy? New evidence from genetic analysis. Curr Opin Ophthalmol 13: 362–370.
51. Aung T, Ocaka L, Ebenezer ND, Morris AG, Brice G, et al. (2002) Investigating the association between OPA1 polymorphisms and glaucoma: comparison between normal tension and high tension primary open angle glaucoma. Hum Genet 110: 513–514.
52. Mabuchi F, Tang S, Kashiwagi K, Yamagata Z, Iijima H, et al. (2007) The OPA1 gene polymorphism is associated with normal tension and high tension glaucoma. Am J Ophthalmol 143: 125–130.
53. Powell BL, Toomes C, Scott S, Yeung A, Marchbank NJ, et al. (2003) Polymorphisms in OPA1 are associated with normal tension glaucoma. Mol Vis 9: 460–464.
54. Woo SJ, Kim DM, Kim JY, Park SS, Ko HS, et al. (2004) Investigation of the association between OPA1 polymorphisms and normal-tension glaucoma in Korea. J Glaucoma 13: 492–495.
55. Yao W, Jiao X, Hejtmancik JF, Leske MC, Hennis A, et al. (2006) Evaluation of the association between OPA1 polymorphisms and primary open-angle glaucoma in Barbados families. Mol Vis 12: 649–654.
56. Liu Y, Schmidt S, Qin X, Gibson J, Munro D, et al. (2007) No association between OPA1 polymorphisms and primary open-angle glaucoma in three different populations. Mol Vis 13: 2137–2141.
57. Wolf C, Gramer E, Muller-Myhsok B, Pasutto F, Reinthal E, et al. (2009) Evaluation of nine candidate genes in patients with normal tension glaucoma: a case control study. BMC Med Genet 10: 91.
58. Fan BJ, Liu K, Wang DY, Tham CC, Tam PO, et al. (2010) Association of polymorphisms of tumor necrosis factor and tumor protein p53 with primary open-angle glaucoma. Invest Ophthalmol Vis Sci 51: 4110–4116.
59. Yu-Wai-Man P, Stewart JD, Hudson G, Andrews RM, Griffiths PG, et al. (2010) OPA1 increases the risk of normal but not high tension glaucoma. J Med Genet 47: 120–125.
60. Fan BJ, Wang DY, Lam DS, Pang CP (2006) Gene mapping for primary open angle glaucoma. Clin Biochem 39: 249–258.
61. Thiselton DL, Alexander C, Taanman JW, Brooks S, Rosenberg T, et al. (2002) A comprehensive survey of mutations in the OPA1 gene in patients with autosomal dominant optic atrophy. Invest Ophthalmol Vis Sci 43: 1715–1724.
62. Lenaers G, Reynier P, Elachouri G, Soukkarieh C, Olichon A, et al. (2009) OPA1 functions in mitochondria and dysfunctions in optic nerve. Int J Biochem Cell Biol 41: 1866–1874.
63. Ioannidis JP, Ntzani EE, Trikalinos TA, Contopoulos-Ioannidis DG (2001) Replication validity of genetic association studies. Nat Genet 29: 306–309.
64. Munafo M (2004) Replication validity of genetic association studies of smoking behavior: what can meta-analytic techniques offer? Nicotine Tob Res 6: 381–382.
65. Attia J, Thakkinstian A, D'Este C (2003) Meta-analyses of molecular association studies: methodologic lessons for genetic epidemiology. J Clin Epidemiol 56: 297–303.

9

Generating Embryonic Stem Cells from the Inbred Mouse Strain DBA/2J, a Model of Glaucoma and Other Complex Diseases

Laura G. Reinholdt[1¶], Gareth R. Howell[1,2¶], Anne M. Czechanski[1], Danilo G. Macalinao[1], Katharine H. MacNicoll[1], Chyuan-Sheng Lin[3], Leah Rae Donahue[1], Simon W. M. John[1,2,4*]

1 The Jackson Laboratory, Bar Harbor, Maine, United States of America, 2 The Howard Hughes Medical Institute, Bar Harbor, Maine, United States of America, 3 Department of Pathology and Cell Biology, Irving Cancer Research Center, Columbia University, New York, New York, United States of America, 4 Department of Ophthalmology, Tufts University of Medicine, Boston, Massachusetts, United States of America

Abstract

Mouse embryonic stem (ES) cells are derived from the inner cell mass of blastocyst stage embryos and are used primarily for the creation of genetically engineered strains through gene targeting. While some inbred strains of mice are permissive to the derivation of embryonic stem cell lines and are therefore easily engineered, others are nonpermissive or recalcitrant. Genetic engineering of recalcitrant strain backgrounds requires gene targeting in a permissive background followed by extensive backcrossing of the engineered allele into the desired strain background. The inbred mouse strain DBA/2J is a recalcitrant strain that is used as a model of many human diseases, including glaucoma, deafness and schizophrenia. Here, we describe the generation of germ-line competent ES cell lines derived from DBA/2J mice. We also demonstrate the utility of DBA/2J ES cells with the creation of conditional knockout allele for Endothelin-2 (*Edn2*) directly on the DBA/2J strain background.

Editor: Anand Swaroop, National Eye Institute, United States of America

Funding: This work was supported by EY011721 (SWMJ), The Barbara and Joseph Cohen Foundation, The Pew Charitable Trust, Kathryn W. Davis and family, and donors of National Glaucoma Research – a program of the American Health Assistance Foundation (GRH). SWMJ is an Investigator of the Howard Hughes Medical Institute. The funders had no role in study design, data collection and analysis, decision to publish, or preparation of the manuscript.

Competing Interests: The authors have declared that no competing interests exist.

* E-mail: simon.john@jax.org

¶ These authors contributed equally to this work.

Introduction

The development of gene targeting technologies and the availability of a well-annotated mouse genome sequence allows the function of individual gene(s) to be assessed in a temporal and spatial manner. Historically, the resources for genetically engineering mice have been available for a limited number of strains, including C57BL/6J (B6) and 129Sv/ImJ (129), and are more recently emerging for C57BL/6N. Resources include ES cell lines, a vast number of null and conditional alleles through the Knockout Mouse Project (KOMP) and Cre driver lines to ablate the function of individual genes in specific cell types. A major advantage of the mouse as an animal model is the availability of well-characterized inbred strains that enable functional genomics on defined genetic backgrounds. Currently, however, exploiting the full utility of mice to study human diseases is hampered by the lack of gene targeting resources for multiple inbred mouse strains.

DBA/2J is a common inbred mouse strain critical in studying a diverse range of human diseases. For example, it is widely used as an inherited model of glaucoma. Glaucoma is a neurodegenerative disorder that affects 70 million people worldwide. Clinically, no treatments that specifically target retinal ganglion cell (RGC) death are in use, as the mechanisms involved are not well understood. However, we and others have used DBA/2J extensively to identify processes involved in glaucomatous RGC death and to test potential neuroprotective treatments for human glaucoma [1,2,3,4,5,6,7,8,9,10,11,12]. Secondly, DBA/2J is used to model temporal lobe epilepsy (TLE) and schizophrenia (SZ) in combination. Psychotic episodes and cognitive impairment are among the most debilitating and common comorbidities of TLE, while SZ patients are more prone to seizures than the general population. To study the overlap between both disease pathologies animal models that combine epileptic seizures with select endophenotypes of schizophrenia are essential and DBA/2J is one of the few animal models that meet these criteria [13,14]. Finally, DBA/2J is used to model other complex diseases including deafness, cardiovascular disease and host response to infections (e.g. [15,16,17,18,19]).

Phenotypes are often very different between mouse strains with diverse genetic backgrounds and the strain characteristics of DBA/2J are often contrasted with other genetically distinct inbred strains such as C57BL/6J. These defined genetic backgrounds provide an excellent system for mapping modifier genes [20,21,22]. To study these differences a number of DBA/2J-relevant resources have been generated. For instance, a genome-wide panel of congenic strains has been created that contain portions of DBA/2J chromosomes on a C57BL/6J background [23]. These 65 strains contain more than 95% of the DBA/2J genome. Also, DBA/2J is one parent in two sets of recombinant inbred lines that have been generated, AKXD (the other parent being AKR/J) and BXD (the other parent being C57BL/6J). Recombinant inbred (RI) strains such as these are especially useful for mapping complex traits, since they create an immortalized mapping population that allows researchers to phenotype as many animals per genome as desired over extended periods of time. AKXD strains have been used to study a variety of diseases including murine lymphoma and glaucoma [24,25]. The more widely used BXD strains have been used to understand the genetics of a variety of diseases and biological systems including aging, the immune system and iron regulation [26,27,28,29,30]. Much of this work has been made available through *GeneNetwork* (formerly *WebQTL*) an on-line resource to study complex gene networks and phenotypes [31].

Stable ES cell lines for gene targeting are available only for inbred strains from which stable ES cells lines can be consistently derived from the inner cell mass of blastocyst stage embryos. These permissive inbred strains include B6 and 129 derived strains [32,33]. However, DBA/2J is one of many inbred strains that are considered recalcitrant to ES cell derivation because pluripotent embryonic stem cells (ES cells) are not easily derived [32,33] from the inner cell mass of blastocyst stage embryos. Therefore, ES cell lines for gene targeting are simply not available. This severely hampers the ability to use DBA/2J mice to assess the role of specific genes in many human diseases. Previously, introducing mutant alleles into DBA/2J mice required targeting of the allele in an available ES cell line (usually B6- or 129-derived), followed by extensive backcrossing of the mutation to DBA/2J (for greater than 10 generations to replace the ES cell genome with a DBA/2J genome). Even after extensive backcrossing, a substantial interval of ES cell-derived DNA will remain surrounding the targeted gene, potentially confounding analysis of the phenotype.

Previous attempts to derive ES cell lines from DBA/2J mice have failed and therefore the DBA/2J strain is considered to be recalcitrant to ES cell derivation [33]. However, recent advances in stem cell biology have revealed that embryonic stem cells derived from the inner cell mass of some strains and some species (like the laboratory rat) have a limited capacity to maintain pluripotency and self-renewal in culture without consistent inhibition of signaling pathways that promote early differentiation [34,35]. Therefore, addition of small molecule inhibitors of fibroblast growth factor (FGF)/mitogen-activated protein kinase (MEK)/extracellular signal-related kinase pathways and of glycogen synthase kinase 3 (Gsk3) have proven highly effective for successful derivation of ES cells from rats and from a recalcitrant mouse strain (NOD) [36]. Taking advantage of this renewed understanding of ES cell pluripotency, we surmised that recalcitrance in DBA/2J is likely due to the same underlying differentiation pathways. By inhibiting these pathways we successfully derived germ line competent ES cells. Using these cells, we have generated the first engineered allele in the DBA/2J genome.

Methods

Mouse Strains, Breeding and Husbandry

All DBA/2J mice used in this study were obtained from either The Jackson Laboratory production facility (Bar Harbor, ME) or from our research colony. Our DBA/2J colony is routinely crossed with DBA/2J mice from The Jackson Laboratory production facility to prevent genetic drift. Mice were housed in a 14 h light to

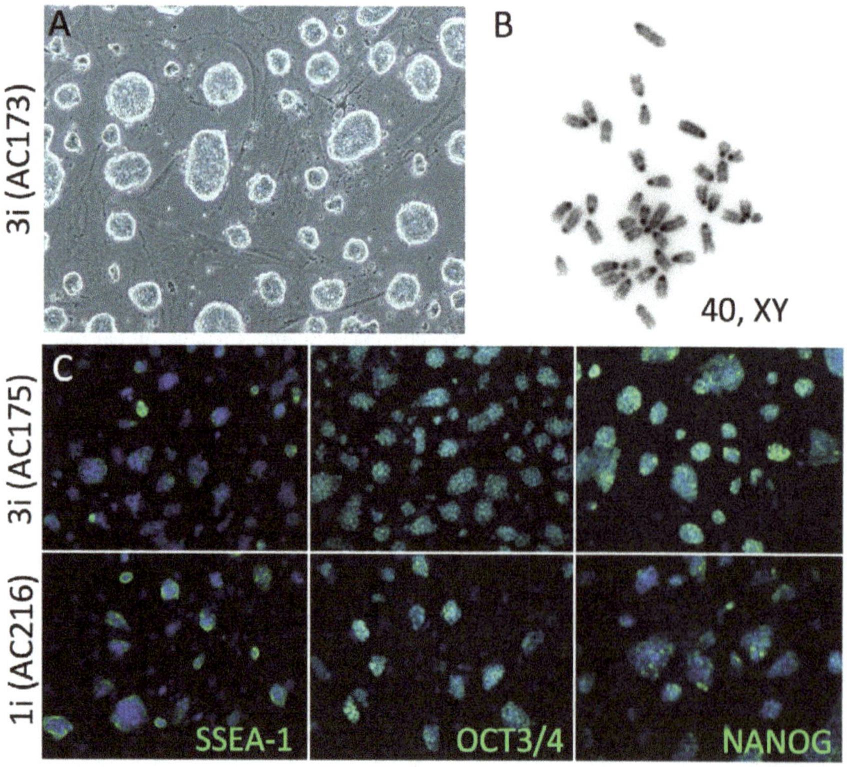

Figure 1. DBA/2J ES cell derivation. (**A**) In each round of derivation, 11–60% of embryos gave rise to stable embryonic stem cell lines (see also Table 1). (**B**) Approximately ~20% of lines were male with normal chromosome counts, regardless of culture conditions. (C) All of the ES cell lines, regardless of culture conditions, expressed the essential pluripotency markers NANOG, SSEA-1 and OCT-3/4 (POU5F1).

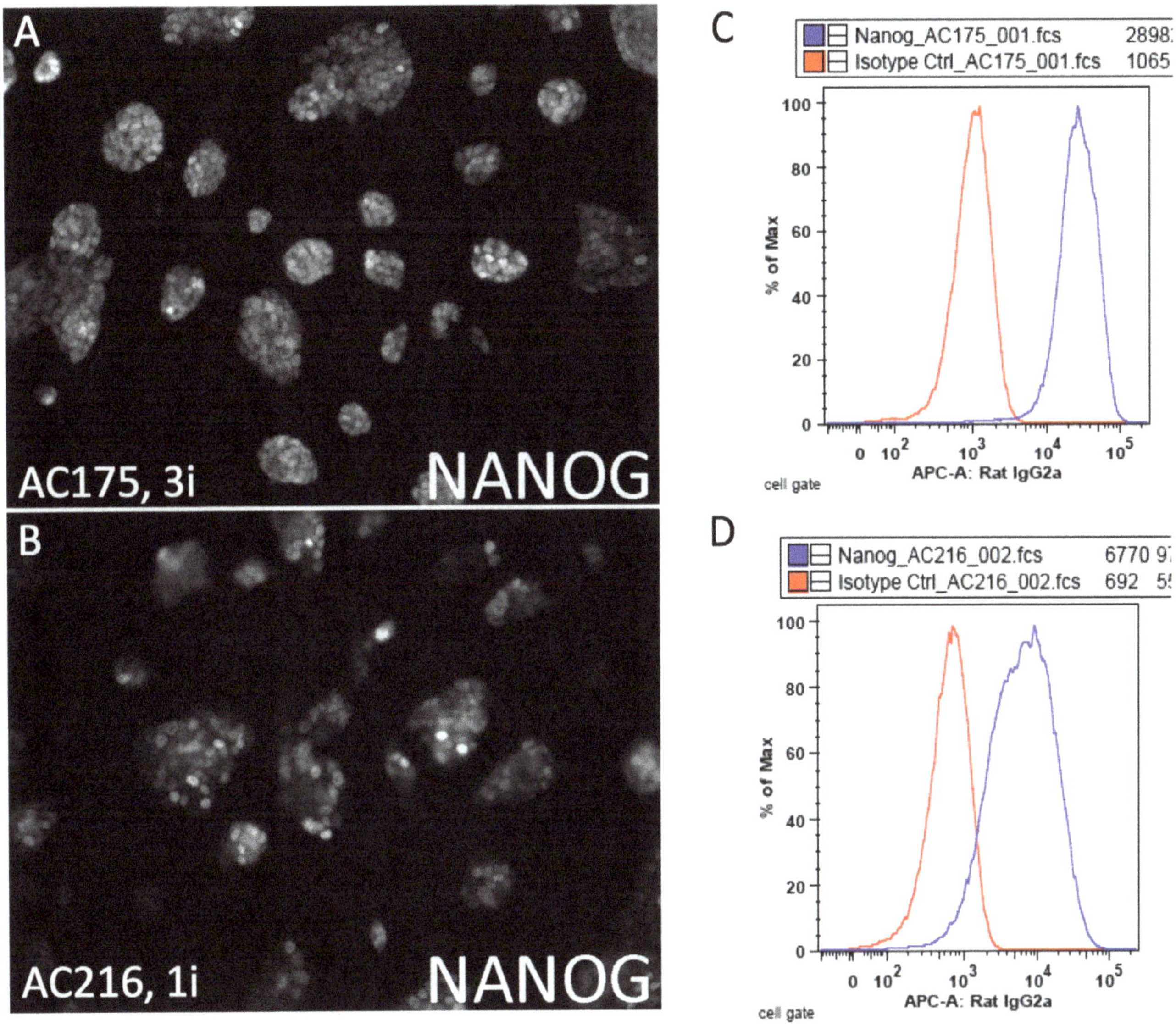

Figure 2. Variable NANOG expression in DBA/2J ES cell lines. (**A–D**) Representative images and FLOW analysis of 3i (AC175, A,C) and 1i lines (AC216, B,D) immunolabeled with an antibody to NANOG. Robust NANOG expression was characteristic of lines derived and cultured in 3i conditions.

10 h dark cycle under previously described conditions [37]. The Jackson Laboratory Animal Care and Use Committee approved all of the experiments in this study.

Generation of DBA/2J-derived ES Cells

Embryo harvest and inner cell mass (ICM) outgrowth. Embryos from natural DBA/2J matings were

Table 1. DBA/2J ES cell derivation.

Media conditions	Number of blastocysts	% blastocytes that gave ES cell lines (n)	Number of euploid, male ES cell lines
3i, derivation 1	36	22% (8)	0
3i, derivation 2	20	60% (12)	4
1i, derivation 1	36	11% (4)	1
1i derivation 2	20	60% (12)	4
1i, C57BL/6J	20	70% (14)	4

Two derivations of two different media types were used to derive DBA/2J ES cell (rows 1–4) and was compared to a control derivation using C57BL/6J blastocysts (row 5). Details are provided for: the total number of blastocyst attempted (column 2); the % of blastocysts that gave ES cell lines (column 3); and the total number of euploid male ES cell lines generated for each derivation (column 4).

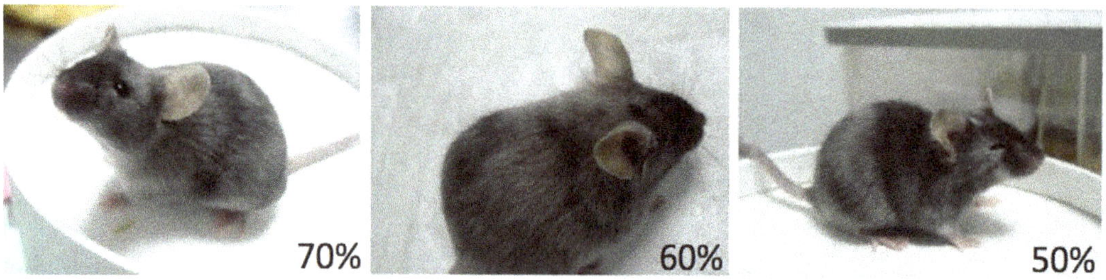

Figure 3. DBA/2J ES cell-derived male chimeras. DBA/2J ES cells were injected into C57BL/6J-derived blastocyst. Estimated percentage of coat derived from DBA/2J ES cells (dilute brown agouti) was used to determine the percent chimerism in each pup.

collected at 3.5 days post coitum by flushing uteri with M2 medium (Millipore). Blastocysts were transferred directly to MEF feeder layers (cell cycle arrested mouse embryonic fibroblasts) in 4-well IVF (in vitro fertilization) culture dishes, 1–2 blastocysts per well. Morulae were cultured overnight in KSOM/M16 (Millipore) medium and the resulting blastocysts were transferred to MEF feeder layers the following day. Blastocysts were then cultured at 37°C, 5% CO_2 for 8–10 days. During the first 4 days, blastocysts were undisturbed to allow for zona hatching and attachment of the embryos to the feeder layers. During days 5–10, the media were replaced every other day and inner cell mass (ICM) outgrowth was observed. The media conditions of ICM outgrowth were either '1i outgrowth media' or '3i media'.

ES cell media. DMEM (Dulbecco's Modified Eagle's Medium, 4500 mg/L glucose and sodium bicarbonate, without L-glutamine and sodium pyruvate, Sigma), 15% fetal calf serum (Lonza), penicillin (100 units)/streptomycin (100 µg) (Life Technologies), Glutamax (1X, Life Technologies), 0.1 mM beta-mercaptoethanol, non-essential amino acids (1X, Life Technologies), sodium pyruvate (1 mM, Life Tecnologies), leukemia inhibitory factor (LIF, ESGRO 1000 U/ml, Chemicon).

1i outgrowth media. ES cell media (as described above) containing KOSR (knockout serum replacement, Life Technologies) in place of fetal calf serum, and PD98059 (MAP kinase inhibitor, 50 µM, Calbiochem [32]) with LIF (1000 U/ml).

3i media. serum free media (as described in [34]] containing 3 inhibitors (PD17304 (FGF receptor tyrosine kinase inhibitor, 100 nM, Stemgent), PD0325901 (MEK kinase inhibitor, 1 µM, Stemgent) and CHIR99021 (glycogen synthase kinase-3 inhibitor, 3 µM)), and LIF (leukemia inhibitory factor, ESGRO 1000 U/ml, Chemicon).

Disaggregation and culture. After 8–10 days, each outgrowth was given a unique identification number (AC###) and mechanically disaggregated. Disaggregated fragments were plated onto new MEF feeder layers in the same media type used for outgrowth (except for 1i media where KOSR was replaced with serum). After ~2 days of growth, each emergent cell line was enzymatically dissociated using 0.05% trypsin EDTA (Life Technologies) and re-plated (P1). Light microscopy was used to monitor cell dissociation and trypsin exposure time was adjusted accordingly (usually 2–4 minutes depending on the culture conditions and cell line).

Emergent cell lines grown in 3i serum free media required less exposure (~2 minutes) to 0.05% trypsin for dissociation and trypsin inhibition (using an equal volume of defined trypsin inhibitor, DTI, Life Technologies). Each cell line was expanded to P4 and any lines with overt differentiation or poor growth were discarded.

ES Cell Line Characterization

Karyotypic analysis. ES cells were grown in 60 mm culture dishes until sub-confluent. Approximately 1–2 hours after media replacement, colcemid (0.02 mg/ml) was added to the media and the cells were incubated at 37°C, 5% CO_2 for three hours. Cells were trypsinized, re-suspended by slow addition 0.56% KCl with constant agitation and incubated for 30–60 minutes. Cells were then fixed with ice-cold 3:1 methanol:glacial acetic acid. Fixed cell suspensions were added dropwise to the surface of clean, moist glass slides and slides were air dried at 37°C for 1–2 days. Slides were mounted with Vectashield® hard set mounting reagent with DAPI (4′, 6-diamidino-2-phenylindole) (Vector Laboratories). A Spectral Karyotyping Microscope (SKY, Applied Spectral Imaging, Ltd.) was used to automatically scan slides for mitotic chromosome spreads and images were digitally captured. Chromosomes were counted in at least 40 well-spread, well-isolated nuclei and sex chromosomes were identified by morphology and

Table 2. Chimerism and germ line transmission of DBA/2J ES cells.

Cell line, culture condition	% of chimeric mice born (n)	% male chimeras	% germline chimeras	transmission rate (male only)
AC203, 1i	16% (19)	67%	100%	100%
AC216, 1i	38% (13)	100%	20%	100%
AC173, 3i	59% (37)	68%	92%	97%
AC175, 3i	46% (13)	100%	67%	100%

Four DBA/2J ES cell lines (two derived from each media type, 1i and 3i) were assessed for capacity to contribute to the germ line. These data are based on standard microinjection of ES cells into C57BL/6J host blastocysts. Additional data, including laser assisted microinjection data can be found in Table S1. Details are provided for: the number of chimeric mice (determined based on coat showing at least partial dilute brown agouti color, column 2); the % of those chimeric mice that were male (column 3); the % of male chimeric mice that sired offspring with 100% dilute brown agouti color (column 4); and the % of offspring that were completely dilute brown agouti (transmission rate, column 5).

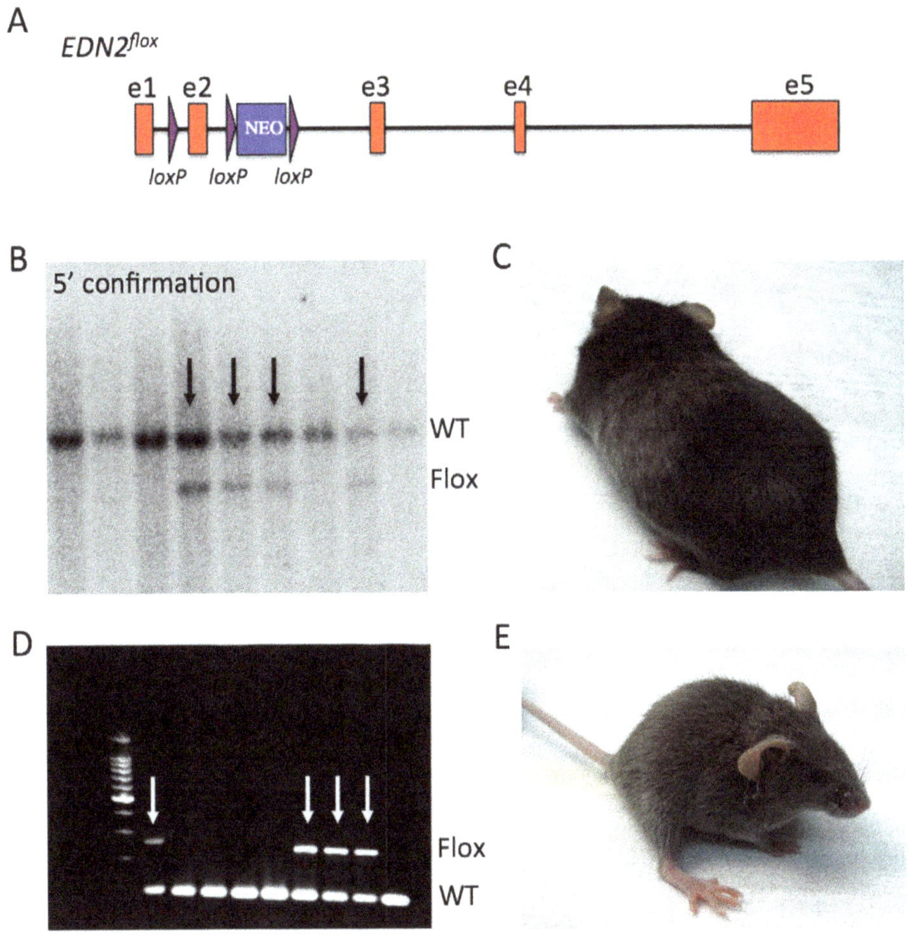

Figure 4. Generating a conditional allele of *Edn2* directly in DBA/2J-derived ES cells. (**A**) A targeting construct was generated that included *loxP* sites flanking exon 2 (e2) of the *Edn2* gene. Exon 2 contains part of the key functional domain for Edn2, and removal of exon 2 induces a frameshift for protein translation (**B**) Correct targeting at the 5′ end of the Edn2 gene was assessed using Xba1 restriction digests and southern blotting. The presence of the Neomycin (NEO) selectable marker incorporates an additional *Xba*1 restriction enzyme site in the targeted allele, generating a 6.6 kb fragment (Flox) compared to the normal 8.7 kb fragment (WT). Black arrows indicate clones correctly targeted at the 5′ end. (**C**) An example of a chimeric mouse generated as a result of injection of targeted DBA/2J ES cell clones into C57BL/6J blastocysts. (**D–E**) Chimeric male mice were mated with DBA/2J females and offspring genotyped for the heterozygous presence of the loxP sites in intron 1 (WT = 481 bp, Flox = 631 bp, see Methods). White arrows indicate mice that carry the floxed allele of *Edn2*. (D). See methods for primer information. As expected, 100% of heterozygous mutant offspring had the DBA/2J coat color (dilute brown agouti, E).

distribution of heterochromatin (as assessed by DAPI, which preferentially binds A-T rich DNA).

Immunolabeling. Sub-confluent ES cells were fixed with 4% paraformaldehyde (PFA) for 20 minutes and washed 3×5 minutes with phosphate buffered saline (PBS). Fixed cells were then blocked with 5% fetal bovine serum (FBS), 0.1% triton-X for 15 minutes, incubated with primary antibody for 4 hours and washed 3×5 minutes with PBS. Secondary antibody incubations were 2 hours, and subsequent washes were 3×5 minutes with PBS, incubation with DAPI (2 mg/ml) for 10 minutes and 2×5 minute washes with PBS. Primary antibodies were anti-OCT 3/4 (1:250, Santa Cruz Biologicals, #sc-5279), anti-NANOG (1:250, Abcam, #ab21603) and anti-SSEA-1 (1:250, Santa Cruz Biologicals, #sc-21702). Secondary antibodies were goat anti-mouse IgG Alexa Fluor® 488 (1:1000, Life Technologies) and goat anti-rabbit IgG Alexa Fluor® 488 (1:1000, Life Technologies). All antibodies were diluted with PBS, 1% FBS. All incubations and washes were performed at room temperature with gentle rocking. Labeled cells were visualized and images were collected with a Zeiss Axio Observer Z1 inverted microscope and a Zeiss AxioCam CCD camera.

To prepare and immunolabel ES cells for flow cytometry, cells were washed, counted and fixed in 4% PFA (100 µl per 1×10^{6} cells) for 15 minutes at room temperature. Cells were then washed 2×5 minutes in PBS, 1% FBS and stored in 1 ml aliquots at 1×10^{6} cells/ml for up to 72 hours at 4°C. For antibody labeling, cells were transferred to 12×75 mm polypropylene tubes, permeabilized for 15 minutes (Perm/Wash Buffer, BD Biosciences), incubated with mouse Fc block (purified rat IgG_{2b} anti-mouse CD16/CD32 monoclonal antibody, BD Biosciences) for 15 minutes, split and then incubated with either rat anti-Nanog Alexa Fluor® 647 (50 µg/ml, eBioscience) or rat IgG2a isotype control Alexa Fluor® 647 (eBioscience). Post-labeling washes were 2×5 minutes in PBS, 1% FBS and cells were resuspended in 400 µl of PBS, 1% FBS. Immunolabeled cells were then analyzed using a FACSCalibur flow cytometer (BD Biosciences).

Microinjection and Chimera Production for Parental ES Cell Lines

Each parental ES cell line (AC203, AC216, AC173 and AC175) was tested for germ line competence by microinjection. For each line, ~12 ES cells were microinjected into 50 C57BL/6J (black, *a/a*, The Jackson Laboratory stock #00664) host blastocysts and 6 ES cells were injected into 8 cell C57BL/6J embryos by the laser assisted method using a Hamilton Thorne XYClone. Male coat color chimeras were generated from both injection methods. Male chimeras were bred to DBA/2J females (dilute brown, *a/a* $Tyrp1^b/Tyrp1^b$ $Myo5a^d/Myo5a^d$, The Jackson Laboratory stock #000671) and germ line transmission of the DBA/2J ES cell line was assessed by calculating the % dilute brown offspring over three litters for each fertile male chimera.

Generation of EDN2 Targeting Construct, pMCS-EDN2-DTA

A Frt-Loxp (FL) was inserted in intron 1 and a LNL (Loxp-Neo-Loxp) cassette was inserted in intron 2 of *Edn2* gene on a BAC clone (RP23-265J18) by BAC recombineering so that exon 2 of *Edn2* gene was flanked by two loxp sites. A gene targeting vector, pMCS-EDN2-DTA, was constructed by retrieving a 10 kb long homology arm (5′ to FL), LNL, and a 2 kb short homology arm (end of LNL to 3′) into a plasmid vector carrying the DTA (Diphtheria toxin alpha chain) negative selection marker.

Targeting DBA/2J ES Cells with *Edn2* Conditional Knockout Construct

Prior to targeting, the following parameters for DBA/2J ES cell line AC173 were established; geneticin sensitivity (150 µg/mL), required working concentration of trypsin inhibitor (0.25 mg/mL), and compatibility of serum free media with available MEF stocks (irradiated at passage 3 or lower). In preparation for electroporation, pMCS-EDN2-DTA was prepared using a mini-prep kit (Qiagen) and DNA linearized with *Not*I. Electroporation was performed using the BTX ECM 830 electroporator. Ten million DBA/2J ES cells (line AC173, P9) were electroporated with 20 µg of DNA at a concentration of 3.8 µg/uL. Cells were plated onto 60 mm dishes in 3i media. Selection with geneticin at 150 µg/mL was started the following day and continued for 9 days. Plates were then switched back to media not containing selection antibiotic until day 12 post electroporation. On day 12, colonies from half the 60 mm plates were picked, selecting each independent colony into a separate 96 well. Colonies from the remaining 60 mm plates were picked on day 13 for a total of 46 colonies. Clones were expanded into two sets of 96 well plates to allow for a stock freeze of one set of 96 well plates and lysate preparation for their duplicates for Southern blot screening. Clones were maintained on MEFs due to poor growth of the DBA/2J line in the absence of MEFs. A total of 43 clones were frozen.

Confirmation of Correct Targeting by Southern Blotting

For each of the 43 clones, Southern blotting was used to assess correct targeting of the 5′ end of the *Edn2* locus. A 622bp 5′ probe was generated upstream of the *Edn2* gene (forward primer, GATGTGGGTGGCCAGTGGC; reverse primer, GCTGGGAGCAGAGGCCAGGTG). DNA from each of the 43 clones was digested with *Xba*1. Correct integration of the targeting construct introduced a novel *Xba*I site to generate a 6.6 kb band after digestion compared to an 8.7 kb band for non-targeted clones. Five of the 43 clones were correctly targeted on the 5′ end (clones 5, 32, 33, 34, and 36), a targeting efficiency of approximately 11.5% of tested clones. For these five clones, Southern blotting was again used to assess correct targeting at the 3′ end. A 1001 bp 3′ probe was generated by PCR (forward primer, AGTAGACAGTGGACAGTTCC; reverse primer, CAAAAGTGTCCCAAGAGAACAGT). Correct integration of the targeting construct at the 3′ end disrupted an *Eco*RI site to generate a 16.2 kb band after digestion compared to a 15.2 kb band for non-targeted clones. Clones 33 and 36 were identified as properly targeted on both ends. (All primers shown 5′ to 3′).

Microinjection of Targeted Clones and Confirmation of Germ Line Transmission

For microinjection of EDN2-targeted AC173 ES cell lines, the correctly targeted clones (33 and 36) were thawed from 96 well plates to 12 well MEF plates using 3i media and injected into C57BL/6J blastocysts (~12 ES cells per embryo). Both clones were at passage 22 at the time of injection. Passage number indicates the total number of trypsin exposures from the emergence of the ES cell line (see *Disaggregation and culture* above). In total, 149 injected blastocysts (approximately half from each of clone 33 and 36) were transferred into 13 pseudopregnant B6(Cg)-*Tyr*<c-2J>/J recipients (albino). For clone 33, 3 chimeric pups were produced (all male) and for clone 36, 2 chimeric pups (1 male and 1 female). Percentage chimerism ranged from 20–50% for both clones (based on coat color).

Mouse Genotyping

To determine the presence or absence of the $EDN2^{flox}$ allele, *Edn2*-Intron2-F (CATAGAGCGGTGAGGCCACAG) and *Edn2*-Intron2-R: (AAGTTGGCACCCTTGGTGTTC) primers were used. The primers amplify a region of intron 2 that includes the first *loxP* site ($Edn2^+$ allele, 113bp; $Edn2^{flox}$ allele, 259bp).

Results

DBA/2J ES Cell Derivation

To define the most efficient protocol for derivation of ES cell lines from DBA/2J, we tested two media conditions that have been previously shown to promote ES cell derivation efficiency and ES cell pluripotency for other recalcitrant mouse strains. These media were tested in parallel over two rounds of derivation. The first medium, '1i', was standard mouse ES cell medium, including LIF (leukemia inhibitory factor) and a single inhibitor of MAP kinase/ERK kinase, PD98059. This medium was previously shown to promote ES cell derivation efficiency from the recalcitrant CBA mouse strain [32]. More recently, several laboratories have had great success deriving ES cells not only from recalcitrant mouse strains (e.g. NOD), but also recalcitrant species (rat) by using defined serum free culture conditions combined with inhibitors of MEK kinase, FGF receptor tyrosine kinase and glycogen synthase kinase-3 [34,35,38]. Therefore, the second media condition, '3i' was serum free media, including LIF and 3 inhibitors, PD17304 (FGF receptor tyrosine kinase inhibitor), PD0325901 (MEK kinase inhibitor, 1 µM, Stemgent) and CHIR99021 (glycogen synthase kinase-3 inhibitor) [34]. Finally, to promote growth of the inner cell mass and to minimize trophoblast differentiation, FBS was excluded from the 1i media during the inner cell mass (ICM) outgrowth stage.

Comparing Derivation Media

ES cell lines were derived from a total of 112 DBA/2J embryos over 2 rounds of derivation (derivation 1 and derivation 2) as shown in Table 1. Regardless of the media used, ES cell derivation efficiency (number of established ES cell lines/number of embryos) was comparable to permissive strains like C57BL/6J and significantly better than has been previously reported for DBA/2J, 1–6% [33]. From a total of 36 ES cell lines, 9 were euploid (>70% normal chromosome counts over 40 nuclei) male lines. These 9 lines were further characterized to select a subset of lines for germ line testing (Figure 1). All 9 ES cell lines showed expression of alkaline phosphatase and the pluripotency markers NANOG, SSEA-1 and OCT 3/4 (POU5F1), however ES cell lines that were derived and cultured in 1i medium showed variable expression of NANOG compared to ES cell lines derived and cultured in 3i medium. This variable expression was evident both qualitatively by immunofluorescence microscopy and quantitatively by flow cytometry, where a broad range of NANOG expression was consistently present in 1i cultures, including a fraction of ES cells with NANOG expression as low as background (Figure 2).

Assessing Chimerism and Germ Line Efficiency

The capacity of an ES cell line to contribute to the germ line of a chimeric animal is the gold standard test of pluripotency for mouse ES cell lines and a pre-requisite for any ES cell line to be used to generate genetically engineered mice. Four DBA/2J ES cell lines were selected for germ line testing based on media conditions (two 1i ES cell lines and two 3i ES cell lines), NANOG expression, and chromosome counts (those with the highest percent of euploid nuclei were favored). These were AC203 (1i, 86% euploid), AC216 (1i, 86% euploid), AC175 (3i, 78% euploid) and AC173 (3i, 86% euploid). All four ES cell lines successfully contributed to chimeras and to the germ line, as determined by coat color (Table 2, Figure 3). The 2 ES cell lines derived and grown in 3i conditions (AC175 and AC173) produced larger percentages of coat color chimeras upon injection into C57BL/6J host embryos, consistent with the more robust expression of the pluripotency factor NANOG in these ES cell lines (Table S1).

Testing Gene Targeting Efficiency in DBA/2J ES Cells

The DBA/2J strain is a widely used mouse model of glaucoma. Glaucoma is characterized by the degeneration of retinal ganglion cells and the degeneration of the optic nerve. We have shown previously that Endothelin-2 (*Edn2*), a component of the endothelin system is upregulated in monocytes and microglia-like cells in the retina and optic nerve during glaucoma [4,5]. Given that no conditional allele was available for *Edn2* on a DBA/2J background, *Edn2* was selected as the gene of interest to assess targeting capabilities for the newly derived DBA/2J ES cells. A targeting construct was generated and used to target the AC173 ES cell line (one of the parental lines with robust NANOG expression and a high degree of chimerism in earlier tests, Figure 4). After targeting and subsequent colony expansion, 43 clones were assessed for correct targeting of the *Edn2* locus. Five of the 43 clones (11%) were correctly targeted on the 5′ end, two of which were also correctly targeted on the 3′ end. These two clones (*Edn2*-clone33 and *Edn2*-clone36) were injected into C57BL/6J blastocysts and chimeric pups obtained. Chimerism for mice derived from either clone ranged from 20–50% (Table S1). Male chimeric mice were bred to DBA/2J females and approximately 50% of offspring were heterozygous for the conditional *Edn2* allele. More than 20 mice heterozygous have been aged for 6–12 months. They have a healthy appearance with no gross adverse phenotypes or premature death.

Discussion

We have demonstrated that ES cells can be derived from DBA/2J mice and that these ES cells are competent to contribute to the germ line both at low passages and higher passages, post-targeting. Moreover, we report the first use of these DBA/2J ES cells to generate a genetically engineered mouse strain. While both media conditions used to derive DBA/2J ES cells favored successful derivation of germ line competent cells, serum free 3i media promoted more robust NANOG expression and higher percentages of coat color chimeras. This is likely due to inhibition of FGF signaling through more efficient inhibition of phospho-ERK combined with the restorative effects of glycogen synthase kinase inhibition [34]. A recent study indicates that inhibition of the FGF receptor tyrosine kinase through PD173074 is not necessary in combination with PD0325901, hence 2i media was equally effective for maintenance of pluripotency in ES cells [39]. Efficient inhibition of FGF signaling promotes the pluripotent ground state of embryonic stems cells, the hallmark of which is NANOG expression [40].

Serum free, 3i culture conditions are frequently used in the absence of MEFs feeder layers since the leukemia inhibitory factor provided by the MEF's can instead be added to the culture medium. However, we found that in the absence of feeders, emergent ES cell lines in serum free, 3i medium were loosely adherent, despite the use of gelatin-coated plates. This made them subsequently difficult to manipulate during gene targeting. Therefore, MEF feeder layers were used throughout our derivation, culture and targeting of DBA/2J ES cells regardless of the culture media used. We found that use of low passage MEFs that have been previously screened for tolerance to serum free culture was critical for maintenance of our serum free, 3i DBA/2J ES cells, especially during drug selection post-targeting where feeder layers are exposed, long term to serum free culture conditions.

The availability of DBA/2J ES cells will enable genetic manipulation of genes of interest directly on a DBA/2J background. As we have shown with the *Edn2* gene, it is possible to generate conditional alleles without the need for costly and time-consuming backcrossing from other genetic backgrounds (commonly C57BL/6J or 6N). Targeting constructs for many genes are available through the Knockout Mouse Project. Although many constructs were generated using C57BL/6N, many will be useful for generation of conditional alleles directly in DBA/2J ES cells. This will greatly aid in the ability to test the role(s) of specific genes of interest. Importantly, this ability means that no congenic interval that is derived from the original strain and that can confound experiments will surround the targeted gene.

In summary, the derivation of ES cells from DBA/2J mice will accelerate the ability to generate genetically engineered DBA/2J mice. These resources will aid in the understanding of and the development of improved therapies for a wide variety of human diseases including glaucoma, deafness and schizophrenia.

Acknowledgments

The authors would like to thank Scientific Services at The Jackson Laboratory, in particular John Kulik, Stephanie Dion and Charles Lerner from Microinjection and Leslie Goodwin from Molecular Biology.

Author Contributions

Conceived and designed the experiments: LR GRH LRD SJ. Performed the experiments: LR GRH AC DM KM CSL. Analyzed the data: LR GRH SWMJ. Contributed reagents/materials/analysis tools: LR GH CSL LRD SWMJ. Wrote the paper: LR GH LRH SWMJ.

References

1. Anderson MG, Smith RS, Hawes NL, Zabaleta A, Chang B, et al. (2002) Mutations in genes encoding melanosomal proteins cause pigmentary glaucoma in DBA/2J mice. Nat Genet 30: 81–85.
2. Bosco A, Inman DM, Steele MR, Wu G, Soto I, et al. (2008) Reduced retina microglial activation and improved optic nerve integrity with minocycline treatment in the DBA/2J mouse model of glaucoma. Invest Ophthalmol Vis Sci 49: 1437–1446.
3. Calkins DJ, Horner PJ, Roberts R, Gradianu M, Berkowitz BA (2008) Manganese-enhanced MRI of the DBA/2J mouse model of hereditary glaucoma. Invest Ophthalmol Vis Sci 49: 5083–5088.
4. Howell GR, Macalinao DG, Sousa GS, Walden M, Soto I, et al. (2011) Molecular clustering identifies complement and endothelin induction as early events in a mouse model of glaucoma. Journal of Clinical Investigation 121: 1429–1444.
5. Howell GR, Soto I, Zhu X, Ryan M, Macalinao DG, et al. (2012) Radiation treatment inhibits monocyte entry into the optic nerve head and prevents neuronal damage in a mouse model of glaucoma. The Journal of clinical investigation 122: 1246–1261.
6. Inman DM, Horner PJ (2007) Reactive nonproliferative gliosis predominates in a chronic mouse model of glaucoma. Glia 55: 942–953.
7. Libby RT, Anderson MG, Pang IH, Robinson ZH, Savinova OV, et al. (2005) Inherited glaucoma in DBA/2J mice: pertinent disease features for studying the neurodegeneration. Vis Neurosci 22: 637–648.
8. May CA, Mittag T (2006) Optic nerve degeneration in the DBA/2NNia mouse: is the lamina cribrosa important in the development of glaucomatous optic neuropathy? Acta Neuropathol (Berl) 111: 158–167.
9. Nagaraju M, Saleh M, Porciatti V (2007) IOP-dependent retinal ganglion cell dysfunction in glaucomatous DBA/2J mice. Invest Ophthalmol Vis Sci 48: 4573–4579.
10. Panagis L, Zhao X, Ge Y, Ren L, Mittag TW, et al. (2009) Gene Expression Changes in Areas of Focal Loss of Retinal Ganglion Cells (RGC) in the Retina of DBA/2J Mice. Invest Ophthalmol Vis Sci 51: 2024–2034.
11. Schlamp CL, Li Y, Dietz JA, Janssen KT, Nickells RW (2006) Progressive ganglion cell loss and optic nerve degeneration in DBA/2J mice is variable and asymmetric. BMC Neurosci 7: 66.
12. Schuettauf F, Rejdak R, Walski M, Frontczak-Baniewicz M, Voelker M, et al. (2004) Retinal neurodegeneration in the DBA/2J mouse-a model for ocular hypertension. Acta Neuropathol (Berl) 107: 352–358.
13. Chung SH, Johnson MS (1984) Studies on sound-induced epilepsy in mice. Proceedings of the Royal Society of London Series B, Containing papers of a Biological character Royal Society 221: 145–168.
14. Connolly PM, Maxwell CR, Kanes SJ, Abel T, Liang Y, et al. (2003) Inhibition of auditory evoked potentials and prepulse inhibition of startle in DBA/2J and DBA/2Hsd inbred mouse substrains. Brain research 992: 85–95.
15. Alberts R, Srivastava B, Wu H, Viegas N, Geffers R, et al. (2010) Gene expression changes in the host response between resistant and susceptible inbred mouse strains after influenza A infection. Microbes and infection/Institut Pasteur 12: 309–318.
16. Drake TA, Schadt E, Hannani K, Kabo JM, Krass K, et al. (2001) Genetic loci determining bone density in mice with diet-induced atherosclerosis. Physiol Genomics 5: 205–215.
17. Nedelko T, Kollmus H, Klawonn F, Spijker S, Lu L, et al. (2012) Distinct gene loci control the host response to influenza H1N1 virus infection in a time-dependent manner. BMC genomics 13: 411.
18. Paigen B (1995) Genetics of responsiveness to high-fat and high-cholesterol diets in the mouse. Am J Clin Nutr 62: 458S–462S.
19. Willott JF, Bosch JV, Shimizu T, Ding DL (2006) Effects of exposing DBA/2J mice to a high-frequency augmented acoustic environment on the cochlea and anteroventral cochlear nucleus. Hear Res 216–217: 138–145.
20. Philip VM, Duvvuru S, Gomero B, Ansah TA, Blaha CD, et al. (2009) High-throughput behavioral phenotyping in the expanded panel of BXD recombinant inbred strains. Genes Brain Behav.
21. Pichard C, Gorwood PA, Hamon M, Cohen-Salmon C (2009) Differential effects of free versus imposed motor activity on alcohol consumption in C57BL/6J versus DBA/2J mice. Alcohol 43: 593–601.
22. Wang X, Chen Y, Lu L Genetic regulatory network analysis for app based on genetical genomics approach. Exp Aging Res 36: 79–93.
23. Davis RC, Schadt EE, Smith DJ, Hsieh EW, Cervino AC, et al. (2005) A genome-wide set of congenic mouse strains derived from DBA/2J on a C57BL/6J background. Genomics 86: 259–270.
24. Anderson MG, Smith RS, Savinova OV, Hawes NL, Chang B, et al. (2001) Genetic modification of glaucoma associated phenotypes between AKXD-28/Ty and DBA/2J mice. BMC genetics 2: 1.
25. Gilbert DJ, Neumann PE, Taylor BA, Jenkins NA, Copeland NG (1993) Susceptibility of AKXD recombinant inbred mouse strains to lymphomas. Journal of virology 67: 2083–2090.
26. Boughter JD, Jr., Mulligan MK, St John SJ, Tokita K, Lu L, et al. (2012) Genetic Control of a Central Pattern Generator: Rhythmic Oromotor Movement in Mice Is Controlled by a Major Locus near Atp1a2. PloS one 7: e38169.
27. Hsu HC, Lu L, Yi N, Van Zant G, Williams RW, et al. (2007) Quantitative trait locus (QTL) mapping in aging systems. Methods in molecular biology 371: 321–348.
28. Jellen LC, Beard JL, Jones BC (2009) Systems genetics analysis of iron regulation in the brain. Biochimie 91: 1255–1259.
29. McKnite AM, Perez-Munoz ME, Lu L, Williams EG, Brewer S, et al. (2012) Murine gut microbiota is defined by host genetics and modulates variation of metabolic traits. PloS one 7: e39191.
30. Mountz JD, Van Zant GE, Zhang HG, Grizzle WE, Ahmed R, et al. (2001) Genetic dissection of age-related changes of immune function in mice. Scandinavian journal of immunology 54: 10–20.
31. Chesler EJ, Lu L, Wang J, Williams RW, Manly KF (2004) WebQTL: rapid exploratory analysis of gene expression and genetic networks for brain and behavior. Nature neuroscience 7: 485–486.
32. Buehr M, Smith A (2003) Genesis of embryonic stem cells. Philos Trans R Soc Lond B Biol Sci 358: 1397–1402; discussion 1402.
33. Gardner RL, Brook FA (1997) Reflections on the biology of embryonic stem (ES) cells. Int J Dev Biol 41: 235–243.
34. Ying QL, Wray J, Nichols J, Batlle-Morera L, Doble B, et al. (2008) The ground state of embryonic stem cell self-renewal. Nature 453: 519–523.
35. Hanna J, Markoulaki S, Mitalipova M, Cheng AW, Cassady JP, et al. (2009) Metastable pluripotent states in NOD-mouse-derived ESCs. Cell Stem Cell 4: 513–524.
36. Nichols J, Jones K, Phillips JM, Newland SA, Roode M, et al. (2009) Validated germline-competent embryonic stem cell lines from nonobese diabetic mice. Nat Med 15: 814–818.
37. Smith RS, Zabaleta A, Kume T, Savinova OV, Kidson SH, et al. (2000) Haploinsufficiency of the transcription factors FOXC1 and FOXC2 results in aberrant ocular development. Hum Mol Genet 9: 1021–1032.
38. Buehr M, Meek S, Blair K, Yang J, Ure J, et al. (2008) Capture of authentic embryonic stem cells from rat blastocysts. Cell 135: 1287–1298.
39. Silva J, Barrandon O, Nichols J, Kawaguchi J, Theunissen TW, et al. (2008) Promotion of reprogramming to ground state pluripotency by signal inhibition. PLoS Biol 6: e253.
40. Silva J, Nichols J, Theunissen TW, Guo G, van Oosten AL, et al. (2009) Nanog is the gateway to the pluripotent ground state. Cell 138: 722–737.

10

An Alteration in the Lateral Geniculate Nucleus of Experimental Glaucoma Monkeys: *In vivo* Positron Emission Tomography Imaging of Glial Activation

Masamitsu Shimazawa[1], Yasushi Ito[1], Yuta Inokuchi[1], Hajime Yamanaka[2], Tomohiro Nakanishi[1], Takuya Hayashi[2], Bin Ji[3], Makoto Higuchi[3], Tetsuya Suhara[3], Kazuyuki Imamura[4], Makoto Araie[5], Yasuyoshi Watanabe[2], Hirotaka Onoe[2], Hideaki Hara[1]*

1 Molecular Pharmacology, Department of Biofunctional Evaluation, Gifu Pharmaceutical University, Gifu, Japan, **2** RIKEN Center for Molecular Imaging Science, Kobe, Japan, **3** Molecular Imaging Center, National Institute of Radiological Sciences, Chiba, Japan, **4** Department of Systems Life Engineering, Maebashi Institute of Technology, Maibashi, Japan, **5** Department of Ophthalmology, University of Tokyo School of Medicine, Tokyo, Japan

Abstract

We examined lateral geniculate nucleus (LGN) degeneration as an indicator for possible diagnosis of glaucoma in experimental glaucoma monkeys using positron emission tomography (PET). Chronic intraocular pressure (IOP) elevation was induced by laser trabeculoplasty in the left eyes of 5 cynomolgus monkeys. Glial cell activation was detected by PET imaging with [^{11}C]PK11195, a PET ligand for peripheral-type benzodiazepine receptor (PBR), before and at 4 weeks after laser treatment (moderate glaucoma stage). At mild, moderate, and advanced experimental glaucoma stages (classified by histological changes based on the extent of axonal loss), brains were stained with cresyl violet, or antibodies against PBR, Iba-1 (a microglial marker), and GFAP (an activated astrocyte marker). In laser-treated eyes, IOP was persistently elevated throughout all observation periods. PET imaging showed increased [^{11}C]PK11195 binding potential in the bilateral LGN at 4 weeks after laser treatment; the increase in the ipsilateral LGN was statistically significant ($P<0.05$, $n=4$). Immunostaining showed bilateral activations of microglia and astrocytes in LGN layers receiving input from the laser-treated eye. PBR-positive cells were observed in LGN layers receiving input from laser-treated eye at all experimental glaucoma stages including the mild glaucoma stage and their localization coincided with Iba-1 positive microglia and GFAP-positive astrocytes. These data suggest that glial activation occurs in the LGN at a mild glaucoma stage, and that the LGN degeneration could be detected by a PET imaging with [^{11}C]PK11195 during the moderate experimental glaucoma stage after unilateral ocular hypertension. Therefore, activated glial markers such as PBR in the LGN may be useful in noninvasive molecular imaging for diagnosis of glaucoma.

Editor: Rafael Linden, Universidade Federal do Rio de Janeiro, Brazil

Funding: This study was supported in part by grants from the Molecular Imaging Program on "Research Base for Exploring New Drugs" from the Ministry of Education, Culture, Sports, science, and Technology, Japan, and from Grant-in-Aid for Scientific Research (C) (No. 21592262) from the Ministry of Education, Culture, Sports, Science, and Technology, Japan. The funders had no role in study design, data collection and analysis, decision to publish, or preparation of the manuscript. No additional external funding received for this study.

Competing Interests: The authors have declared that no competing interests exist.

* E-mail: hidehara@gifu-pu.ac.jp

Introduction

Open-angle glaucoma (OAG) is a slowly progressive and irreversible ocular disease that is one of the leading causes of blindness worldwide. Therefore, increasing attention is being paid to evaluation of the appearance of the optic nerve head and peripapillary retina in the diagnosis of OAG, especially in its early stage. Glaucoma pathology has been extensively studied at the level of the retinal ganglion cells (RGC) and optic nerve, with diagnosis resulting primarily from intraocular pressure (IOP), ophthalmoscopic, and visual field measurements. On the other hand, we and several investigators [1,2,3,4] reported that neuronal degeneration in the lateral geniculate nucleus (LGN), which is the primary processing center for visual information received from the retina, occurred in experimental glaucoma models. Briefly, in experimental glaucoma monkeys, neuronal atrophy in the LGN appeared to occur at an early stage after IOP elevation, and LGN neurons were apparently more susceptible to the effects of IOP elevation than optic nerve axons [1,2]. Furthermore, Gupta and her colleagues [5,6] firstly reported that the death of the RGC in glaucoma patients is accompanied by transsynaptic degradation of neurons in the LGN. These findings strongly suggest that LGN degeneration may become new diagnostic and/or therapeutic targets for glaucoma.

Recently, we demonstrated that glial fibrillary acidic protein (GFAP) immunoreactivity as well as neuronal cell loss was increased in the LGN of cynomolgus monkeys at 4 months after unilateral ocular hypertension [7], and that microglial activation was detectable by positron emission tomography (PET) imaging with [^{11}C]PK11195, a PET ligand for the peripheral-type benzodiazepine receptor (PBR), at 4 to 12 months after unilateral ocular hypertension [8]. PBR, also known as translocator protein

(18 kDa) (TSPO) [9], is a highly hydrophobic protein located primarily on the outer mitochondrial membrane [10]. Although PBR is expressed at low or reduced levels in resting microglial cells and astrocytes of the normal brain, it is upregulated in activated microglial cells and astrocytes [11,12,13]. Thus, noninvasive molecular imaging of the LGN targeted against activated glial markers such as PBR may be helpful in the early diagnosis of glaucoma. However, the courses of glial activation and PBR expression that accompany LGN degeneration in glaucoma are as yet unknown.

In the present study, we examined LGN degeneration secondary to experimental hypertensive glaucoma as an indicator for glaucoma in ocular hypertensive monkeys using PET, and validated glial activation by morphological and immunohistochemical examinations.

Materials and Methods

Animals

The 5 adult cynomolgus monkeys (*Macaca fascicularis*) in this study, aged 4 to 6 years (Japan SLC Co. Ltd, Hamamatsu, Japan), were housed in an air-conditioned room at 24±2°C with 60±10% humidity, and given food and water *ad libitum*. The animal welfare and steps taken to ameliorate suffering were in accordance with the recommendations of the Weatherall report on the use of non-human primates in research, and all investigations were approved and monitored by the Institutional Animal Care and Use Committee of Kobe Institute in RIKEN (Permit Number: MAH18-05-15).

Argon-Laser Photocoagulation (Experimental Glaucoma Model)

An elevation of intraocular pressure (IOP) was induced in each monkey by applying argon-laser burns to the mid portion of the trabecular meshwork of the left eye, with the right eye being used as an untreated control, as previously described [14,15]. The laser irradiation was performed only on the left eyes, because we considered that laser irradiation on the ipsilateral eyes under the same conditions would facilitate accurate irradiation without technical dispersion. For the laser treatment, the animals were anesthetized with an intramuscular injection of ketamine (8.75 mg/kg, Ketalar 50®; Sankyo, Tokyo, Japan) plus xylazine (0.5 mg/kg, Celactal®; Bayer, Leverkusen, Germany). A single-mirror Goldmann lens (OSMGA, Ocular Instruments, Inc., Bellevue, WA, USA) filled with a hydroxyethylcellulose solution (Scopisol®15; Senjyu Pharmaceutical, Osaka, Japan) was then placed on the eye to be treated. An argon blue/green laser was focused on the mid-portion of the trabecular meshwork, and a total of 100 to 150 laser-beam spots was applied around 360° (spot size, 100 μm; power, 1000 mW; exposure time, 0.2 sec) using an argon-laser photo-coagulator (Ultima 2000 SE®; Coherent, Inc., CA, USA) attached to a standard slit-lamp microscope (BQ 900; Haag-Streit, Köniz, Switzerland). Two weeks after the first treatment, the laser treatment was repeated, except for monkey #5, so as to produce a maintained elevation in IOP. Time (in weeks) "after the laser treatment" was defined as dating from the first of these treatments.

IOP and Ophthalmoscopy

IOP was measured in both eyes of each animal using a calibrated pneumatonometer (Model 30 Classic Pneumatonometer; Medtronic Solan, FL, USA) under ketamine anesthesia (8.75–10 mg/kg, i.m.), with local anesthesia using 0.4% oxibuprocaine hydrochloride (Benoxil® 0.4% solution; Santen Pharmaceutical Co. Ltd.). IOP was measured between 2 p.m. and 4 p.m. at 1- or 2-weeks intervals.

Then, fundus photographs (AFC-210; NIDEK Co. Ltd. Gamagori, Japan) were obtained under additive injection of xylazine (0.5 mg/kg, i.m.), and cup/disc (C/D) area ratio was assessed using data filing and analysis software (NAVIS-Lite ver 1.0.4.1, NIDEK Co. Ltd.). All measurements were taken at one- or two-week intervals.

PET Imaging for [^{11}C]PK11195

PET imaging was performed in 4 monkeys (#2 to #5) at 4 weeks after the first laser treatment, but monkey #1 was not measured the PET imaging, because monkey #1 showed IOP elevation, but did not change the optic disc. Before PET, a venous cannula was placed into a radial vain. For the scan, the animals were placed on the bed in a small animal PET scanner (microPET Focus220; Siemens Medical Solutions, Knoxville, TN, USA) under anesthesia with a continuous intravenous infusion of propofol (10 mg/kg/h, Hospira Japan Co. Ltd., Osaka, Japan). The spatial resolution at the center of the field of view was ~1.35 mm in full width at half maximum (FWHM). The [^{11}C]PK11195 was prepared according to previously described methods, using the reaction of (R)-*N*-desmethyl precursor (1 mg) in dimethylsulfoxide (200 μl) containing 1 mg of KOH, with [^{11}C]-CH_3I produced by a cyclotron (HM12; Sumitomo Heavy Industry, Tokyo, Japan) [16]. Radiochemical purities were >99.5%, and the mean (± SD) specific activity was 65.9 (±29.4) GBq/μmol. After a transmission scan for 30 min with ^{68}Ga-^{68}Ge pin source, [^{11}C]PK11195 (187.6±22.9 MBq) was injected as an intravenous bolus, and PET scanning was performed for 90 min. PET images were acquired with three-dimensional list mode reconstructed by an algorithm of filtered back projection (FBP), and were smoothed by a Hanning filter with a cutoff of 0.4. Attenuation correction, but not scatter fraction correction, using blank and transmission images, was performed to obtain quantitative images. A dynamic histogram acquired during 90 min (6×10 sec, 6×30 sec, 11×60 sec, 15×180 sec, 3×600 sec) was used for data analysis.

Reconstructed images were processed with PMOD version 3.0 image analysis software (PMOD Technologies, Zürich, Switzerland). To elucidate the quantitative [^{11}C]PK11195 binding to PBR in the brain, the cerebellum was used as a reference region to calculate binding potential value in a simplified reference tissue model (SRTM) developed by Lammertsma and Hume [17]. Regional binding potential values were obtained by applying some regions of interest (ROI) to the individual PET images aligned on individual magnetic resonance imaging (MRI). ROIs were manually drawn with reference to the stereotaxic brain atlas of the cynomolgus monkey for the cerebellum and LGN.

MRI was performed for all animals using a 3-T MRI scanner (Signa Horizon Lx VH3; General Electric Healthcare, Milwaukee, WI) under pentobarbital anesthesia to define anatomical ROIs in a separate session from PET imaging.

Histological Examination

After the last measurements, animals were transcardially perfused to the bilateral common carotid arteries with 2.0 liters of 0.9% saline containing 10 U/ml heparin at 4°C after ligation of thoracic aorta., under deep sodium pentobarbital anesthesia (30 mg/kg, i.v.; Nembutal; Abbott, North Chicago, IL, USA), followed by 2.0 liters of 4% paraformaldehyde in 0.1 M phosphate buffer (pH 7.4). The brains and eyeballs with optic nerve were removed after the perfusion. The brains and eyes were cut into several sections and immersed in the same fixative solution for at least 24 h, soaked in 10 to 30% (w/v) sucrose, then frozen in embedding compound (Tissue-Tek; Sakura Finetechnical Co. Ltd., Tokyo, Japan). Next, 20-μm thick coronal sections of the LGN and retina were serially cut, then stained with cresyl violet or hematoxylin and eosin, respectively. Retinal damage was evaluated as follows: six sections stained with hematoxylin and eosin from each eye being used for the morphometric analysis. Light-microscope photographs were taken using a digital camera a charge-coupled device camera (MicroPublisher 5.0RTV, QIMAGING, Burnaby, BC, Canada), and the cell counts in the ganglion cell layer (GCL) and inner nuclear layer (INL) at a distance between 1750 and 2200 μm from the optic disc were measured on the images in a masked fashion by a single observer (Y. I.). Data from six sections were averaged for each eye, and the values obtained were used to evaluate the GCL and INL cell counts.

To assess number and size of neurons in the LGN, sections stained with cresyl violet were used for these measurements: The measurements were performed on three sections representative of the anterior, middle, and posterior parts of each LGN. The volume used for the measurements was 216×162×20 μm (section thickness) of each side in the LGN. Care was taken to count only neurons with clearly visible nuclei and cytoplasm. For quantification of cresyl violet-stained sections, neuron numbers in the M- and P-layers were estimated by counting under objective ×40 with brightfield microscope in a masked fashion by a single observer (Y.I.). The number on each section was measured using image-processing software (Image-J ver. 1.33f; National Institutes of Health, USA). Neuron counts were derived from three regions per layer in each of the three LGN sample sections. The effects of elevated IOP on neuronal cell size were studied by measuring 1200 geniculate neurons in each animal. Neuron samples (100 neurons/layer) were taken randomly from the full width of each lamina and included only those neurons with clearly visible nucleoli, and measured soma area. Average neuronal cell size for each layer was calculated on the basis of data from 100 neurons.

Segments of optic nerve from 3 mm behind the eye were postfixed by immersion in 1.25% glutaraldehyde with 2% paraformaldehyde in PBS for at least 1 week at 4°C. After three washes with PBS, the nerve segments were placed in 2% osmium tetroxide in saline for 2 h, then washed with PBS at room temperature. Subsequently, they were dehydrated in alcohol and embedded as cross-sections in epoxy resin for sectioning. Cross-sections (1 μm thickness) were cut with an ultramicrotome, mounted on glass slides, and stained for myelin using 1% toluidine blue. For counting of the numbers of RGC axons, the optic nerve area was divided into five segments (nasal, temporal, superior, inferior and central) in each optic nerve sections. We captured thirteen images from these segments in each optic nerve at high power using an oil immersion objective ×100 with bright-field microscope completed with wide field and high resolution CCD camera (BZ-9000, KEYENCE CORPORATION, Osaka, Japan),. In each image (145×109 μm), every myelinated axon was counted in masked fashion by a single observer (T.N.) and the data from the thirteen images were summed. Estimated total area was covered more than 3% per nerve, according to the previous report [18]. Axon number was expressed as (healthy axon number on left side)/(healthy axon number on right side)×100% for each animal. Glaucoma stages were classified by the extent of axonal loss as mild (0–20%), moderate (20–50%), and advanced (50–100%) (Table 1).

Immunohistochemistry

During the immunostaining procedures, coronal sections containing LGN were washed with 0.01 M phosphate-buffered saline (PBS, pH 7.4), then treated with 0.3% hydrogen peroxide in 0.01 M PBS. They were then preincubated with 10% normal goat serum (Vector, Burlingame, CA, USA) in 0.01 M PBS for 30 min and incubated for one day at 4°C with specific mouse anti-glial fibrillary acidic protein (GFAP) monoclonal antibody (1:800 dilution) (MAB360; Chemicon, Temecula, CA, USA), rabbit anti-ionized calcium-binding adaptor molecule 1 (Iba-1) polyclonal antibody (1: 600 dilution) (019-19741;Wako, Osaka, Japan) in a solution of 10% normal goat serum in 0.01 M PBS containing 0.3% (v/v) Triton X-100. The coronal sections were then washed with PBS and incubated with biotinylated anti-mouse or anti-rabbit IgG before being incubated with avidin-biotin-peroxidase complex for 30 min at room temperature. Finally, diaminobenzidine was used as a peroxidase substrate for visualization. To assess area of GFAP and Iba-1 immunoreactivity in the LGN, sections immunostained with GFAP or Iba-1 were used for the area measurements: The measurements were performed on three sections representative of the anterior, middle, and posterior parts of each LGN. The volume used for the area measurements was 216×162×20 μm (section thickness) of each side in the LGN. The measurements were carried out under objective ×40 with brightfield microscope in a masked fashion by a single observer (Y.I.). The area on each section was

Table 1. Changes in IOP and the optic disc in cynomolgus monkeys after laser-photocoagulation.

No.	Baseline IOP (mmHg) R	Baseline IOP (mmHg) L	D (weeks)	Glaucomatous left eye: Mean IOP (mmHg)	Max. IOP (mmHg)	Integral ΔIOP	C/D area ratio (left eye) Pre	C/D area ratio (left eye) End	Glaucoma stages
#1	22.6	24.3	9	40.2	52.7	1109.5	0.19	0.20	Mild
#2	21.7	23.4	4	61.3	72.0	475.7	0.25	0.40	Moderate
#3	21.0	20.3	11	60.2	73.3	2501.9	0.17	0.64	Advanced
#4	24.3	24.7	15	62.1	70.7	3267.8	0.19	0.56	Advanced
#5	24.8	22.4	24	50.8	60.0	4450.8	0.23	0.77	Advanced

C/D area ratio: cup/disc area ratio, ONH: Optic nerve head, IOP: Intraocular pressure, R: right eye, L: left eye, D: Duration, Max IOP: Maximum IOP, Integral ΔIOP: Integral IOP to right eye (Δ mmHg/day). Glaucoma stages were classified by histological changes based on the extent of axonal loss as mild (0–20%), moderate (20–50%), and advanced glaucoma (50–100%).

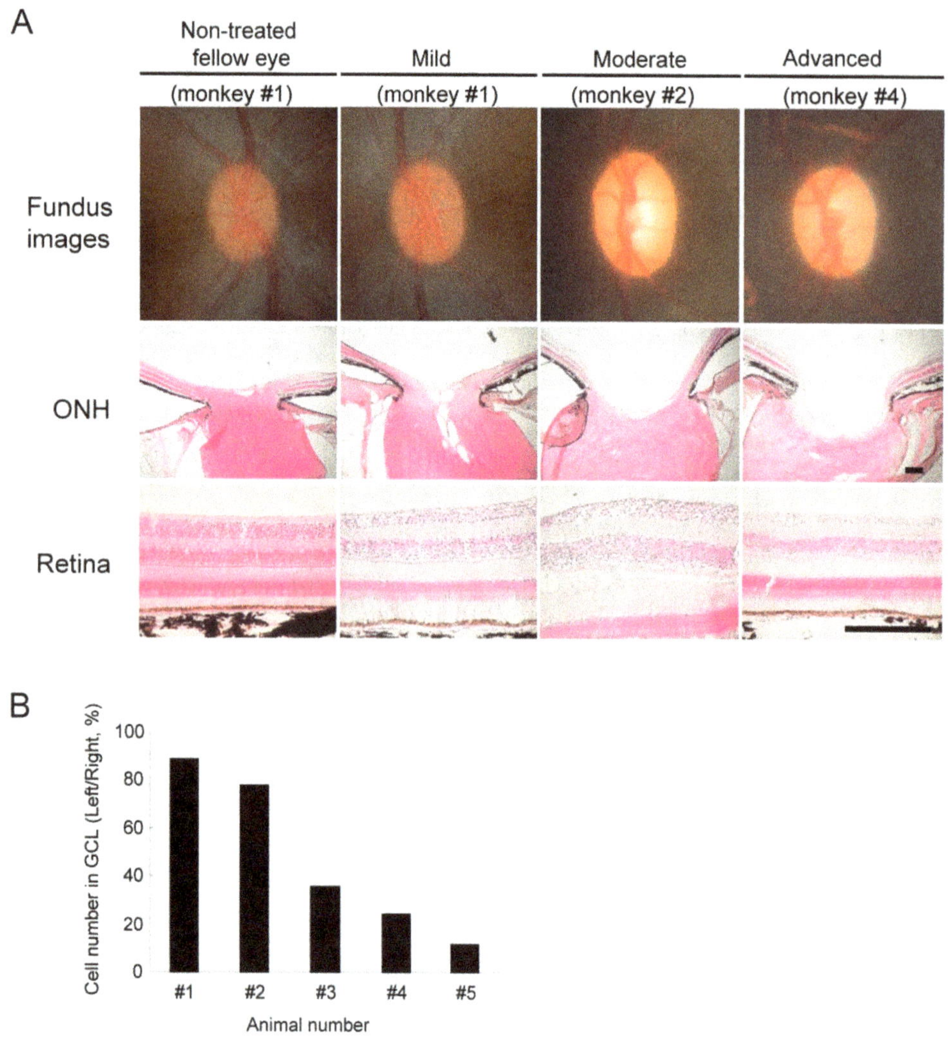

Figure 1. Ocular fundus photographs and histological sections of the retina at each experimental glaucoma stage in laser-treated eyes of cynomolgus monkeys. (A) Ocular fundus photographs were taken just before the end of the experiment for each monkey Each scale bar indicates 200 μm for ONH and retina. (B) The cell numbers in ganglion cell layers (GCL) of each experimental glaucoma stage were estimated by counting GCL cells at a distance between 1750 and 2200 μm from the optic disc. Cell number was expressed as (healthy cell number on GCL of left eye)/(healthy cell number on GCL of right eye)×100% for each animal.

measured using MetaMorph software (Molecular Devices, Sunnyvale, CA , USA). Data from each section was averaged for each LGN, and the values obtained were used to evaluate the area of GFAP and Iba-1 immunoreactivity.

Immunofluorescence Staining

During the immunofluorescence staining procedures, coronal sections containing LGN were subjected to antigen retrieval by autoclaving in 0.01 M sodium citrate buffer, pH 6.0, at 121°C for 15 min. Next, they were preincubated with 10% normal goat serum (Vector) in 0.01 M PBS for 30 min, then incubated for one day at 4°C with specific rabbit anti-peripheral benzodiazepine receptor (PBR) polyclonal antibody (1:1000 dilution) in a solution of 10% normal goat serum in 0.01 M PBS containing 0.3% (v/v) Triton X-100. We raised a rabbit polyclonal antibody against the peptide residues 36–47 of mouse PBR (SLQKPSWHPPRW), designated NP36, and purified it with an antigen peptide affinity-column to ensure reactivity against the antigen. After washing with 0.01 M PBS, the sections were incubated for 3 h at room

Table 2. Pathological changes in cynomolgus monkeys after laser-photocoagulation.

No.	Glaucoma stages	RGC loss	Neuronal loss in LGN layers	Immunoreactivity in LGN layers		
				GFAP	Iba-1	PBR
#1	Mild	+	−	+	+	+++
#2	Moderate	++	+	+++	++	+++
#3	Advanced	+++	+++	+++	+++	+++
#4	Advanced	+++	+++	+++	+++	+++
#5	Advanced	+++	+++	+++	++	+++

LGN: lateral geniculate layer, ONH: optic nerve head, ON: optic nerve, GFAP: glial fibrillary acidic protein, Iba-1: ionized calcium-binding adaptermolecule-1, PBR: peripheral benzodiazepine receptor. Glaucoma stages were classified by histological changes based on the extent of axonal loss as mild (0–20%), moderate (20–50%), and advanced glaucoma (50–100%). Neuronal atrophy, RGC loss and immunoreactivity were classified based on the quantitative data as follows: no changes; −, mild; +, moderate; ++, robust; +++.

temperature with a mixture of an Alexa Fluor 488 F(ab′)$_2$ fragment of goat anti-rabbit IgG (H+L) (1:1000 dilution) (A11070; Invitrogen, Carlsbad, CA, USA). To assess number of PBR-positive cell in the LGN, sections immunostained with PBR were used for the number measurement: The Measurement were performed on three sections representative of the anterior, middle, and posterior parts of each LGN. The volume used for the measurements was 216×162×20 μm (section thickness) of each side in the LGN. The measurements were carried out under objective ×40 with brightfield microscope in a masked fashion by a single observer (Y.I.). The number on each section was measured using image-processing software (Image-J ver. 1.33f; National Institutes of Health, USA). Data from each section was averaged for each LGN, and the values obtained were used to evaluate the number of PBR-positive cell.

Retinal sections were preincubated with 10% normal horse serum and (Vector) and 0.3% TritonX100 in 0.01 M PBS for 30 min, then incubated for one day at 4°C with mouse anti-calbindin mAb (1:200 dilution) (Abcam, Cambridge, MA, USA), rabbit anti-calretinin mAb (1:200 dilution) (Abcam), mouse anti-parvalbumin mAb (1:1000 dilution) (Millipore, Temecula, CA, USA) or and goat anti-Brn3a (1:1000 dilution) (Santa Cruz Biotechnology, Santa Cruz, CA, USA), in a solution of 10% normal horse serum in 0.01 M PBS containing 0.3% (v/v) Triton X-100. After washing with 0.01 M PBS, the sections were incubated for 3 h at room temperature with a mixture of AlexaFluor 546 labeled rabbit anti-goat IgG (1:1000 dilution) (Invitrogen) and AlexaFluor 488 labeled rabbit anti-mouse IgG(F(ab′)$_2$) (1:1000 dilution) (Invitrogen), or with a mixture of AlexaFluor 546 labeled donkey anti-rabbit IgG (1:1000 dilation) (Invitrogen) and AlexaFluor 488 labeled donkey anti-goat IgG (1:1000 dilution) (Invitrogen) in PBS with 10% normal horse serum and 0.3% TritonX100 and Hoechst33342 (1:5000 dilution) (Invitrogen) for 3 h at room temperature. Immunofluorescence

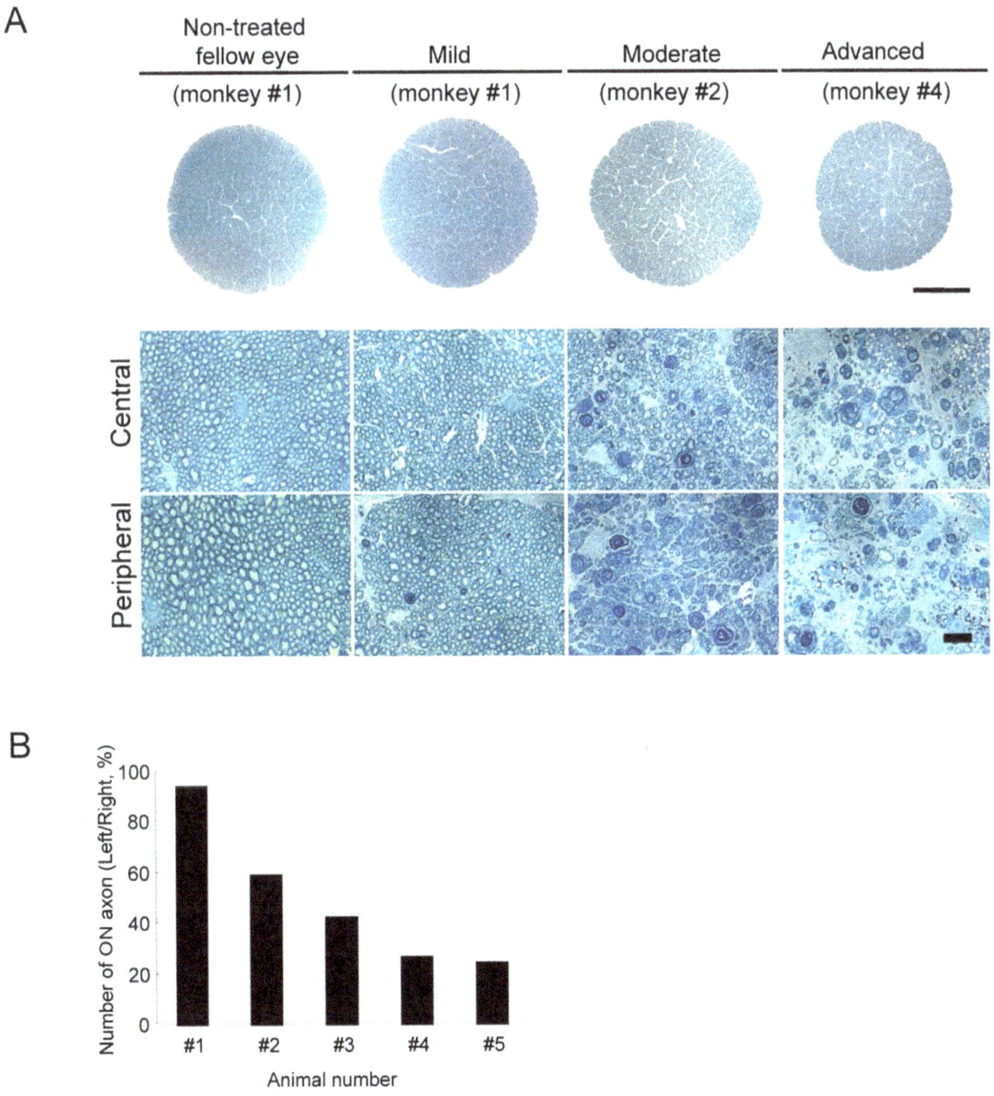

Figure 2. Optic nerve degeneration at each experimental glaucoma stage in laser-treated eyes of cynomolgus monkeys. (A) Optic nerve were cut with an ultramicrotome, mounted on glass slides, and stained for myelin using 1% toluidine blue. Each scale bar indicates 1000 μm (low magnification images) and 10 μm (high magnification images), respectively. (B) The axonal numbers in optic nerve (ON) of each experimental glaucoma stage were estimated by counting myelinated axons in each segment 145×109×1 μm (section thickness). Axon number was expressed as (healthy axon number on left side)/(healthy axon number on right side)×100% for each animal.

images were taken using a microscope (BX50; Olympus, Tokyo, Japan) with a cooled charge-coupled device camera (DP30BP; Olympus) at 1360×1024 pixels via MetaMorph software (Molecular Devices), and the calbindin-positive cells were counted in the inner part of inner nuclear layer (INL) at a distance between 1750 and 2200 μm from the optic disc on the images in a masked fashion by a single observer (M.S.).

Double Immunofluorescence Staining

To confirm the cell phenotypes containing PBR, we performed double immunofluorescence staining for PBR and GFAP or Iba-1 on LGN sections. Coronal sections containing LGN were prepared as described above.

To visualize co-localization of PBR with GFAP, the sections were incubated overnight at 4°C with rabbit anti-PBR polyclonal antibody (1:1000 dilution) and mouse anti-GFAP monoclonal antibody (1:800 dilution) in a solution of 10% normal goat serum in 0.01 M PBS with 0.3% (v/v) Triton X-100. Next, they were washed with 0.01 M PBS and then incubated for 3 h at room temperature with a mixture of an Alexa Fluor 488 $F(ab')_2$ fragment of goat anti-rabbit IgG (H+L) (1:1000 dilution) (Molecular Probes) and an Alexa Fluor 546 $F(ab')_2$ fragment of goat anti-mouse IgG (H+L) (1:1000 dilution) (A-11018; Molecular Probes). Co-localization of PBR with Iba-1 was visualized by double immunofluorescence staining on LGN sections. The sections were incubated with a primary antibody for PBR (1:500 dilution) labeled with Zenon Alexa Fluor 488 (Z25302; Molecular Probes), and with a primary antibody for Iba-1 (1:300 dilution) with Zenon Alexa Fluor 594 (Z25207; Molecular Probes,) for 3 h at room temperature.

Data Analysis

Data are expressed as mean ± S.E.M. A paired t-test was used to compare [^{11}C]PK11196 binding potential between before and 4 weeks after the laser treatment. Pearson correlation coefficient was calculated between the mean PBR-positive cell numbers in LGN layers receiving input from glaucoma eye and the percent changes of GFAP-, Iba-1-immunoreactivities, soma size in LGN, or percent change of axon numbers in optic nerve in each of five glaucoma monkeys. Results were considered significantly different if $P<0.05$.

Results

Fundus Images and Retinal Damage after IOP Elevation

The mean IOP value in 10 eyes of 5 normal cynomolgus monkeys examined in this study was 22.9±0.7 mmHg ($n=5$) in the right eye and 23.0±0.8 mmHg ($n=5$) in the left eye. The IOP data are summarized in Table 1. There were no significant changes ($p>0.05$) between the two eyes. The IOP of the monkeys was elevated and remained above baseline throughout the observation period (4–24 weeks) after the first laser treatment.

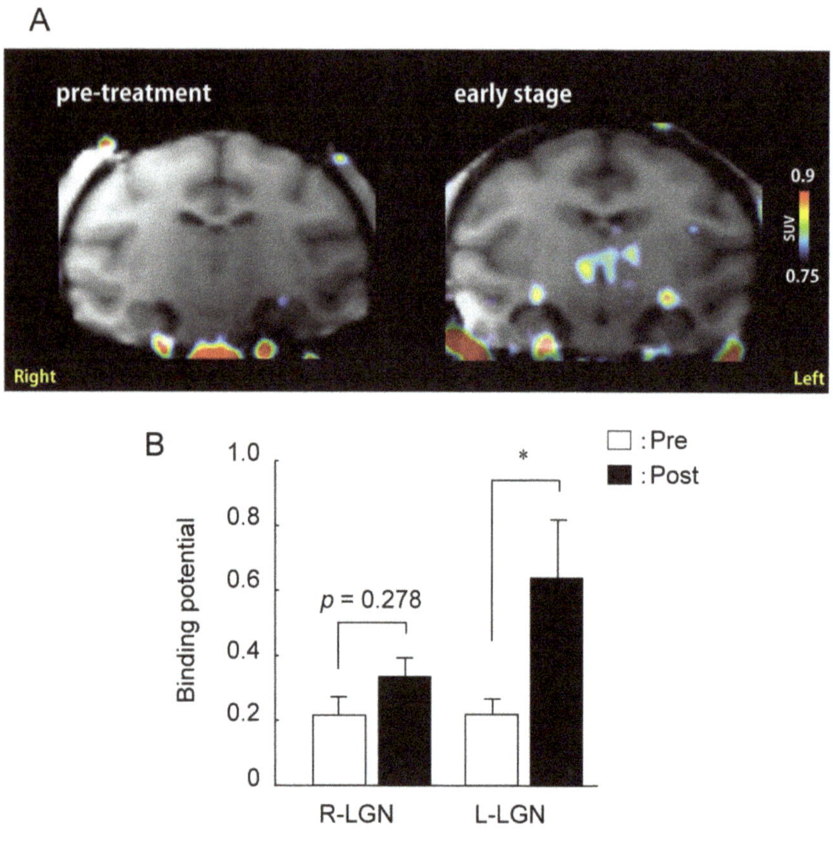

Figure 3. Changes in optic disc and [^{11}C]PK11195 PET image in coronal slices from cynomolgus monkeys at a moderate stage after laser photocoagulation. (A) Accumulation of [^{11}C]PK11195 binding potential in the LGN before and 4 weeks after laser photocoagulation. Coronal planes at the level of the LGN are shown. The PET images are shown in color, overlaid on the template MRIs is shown in gray scale. The color scale on the right represents standard uptake value (SUV). (B) Binding potential values of the right and left LGN obtained from 4 different individuals (4 monkeys; #2, #3, #4, #5, seen in tables 1 and 2). White and black column indicate pretreatment (pre) and post treatment (post) periods, respectively, for the laser photocoagulation. Each column represents the mean ± S.E.M. ($n=4$). *$p<0.05$ versus the pretreatment.

The extent of IOP elevation was similar among monkey #2 to #5, but it was lower in monkey #1 than other 4 monkeys. No obvious retinal lesions, nerve fiber layer defects, or abnormalities of either the optic nerve head or vascular structures were observed in any of the eyes before laser irradiation. Ocular fundus photographs of laser-treated eyes at each glaucoma stage are shown in Fig. 1A.

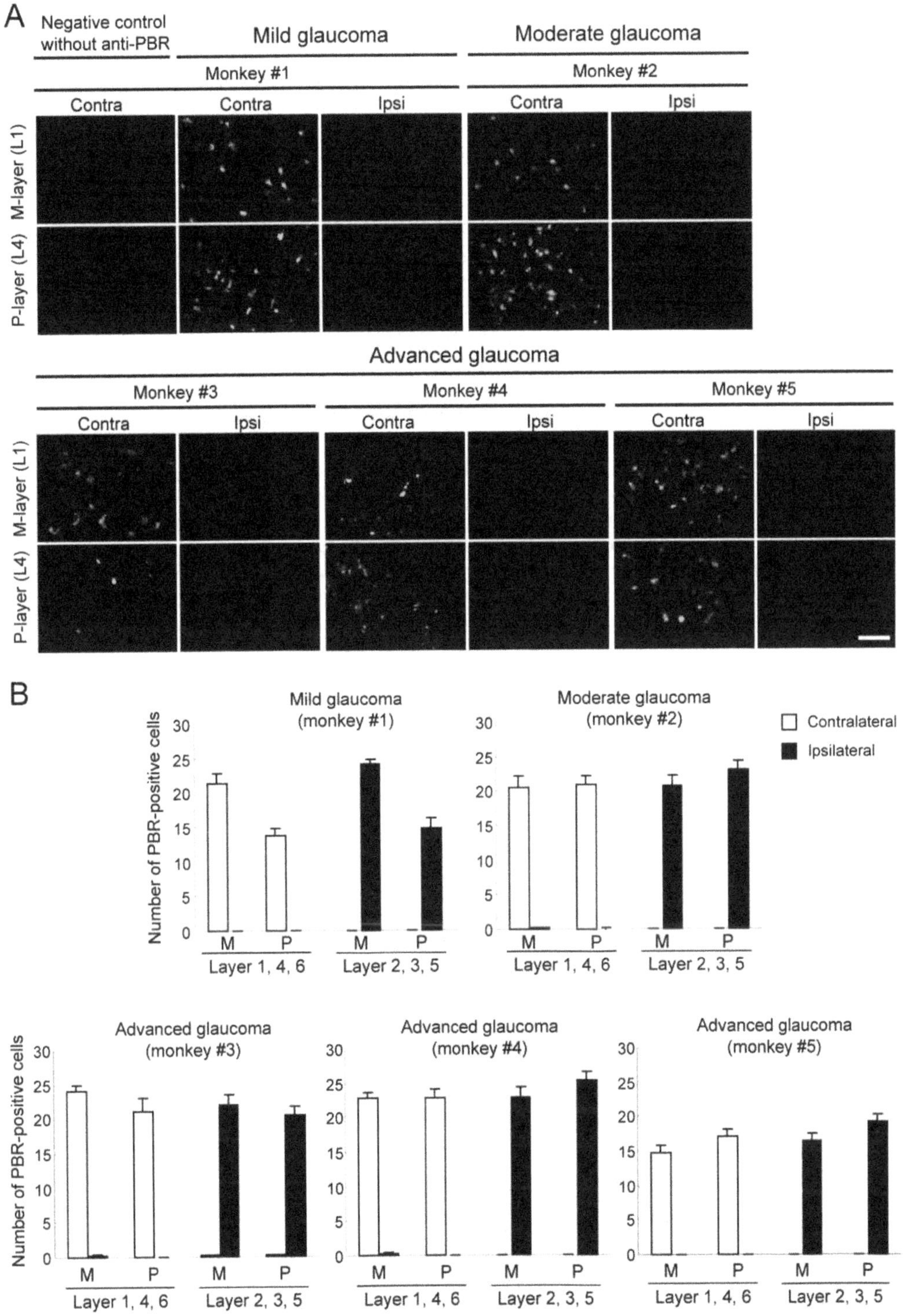

Figure 4. The expression of peripheral benzodiazepine receptor (PBR) in LGN layers receiving input from a glaucomatous eye. Each experimental glaucoma stage was classified by the glaucoma severity based on the extent of axonal loss as mild (0–20%), moderate (20–50%), and advanced (50–100%). (A) Representative photographs of PBR-positive cells in LGN layers of the contralateral (Contra) and ipsilateral (Ipsi) sides are shown for each experimental glaucoma stage. Layers 1 (L1) and 4 (L4) on the contralateral side receive their innervations from the glaucomatous (left) eye, whereas L1 and L4 on the ipsilateral side receive their retinal inputs from the non-treated fellow (right) eye. Each scale bar indicates 50 μm. (B) The numbers of PBR-positive cells on each section were measured, and averaged for each LGN as mean ± S.E.M. at each M-(layers 1 and 2) and the P-(layers 3–6) layers.

Optic disc cupping was seen and increased depending on the extent of IOP elevation and duration after laser irradiation (Fig. 1A and Table 1). The cell numbers in GCL and myelinated axon in the optic nerve (ON), but not the cell number in INL, were also decreased depending on the extent of IOP elevation and duration (Figs. 1B, 2 and Table 2): the cell number of GCL was 88.5, 77.9, 35.8, 24.0, and 11.7% of that in the contralateral control GCL of monkey #1 to #5, respectively, the cell number of INL was 102.3, 104.8, 97.9, 99.1, 98.9% of that in the contralateral control INL of monkey #1 to #5, respectively , and the mean axonal number in the (left) ON was 93.7, 58.9, 42.2, 26.8, and 24.4% of that in the contralateral control (right) ON of monkey #1 to #5, respectively. On the other hand, a monkey #1 defined as mild glaucoma stage (Table 1) showed a persistent IOP elevation, but there was slight optic disc change based on ophthalmoscopy during 9 weeks. Therefore, histological analysis was performed in this monkey at 9 weeks after the laser treatment, and focal degeneration of the optic nerve was observed at the peripheral region (89.1% of the axon number in the fellow ON), but not at the central region (102.4% of the axon number in the fellow ON) (Fig. 2).

[^{11}C]PK11195 Binding in LGN before and during the moderate stage of glaucoma after Laser Treatment

We measured binding potential value of [^{11}C]PK11195 in the brain before and during the moderate stage of glaucoma based on ophthalmoscopy (at 4 weeks) after the laser treatment in 4 cynomolgus monkeys. Representative PET images in a moderate glaucoma monkey are shown in Fig. 3A. At the moderate stage of glaucoma, mean cup/disc area ratio was 0.43±0.02 (monkeys #2 to #5, $n=4$) against 0.21±0.02 ($n=4$) before the laser treatment. In the PET study, [^{11}C]PK11195 binding potential value was significantly increased in the ipsilateral LGN during the moderate glaucoma stage after unilateral ocular hypertension compared to before the laser treatment (Fig. 3B). In contrast, in the contralateral LGN, [^{11}C]PK11195 binding potential value tended to increase but the differences were not statistically significant ($p=0.278$, Fig. 3B).

Expression of the Peripheral Benzodiazepine Receptor (PBR) in the LGN at Each Experimental Glaucoma Stage

To examine the expression of PBR in the LGN at each experimental glaucoma stage, we used antibodies against PBR (Fig. 4). PBR-positive cells were observed in the LGN layers (including both magnocellular- and parvocellular-layers) receiving input from laser-treated eyes at all experimental glaucoma stages, and PBR was expressed even at the mild glaucoma stage (Fig. 4 and Table 2). On the other hand, no PBR-positive cells were observed in the LGN layers receiving input from non-treated fellow eyes. Furtheremore, there was no fluorescence detected from negative controls without anti-PBR antibody (Fig. 4A).

To identify PBR-positive cells in the LGN, double immunofluorescence staining was performed for PBR and Iba-1 or for PBR and GFAP (Fig. 5). PBR-positive cells were co-labeled in a portion of the Iba-1-positive microglial cells and GFAP-positive astroglial cells in the LGN at both moderate (monkey #2) and advanced glaucoma (monkey #5) stages (Fig. 5).

Histological Changes and Glial Activation in LGN at Each Experimental Glaucoma Stage

To examine the histological and pathological changes in the LGN at each stage of experimental glaucoma, coronal sections including the LGN were stained with cresyl violet, and for antibodies against PBR, ionized calcium-binding adaptor molecule 1 (Iba-1; a microglial marker), and glial fibrillary acidic protein (GFAP; an activated astrocyte marker) (Figs. 6, 7, 8 and Table 2). Cresyl violet staining showed that the number of neuron and neuronal size in the LGN layers (1, 4 and 6 on the contralateral, and 2, 3 and 5 on the ipsilateral) receiving input from the laser-treated eyes were decreased at advanced glaucoma stages (monkeys #3, #4, and #5), but no changes were seen in the LGN layers receiving input from the fellow eye (Fig. 6). No morphological changes including cell number and cellsize were seen in any LGN layers receiving input from eye in the mild

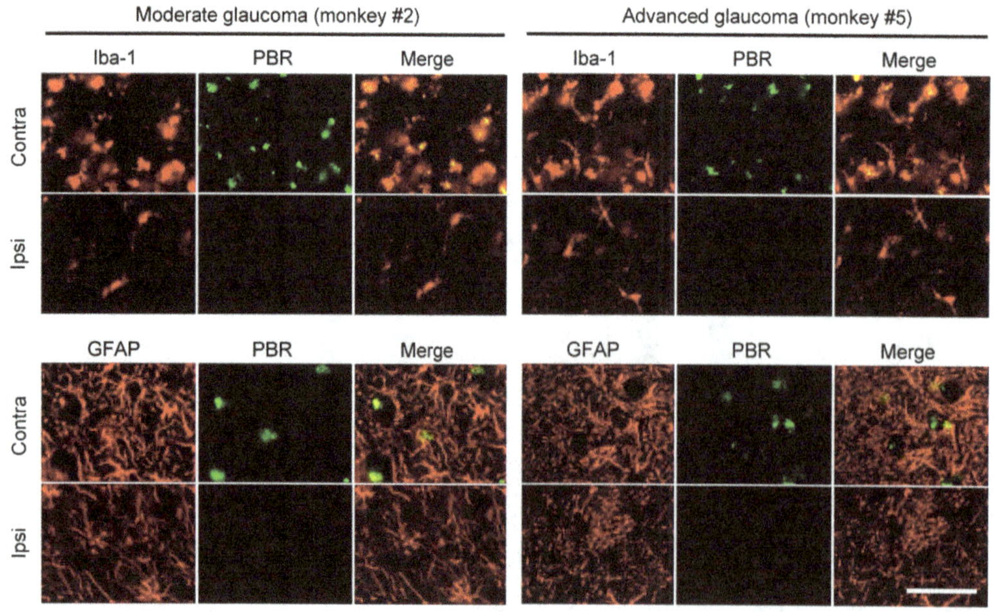

Figure 5. Double-immunofluorescence staining for PBR with a microglial marker (Iba-1) or a reactive astrocyte marker (GFAP). Layer 1 (L1) on the contralateral side receive their innervations from the glaucomatous (left) eye, whereas L1 on the ipsilateral side receive their retinal inputs from the non-treated fellow (right) eye. Each scale bar indicates 50 μm.

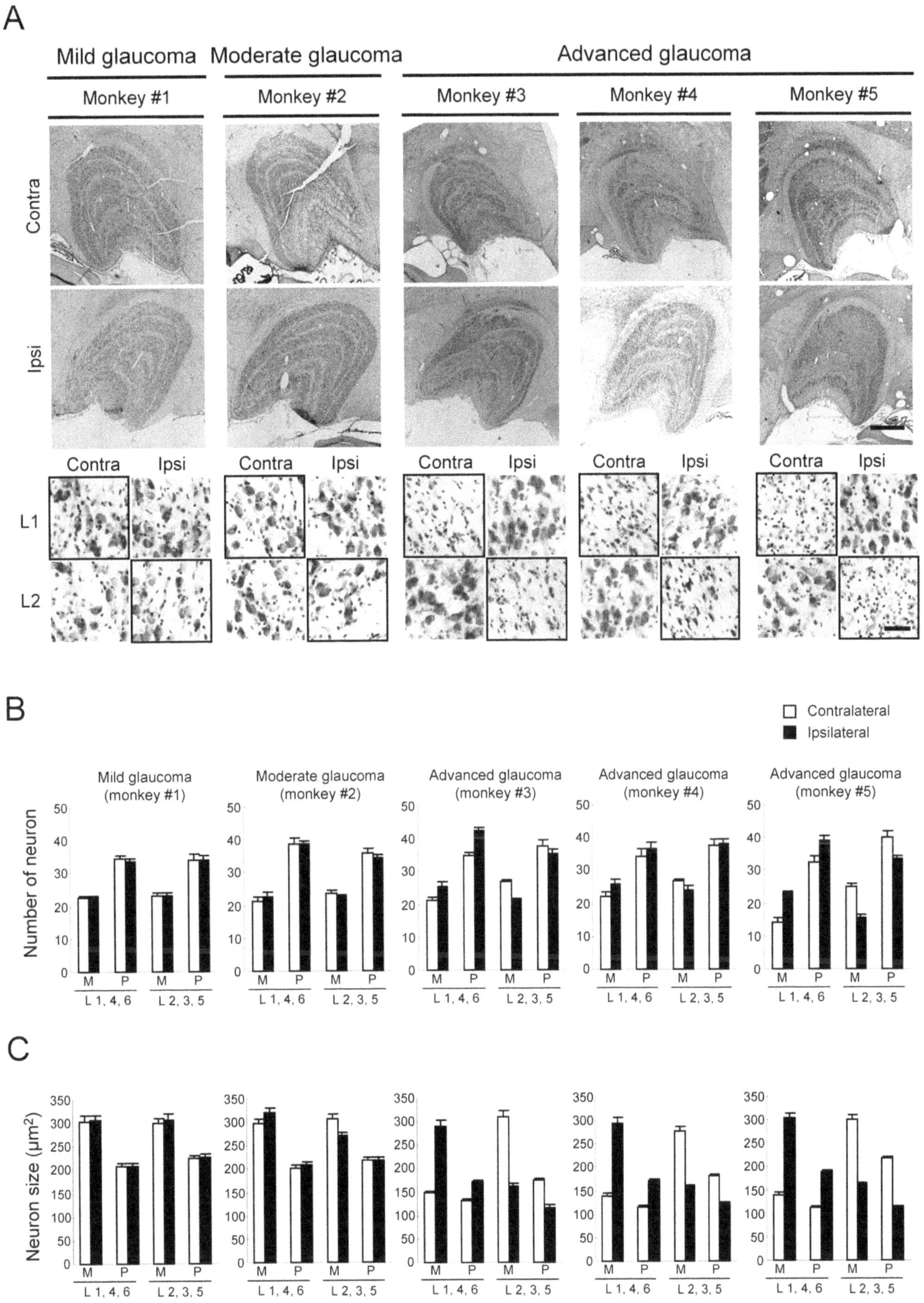
A
Mild glaucoma
Moderate glaucoma
Advanced glaucoma
Monkey #1
Monkey #2
Monkey #3
Monkey #4
Monkey #5
Contra
Ipsi
L1
L2
B
Contralateral
Ipsilateral
Mild glaucoma (monkey #1)
Moderate glaucoma (monkey #2)
Advanced glaucoma (monkey #3)
Advanced glaucoma (monkey #4)
Advanced glaucoma (monkey #5)
Number of neuron
M
P
L 1, 4, 6
L 2, 3, 5
C
Neuron size (μm²)

Figure 6. Histological changes in LGN neurons of cynomolgus monkeys after laser photocoagulation. (A) Representative microphotographs of cresyl violet-stained coronal sections of LGN on the contralateral and ipsilateral sides for each experimental glaucoma stage. Each experimental glaucoma stage was classified by the glaucoma severity based on the extent of axonal loss as mild (0–20%), moderate (20–50%), and advanced (50–100%). Layer 1 on the contralateral side and layer 2 on the ipsilateral side receive their innervations from the glaucomatous (left) eye (shown in bold frame), whereas layer 1 on the ipsilateral side and layer 2 on the contralateral side receive their retinal inputs from the non-treated fellow (right) eye. L1 and L2: layer 1 and 2. Scale bars indicate 1000 μm in whole LGN image and 50 μm in enlarged image. Neuron number (B) and mean neuronal cell size (C) in each layer of LGN were measured and averaged as mean ± S.E.M. at each M-(layers 1 and 2) and the P-(layers 3–6) layers.

glaucoma (monkey #1), but neuronal size was slightly decrease in the magnocellular (M) layer, but not parvocellular (P-) layer, of LGN receiving input from eye in the moderate glaucoma (monkey #2) stage (Fig. 6).

We next tested glial activation in the LGN after laser irradiation (Figs. 7, 8 and Table 2). Numbers of GFAP-positive astroglial cells (Fig. 7) and Iba-1-positive microglial cells (Fig. 8) were increased in the LGN layers receiving input from laser-treated eyes compared to the LGN layers receiving input from the fellow eyes. These changes depended on the extents of RGC and optic nerve losses after laser irradiation (Figs. 1, 2 and Table 2). Even at the mild glaucoma stage, GFAP-positive astroglial cells and Iba-1-positive microglial cells were increased in the bilateral LGN (Figs. 7 and 8).

Next, we performed Pearson correlation coefficient analysis between PBR and GFAP, Iba-1, LGN degeneration (soma size), or optic nerve axons (a glaucoma severity) in each of five glaucoma monkeys. The correlation coefficients between the mean PBR-positive cell numbers in LGN layers receiving input from glaucoma eye and percent changes of GFAP-, Iba-1-immunoreactivity, or soma size in LGN, or optic nerve axons were 0.512 ($P = 0.378$, $n = 5$), 0.064 ($P = 0.918$, $n = 5$), −0.199 ($P = 0.748$, $n = 5$), and −0.426 ($P = 0.475$, $n = 5$), respectively. In these comparisons, some parameters showed higher correlation coefficients of 0.512 (between PBR and GFAP) and −0.426 (between PBR and optic nerve axons) than other parameters, but did not show any significance. On the other hand, there was a significant correlation ($r = 0.923$, $P = 0.025$, $n = 5$) between percent changes of axon numbers in optic nerve and soma size in LGN.

Discussion

In the present study, we demonstrated that binding potential value for [^{11}C]PK11195 was increased in the LGN of unilateral hypertensive monkeys at a moderate experimental glaucoma stage (at 4 weeks after laser treatment). PBR was persistently expressed in glial cells of the LGN receiving input from laser-treated eye in mild through advanced stages of experimental glaucoma.

In experimental glaucoma, axonal injury in the lamina results in rapid Wallerian degeneration of the distal axon prior to the death of the RGC cells [19]. Howell et al. [20] have also reported that the distal axons are more vulnerable than the RGC soma and proximal axons in a mouse model of glaucoma (DBA/2J). In the present study, a mild glaucoma monkey with slight increase of disc cupping and a moderate glaucoma monkey with mild increase of disc cupping showed mild and moderate axonal degeneration, respectively, in the optic nerve, but RGC losses were a modest. Thus, the axonal injury is more severe than RGC loss during moderate glaucoma stage. These data strongly support the idea that the axonal injury is an initial key step in glaucoma, and therefore the loss of the RGC soma may be preceded by axonal degeneration. The RGC is known to die by apoptosis in glaucoma [21,22], but the precise mechanism underlying the transsynaptic degeneration of the retinogeniculate pathways remains unknown.

Recently, evidences have been growing that the atrophy of the LGN neuron occurs in experimental primate [1,2,3] and human glaucoma [5,6]. In primate glaucoma, we and others have reported that the neuronal shrinkage within LGN occurs at an early phase after IOP elevation [1,2,3]. In the present study, there was a significant correlation ($r = 0.923$, $P = 0.025$) between axonal degeneration in optic nerve and neuronal atrophy in LGN. These findings indicate that the decreased input from the retina to LGN is caused by optic nerve dysfunction and/or degeneration. This type of neurodegeneration starts at the axon terminals and progresses to the cell bodies. In the present study, activation of microglia and astrocytes was observed bilaterally in the LGN layers receiving input from the treated eye and even at the mild glaucoma stage. These results were also consistent with our previous reports that showed immunoreactivity with GFAP and major histocompatibility complex Class II CR3/43 [23], which are antigens specifically expressed in activated microglia, were elevated in the bilateral LGN and confined to the LGN layers receiving input from the affected eye [7,8]. On the other hand, Lam et al. [24] have reported that GFAP immunoreactivity was elevated in the LGN layers receiving input from the treated eye after unilateral optic nerve transection or ocular hypertension in monkeys, but found no microglial activation with Mac-1 immunoreactivity in the LGN after ocular hypertension. In this study, we used an antibody which recognized Iba-1 as a microglia marker, and demonstrated microglia activation in the bilateral LGN receiving input from the laser-treated eye as well. Iba-1 is specifically expressed in macrophages/microglia and is upregulated during the activation of these cells. Unlike CR3/43 or Mac-1, Iba-1 is also expressed in ramified microglia (resting form). Therefore, this antibody could be highly sensitive and morphologically distinguish between activated and resting microglia. Accordingly, this discrepancy may be due to the differences of sensitivity among antibodies used in each experiment, but further study is needed. Nevertheless, the findings suggest that the glial activation may become a promising hallmark for early diagnosis and determination of severity of glaucoma.

A non-invasive PET imaging with [^{11}C]PK11195 for activated microglial cells has been extensively used in several neurodegenerative disorders, such as multiple sclerosis [25], Alzheimer disease [26], Parkinson disease [27], and Huntington disease [28]. Although PBR is expressed at low levels in resting microglial cells and astrocytes of the normal brain, it is upregulated in activated microglial cells and astrocytes [11,12,13]. Previously, we found that [^{11}C]PK11195 binding potential value in PET imaging was detected in the bilateral LGN during the advanced glaucoma stage (4 to 12 months) after unilateral ocular hypertension in cynomolgus monkeys [8]. In the present study, we could detect the increase of [^{11}C]PK11195 binding potential value in the LGN during the moderate stage of glaucoma after unilateral ocular hypertension. Briefly, [^{11}C]PK11195 binding potential values in 4 cynomolgus monkeys were significantly increased in the ipsilateral LGN at 4 weeks after unilateral ocular hypertension compared to before the laser treatment. In the contralateral LGN, [^{11}C]PK11195 binding potential values tended to increase, but the

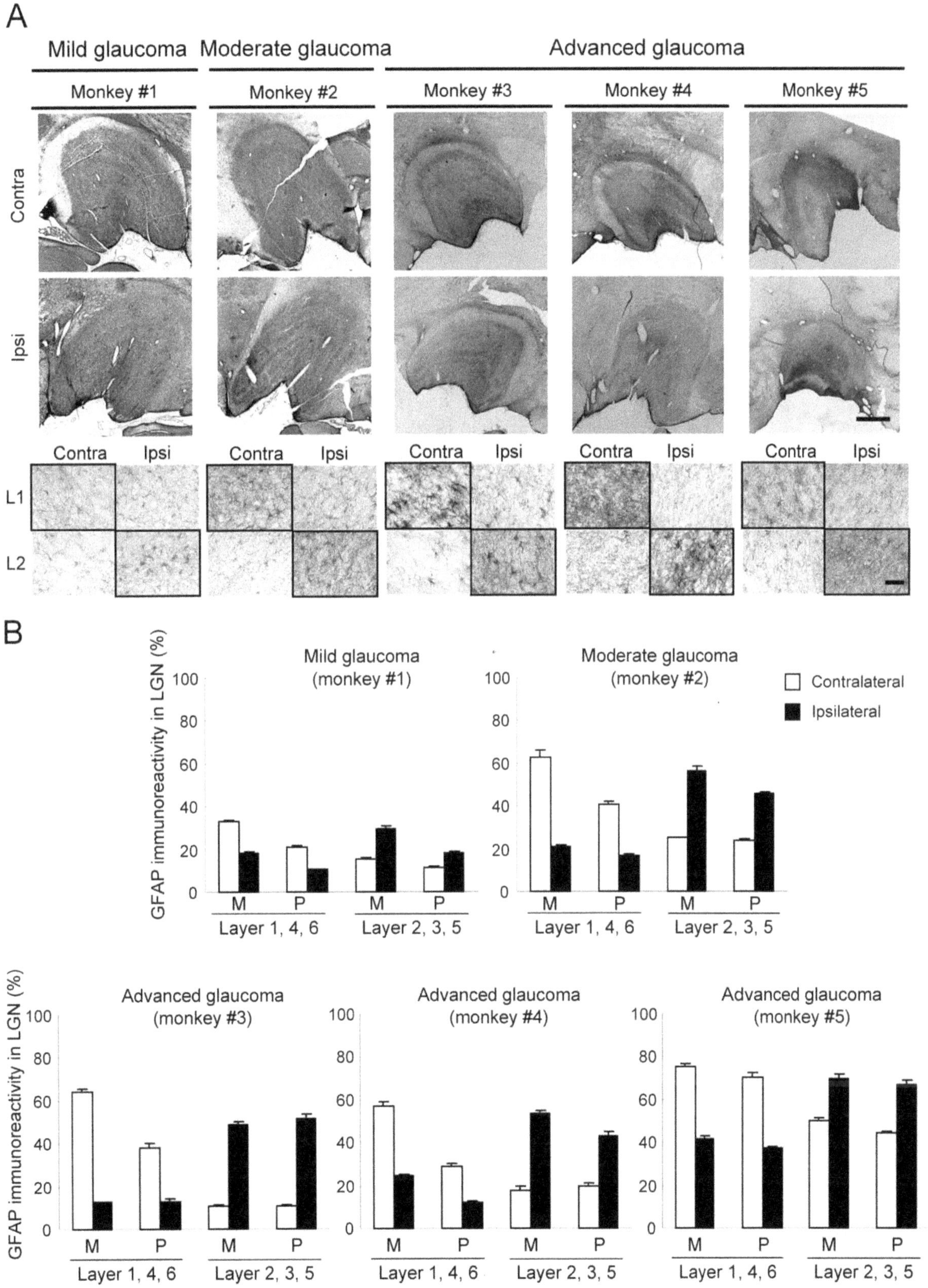

Figure 7. Astrocyte activation in LGN layers receiving input from a glaucomatous eye. (A) Representative photographs of GFAP immunoreactivity in LGN of the contralateral and ipsilateral sides are shown for each experimental glaucoma stage. Each experimental glaucoma stage was classified by the glaucoma severity based on the extent of axonal loss as mild (0–20%), moderate (20–50%), and advanced (50–100%). Layer 1 on the contralateral side and layer 2 on the ipsilateral side receive their innervations from the glaucomatous (left) eye (shown in bold frame), whereas layer 1 on the ipsilateral side and layer 2 on the contralateral side receive their retinal inputs from the non-treated fellow (right) eye. L1 and L2: layer 1 and 2. Scale bars indicate 1000 μm in whole LGN image and 50 μm in enlarged image. (B) The GFAP-immunoreactive area on each section was measured, and averaged for each LGN as mean ± S.E.M. at each M-(layers 1 and 2) and the P-(layers 3–6) layers.

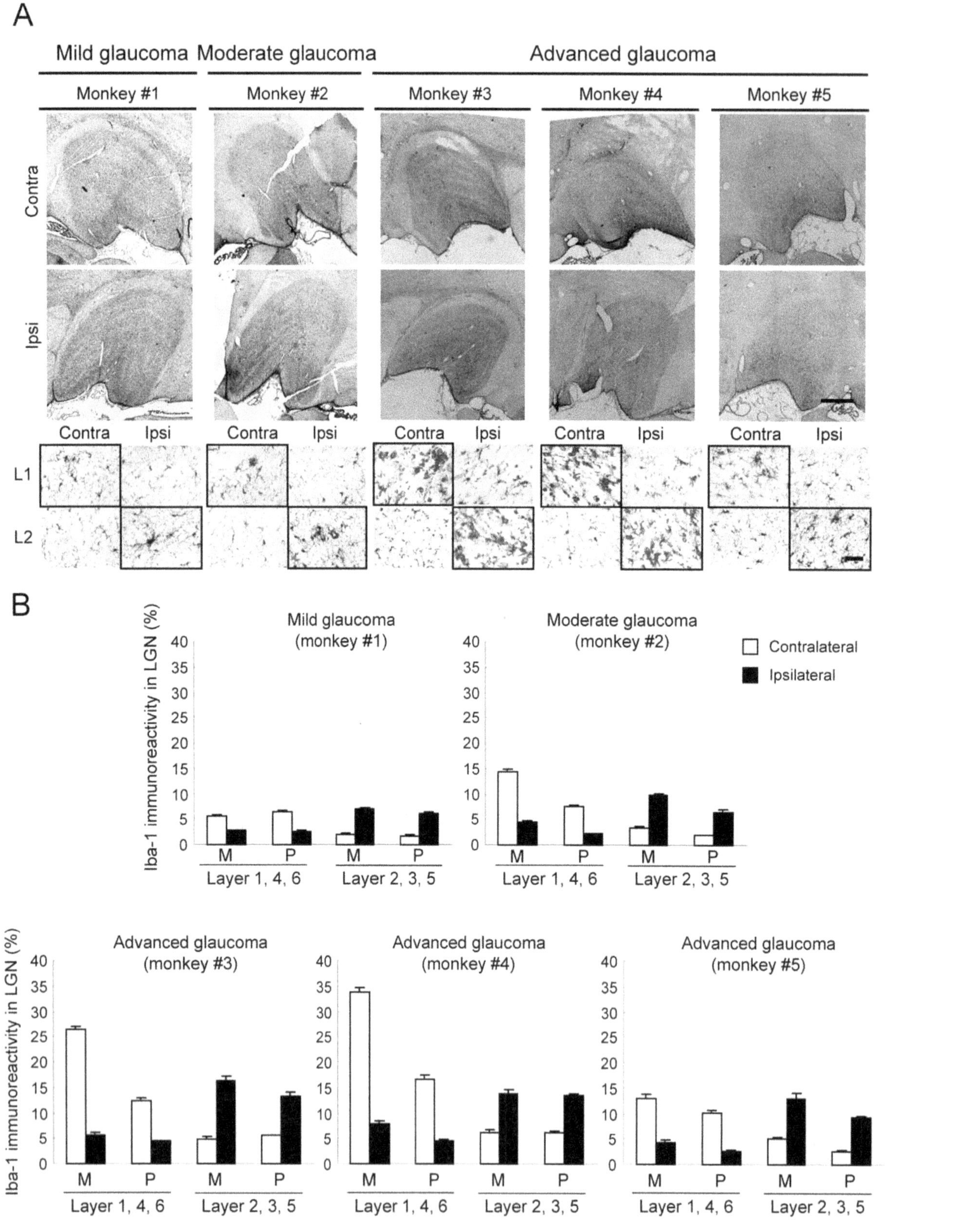

Figure 8. Microglial activation in LGN layers receiving input from a glaucomatous eye. (A) Representative photographs of Iba-1 immunoreactivity in LGN of the contralateral and ipsilateral sides are shown for each experimental glaucoma stage. Each experimental glaucoma stage was classified by the glaucoma severity based on the extent of axonal loss as mild (0–20%), moderate (20–50%), and advanced (50–100%). Layer 1 on the contralateral side and layer 2 on the ipsilateral side receive their innervations from the glaucomatous (left) eye (shown in bold frame), whereas layer 1 on the ipsilateral side and layer 2 on the contralateral side receive their retinal inputs from the non-treated fellow (right) eye. L1 and L2: layer 1 and 2. Scale bars indicate 1000 μm in whole LGN image and 50 μm in enlarged image. (B) The Iba-1-immunoreactive area on each section was measured, and averaged for each LGN as mean ± S.E.M. at each M-(layers 1 and 2) and the P-(layers 3–6) layers.

differences were not statistically significant. We previously reported that metabolic activity using 2-[^{18}F]fluoro-2-deoxy-glucose (^{18}FDG) uptake during monocular viewing was significantly reduced in the ipsilateral visuocortical areas of the glaucoma eye [8]. Taken together, this asymmetry might suggest that visual field defects in the nasal area and the corresponding RGC and optic nerve damage in the temporal retina are more severe than are those on the opposite side.

In the present study, we demonstrated for the first time that PBR-positive cells occurred in the LGN layers (including both magnocellular- and parvocellular-layers) that received input from laser-treated eyes at all glaucoma stages. Interestingly, PBR expression was even observed at the mild glaucoma stage with slight increase of disc cupping based on ophthalmoscopy. A portion of the PBR-expressing cells were also with Iba-1-positive microglial cells and GFAP-positive astroglial cells. These data provide further evidence that PBR is persistently expressed in glial cells of the LGN that receive input from the laser-treated eye in mild through advanced stages of glaucoma. In contrast to the asymmetry seen for [^{11}C]PK11195 binding potential values between bilateral LGN, Iba-1- , GFAP-, or PBR-positive glial cells showed no similar asymmetry in the bilateral LGN. In the PET imaging, living monkeys were used and, therefore, some differences of biological or haemodynamic activities such as cellular activity and blood flow between the bilateral LGN might be affected to PK11195 binding potentials, but further studies will be needed to explain this discrepancy.

Recently, reduction of functional activity in the primary visual cortex has been reported in open-angle glaucomatous patients with asymmetric visual field damage by using fMRI technique [29,30], though the result of the correlation between fMRI responses and measurements of optic disc damage is still controversial in these studies. There may be strong plasticity and compensatory mechanism of the visual pathway during early stage of diagnosis progression, which makes difficult to use the activity related fMRI signal for identifying the early indicators of glaucoma. Though MRI scans have generally higher spatial and temporal resolutions than PET, and allows functional assessment of the region brain without any imaging agents, the PET imaging technique has higher sensitivity and specificity to the biological process in the specific cell, PBR in the activated glial cells in this case, which has not been available by MRI technique yet. Therefore, at present PET imaging has more reliable with sensitive and specific values for diagnosing glaucoma especially in the early stage. Furthermore, PET imaging may have more sensitive and specific value for diagnosing glaucoma especially in the early stage.

In conclusion, these findings indicate that non-invasive molecular imaging of the LGN targeted against activated glial markers such as PBR may be useful in diagnosis of glaucoma and in the development of neuroprotective agents. However, in the present study the sample size was small at each stage of glaucoma and, therefore, further additional studies will be needed.

Acknowledgments

The authors thank M. Goto for PET tracer production, and C. Takeda for technical assistance.

Author Contributions

Conceived and designed the experiments: MS HH MI MA YW HO KI. Performed the experiments: MS Y. Inokuchi Y. Ito HY TN TH. Analyzed the data: MS Y. Inokuchi Y. Ito HY TN. Contributed reagents/materials/analysis tools: BJ MH TS. Wrote the paper: MS.

References

1. Ito Y, Shimazawa M, Chen YN, Tsuruma K, Yamashima T, et al. (2009) Morphological changes in the visual pathway induced by experimental glaucoma in Japanese monkeys. Exp Eye Res 89: 246–255.
2. Weber AJ, Chen H, Hubbard WC, Kaufman PL (2000) Experimental glaucoma and cell size, density, and number in the primate lateral geniculate nucleus. Invest Ophthalmol Vis Sci 41: 1370–1379.
3. Yücel YH, Zhang Q, Gupta N, Kaufman PL, Weinreb RN (2000) Loss of neurons in magnocellular and parvocellular layers of the lateral geniculate nucleus in glaucoma. Arch Ophthalmol 118: 378–384.
4. Yücel YH, Zhang Q, Weinreb RN, Kaufman PL, Gupta N (2001) Atrophy of relay neurons in magno- and parvocellular layers in the lateral geniculate nucleus in experimental glaucoma. Invest Ophthalmol Vis Sci 42: 3216–3222.
5. Gupta N, Ang LC, Noel de Tilly L, Bidaisee L, Yücel YH (2006) Human glaucoma and neural degeneration in intracranial optic nerve, lateral geniculate nucleus, and visual cortex. Br J Ophthalmol 90: 674–678.
6. Gupta N, Greenberg G, de Tilly LN, Gray B, Polemidiotis M, et al. (2009) Atrophy of the lateral geniculate nucleus in human glaucoma detected by magnetic resonance imaging. Br J Ophthalmol 93: 56–60.
7. Sasaoka M, Nakamura K, Shimazawa M, Ito Y, Araie M, et al. (2008) Changes in visual fields and lateral geniculate nucleus in monkey laser-induced high intraocular pressure model. Exp Eye Res 86: 770–782.
8. Imamura K, Onoe H, Shimazawa M, Nozaki S, Wada Y, et al. (2009) Molecular imaging reveals unique degenerative changes in experimental glaucoma. Neuroreport 20: 139–144.
9. Papadopoulos V, Baraldi M, Guilarte TR, Knudsen TB, Lacapere JJ, et al. (2006) Translocator protein (18 kDa): new nomenclature for the peripheral-type benzodiazepine receptor based on its structure and molecular function. Trends Pharmacol Sci 27: 402–409.
10. Anholt RR, Pedersen PL, De Souza EB, Snyder SH (1986) The peripheral-type benzodiazepine receptor. Localization to the mitochondrial outer membrane. J Biol Chem 261: 576–583.
11. Benavides J, Guilloux F, Rufat P, Uzan A, Renault C, et al. (1984) In vivo labelling in several rat tissues of 'peripheral type' benzodiazepine binding sites. Eur J Pharmacol 99: 1–7.
12. Vowinckel E, Reutens D, Becher B, Verge G, Evans A, et al. (1997) PK11195 binding to the peripheral benzodiazepine receptor as a marker of microglia activation in multiple sclerosis and experimental autoimmune encephalomyelitis. J Neurosci Res 50: 345–353.
13. Chen MK, Baidoo K, Verina T, Guilarte TR (2004) Peripheral benzodiazepine receptor imaging in CNS demyelination: functional implications of anatomical and cellular localization. Brain 127: 1379–1392.
14. Quigley HA, Hohman RM (1983) Laser energy levels for trabecular meshwork damage in the primate eye. Invest Ophthalmol Vis Sci 24: 1305–1307.
15. Shimazawa M, Tomita G, Taniguchi T, Sasaoka M, Hara H, et al. (2006) Morphometric evaluation of changes with time in optic disc structure and thickness of retinal nerve fibre layer in chronic ocular hypertensive monkeys. Exp Eye Res 82: 427–440.
16. Shah F, Hume SP, Pike VW, Ashworth S, McDermott J (1994) Synthesis of the enantiomers of [N-methyl-^{11}C]PK 11195 and comparison of their behaviours as radioligands for PK binding sites in rats. Nucl Med Biol 21: 573–581.
17. Lammertsma AA, Hume SP (1996) Simplified reference tissue model for PET receptor studies. Neuroimage 4: 153–158.
18. Sanchez RM, Dunkelberger GR, Quigley HA (1986) The number and diameter distribution of axons in the monkey optic nerve. Invest Ophthalmol Vis Sci 27: 1342–1350.
19. Whitmore AV, Libby RT, John SW (2005) Glaucoma: thinking in new ways-a role for autonomous axonal self-destruction and other compartmentalised processes? Prog Retin Eye Res 24: 639–662.
20. Howell GR, Libby RT, Jakobs TC, Smith RS, Phalan FC, et al. (2007) Axons of retinal ganglion cells are insulted in the optic nerve early in DBA/2J glaucoma. J Cell Biol 179: 1523–1537.
21. Kerrigan LA, Zack DJ, Quigley HA, Smith SD, Pease ME (1997) TUNEL-positive ganglion cells in human primary open-angle glaucoma. Arch Ophthalmol 115: 1031–1035.
22. Quigley HA, Nickells RW, Kerrigan LA, Pease ME, Thibault DJ, et al. (1995) Retinal ganglion cell death in experimental glaucoma and after axotomy occurs by apoptosis. Invest Ophthalmol Vis Sci 36: 774–786.
23. McGeer PL, Schwab C, Parent A, Doudet D (2003) Presence of reactive microglia in monkey substantia nigra years after 1-methyl-4-phenyl-1,2,3,6-tetrahydropyridine administration. Ann Neurol 54: 599–604.
24. Lam D, Jim J, To E, Rasmussen C, Kaufman PL, et al. (2009) Astrocyte and microglial activation in the lateral geniculate nucleus and visual cortex of glaucomatous and optic nerve transected primates. Mol Vis 15: 2217–2229.
25. Banati RB, Newcombe J, Gunn RN, Cagnin A, Turkheimer F, et al. (2000) The peripheral benzodiazepine binding site in the brain in multiple sclerosis: quantitative in vivo imaging of microglia as a measure of disease activity. Brain 123(Pt 11): 2321–2337.

26. Cagnin A, Brooks DJ, Kennedy AM, Gunn RN, Myers R, et al. (2001) In-vivo measurement of activated microglia in dementia. Lancet 358: 461–467.
27. Gerhard A, Pavese N, Hotton G, Turkheimer F, Es M, et al. (2006) In vivo imaging of microglial activation with $[^{11}C](R)$-PK11195 PET in idiopathic Parkinson's disease. Neurobiol Dis 21: 404–412.
28. Pavese N, Gerhard A, Tai YF, Ho AK, Turkheimer F, et al. (2006) Microglial activation correlates with severity in Huntington disease: a clinical and PET study. Neurology 66: 1638–1643.
29. Duncan RO, Sample PA, Weinreb RN, Bowd C, Zangwill LM (2007) Retinotopic organization of primary visual cortex in glaucoma: a method for comparing cortical function with damage to the optic disk. Invest Ophthalmol Vis Sci 48: 733–744.
30. Qing G, Zhang S, Wang B, Wang N (2010) Functional MRI signal changes in primary visual cortex corresponding to the central normal visual field of patients with primary open-angle glaucoma. Invest Ophthalmol Vis Sci 51: 4627–4634.

11

Mitochondrial Damage in the Trabecular Meshwork Occurs Only in Primary Open-Angle Glaucoma and in Pseudoexfoliative Glaucoma

Alberto Izzotti[1], Mariagrazia Longobardi[1], Cristina Cartiglia[1], Sergio Claudio Saccà[2]*

1 Department of Health Sciences, University of Genoa, Genoa, Italy, **2** Department of Head/Neck Pathologies, Ophthalmology Unit, St. Martino Hospital, Genoa, Italy

Abstract

Background: Open-angle glaucoma appears to be induced by the malfunction of the trabecular meshwork cells due to injury induced by oxidative damage and mitochondrial impairment. Here, we report that, in fact, we have detected mitochondrial damage only in primary open-angle glaucoma and pseudo-exfoliation glaucoma, among several glaucoma types compared.

Methodology/Principal Findings: Mitochondrial damage was evaluated by analyzing the common mitochondrial DNA deletion by real-time PCR in trabecular meshwork specimens collected at surgery from glaucomatous patients and controls. Glaucomatous patients included 38 patients affected by various glaucoma types: primary open-angle, pigmented, juvenile, congenital, pseudoexfoliative, acute, neovascular, and chronic closed-angle glaucoma. As control samples, we used 16 specimens collected from glaucoma-free corneal donors. Only primary open-angle glaucoma (3.0-fold) and pseudoexfoliative glaucoma (6.3-fold) showed significant increases in the amount of mitochondrial DNA deletion. In all other cases, deletion was similar to controls.

Conclusions/Significance: Despite the fact that the trabecular meshwork is the most important tissue in the physiopathology of aqueous humor outflow in all glaucoma types, the present study provides new information regarding basic physiopathology of this tissue: only in primary open-angle and pseudoexfoliative glaucomas oxidative damage arising from mitochondrial failure play a role in the functional decay of trabecular meshwork.

Editor: Alfred Lewin, University of Florida, United States of America

Funding: This study was supported by the United States Glaucoma Foundation (New York, NY). The funders had no role in study design, data collection and analysis, decision to publish, or preparation of the manuscript.

Competing Interests: The authors have declared that no competing interests exist.

* E-mail: sergio.sacca@hsanmartino.it

Introduction

Glaucoma is a neurodegenerative eye disease, the affected regions of which are (a) the retina, particularly the optic nerve; (b) the central nervous system, especially the lateral geniculate nucleus of the brain [1]; and (c) the eye anterior chamber, specifically the trabecular meshwork (TM). TM is crucial in glaucoma pathogenesis because its malfunction causes intraocular pressure (IOP) increases, as occur during open-angle glaucoma [2]. Indeed, TM cellularity, in particular the number of endothelial cells, plays a fundamental role in regulating the passage of fluids from the anterior chamber (AC) to Schlemm's canal [3]. Moreover, TM endothelial cells regulate the permeability of endothelial cells in Schlemm's canal, giving them a major role in the regulation of aqueous outflow [4]. The number of TM endothelial cells decreases with age [5]. During a patient's lifetime, TM cells are constantly exposed by free radicals in the AC, where a precarious balance between antioxidant defenses and oxidative free radicals exists [6]. Free radicals and reactive oxygen species are able to affect the cellularity of the human TM (HTM). These findings suggest that an intraocular pressure increase, which characterizes most glaucomas, is related to oxidative and degenerative processes affecting the HTM and, more specifically, its endothelial cells [7]. Furthermore, HTM is more sensitive to oxidative stress than other tissues around the AC [8]. Indeed, oxidative damage caused by reactive oxygen species (ROS) is greater in primary open-angle glaucoma (POAG) and pseudoexfoliative glaucoma (PEXG) patients than in healthy subjects [9]. TM endothelial cells secrete a number of factors, such as enzymes and cytokines, which modulate the functions of the cells and the extracellular matrix of the conventional aqueous outflow pathway [10] Damage to TM endothelial cells causes malfunction in the homeostasis of the outflow of the aqueous humor. The exact molecular mechanism underlying TM cell loss in glaucoma patients is still unclear. Indeed, chronic oxidative stress leads to the endogenous production of ROS by mitochondria in TM cells, thereby increasing the level of oxidative damage in the tissue [11]. In glaucomatous patients, a spectrum of mitochondrial abnormalities involving oxidative stress and implying mitochondrial dysfunction has been found [12]. The composition of aqueous humor proteins changes dramatically [13], and antioxidant proteins undergo down-regulation, in glaucoma; this leads to increased concentrations of nitric oxide synthase 2 and other proteins that, in physiological conditions, are segregated inside the functional mitochondria of TM cells [14]. Mitochondria are endowed with a specific DNA of maternal origin, mitochondrial DNA (mtDNA). This encodes only 13 structural proteins, all of which are involved in the respiratory chain. Most mitochondrial proteins are encoded by nuclear DNA. A complex interaction between the two genomes is therefore at the basis of mitochondrial protein synthesis and of mtDNA replication [15]. Mitochondria produce up to 90% of the cellular energy and also play a critical role in mediating cell death through the apoptotic pathway [16]. Damage accruing to the mitochondrial genome is associated with increased cellular stress and organelle dysfunction [17]. He and colleagues showed that TM cells of patients with POAG undergo ATP diminution, as their functionality is endangered by an intrinsic mitochondrial complex I defect, causing a respiratory chain deficit in these cells [18]. Recently, we reported that in TM of POAG patients, as compared with control subjects, mtDNA deletion is dramatically increased and the ratio between mtDNA and nuclear DNA is reduced. The amount of nuclear DNA in relation to wet tissue weight is also decreased [14]. These findings provide evidence that mitochondrial damage is severe in the TM of POAG patients.

Besides POAG, many other glaucoma types exist, including pigmented (PG), juvenile (JG), congenital (CG), acute closed-angle (ACG), neovascular (NVG), and chronic closed-angle glaucoma (CCAG), each one characterized by different and specific pathogenic mechanisms. The aim of the present paper is to establish whether there are biomolecular differences between mtDNA deletions in POAG and those found in other glaucoma types.

Results

The extent of mitochondrial DNA deletion in various glaucoma types as detected by QPCR is reported in Figure 1. These findings are paralleled by the amount of oxidative nuclear DNA damage (8-hydroxy-2′-deoxyguanosine) of the same samples by ^{32}P-postlabeling (Figure 1).

Furthermore, a variety of parameters reflecting the occurrence of molecular alterations in mitochondria were considered, including (a) %mtDNA deletion/mtDNA, which is the amount of deleted mtDNA compared to total mtDNA and thus directly expresses the extent of the 4977 mtDNA common lesion; (b) total mtDNA/mg wet tissue, which represents the amount of mitochondria in the analyzed TM biopsy; (c) total nDNA/mg wet tissue, which represents the number of cells in the analyzed TM biopsy. As reported in Table 1, only POAG and PEXG showed a high level of mitochondrial deletion as compared to controls. The mtDNA 4977 deletion values observed in PEXG were more than double those detected in POAG.

In all glaucoma types other than POAG and PEXG, the amount of mitochondrial deletion did not significantly vary from that observed in control TM samples (Table 1).

Similar findings were obtained for oxidative damage to nuclear DNA, which significantly increased only in POAG and PEXG and not in other glaucoma types.

TM cellularity, expressed as total nDNA/mg wet tissue, was dramatically decreased in all glaucoma types, indicating that cell loss in TM is a non-specific event occurring in many glaucoma types. Similarly, the total number of mitochondria in TM decreased in all glaucoma types, a finding related to the cell loss observed. Conversely, the number of mitochondria per cell (mtDNA/nDNA ratio) was significantly decreased only in POAG and PEXG (Table 1).

A non-significant trend towards a lower level of mtDNA deletion in some glaucoma types (juvenile, congenital,) than in controls was observed, probably due to the younger age of these patients as compared to controls.

A significant correlation between the amount of mtDNA deletion and the level of oxidative DNA damage detected in different glaucoma types was observed ($r = +0.942$, $P < 0.001$). This finding indicates that mitochondrial damage is tightly correlated with the development of oxidative damage in TM cells. A significantly inverse relationship was observed between the number of mitochondria per TM cell and oxidative damage ($r = -0.780$, $P < 0.05$). This finding indicates that accumulation of oxidative damage inside TM cells results in severe mitochondrial loss.

Together, our results provide evidence of the strong connection existing in TM between oxidative stress and mitochondrial damage in degenerative forms of glaucoma (POAG and PEXG).

Discussion

Our results indicate that mitochondrial damage and related oxidative stress specifically occur in POAG and PEXG and not in other glaucoma types.

A high level of mitochondrial alterations was observed, particularly in PEXG, which had the highest levels of mtDNA deletion, oxidative nDNA damage, and mitochondrial loss per cell. These results justify the clinical features of PEXG, which is more aggressive than POAG and typically displays higher intraocular pressure [19]; moreover, tonometric compensation is also more difficult in PEXG.

These results indicate that POAG and PEXG are characterized by specific mechanisms involving mitochondrial damage, oxidative stress, and mitochondrial loss, finally resulting in TM cell loss. Conversely, in other glaucoma types, TM cell loss is independent of mitochondrial damage and loss.

The observed specific role of mitochondria damage in the degenerative glaucomas (i.e., POAG and PEXG) is in line with the important function of this organelle. Human cells depend on ATP for growth, differentiation and responses to physiological and environmental stimuli. Mitochondria are cytoplasmic organelles, the main role of which is to synthesize ATP. They play crucial roles in other cell processes, the most important of which include development, calcium homeostasis, cell cycle regulation, thermogenesis, free radical production and apoptosis. The respiratory chain is composed of five multiheteromeric enzymatic complexes (I, II, III, IV and V) embedded in the inner membrane of mitochondria. The respiratory chain is under the control of two separate genetic systems, i.e. mtDNA and nDNA behaving differently in many respects [20]. The mitochondrial genome regularly replicates in postmitotic cells, about once per month. The mitochondria divide mainly in response to the energy needs of the cell, i.e., independently of the cell cycle [21]. The mitochondria continuously fuse with one another, and the cells may therefore contain both normal and possibly modified mitochondrial genes. After cell division, the proportions of mutant genomes differ in the individual descendant cells. The frequency and proportion of the deleted mtDNA in human tissues increase with age. mtDNA deletions occur more frequently and abundantly in high energy-demanding tissues during the aging process [22]. mtDNA is more vulnerable to oxidative stress, its mutation rate being about 10-fold higher than that of nDNA [23]. All tissues from adult subjects show the presence of mitochondrial DNA molecules with deletions [24], and the accumulation of mtDNA mutations in aging contributes significantly to the decline of mitochondrial energy production that characterizes the aging process in many tissues [25–26].

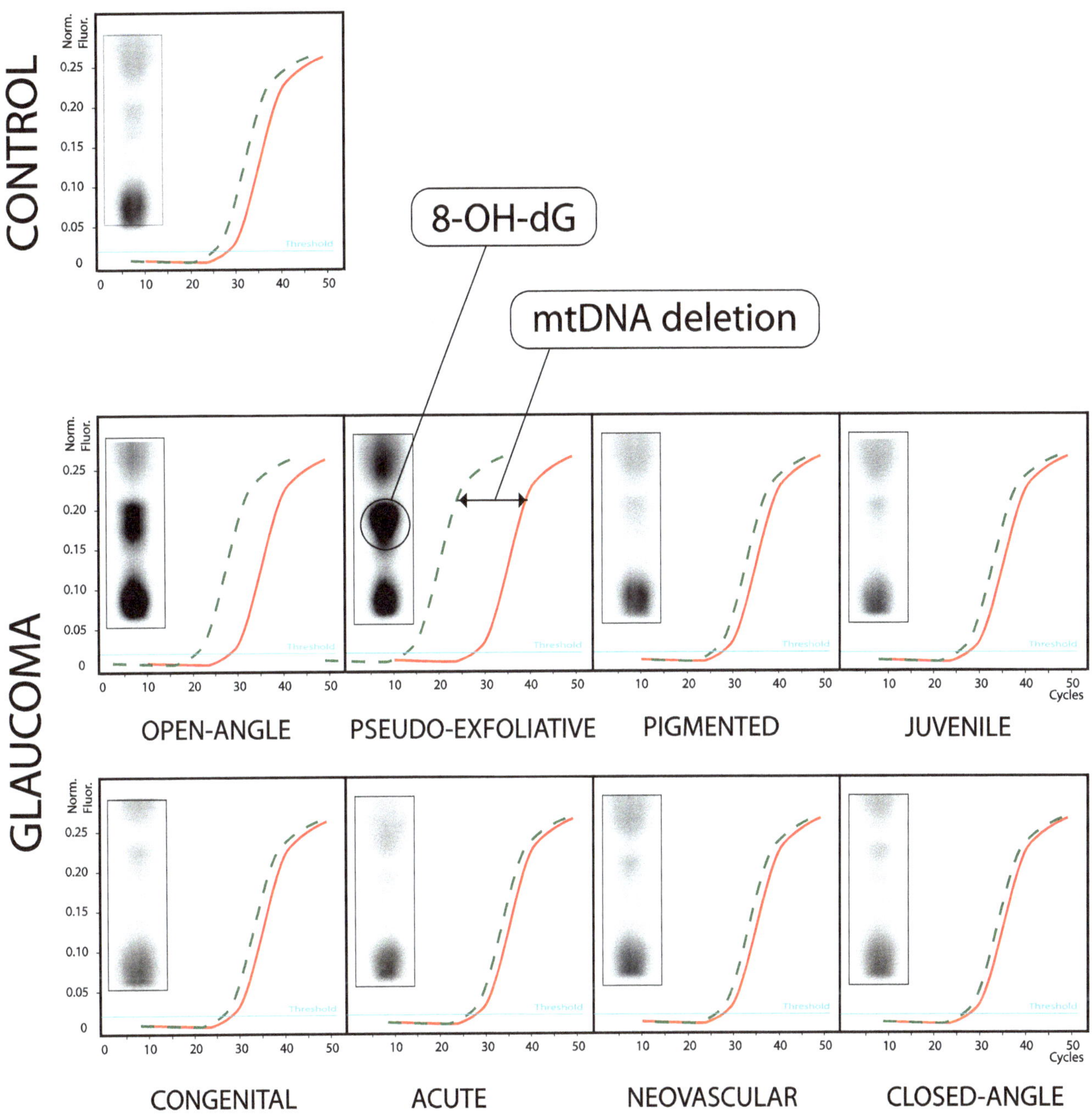

Figure 1. Normalized QPCR evaluation of the common 4977-bp mtDNA deletion in TM of patients with different glaucoma types. The horizontal axis shows the number of QPCR cycles, the vertical axis the amount of amplified DNA as inferred from the intensity of the fluorescence signal. The continuous curve indicates the normalized quantity of total mtDNA, the dashed curve indicates the relative amount of 4977 bp–deleted mtDNA. Samples in which the dashed curve intercepts the threshold horizontal line at lower QPCR cycles (left side) have a greater amount of 4977 bp–deleted mtDNA. For each sample, the box on the left shows oxidative nuclear DNA damage (8-oxo-dG) as detected by ^{32}P-postlabeling.

In mitochondria, the production of reactive oxygen species (ROS) increases, as do the by-products of aerobic metabolism in aging tissues. Indeed, the mitochondrial respiratory chain is one of the main sources of deleterious free radicals in the human organism. Under normal physiological conditions, a small fraction of the oxygen consumed by mitochondria is constantly converted to superoxide anions, hydrogen peroxide, hydroxyl radicals and other ROS [27]. The age-dependent decline in the capacity of mitochondria to dispose of these oxy-radicals renders mtDNA more vulnerable to mutations during the ageing process [28]. In this light, the mtDNA deletions in the human TM that accumulate during the aging process are the result of this reduced capability. Mitochondrial decay, as evaluated by cytochrome *c* oxidase analysis, is associated with apoptotic activation in TM cells in patients with POAG [18], in that oxidative stress causes activation of mitochondrial matrix caspase activity, which is secondary to cytochrome *c* release [28]. In addition to the endogenous formation and accumulation of mtDNA deletions in human tissues during the normal aging process, physiological and environmental factors such as light may also play important roles

Table 1. Mitochondrial DNA damage detected in TM of various glaucoma types.

Disease status	Age (years)	mtDNA deletion amount (%mtDNA deletion/mtDNA)	Mitochondrial number (mtDNA/mg wet tissue)	TM cell number (nDNA/mg wet tissue)	Oxidative nDNA damage (8-oxo-dG/105 nucleotides)
Controls N=16	65±12	12.9±5.1	18.7±1.6	9.1±1.6	2.3±2.5
POAG n=16	71±9	38.7±21.8*	2.9±0.5*	0.5±0.1*	8.0±4.2*
PEXG n=5	72±4	82.1±39.0*	0.1±0.0*	0.1±0.1*	9.8±3.7*
PG n=2	36±14	5.0±4.1	3.5±3.2	0.7±0.5*	NT
JG n=4	43±2	2.7±1.3	0.7±0.6*	0.1±0.1*	3.0±2.8
CG n=4	21±10	0.3±0.1	0.9±0.4*	0.2±0.1*	1.5±0.4
ACG n=3	60±2	0.9±0.8	4.1±2.4*	0.9±0.7*	2.8±1.0
NvG n=2	70±4	0.1±0.0	4.7±0.7*	0.7±0.3*	3.2±1.2
CCAG n=2	64±2	0.4±0.3	1.8±1.5*	3.3±3.1*	2.1±0.4

*P<0.05 compared to controls.

in eliciting the deposition of deleted mtDNA molecules in cells [29]. Such mutations are induced through a similar mechanism as the endogenous mutations, although the absolute extent of accumulation differs among tissues [30]. Our results show that the generalized relative abundance of particular mtDNA mutations in specific tissues is associated with specific TM pathologies, i.e., PEXG and POAG.

Exfoliation syndrome, associated with PEXG, is an age-related disorder of the extracellular matrix characterized by the production and progressive accumulation of a fibrillar material not only in ocular tissues but also in skin and connective tissue portions of various visceral organs. From a histopathological point of view, PEXG is different from POAG. Whereas POAG is characterized by increased juxtacanalicular plaque material and decreased TM cellularity [5], in pseudoexfoliative glaucoma, both plaque material and cellularity are unchanged compared with normal eyes; the characteristic exfoliation material is deposited instead [31]. Although these histopathological differences suggest completely different pathogenetic mechanisms [32], our results show that POAG and PEXG share one mechanism in common. They both produce a decrease in TM cellularity through mitochondrial damage and apoptosis, which is stimulated by the ROS circulating in the AC and produced in TM by damaged mitochondria. Oxidative DNA damage in pseudoexfoliative patients is greater than that which occurs in POAG patients in the TM region. However, the accumulation of locally produced pseudoexfoliative material in the juxtacanalicular tissue, and the consequent dysfunction of endothelial cells and disorganization of juxtacanalicular tissue and Schlemm's canal, are causative factors in the development of a special type of secondary open-angle glaucoma in exfoliation syndrome [31]. Decreased cellularity of the trabecular meshwork appears to be a particular characteristic of POAG, but other authors reported that it does not seem to play a role in the pathogenesis of PEX glaucoma [31].

Interestingly, other types of glaucoma have not shown signs of mitochondrial deletion increases. In neovascular glaucoma, the TM is damaged by neo-vessels that invade the tissue, causing its malfunctioning and increasing IOP. Indeed, if neovascularization regresses, a rapid IOP decrease results [33]. Both chronic and acute closed-angle glaucomas present structural similarities: pupil-blocking force, status of angle synechia closure, and shallow depth of the anterior chamber; however, the former is asymptomatic, whereas the latter is symptomatic. In any case, both glaucomas share a final pathway involving the formation of irreversible synechial adhesion between the peripheral iris and the TM [34]. In closed-angle glaucomas, the TM is obstructed by the iris, which prevents TM cells from functioning, thereby impeding the normal flow of aqueous humor across this region. The duration of contact closure necessary to cause synechial closure appears to vary greatly from patient to patient. If the obstacle to outflow is promptly removed, IOP may return to normal values. However, prolonged contact between the iris or iris/lens and the TM may lead to permanent damage to TM functionality and produce a permanent IOP increase.

In congenital and juvenile glaucoma, there are several pathogenic factors that come into play, spanning from arrested development of the anterior chamber angle structures, which is characterized by incomplete maturation of the TM and Schlemm's canal [35], to mesodermal dysgenesis of the iris and cornea characterized by abnormalities of the anterior chamber cleavage [36] and from congenital hereditary endothelial dystrophy [37] to arginase deficit [38]. The increased resistance to aqueous humor outflow in congenital glaucoma may stem from abnormalities of the TM and the internal wall of Schlemm's canal [39]. It is possible that both congenital and juvenile glaucoma occur because of developmental immaturity of the TM in anterior chamber angle tissues [40]. Ultrastructural examination of TM shows that the inner cribriform area is greatly thickened and the amount of sheath-derived plaque material is increased in the subendothelial layer adjacent to Schlemm's canal [41]; there are no vacuoles in the endothelium of Schlemm's canal, and there is a broad layer of collagen and amorphous material in the juxtacanalicular connective tissue [42]. The class and distribution of proteoglycans in the goniodsygenetic trabecular tissues are virtually the same as in normal tissues [43], and there are no significant differences between the morphological picture of primary congenital glaucoma and that found in Axenfeld and Rieger anomalies [44]. Accordingly, the pathogenesis of all these glaucoma types does not require the occurrence of mitochondrial damage, as demonstrated by the data reported here.

The lack of mitochondrial deletion was also confirmed in the cases of pigmentary glaucoma. In this situation, the development of the chronic glaucomatous condition cannot be directly attributed to pigment accumulation in the juxtacanalicular tissue [45]. However, many TM alterations have been described: loss of trabecular cells, fusion of trabecular lamellae and collapse of intertrabecular spaces, increase in extracellular material, and obliteration of the canal have been found to varying degrees around the circumference of eyes with pigment dispersion syndrome and elevated intraocular pressure and in pigmentary glaucoma. These probably all contribute to the development of increased intraocular pressure in pigmentary glaucoma [46]. Macrophages are the main cell type responsible for TM clearance of pigment and debris [47]. It is possible that, on a genetic basis, they play a central role in the pathophysiology of pigmentary glaucoma.

In conclusion, our findings demonstrate that in all types of glaucoma in which IOP is high, TM malfunction resulting from cellularity decrease is the key to the development of the disease. However, only in primary open angle and pseudo-exfoliation glaucoma was mitochondrial damage detected, as the outflow dysfunction in the other glaucomas studied may have a different underlying basis.

Materials and Methods

Patient recruitment and sample collection

Between January 2007 and July 2009, 38 consecutive glaucoma patients (21 women, 17 men) aged 55–82 years (70±7.15 years, mean ± SE) were enrolled. They included 16 cases of primary open-angle (POAG), 2 pigmented (PG), 4 juvenile (JG), 4 congenital (CG), 5 pseudoexfoliative (PEXG), 3 acute (ACG), 2 neovascular (NvG), and 2 chronic closed-angle (CCAG) glaucoma.

Various glaucoma diagnosis were performed on a clinical basis. Both NVG patients were suffering from systemic hypertension and both have had a thrombosis of central vein of the retina.

Glaucoma was diagnosed and classified on the basis of clinical characteristics (slit-lamp examination, gonioscopy, intraocular pressure (IOP) increase, pachymetry, perimetric test and optic nerve morphometric or nerve fiber layer analysis with GDx or HRT) according to the classification of Shields, Ritch and Krupin [48]. GDx-VCC software version 5.2.3 (Laser Diagnostic Technologies, San Diego, CA) was used to evaluate the parapapillary RNFL. Confocal scanning laser ophthalmoscopy was performed with the Heidelberg Retina Tomograph II and analyzed with HRT III software (Heidelberg Engineering GmbH, Heidelberg, Germany). Visual-field testing was performed with the Humphrey Field Analyzer 750 (Allergan Humphrey, San Leandro, CA). The presence of perimetric glaucomatous defects was assessed by computerized visual-field testing (Humphrey 30-2 computerized visual-field examination) and graded according to the criteria proposed by Caprioli [49]. A visual-field defect score was assigned according to Brusini and Tosoni [50]. The study adhered to the tenets of the Declaration of Helsinki and was approved by the Ethical Board of the Ophthalmologic Division. The glaucoma patients, after having provided written informed consent, underwent ocular filtration surgery for therapeutic purposes. Trabeculectomy specimens were collected at surgery from the 38 glaucomatous patients. For each patient, we considered only one eye with an established diagnosis of POAG showing failed tonometric compensation and worsening of perimetric and optic disc conditions. All patients were treated with maximal therapy, including prostaglandin F2 analogs (92.1% [35 patients]), systemic carbonic anhydrase inhibitors (86.8% [33 patients]), topical beta-blockers (84.2% [32 patients]), topical carbonic anhydrase inhibitors (84.2% [32 patients]), α_2-agonists (76.3% [29 patients]), and pilocarpine (28.9% [11patients]). Despite using the maximal tolerated therapy, all patients showed elevated IOP on entry to the hospital department (min 25 mmHg; max 41 mmHg; mean 31.3±4.62). Patients underwent ocular filtration surgery for therapeutic purposes at the Ophthalmology Unit of S. Martino Hospital in Genoa from 2007 to 2009. Samples were collected by standard surgical trabeculectomy as previously described [5–9]. Inclusion criteria were the presence of glaucoma with no tonometric compensation and the absence of any other ocular, systemic or neurological diseases other than optic nerve damage.

As control samples, we used trabeculectomy and iris specimens collected from 16 subjects aged 66.1±1.27 years who were gender-matched with patients. These samples were provided by the Melvin Jones Eye Bank in Genoa from 2007 to 2009. The control samples had been obtained immediately after death from glaucoma-free subjects undergoing eye removal for cornea transplantation, as previously described [9]. Every effort was made to ensure that the sampling times in donors were the same as in the patients studied. Control samples were taken no later than 1 hour after death, thus ensuring cell viability, which is obviously very important in cornea transplantation. Samples were immersed in stabilizing buffers containing antioxidants and stored at −80°C until DNA purification, which was performed with proteinase K and solvent extraction in an oxygen-free atmosphere, as previously described [9].

Approval for this study was given by the Ethics Committee of the Ophthalmologic Unit of the Head/Neck Department of San Martino Hospital, Genoa, Italy, and all study patients provided written informed consent. The research followed the tenets of the Declaration of Helsinki.

Detection of mitochondrial DNA damage

Mitochondrial DNA damage was evaluated in terms of the common 4977-bp deletion, which is a large mtDNA deletion involving the loss of almost one third of the mitochondrial genome.

To evaluate the frequency of the common 4977-bp deletion in mtDNA, we performed two real-time QPCR reactions for each sample, one aimed at detecting the amount of total mtDNA (TMDQ) and one to quantify the deleted mtDNA (DMDQ). The TMDQ evaluation was carried out by using two primers (tot mt S: CCATCTTTGCAGGCACACTCATC and tot mt A: ATC-CACCTCAACTGCCTGCTATG) flanking a sequence of mt DNA known not to be susceptible to deletion [51] and an *ad hoc*–designed FAM-labeled molecular beacon (mt tot: CGCGATCT-CACGCAAGCAACCGCATCCATGATCGCG). The DMDQ evaluation was performed using two primers (del mt S: GGCCCGTATTTACCCTATAG and del mt A: GGTGAGAA-GAATTATTCGAGTG) flanking the region susceptible to deletion and a second *ad hoc* FAM-labeled molecular beacon (mt del: CGCGATCCAGCCTAGCATTAGCAGGAATACCTT-GATCGCG). Because of the short elongation time, only deleted mtDNA can efficiently give rise to an amplicon containing the target sequence for the mt del molecular beacon. DNA for TMDQ quantification was diluted 10-fold more than for DMDQ. The reaction conditions were 5 µl 10x PCR buffer, 0.4 µl 100 mM dNTP mix, 2 µl 50 mM $MgCl_2$, 0.5 µl Platinum *Taq* DNA polymerase (Invitrogen Corporation, Carlsbad, CA), 37.1 µl sterile water, 1 µl 10 mM sense primer, 1 µl 10 mM anti-sense primer, 2 µl molecular beacon, and 1 µl DNA. The mixture was split into two 200-µl flat-cap transparent tubes.

The reactions were performed in a Rotorgene 3000 (Corbett Research, Mortlake NSW 2137, Australia) as follows: 94°C for 2 min, followed by 45 cycles at 94°C for 30 sec, room temperature for 30 sec, and 72°C for 30 sec. The FAM channel was acquired at the end of the annealing step. The annealing temperature for mt tot was 54°C and for mt del 51°C.

The del-mtDNA/tot-mtDNA ratio was assessed for each sample and normalized to the number of cells and to the quantitiy of nuclear DNA, as assessed by a further QPCR reaction quantifying the housekeeping gene GAPDH.

Primer sequences and PCR conditions were determined by using Beacon Designer 6.0 software (Premier Biosoft International, Palo Alto, CA). Result specificity was checked by analyzing the melting curves of PCR products.

The relative amount of total nuclear DNA in each sample was evaluated by quantifying the copies of GAPDH mRNA by means of quantitative real-time PCR (QPCR). This parameter was compared both to the number of mitochondrial DNA copies (nuclear/mitochondrial DNA ratio) and to the amount of wet tissue processed (DNA/g wet tissue). This last parameter was taken as an indicator of TM cellularity. The following primers and the molecular beacon specific for a 149-bp DNA sequence of human GAPDH were designed with Beacon Designer and purchased from TIB (Molbiol, Berlin, Germany): Sense TGTCTGCT-TCTCTGCTGTAG, Anti-sense CTGCCTTCCTCACCT-GATG, Probe 5′ – FAM – CGCGATCCATGTTCGTCAT-GGGTGTGAACCAGATCGCG – BHQ1.

The QPCR reaction was carried out in a rotating real-time thermocycler (Corbett Life Science, Sydney, Australia) in a mixture containing 0.1 µg DNA, 0.2 mM each of ATP, GTP, TTP and CTP, 1.5 mM $MgCl_2$, 2 U Platinum *Taq* DNA polymerase, 0.2 µM primer Sense, 0.2 µM primer Anti-sense, 0.4 µm Probe and water to 50 µl. Polymerase was hot start-activated at 94°C for 2 min, and 40 amplification cycles of 94°C for 40 sec, 53°C for 30 sec and 72°C for 30 sec followed. The fluorescent signal was detected at every annealing step.

Relative quantification was performed by comparing the cycle threshold of every sample with that of a standard dilution of a DNA sample of known concentration.

Detection of oxidative DNA damage to nuclear DNA

Oxidative DNA damage was analyzed in terms of 8-hydroxy-2′-deoxyguanosine (8-oxo-dG) by ^{32}P-postlabeling as previously reported [9].

Statistical analyses

Comparisons of quantitative variables among different groups were performed by ANOVA and Student's *t* test for unpaired data after checking the normality of the distribution by kurtosis skew analysis. The accepted level of significance in all cases was $P<0.05$. In the case of non-normal distribution of data, non-parametric Mann-Whitney U and Kruskal-Wallis tests were used. Correlations between continuous variables were tested by linear regression analysis. Differences in frequency distributions among nominal variables were tested by the chi-square test. All statistical analyses were performed with the Statview software (Abacus Concepts, Berkeley, CA).

Author Contributions

Conceived and designed the experiments: AI SCS. Performed the experiments: ML CC. Analyzed the data: AI. Contributed reagents/materials/analysis tools: ML CC. Wrote the paper: AI SCS.

References

1. Gupta N, Ly T, Zhang Q, Kaufman PL, Weinreb RN, et al. (2007) Chronic ocular hypertension induces dendrite pathology in the lateral geniculate nucleus of the brain. Exp Eye Res 84: 176–84.
2. Saccà SC, Pascotto A, Camicione P, Capris P, Izzotti A (2005) Oxidative DNA damage in the human trabecular meshwork: clinical correlation in patients with primary open-angle glaucoma. Arch Ophthalmol 123: 458–63.
3. Alvarado JA, Yeh RF, Franse-Carman L, Marcellino G, Brownstein MJ (2005) Interactions between endothelia of the trabecular meshwork and of Schlemm's canal: a new insight into the regulation of aqueous outflow in the eye. Trans Am Ophthalmol Soc 103: 148–62.
4. Alvarado JA, Alvarado RG, Yeh RF, Franse-Carman L, Marcellino GR, et al. (2005) A new insight into the cellular regulation of aqueous outflow: how trabecular meshwork endothelial cells drive a mechanism that regulates the permeability of Schlemm's canal endothelial cells. Br J Ophthalmol 89: 1500–5.
5. Alvarado JA, Murphy CG, Juster R (1984) Trabecular meshwork cellularity in primary open-angle glaucoma and nonglaucomatous normals. Ophthalmology 91: 564–579.
6. Saccà SC, Izzotti A, Rossi P, Traverso C (2007) Glaucomatous outflow pathway and oxidative stress. Exp Eye Res 84: 389–99.
7. Saccà SC, Izzotti A (2008) Oxidative stress and glaucoma: injury in the anterior segment of the eye. Prog Brain Res 173: 385–407.
8. Izzotti A, Sacca SC, Longobardi M, Cartiglia C (2009) Sensitivity of ocular anterior chamber tissues to oxidative damage and its relevance to glaucoma pathogenesis. Invest Ophthalmol Vis Sci 50: 5251–8.
9. Izzotti A, Saccà SC, Cartiglia C, De Flora S (2003) Oxidative deoxyribonucleic acid damage in the eyes of glaucoma patients. Am J Med 114: 638–46.
10. Shifera AS, Trivedi S, Chau P, Bonnemaison LH, Iguchi R, et al. (2010) Constitutive secretion of chemokines by cultured human trabecular meshwork cells. Exp Eye Res 91: 42–7.
11. Li G, Luna C, Liton PB, Navarro I, Epstein DL, et al. (2007) Sustained stress response after oxidative stress in trabecular meshwork cells. Mol Vis 13: 2282–8.
12. Abu-Amero KK, Morales J, Bosley TM (2006) Mitochondrial abnormalities in patients with primary open-angle glaucoma. Invest Ophthalmol Vis Sci 47: 2533–41.
13. Tane N, Dhar S, Roy S, Pinheiro A, Ohira A, et al. (2007) Effect of excess synthesis of extracellular matrix components by trabecular meshwork cells: possible consequence on aqueous outflow. Exp Eye Res 84: 832–42.
14. Izzotti A, Saccà SC, Longobardi M, Cartiglia C (2010) Mitochondria loss and damage in the trabecular meshwork of primary open angle glaucomatous patients. Arch Ophthalmol 128: 724–30.
15. Di Mauro S, Schon EA (1998) Mitochondrial DNA and diseases of the nervous system: the spectrum. Neuroscientist 4: 53–63.
16. Brenner C, Kroemer G (2000) Apoptosis: mitochondria; the death signal integrators. Science 289: 1150–1151.
17. Van Houten B, Woshner V, Santos JH (2006) Role of mitochondrial DNA in toxic responses to oxidative stress. DNA Repair (Amst) 5: 145–152.
18. He Y, Leung KW, Zhang YH, Duan S, Zhong XF, et al. (2008) Mitochondrial Complex I Defect Induces ROS Release andDegeneration in Trabecular Meshwork Cells of POAG Patients: Protection by Antioxidants. Invest Ophthalmol Vis Sci 49: 1447–58.
19. Konstas AG, Mantziris DA, Stewart WC (1997) Diurnal intraocular pressure in untreated exfoliation and primary open-angle glaucoma. Arch Ophthalmol 115: 182–5.
20. Krieger C, Duchen MR (2002) Mitochondria, Ca2+ and neurodegenerativa disease. Eur J Pharmacol 447: 177–88.
21. Sas K, Robotka H, Toldi J, Vécsei L (2007) Mitochondria, metabolic disturbances, oxidative stress and the kynurenine system, with focus on neurodegenerative disorders. J Neurol Sci 257: 221–39.
22. Lee HC, Pang CY, Hsu HS, Wei YH (1994) Differential accumulations of 4,977 bp deletion in mitochondrial DNA of various tissues in human ageing. Biochim Biophys Acta 1226: 37–43.
23. Yakes FM, Van Houten B (1997) Mitochondrial DNA damage is more extensive and persists longer than nuclear DNA damage in human cells following oxidative stress. Proc Natl Acad Sci USA 94: 514–9.
24. Linnane AW, Baumer A, Maxwell RJ, Preston H, Zhang CF, et al. (1990) Mitochondrial gene mutation: the ageing process and degenerative diseases. Biochem Int 22: 1067–76.

25. Trounce I, Byrne E, Marzuki S (1989) Decline in skeletal muscle mitochondrial respiratory chain function: possible factor in ageing. Lancet 1: 637–639.
26. Yen TC, Chen YS, King KL, Yeh SH, Wei YH (1989) Liver mitochondrial respiratory functions decline with age. Biochem Biophys Res Commun 165: 994–1003.
27. Wei YH, Lee HC (2002) Oxidative stress, mitochondrial DNA mutation, and impairment of antioxidant enzymes in aging. Exp Biol Med (Maywood) 227: 671–82.
28. Takahashi A, Masuda A, Sun M, Centonze VE, Herman B (2004) Oxidative stressinduced apoptosis is associated with alterations in mitochondrial caspase activity and Bcl-2-dependent alterations in mitochondrial pH (pHm). Brain Res Bull 62: 497–504.
29. Pang CY, Lee HC, Yang JH, Wei YH (1994) Human skin mitochondrial DNA deletions associated with light exposure. Arch Biochem Biophys 312: 534–8.
30. Liu VW, Zhang C, Nagley P (1998) Mutations in mitochondrial DNA accumulate differentially in three different human tissues during ageing. Nucleic Acids Res 26: 1268–75.
31. Schlotzer-Schrehardt U, Naumann GOH (1995) Trabecular meshwork in pseudoexfoliation syndrome with and without open-angle glaucoma. A morphometric, ultrastructural study. Invest. Ophthalmol Visual Sci 36: 1750–1764.
32. Ritch R, Schlötzer-Schrehardt U, Konstas AG (2003) Why is glaucoma associated with exfoliation syndrome? Prog Retin Eye Res 22: 253–75.
33. Ehlers JP, Spirn MJ, Lam A, Sivalingam A, Samuel MA, et al. (2008) Combination intravitreal Bevacizumab/panretinal photocoagulation versus panretinal photocoagulation alone in the treatment of neovascular glaucoma. Retina 28: 696–702.
34. Ritch R, Liebmann J, Tello C (1995) A construct for understanding angle-closure glaucoma, The ultrasound biomicroscopy role of. In: Lee DA, ed. New Developments in Glaucoma, Ophthalmologic Clinics of North America. Philadelphia: WB Saunders. pp 281–93.
35. Shields MB (1983) Axenfeld-Rieger syndrome a theory of mechanism and distinctions from the iridocorneal endothelial syndrome. Trans Am Ophthalmol Soc 81: 736–84.
36. Waring GO, Rodrigues MM, Laibson PR (1975) Anterior chamber cleavage syndrome. A stepladder classification. Surv Ophthalmol 20: 3–27.
37. Ramamurthy B, Sachdeva V, Mandal AK, Vemuganti GK, Garg P, et al. (2007) Coexistent congenital hereditary endothelial dystrophy and congenital glaucoma. Cornea 26: 647–9.
38. Saccà SC, Campagna P, Ciurlo G (1996) Congenital glaucoma associated with an arginase deficit: a case report. Eur J Ophthalmol 6: 421–6.
39. Maul E, Strozzi L, Muñoz C, Reyes C (1980) The outflow pathway in congenital glaucoma. Am J Ophthalmol 89: 667–73.
40. Tawara A, Inomata H (1984) Developmental immaturity of the trabecular meshwork in juvenile glaucoma. Am J Ophthalmol 98: 82–97.
41. Furuyoshi N, Furuyoshi M, Futa R, Gottanka J, Lütjen-Drecoll E (1997) Ultrastructural changes in the trabecular meshwork of juvenile glaucoma. Ophthalmologica 211: 140–6.
42. Anderson DR (1981) The development of the trabecular meshwork and its abnormality in primary infantile glaucoma. Trans Am Ophthalmol Soc 79: 458–85.
43. Tawara A, Inomata H (1994) Distribution and characterization of sulfated proteoglycans in the trabecular tissue of goniodysgenetic glaucoma. Am J Ophthalmol 117: 741–55.
44. Bakunowicz-Lazarczyk A, Sulkowska M, Sulkowski S, Urban B (2001) Ultrastructural changes in the trabecular meshwork of congenital glaucoma. J Submicrosc Cytol Pathol 33: 17–22.
45. Murphy CG, Johnson M, Alvarado JA (1992) Juxtacanalicular tissue in pigmentary and primary open angle glaucoma. The hydrodynamic role of pigment and other constituents. Arch Ophthalmol 110: 1779–85.
46. Gottanka J, Johnson DH, Grehn F, Lütjen-Drecoll E (2006) Histologic findings in pigment dispersion syndrome and pigmentary glaucoma. J Glaucoma 15: 142–51.
47. Alvarado JA, Murphy CG (1992) Outflow obstruction in pigmentary and primary open angle glaucoma. Arch Ophthalmol 110: 1769–78.
48. Shields MB, Ritch R, Krupin T (1996) Classifications of the glaucomas. In The glaucomas St Louis, Missouri: Mosby. pp 717–725.
49. Caprioli J (1994) Clinical evaluation of the optic nerve in glaucoma. Trans Am Ophthalmol Soc 92: 589–641.
50. Brusini P, Tosoni C (2003) Staging of functional damage in glaucoma using frequency doubling technology. J Glaucoma 12: 417–26.
51. Hamblet NS, Castora FJ (1995) Mitochondrial DNA deletion analysis: a comparison of PCR quantitative methods. Biochem Biophys Res Commun 207: 839–47.

12

Association of *HK2* and *NCK2* with Normal Tension Glaucoma in the Japanese Population

Dong Shi[1,2], Tomoyo Funayama[3], Yukihiko Mashima[4], Yoshimasa Takano[1], Ai Shimizu[1], Kotaro Yamamoto[1], MinGe Mengkegale[1], Akiko Miyazawa[1], Noriko Yasuda[5], Takeo Fukuchi[6], Haruki Abe[6], Hidenao Ideta[7], Kohji Nishida[8], Toru Nakazawa[1], Julia E. Richards[9,10], Nobuo Fuse[1,11]*

1 Department of Ophthalmology, Tohoku University Graduate School of Medicine, Sendai, Miyagi, Japan, **2** Department of Ophthalmology, the Fourth Affiliated Hospital, China Medical University, Shenyang, Liaoning, China, **3** Department of Chemistry, Faculty of Education, Bunkyo University, Koshigaya, Saitama, Japan, **4** Department of Ophthalmology, Keio University School of Medicine, Shinjuku-ku, Tokyo, Japan, **5** Department of Ophthalmology, Tokyo Metropolitan Police Hospital, Tokyo, Japan, **6** Division of Ophthalmology and Visual Science, Graduate School of Medical and Dental Sciences, Niigata University, Niigata, Japan, **7** Ideta Eye Hospital, Kumamoto, Japan, **8** Department of Ophthalmology, Osaka University Graduate School of Medicine, Suita, Osaka, Japan, **9** Department of Ophthalmology and Visual Sciences, W. K. Kellogg Eye Center, University of Michigan, Ann Arbor, Michigan, United States of America, **10** Department of Epidemiology, University of Michigan, Ann Arbor, Michigan, United States of America, **11** Department of Integrative Genomics, Tohoku Medical Megabank Organization, Sendai, Miyagi, Japan

Abstract

Although family studies and genome-wide association studies have shown that genetic factors play a role in glaucoma, it has been difficult to identify the specific genetic variants involved. We tested 669 single nucleotide polymorphisms (SNPs) from the region of chromosome 2 that includes the GLC1B glaucoma locus for association with primary open-angle glaucoma (POAG) and normal tension glaucoma (NTG) in the Japanese population. We performed a two-stage case-control study. The first cohort consisted of 123 POAG cases, 121 NTG cases and 120 controls: the second cohort consisted of 187 POAG cases, 286 NTG cases, and 271 controls. Out of six SNPs showing significant association with POAG in the first round screening, seven SNPs were tested in the second round. Rs678350 in the *HK2* gene coding sequence showed significant allelic ($p = 0.0027$ in Stage Two, 2.7XE-4 in meta-analysis) association with POAG, and significant allelic ($p = 4.7XE\text{-}4$ in Stage Two, 1.0XE-5 in meta-analysis) association with NTG. Although alleles in the *TMEM182* gene did not show significant association with glaucoma in the second round, subjects with the A/A allele in *TMEM182* rs869833 showed worse visual field mean deviation ($p = 0.01$). Even though rs2033008 in the *NCK2* gene coding sequence did not show significant association in the first round, it had previously shown association with NTG so it was tested for association with NTG in round 2 ($p = 0.0053$ in Stage Two). Immunohistochemistry showed that both *HK2* and *NCK2* are expressed in the retinal ganglion cell layer. Once multi-testing was taken into account, only *HK2* showed significant association with POAG and NTG in Stage Two. Our data also support previous reports of *NCK2* association with NTG, and raise questions about what role *TMEM182* might play in phenotypic variability. Our data suggest that *HK2* may play an important role in NTG in the Japanese population.

Editor: Rajiv R. Mohan, University of Missouri-Columbia, United States of America

Funding: This study was supported in part by a Grant-In-Aid for Scientific Research from the Ministry of Education, Science, and Culture of the Japanese Government (C-22591928), Tokyo, Japan (NF); by a grant from the Ministry of Health, Labor and Welfare of Japan (NF); by Tohoku Medical Megabank Project (NF); by a grant from the Japan-China Medical Association (DS); by a grant R01-EY011671 from the National Eye Institute at the National Institutes of Health (JER), Bethesda, MD, USA; and a grant from Research to Prevent Blindness, New York, NY, USA (JER). The funders had no role in study design, data collection and analysis, decision to publish, or preparation of the manuscript.

Competing Interests: The authors have declared that no competing interests exist.

* E-mail: fusen@oph.med.tohoku.ac.jp

Introduction

Glaucoma is a complex, heterogeneous disease characterized by a progressive degeneration of the optic nerve fibers, and is the second highest cause of blindness worldwide affecting approximately 70 million people [1]. The most common type of open-angle glaucoma, primary open-angle glaucoma (POAG), is associated with elevated intraocular pressure (IOP) [2], and another less-common subgroup of open-angle glaucoma, called low-tension glaucoma (LTG) [3,4] or normal tension glaucoma (NTG) is associated with IOP that does not rise outside of the normal range [5]. The prevalence of NTG is reported to be higher among the Japanese than among Caucasians [6,7]. This is an important medical and public health problem because simple screening programs based on detection of elevated IOP are not effective in a population where NTG is highly prevalent. Thus, an accurate diagnostic test for presymptomatic detection of individuals at risk for glaucoma, especially NTG in Japan, is urgently needed.

Open-angle glaucoma is a genetically heterogeneous disorder attributed to the interaction of multiple genes and environmental factors [8,9]. More than 15 POAG loci have been identified by linkage, and five open-angle glaucoma genes located within those loci have been identified [10,11]. More recently, genome-wide association studies (GWAS) using high-density single nucleotide polymorphism (SNP) arrays have been used to identify genetic risk factors involved in the common, complex forms of open-angle glaucoma that do not show classical Mendelian inheritance patterns. Burdon et al. identified susceptibility loci at TMCO1 and CDKN2B-AS1 that contribute to severe forms of glaucoma [12]. Ramdas et al. used meta-analysis of data from six separate studies to find significant evidence that three common variants of CDKN2B, ATOH7 and SIX1 are associated with POAG [13]. Wiggs et al. found significant evidence that genetic variants in CDKN2B-AS1 and a gene desert on 8q22 are associated with optic nerve damage in glaucoma [14].

Based on a linkage study involving 6 Caucasian families in the UK, the *GLC1B* locus for adult-onset open-angle glaucoma was identified at chromosome 2cen–q13 [15]. The patients in these families had clinical characteristics of low to moderate IOP, disease onset in their late 40 s, and a good response to medical therapy, and those phenotypes mimic the majority of Japanese NTG cases. Thus, the screening of the gene around GLC1B locus may be useful for diagnosis of POAG and NTG in the general Japanese population.

The purpose of this study was to screen for candidate genes for POAG and NTG on chromosome 2, around the GLC1B (glaucoma 1, open angle, B) locus in unrelated Japanese patients, using high density SNP scanning and case-control association. Here we report one gene that shows significant association with POAG and NTG, support for a previously reported association with NTG, and a gene for which genotype is predictive of severity of mean deviation on the visual field test.

Results

A Two-stage Case-control Study of SNPs on Chromosome2

To identify a gene associated with glaucoma we did a high-density scan of the region around GLC1B on chromosome 2 by screening 669 SNPs on chromosome 2 in a two-stage case-control study design (Figure 1). We were especially interested in whether any SNPs that fall within genes in the GLC1B region might be associated with POAG or NTG (Table 1). Among genes from this region we found fourteen SNPs that show significant evidence of association with POAG, and nine SNPs that show significant evidence of association with NTG. Four of the SNP alleles which show significant evidence of association are identical between the POAG and NTG subjects.

We identified six SNPs in Stage One that showed evidence of association with POAG (rs1239066, rs1529385, rs869833, rs960011, rs1027003) and two SNPs (rs678350, rs2033008) that showed association with NTG (Figure 2 and Table 2). The SNPs rs869833 and rs960011 are located within the *TMEM182* gene, which contains 5 exons and 229 amino acids. The amino acid sequence of *TMEM182* predicts an evolutionarily-conserved novel transmembrane protein, which consists of four putative membrane-spanning regions indicative of an integral membrane topology. The SNP rs678350 is located within the *Hexokinase 2 (HK2)* gene which contains 18 exons and 917 amino acids. The SNP rs678350 exists on intron1 of *HK2* gene. The *HK2* gene produces a protein product localizes on the outer membrane of mitochondria and plays an important role in intracellular glucose metabolism by catalyzing the conversion of glucose to glucose-6-phosphate. There are no known genes closely neighboring the SNP rs1239066 and rs1027003. We have checked the SNPs near rs1529385 within LOC129293 and TMSB10 and did not find get any positive polymorphisms.

We selected three genes for second stage mutation screening. *TMEM182* and *HK2* genes were selected because they contain SNPs that showed significant evidence of association in Stage One in this study. Even though SNPs in the *NCK2* gene showed significant evidence of association ($p = 0.014$), the *NCK2* gene was selected for second stage mutation screening based of the previous report that it is associated with NTG [16].

The SNP rs1239066 showed significant evidence of association in both Stage One and Stage Two screenings. In the meta-analysis it showed significant evidence of association (POAG, NTG; P = 0.001, 0.005), as did rs1027003 (POAG; P = 0,010) (Table 2).

HK2 Variants Detected in this Study

The SNP rs678350 in the *HK2* gene coding sequence showed significant allelic ($p = 0.0027$ in Stage Two, 2.7XE-4 in meta-analysis) association with POAG, and significant allelic ($p = 4.7XE\text{-}4$ in Stage Two, 1.0XE-5 in meta-analysis) association

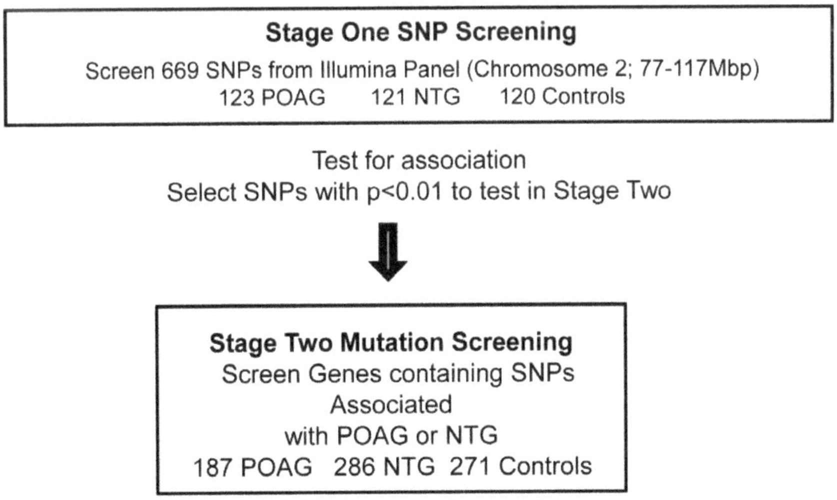

Figure 1. Experimental Study Design. The study used a first stage of SNP screening in one population to identify SNPs and genes to be tested in a second population through SNP association testing and mutation screening of genes containing SNPs associated with glaucoma. Stage Two tested SNPs for association in a second population and did mutation screening in that second population in genes containing SNPs that showed significant association with POAG or NTG ($p < 0.01$) in Stage One of our study or that had been previously reported to show significant evidence of association [16].

Table 1. Stage one Test of SNPs in GLC1B-Region Genes for Association with POAG or NTG.

Genomic Information			POAG			NTG			Control
rs number	**Location**	**Gene Symbol**	**MAF**	**Odds ratio (CI)**	**p value***	**MAF**	**Odds ratio (CI)**	**p value***	**MAF**
rs741788	2p13	*DCTN1*	0.455	1.47 (1.02–2.12)	0.038	0.455	1.47 (1.02–2.11)	0.040	0.363
rs909177		*DCTN1*	0.455	1.44 (1.00–2.08)	0.047	0.463	1.49 (1.03–2.14)	0.032	0.367
rs740277		*DCTN1*	0.455	1.44 (1.00–2.08)	0.047	0.463	1.49 (1.03–2.14)	0.032	0.367
rs678350	2p13	*HK2*	0.333	1.50 (1.01–2.23)	0.043	0.371	1.77 (1.19–2.62)	0.004	0.250
rs651071		*HK2*	0.199	0.60 (0.40–0.92)	0.018	0.256	0.84 (0.56–1.25)	0.383	0.292
rs1807090		*HK2*	0.268	1.59 (1.03–2.44)	0.034	0.238	1.35 (0.87–2.10)	0.181	0.188
rs1239066	2p12		0.293	3.04 (1.95–4.72)	0.009	0.269	1.55 (1.01–2.38)	0.045	0.192
rs53915	2p12-p11.1	*CTNNA2*	0.199	0.64 (0.42–0.98)	0.039	0.260	0.91 (0.61–1.36)	0.641	0.279
rs1529385	2p11.2	*LOC129293 (C2orf89)*	0.053	0.39 (0.20–0.77)	0.005	0.087	0.66 (0.37–1.20)	0.173	0.125
rs1053561	2p11.2	*TGOLN2*	0.114	0.53 (0.32–0.88)	0.012	0.178	0.89 (0.56–1.40)	0.609	0.196
rs1562322	2p11.2	*LOC51255 (RNF181)*	0.321	0.88 (0.61–1.29)	0.520	0.256	0.64 (0.43–0.95)	0.027	0.349
rs3024831	2p12-p11.2	*SFTPB*	0.250	0.92 (0.61–1.38)	0.675	0.190	0.65 (0.42–0.99)	0.045	0.267
rs6875	2q11.2	*RW1 (TMEM131)*	0.008	0.21 (0.05–0.98)	0.030	0.025	0.66 (0.23–1.88)	0.431	0.038
rs1982336		*RW1 (TMEM131)*	0.008	0.23 (0.05–1.05)	0.027	0.029	0.75 (0.28–2.05)	0.576	0.038
rs718159		*RW1 (TMEM131)*	0.008	0.21 (0.05–0.98)	0.028	0.029	0.76 (0.28–2.07)	0.587	0.038
rs222	2q11.2	*INPP4A*	0.183	0.69 (0.44–1.06)	0.091	0.161	0.59 (0.38–0.93)	0.021	0.246
rs1530028	2q11.2	*FLJ45273 (LONRF2)*	0.228	0.66 (0.44–0.99)	0.045	0.306	0.99 (0.67–1.46)	0.952	0.308
rs1030902	2q11.2	*ALS2*	0.225	0.65 (0.44–0.98)	0.039	0.314	1.03 (0.70–1.51)	0.892	0.308
rs1369482	2q11.2	*NPAS2*	0.244	0.65 (0.43–0.96)	0.030	0.298	0.85 (0.58–1.24)	0.398	0.333
rs871656	2q12	*IL1R1*	0.337	0.70 (0.49–1.01)	0.058	0.322	0.66 (0.45–0.95)	0.025	0.421
rs878539	2q11.2	*SLC9A2 (NHE2)*	0.463	1.52 (1.06–2.18)	0.024	0.422	1.28 (0.89–1.85)	0.185	0.363
rs869833	2q12.1	*TMEM182*	0.467	1.66 (1.15–2.40)	0.006	0.376	1.14 (0.79–1.65)	0.490	0.346
rs960011		*TMEM182*	0.415	0.57 (0.40–0.82)	0.001	0.512	0.85 (0.60–1.21)	0.232	0.554**
rs2033008	2q12	*NCK2*	0.293	0.76 (0.51–1.11)	0.147	0.252	0.62 (0.42–0.91)	0.015	0.354
rs1027003	2q12		0.110	3.16 (1.46–6.88)	0.002	0.058	1.58 (0.67–3.71)	0.295	0.038
rs1474220	2q12.3	*GCC2*	0.106	0.59 (0.35–1.00)	0.050	0.136	0.79 (0.48–1.30)	0.353	0.167
rs899259	2q13	*EDAR*	0.098	0.66 (0.38–1.14)	0.134	0.075	0.49 (0.28–0.90)	0.019	0.142
rs1509414	2q13	*BENE(MALL)*	0.037	0.40 (0.18–0.88)	0.020	0.041	0.45 (0.21–0.98)	0.039	0.096
rs1567366	2q13	*NPHP1*	0.561***	1.34 (0.94–1.92)	0.105	0.576***	1.44 (1.01–2.07)	0.045	0.488
rs2119112	2q14.2	*MARCO*	0.110	0.57 (0.34–0.95)	0.029	0.107	0.55 (0.33–0.93)	0.025	0.179

*chi-square test.
**minor allele frequency in stage 2 control was 0.494.
***minor allele in control was major allele in POAG and NTG subjects.
MAF; minor allele frequency, CI; confidence interval.

with NTG (Table 2). The rs678350 showed also a significant difference in genotype frequency (p = 0.0046 and 0.0039) in the POAG and NTG groups (Table 3). In the second round, we screened the *HK2* coding sequence and intron-exon boundaries for mutations in POAG and NTG patients. After direct sequencing, we found 2 coding SNPs; p.Gln142His (A/T at the third nucleotide; rs2229621) in exon 4 and p.Arg844Lys (G/A at the second nucleotide; rs2229629) in exon 17. The allelic frequency of the p.Gln142His (A/T) variant was significantly higher in the NTG group than in the control group (p = 0.025), but it was not higher in the POAG group than in the control group (p = 0.181). The genotype frequency of the p.Gln142His (A/T) variant (dominant model) was significantly higher in the NTG group than in the control group (p = 0.019) but we did not find evidence that the frequency in the POAG group was different from the control group (p = 0.179). There was no evidence of a significant difference between POAG and NTG for p.Arg844Lys. No other mutation was found. We tested the LD block and found no linkage disequilibrium between SNPs rs678350 and rs2229621 (D′ = 0.08). We tested the correlation between the phenotypes POAG or NTG and the genotypes screened in the second stage screening of HK2, and found no association with any phenotypes including age at diagnosis, maximum IOP under medication, and MD value of the visual field (Table 4). None of the polymorphisms showed deviation from Hardy–Weinberg equilibrium ($P<0.05$).

NCK2 Variants Detected in this Study

The SNP rs2033008 in the *NCK2* gene showed a significant difference in allelic frequency (p = 0.015 in Stage One, p = 0.0053 in Stage Two, and 2.2XE-4 in meta-analysis) between controls and NTG, but not between control and POAG status (p = 0.147 in Stage One, 0.35 in Stage Two, 0.12 in meta-analysis) (Table 2 and

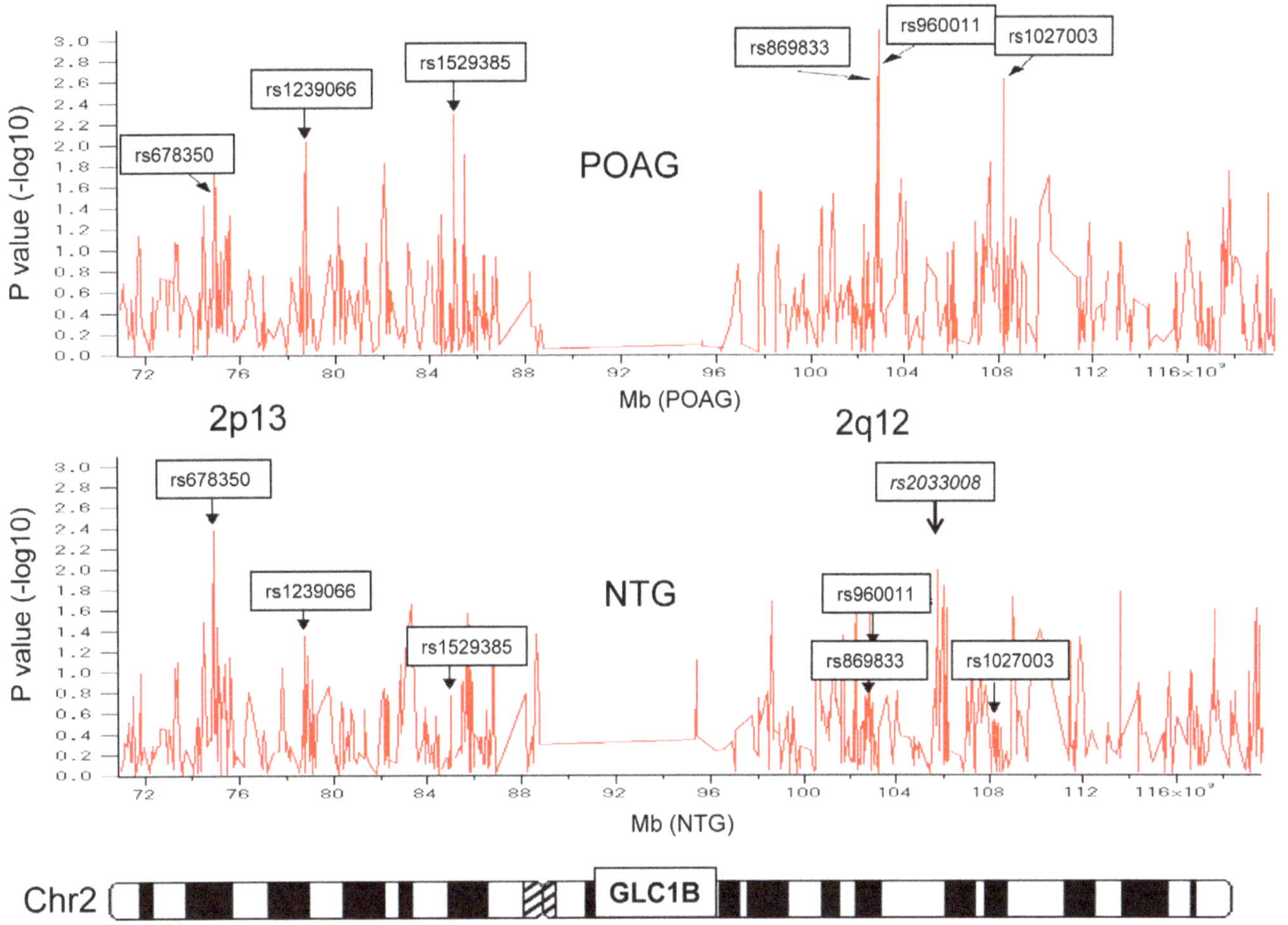

Figure 2. High-density scan of the GLC1B region on chromosome 2 to identify candidate glaucoma genes. Six SNPs that showed significant evidence of association with POAG or NTG ($p<0.01$) and the previously-reported candidate *NCK2* gene are shown. Vertical line shows p value (−log10), and horizontal line shows chromosomal location (kb).

Table 5). The odds ratio for association with NTG supports a model in which *NCK2* is associated with NTG; OR = 0.69 (0.53–0.89), but the odds ratio for association with POAG was not significant; 0.87 (0.65–1.16) in Stage Two. Only this rs2033008 polymorphism in Stage One showed deviation from Hardy–Weinberg equilibrium ($p = 0.030$).

We screened the sequence of the *NCK2* coding sequence and intron-exon boundaries for mutations in POAG and NTG patients and found 1 synonymous coding base change: Thr14Thr (ACC >ACT) in one NTG subject. Although SNP rs2033008 showed significant association but the Thr14Thr variant showed no statistical difference in allele frequency between NTG and normal subjects ($p = 0.33$). The Thr14Thr heterozygotes (A/A) in the NTG subjects have the worse Mean Deviation value of the visual field compared with human reference sequence (T/T) ($p = 0.05$) (Table 6).

The single NTG subject with the Thr14Thr variant was a 50 year old woman whose father also had NTG. Her age at diagnosis was 40 years old. Her initial IOP was 15 mmHg in each eye. The mean deviation (MD) of the visual field test was −3.87 dB in the right eye, and −1.97 dB in the left eye, reflecting a mild NTG phenotype.

TMEM182 Variants Detected in this Study

We found no mutations in *TMEM182* coding sequence and intron-exon boundaries, for mutations in POAG and NTG patients. After finding association for SNPs rs869833 and rs960011 in the POAG and NTG subjects in Stage One, we did not find this association confirmed in Stage Two SNP testing (Table 7). When we tested for correlation between Stage Two case endophenotypes and TMEM182 genotype, we found association with the MD value of the visual field in POAG subjects. The POAG subjects homozygous for the A/A allele of SNP rs869833 have worse Mean Deviation value of the visual field test compared with those who carry the G/G genotype in Stage Two subjects ($p = 0.01$) (Table 8).

Immunohistochemistory of the *HK2* and *NCK2*

Representative immunohistochemistory (IHC) photographs with *Hk2*, *Nck2*, astrocyte marker (GFAP) and retinal ganglion cell marker (C38) on the retinas of untreated mice were shown (Fig. 3, A, B). *Hk2* and *Nck2* were strongly immunoreactive in the ganglion cell layer. C38 signals co-localized with *Hk2* or *Nck2* in the ganglion cell layer, as indicated by arrows (Fig. 3 A, B). *Hk2* expression is only located in the ganglion cell layer. *Nck* is expressed in the ganglion cell layer, inner nuclear layer, and outer plexiform layer, with the highest level of expression in the ganglion cell layer.

Discussion

HK2 in POAG and NTG subjects

The rs678350 in the *HK2* gene coding sequence showed significant allelic ($p = 0.043$ in Stage One, $p = 0.0027$ in Stage

Table 2. Stage One and Stage Two Association Test Results.

Stage One Screening

		POAG			NTG			CNTL
SNP	**Minor Allele**	**MAF**	**Odds ratio**	**p value***	**MAF**	**Odds ratio**	**p value***	**MAF**
rs1239066	C	0.293	3.04 (1.95–4.72)	0.009	0.269	1.55 (1.01–2.38)	0.045	0.192
rs1529385	T	0.053	0.39 (0.20–0.77)	0.005	0.087	0.66 (0.37–1.20)	0.173	0.125
rs869833	G	0.467	1.66 (1.15–2.40)	0.006	0.376	1.14 (0.79–1.65)	0.490	0.346
rs960011	T	0.415	0.57 (0.40–0.82)	0.001	0.512	0.85 (0.60–1.21)	0.232	0.554
rs1027003	G	0.110	3.16 (1.46–6.88)	0.002	0.058	1.58 (0.67–3.71)	0.295	0.038
rs678350	G	0.333	1.50 (1.01–2.23)	0.043	0.371	1.77 (1.19–2.62)	0.004	0.250
rs2033008	A	0.293	0.76 (0.51–1.11)	0.147	0.252	0.62 (0.42–0.91)	0.015	0.354

Stage Two Screening

		POAG			NTG			CNTL
SNP	**Minor Allele**	**MAF**	**Odds ratio**	**p value***	**MAF**	**Odds ratio**	**p value***	**MAF**
rs1239066	C	0.246	1.70 (1.09–2.65)	0.019	0.240	1.64 (1.06–2.51)	0.024	0.161
rs1529385	T	0.122	1.42 (0.73–2.77)	0.305	0.072	0.79 (0.37–1.68)	0.543	0.089
rs869833	G	0.409	0.98 (0.75–1.28)	0.855	0.421	1.03 (0.81–1.30)	0.834	0.415
rs960011	T	0.497	1.13 (0.86–1.47)	0.363	0.481	1.06 (0.84–1.34)	0.641	0.467
rs1027003	G	0.049	1.10 (0.42–2.90)	0.840	0.047	1.04 (0.30–2.83)	0.944	0.045
rs678350	G	0.334	1.58 (1.18–2.11)	0.0027	0.337	1.60 (1.23–2.08)	4.7XE-4	0.242
rs2033008	A	0.297	0.87 (0.65–1.16)	0.348	0.250	0.69 (0.53–0.89)	0.0053	0.327

Meta-analysis

		POAG			NTG			CNTL
SNP	**Minor Allele**	**MAF**	**Odds ratio**	**p value***	**MAF**	**Odds ratio**	**p value***	**MAF**
rs1239066	C	0.264	1.65 (1.22–2.23)	0.001	0.248	1.52 (1.14–2.04)	0.005	0.178
rs1529385	T	0.082	0.73 (0.46–1.16)	0.20	0.081	0.71 (0.45–1.14)	0.16	0.109
rs869833	G	0.432	1.17 (0.95–1.45)	0.16	0.408	1.06 (0.87–1.30)	0.54	0.393
rs960011	T	0.465	0.89 (0.72–1.10)	0.28	0.490	0.99 (0.81–1.20)	0.92	0.494
rs1027003	G	0.084	2.17 (1.20–3.92)	0.010	0.053	1.32 (0.69–2.53)	0.42	0.041
rs678350	G	0.334	1.56 (1.23–1.96)	2.7XE-4	0.347	1.65 (1.32–2.05)	1.0XE-5	0.244
rs2033008	A	0.295	0.83 (0.66–1.04)	0.12	0.251	0.66 (0.53–0.82)	2.2XE-4	0.335

MAF; Minor allele frequency, CNTL; Control.
*Fisher's exact test.

Table 3. Stage Two *HK2* SNPs Allele Frequencies in Japanese POAG, NTG and Control Subjects.

	Allele frequency				Genotype			
rs678350	**A**	**G**	**Odds ratio (CI)**	**p value***	**A/A**	**A/G**	**G/G**	**p value***
POAG	0.666	0.334	1.58 (1.18–2.11)	0.0027	82/187	85/187	20/187	0.0046
NTG	0.663	0.337	1.60 (1.23–2.08)	4.7XE-4	133/286	113/286	40/286	0.0039
Control	0.758	0.242			161/271	89/271	21/271	
	Allele frequency				**Genotype**			
rs2229621/Q142H	**A**	**T**	**Odds ratio (CI)**	**p value***	**A/A**	**A/T**	**T/T**	**p value***
POAG	0.738	0.262	1.24 (0.92–1.69)	0.181	102/187	72/187	13/187	0.179
NTG	0.719	0.281	1.36 (1.04–1.79)	0.025	146/286	119/286	21/286	0.019
Control	0.777	0.223			165/271	91/271	15/271	

*Fisher's exact test; dominant model.
G/G or T/T is mutant homozygote, A/G or A/T is heterozygote, and A/A is wild homozygote.

Two, 2.7XE-4 in meta-analysis association with POAG, and significant allelic (p = 0.004 in Stage One, p = 4.7XE-4 in Stage Two, 1.0XE-5 in meta-analysis) association with NTG (Table 2). The rs678350 polymorphism showed a significant case-control difference in genotype frequency ($p = 0.0046$ and 0.0039) in the POAG and NTG groups (Table 3). However, there was no association of this SNP with glaucoma endophenotypes including age at diagnosis, maximum intra ocular pressure under medication, and MD value of the visual field. So the *HK2* gene may contribute to disease susceptibility to POAG and NTG, but may not account for all of the phenotypic variability between individuals whose glaucoma results from variants in this gene. Our association findings suggest that the *HK2* gene that contains this polymorphism might play a role in POAG and NTG in the Japanese population, but it remains to be seen whether rs678350 is actually causative, perhaps through altering transcription or splicing, or whether another allele(s) in this gene or its regulatory region might actually be causing the disease. There remains a possibility that the p.Gln142His (A/T) SNP in *HK2* may play a role in disease pathology, but our study can only show association, not causation. Because none of our subjects come from the original families used to map the GLC1B locus, we can only draw conclusions regarding the possible role of this gene in the Japanese population, but this finding raises questions about whether this could be the GLC1B gene.

The HK2 gene product plays an important role in intracellular glucose metabolism by catalyzing the conversion of glucose to glucose-6-phosphate. The *HK2* gene localizes to the outer membrane of mitochondria. Since reduced glucose-6-phosphate content in muscle has been demonstrated in pre-non-insulin-dependent diabetes mellitus (pre-NIDDM) and NIDDM subjects, *HK2* was investigated as a promising candidate gene for noninsulin-dependent diabetes mellitus (NIDDM; OMIM125853) [17,18]; however, those studies concluded that mutations of the *HK2* gene, including a common p.Gln142His polymorphism is not a major etiologic factor for NIDDM in the Finnish [17,18,19,20], British [19], and Danish [20] populations. In brain, mitochondrial-hexokinase activity plays a key antioxidant role protecting against oxidative stress (ROS) [21], and complements the classical antioxidant enzymes that protect against oxidative stress [22]. Hexokinase antagonizes the release of mitochondrial cytochrome C activation of Akt, which is recognized as a potent inhibitor of apoptosis. *HK2* is probably associated with an anti-oxidative reaction and inhibition of apoptosis through Bax/Bak-mediated cytochrome *c* release [23]. Leber's hereditary optic neuropathy (LHON) -associated mitochondrial DNA mutations were found in Japanese patients with POAG [24], so it is reasonable to consider a gene whose product plays a role in mitochondria as a candidate gene for other phenotypes involving optic neuropathy.

NCK2 genes in POAG and NTG subjects

The *NCK2* gene, which was previously reported to be associated with NTG [16], encodes a member of the NCK family of adaptor proteins, and the adaptor protein which associates with tyrosine-phosphorylated growth factor receptors of their cellular substrates. SH2/SH3 domain-containing adapter proteins, such as the NCK family, play a major role in regulating tyrosine kinase signaling [25]. Previously, microsatellite marker D2S176 within the GLC1B locus showed significant association with NTG in the Japanese population, and D2S176 is located 24 kb from the *NCK2* gene [16]. Brain-derived neurotrophic factor (BDNF) binds to and activates the TrkB tyrosine kinase receptor to regulate cell differentiation and survival in the nervous system. BDNF

Table 4. Correlation between the POAG or NTG Endophenotypes and *HK2* SNPs Screened in Stage Two.

Endophenotype	Age at diagnosis (y.o.)				Maximum IOP* (mmHg)				MD value of the visual field (dB)			
rs678350 genotype	**A/A**	**A/G**	**G/G**	**p value****	**A/A**	**A/G**	**G/G**	**p value****	**A/A**	**A/G**	**G/G**	**p value****
POAG	61.6	55.3	59.0	0.83	24.0	23.6	21.9	0.56	−14.82	−15.64	−11.94	0.53
NTG	57.5	54.9	56.9	0.99	17.1	16.0	17.6	0.64	−10.72	−12.10	−7.14	0.37
rs2229621 genotype	**A/A**	**A/T**	**T/T**	**p value****	**A/A**	**A/T**	**T/T**	**p value****	**A/A**	**A/T**	**T/T**	**p value****
POAG	58.5	58.0	55.5	0.93	24.4	22.9	25.5	0.94	−16.42	−11.94	−17.65	0.65
NTG	57.8	55.2	57.4	0.91	16.1	17.5	16.9	0.63	−11.93	−10.34	−11.16	0.95

*IOP; intraocular pressure (under medication).
**Dunnett's test.
G/G or T/T is mutant homozygote, A/G or A/T is heterozygote, and A/A is wild homozygote.

stimulation promotes interaction of *Nck2* with TrkB in cortical neuron [26]. And BDNF signaling in glia is known to play important roles in neural protection and regeneration, particularly in conversion of Muller glia to photoreceptors [27]. In our study, it is interesting that the *NCK2* variant rs2033008 showed a significantly difference from the control population in the NTG group, where the disease pathology seems to be focused on the retinal ganglion cells and the optic nerve, but not in the POAG group, where a substantial disease component localizes to the anterior chamber of the eye (Table 5). Thus although our study falls short of achieving a level of significance needed to identify *NCK2* de novo as a glaucoma gene and this polymorphism showed deviation from Hardy–Weinberg equilibrium ($p = 0.030$ in Stage One), our data do support the prior finding of significant allele frequency differences between NTG cases and normal controls in the Japanese population [16]. It is unclear whether this deviation from Hardy-Weinberg equilibrium in Stage One might represent the absence of some alleles from this population because they are associated with diagnoses specifically excluded from this study, such as ocular hypertension.

Immunohistochemistory of the *Hk2* and *Nck2*

Although KH2 and NCK2 had previously been detected in retina, more precise localization to specific cell types is needed to begin understanding how the gene products might play a role in disease pathology. In the representative IHC photographs, antibody against *Hk2* was strongly immunoreactive in the ganglion cell layer (GCL). The *Hk2* protein localizes to the outer membrane of mitochondria, and interestingly the *Hk2* protein appears in the GCL. *Nck2*, which interacts with BDNF, is expressed in ganglion cell layer (GCL), inner nuclear layer (INL) and outer plexiform layer (OPL), and most expressed in GCL. This localization makes it highly conceivable that the *Hk2 gene products* could each play a role in glaucoma, and there is possibility that *Nck2* could have relationship with glaucoma.

TMEM182 in POAG and NTG

SNPs rs869833 and rs960011 in the TMEM182 gene showed significant association with POAG and NTG in Stage One that was not confirmed in the second stage. The primary amino acid sequence of *TMEM182* predicts an evolutionarily-conserved novel transmembrane protein, which consists of four putative membrane-spanning regions indicative of an integral membrane topology. The *TMEM182* protein sequence lacks homologies with previously-defined protein families. However, the pro-inflammatory cytokine TNFα down-regulates *TMEM182* transcript expression in adipocytes [28]. Its transcript expresses in white adipose tissues, heart, muscle, and lower relative levels of *TMEM182* transcript are found in kidney, testis, and brain. Identification of the intracellular signaling pathway involved in the TNFα-mediated decrease might be one clue offering insights into association between POAG and *TMEM182* function. Failure to confirm the association with POAG in the second stage could be attributable to clinical heterogeneity, but this result still needs to be confirmed in a second population. Nakano et al. demonstrated heterogeneity in the Japanese POAG population when their genome-wide association study of 1,575 Japanese POAG and normal subjects identified significant evidence of association with 6 SNPs on Chromosome 1, 10, 12 [29]. They did not report evidence of association with SNPs on Chromosome 2.

Table 5. Stage Two *NCK2* SNP rs2033008 Allele Frequencies in Japanese POAG, NTG and Controls Subjects.

	Allele frequency				Genotype			
	T	**A**	**Odds ratio (CI)**	**p value***	**T/T**	**T/A**	**A/A**	**p value****
POAG	0.703	0.297	0.87 (0.65–1.16)	0.35	89/187	85/187	13/187	0.069
NTG	0.750	0.250	0.69 (0.53–0.89)	0.0053	159/286	111/286	16/286	0.0056
Control	0.673	0.327			130/271	105/271	36/271	

*Fisher's exact test,
**Chi-square test.
A/A is mutant homozygote, T/A is heterozygote, and T/T is wild homozygote.

Table 6. Correlation between the POAG or NTG Endophenotypes and *NCK2* SNP rs2033008 Screened in Stage Two.

Endophenotype	Age at diagnosis (y.o.)				Maximum IOP* (mmHg)				MD value of the visual field (dB)			
Genotype	**T/T**	**T/A**	**A/A**	**p value****	**T/T**	**T/A**	**A/A**	**p value****	**T/T**	**T/A**	**A/A**	**p value****
POAG	55.8	61.0	54.2	0.94	23.7	24.2	25.0	0.87	−15.38	−14.94	−12.28	0.63
NTG	56.8	56.0	52.2	0.70	16.7	17.0	16.0	0.79	−9.83	−10.95	−16.28	0.05

*IOP; intraocular pressure (under medication).
**Dunnett's test.
A/A is mutant homozygote, T/A is heterozygote, and T/T is wild homozygote.

Thus these SNPs on Chr2 might be the variants for which our study is not well-powered, or clinical heterogeneity might be complicating our ability to detect the association in our limited sample size.

In our data set, *HK2* shows the strongest evidence of association with NTG in the Japanese population out of all of the genes that have SNPs represented on the screening panel we used.

Even when a single simple Mendelian locus causes a disease, variants in other genes may contribute to phenotypic variability, and phenotypic complexity along with locus and allele heterogeneity can complicate the problem of identifying the underlying causes of the disease. Our findings raise questions about whether additional genes in this region may be contributing to phenotypic heterogeneity within the NTG and POAG populations. The MD values of the visual field in these studies indicate middle to advanced stages of the disease, with the range of values possibly resulting from a combination of genetic complexity and genetic heterogeneity.

On the other hand, we also have to consider the importance of apparent gene deserts. The SNP rs1239066 shows significant evidence of association in both Stage One and Stage Two screenings, and in the meta-analysis (POAG, NTG; P = 0.001, 0.005). Significant evidence was also found for rs1027003 (POAG; P = 0,010) (Table 2), but neither one is in the immediate vicinity of a known gene. Wiggs et al. found significant evidence that genetic variants in a gene desert on 8q22 are associated with optic nerve damage in glaucoma [14]. So additional follow up studies will need to explore this gene desert region to determine whether any functional sequences there are playing a role in the disease.

Glaucoma is a complex disease, and it involves genetic variants that confer moderate to low effect sizes (e.g., OR = 1.2–1.5). The OR which was identified in the first stage with the P value cutoff of 0.01 was 1.68. This cutoff value was a bit strict to exclude the false positives.

Further investigations of the structure and function of the *HK2*, *NCK2* and *TMEM182* proteins would be helpful in understanding the pathogenesis of POAG and NTG. Our data suggest that *HK2* may play an important role in NTG in the Japanese population; although our data suggest that *HK2* might be the GLC1B gene, a firm conclusion on the subject awaits screening of members of the families originally used to map the GLC1B locus.

Patients and Methods

Ethics statement

This study was approved by the Institutional Review Board of Tohoku University, Keio University, Tokyo Metropolitan Police Hospital, Niigata University, Ideta Eye Hospital, and all procedures were conducted in accordance with the Declaration of Helsinki. All participants provided written informed consent after an explanation of the purpose and procedures to publish these case details.

Patient Recruitment and Characteristics

The samples used in the first screening (Stage One) were collected in Keio University hospitals, Tokyo Metropolitan Police Hospital, Niigata University, and Ideta Eye Hospital, and the

Table 7. Stage Two *TMEM182* SNP Allele Frequencies in Japanese POAG, NTG and Control Subjects.

	Allele frequency			Genotype			
rs869833	**A**	**G**	**p value***	**A/A**	**A/G**	**G/G**	**p value****
POAG	0.590	0.410	0.855	61/187	99/187	27/187	0.095
NTG	0.579	0.421	0.834	94/286	143/286	49/286	0.269
Control	0.585	0.415		100/271	117/271	54/271	
	Allele frequency			**Genotype**			
rs960011	**C**	**T**	**p value***	**C/C**	**C/T**	**T/T**	**p value****
POAG	0.503	0.497	0.363	45/187	98/187	44/187	0.479
NTG	0.520	0.480	0.641	76/286	145/286	65/286	0.782
Control	0.533	0.467		79/271	131/271	61/271	

*Fisher's exact test,
**Chi-square test.
G/G or T/T is mutant homozygote, A/G or C/T is heterozygote, and A/A or C/C is wild homozygote.

Table 8. Correlation between the POAG or NTG Endophenotypes and *TMEM182* SNPs Screened in Stage Two.

Endophenotype	Age at diagnosis (y.o.)				Maximum IOP* (mmHg)				MD value of the visual field (dB)			
rs869833 Genotype	**A/A**	**A/G**	**G/G**	**p value****	**A/A**	**A/G**	**G/G**	**p value****	**A/A**	**A/G**	**G/G**	**p value****
POAG	54.8	61.1	56.0	0.95	24.7	23.8	23.3	0.80	−17.5	−15.0	−9.95	0.01
NTG	55.8	55.7	59.9	0.40	16.9	16.9	16.4	0.84	−12.60	−9.62	−12.21	0.98
rs960011Genotype	**C/C**	**C/T**	**T/T**	**p value****	**C/C**	**C/T**	**T/T**	**p value****	**C/C**	**C/T**	**T/T**	**p value****
POAG	55.5	57.3	62.0	0.29	24.8	24.4	23.2	0.73	−14.2	−18.5	−9.44	0.37
NTG	53.8	56.4	60.1	0.14	17.1	17.3	15.7	0.16	−10.77	−11.02	−11.76	0.88

*IOP; intra ocular pressure (under medication),
**Dunnett's test.
G/G or T/T is mutant homozygote, A/G or C/T is heterozygote, and A/A or C/C is wild homozygote.

samples used in the second screening (Stage Two) were collected at Tohoku University.

Routine ophthalmic examinations were performed on all subjects. Individuals were included as POAG cases if they fulfilled the following inclusion criteria: 1) applanation IOP greater than 22 mm Hg in each eye; 2) spherical equivalent more than −8 diopter; 3) glaucomatous cupping in each eye including cup-to-disc ratio greater than 0.7; 4) visual field loss measured by Goldmann perimetry or Humphrey automated field analyzer (Carl Zeiss Meditec, Dublin, CA) in Stage One. The severity of the visual field defects was scored from 1 to 5 according to previously reported criteria ref. The data obtained by two types of perimetry were combined using a five-point scale: 1, no alterations; 2, early defects; 3, moderate defects; 4, severe defects; and 5, light perception only or no light perception. The first four groups on this severity scale followed Kozaki's classification based on Goldmann perimetry or the classification was based on results of Humphrey automated field analyzer [30,31]. Kozaki's classification is widely used in Japan. In Stage Two, all of the visual field loss were measured by Humphrey automated field analyzer according to Anderson-Pattela classification [30] consistent with the glaucomatous cupping in at least one eye; and 5) open anterior chamber angles; and exclusion of secondary causes (e.g., trauma, uveitis, or steroid-induced glaucoma). The criteria for NTG were the same as for POAG except that NTG subjects showed applanation IOP less than 22 mm Hg in both eyes at each examination. Baseline clinical parameters including age, gender, spherical equivalent base line visual acuity (VA), IOP measured by Goldmann applanation tonometry were recorded at the time of first diagnosis of POAG or NTG in each patient. Mean deviation (MD) values indicative of visual field damage were obtained by the Swedish interactive threshold algorithm (SITA)-standard strategy of the 30-2 program of HFA (Carl Zeiss Meditec, Dublin, Californuia, USA). MD was used on reliable visual field test results (<20% fixation errors, <33% false-positive results, and <33% false-negative results). Control subjects had these characteristics: IOP less than 22 mm Hg, normal optic discs, and no family history of glaucoma. To decrease the chance of enrolling individuals with pre-symp-

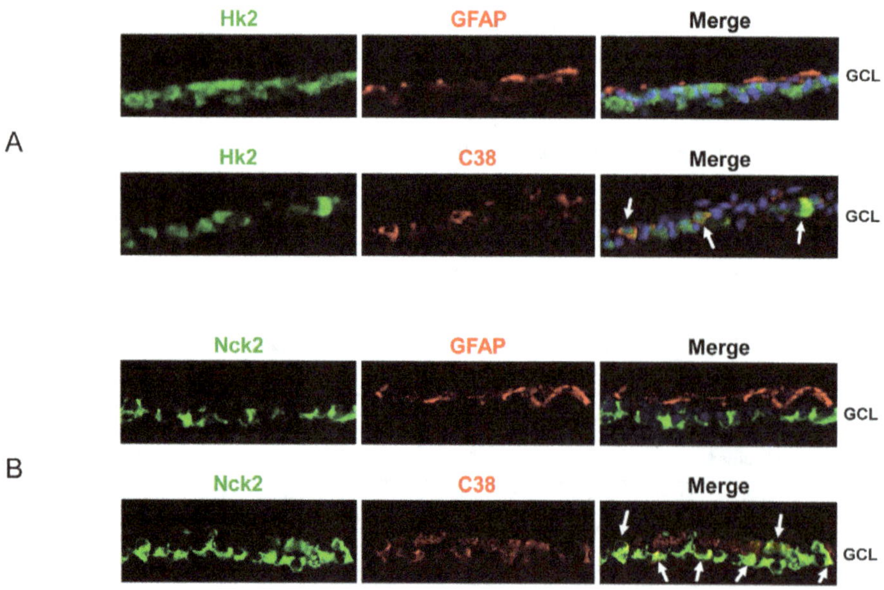

Figure 3. *Hk2* and *Nck2* Immunohistochemistry. Representative IHC photographs showing Hk2, Nck2, astrocyte maker (GFAP) and RGC marker (C38) in the retinas of untreated mice. Arrows indicated the co-localization area.

tomatic glaucoma, we limited this group to individuals older than 60 years.

Two Stage Screening Protocol

The two-stage screening strategy is shown in Figure 1. The first stage screened used 669 SNPs from the GLC1B region, using the Illumina panel #8 (Chromosome 2; 77–117 Mbp) (Illumina, San Diego, CA, USA) carried by Illumina (San Diego, CA, USA), and each SNP was tested for association with POAG or NTG. The first stage used a cohort of 368 unrelated Japanese individuals: 123 POAG cases (63 men and 60 women), 121 NTG cases (61 men and 60 women) and 120 normal subjects (61 men and 59 women). Mean age of POAG cases was 56.9±11.5 years. Mean age of NTG cases was 54.0±12.3 years. Mean age of controls was 70.3±10.2 years. The visual field scores were 2.8±1.0 in POAG cases and 2.7±0.9 in NTG cases (Table 9). Single-nucleotide polymorphisms (SNPs) with a call rate <90% were excluded from the analysis. All of the polymorphisms showed no deviation from Hardy–Weinberg equilibrium ($P>0.05$) except rs2033008 in Stage One ($p = 0.030$).

The second stage screened SNPs that showed significant evidence for association in the first round in this study ($p<0.01$) and in the NCK2 gene, which previously showed association with NTG [16]. The odds ratio which was identified in the first stage with the P value cutoff of 0.01 was 1.68. Second stage screening was carried out using sequencing of DNA PCR amplified by polymerase chain reaction from genomic DNA samples from a population of 473 unrelated Japanese individuals, including 187 POAG cases (119 men and 68 women), 286 cases NTG (139 men and 147 women), and 271 control subjects (145 men and 126 women). Mean age of POAG cases was 57.8±12.0 years. Mean age of NTG cases was 56.4±13.3years. Mean age of controls was 69.7±9.3 years. Maximum intra ocular pressure under medication were 23.5±5.3 mmHg in POAG subjects and 16.8±2.4 mmHg in NTG subjects. Mean deviation (MD) value of the visual field test was −15.0±9.0 dB in POAG cases and −11.0±7.1 dB in NTG cases (Table 9).

Sample Preparation

Genomic DNA was extracted from leukocytes of the peripheral blood. It was purified by the Qiagen QIAamp Blood Kit (Qiagen, Valencia, CA, USA).

Mutation Screening

Mutation screening was carried out in genes that contained SNPs that showed significant evidence of association in the first stage (HK2 and TMEM182) plus the previously-reported NCK2 gene [16]. All of the exons of the *HK2*, *NCK2*, *TMSB10* and *TMEM182* genes, and positive SNPs were amplified by a polymerase chain reaction (PCR) using 0.5 μM concentration of primers in an amplification mixture (25 μl) containing 0.2 mM dNTPs and 0.5 U Ex Taq polymerase (Takara Bio, Shiga, Japan) with 30 ng template DNA. Oligonucleotides for amplification and sequencing were selected using Primer3 software (http://frodo.wi.mit.edu/cgi-bin/primer3/primer3_www.cgi/ provided in the public domain by the Massachusetts Institute of Technology, Cambridge, MA). Primers for amplification and sequencing of coding sequence were placed in introns far enough from the intron/exon junctions to allow for visualization of the splice site sequences. The PCR fragments were purified with ExoSAP-IT (USB, Cleveland, Ohio, USA), sequenced by the BigDye™ Terminator v3.1 Cycle Sequencing Kit (Perkin-Elmer, Foster City, CA, USA) on an automated DNA sequencer (ABI PRISM™ 3100 Genetic Analyzer, Perkin-Elmer, Waltham, MA, USA).

Statistical Analysis

The significance of association was determined by contingency table analysis using Fisher's exact test or Chi-square test, depending on cell counts. In estimation of genotype-phenotype correlation, we used Dunnett's test to compare group means of those carrying the mutant variant being tested against the group means of those carrying the normal, reference sequence. Odds ratios (approximating to relative risk) were calculated as a measure of the association between the allele frequency and the phenotype of POAG/NTG, estimated using the SNPAlyze program version 7.0 (Dynacom, Yokohama, Japan). Hardy–Weinberg equilibrium was analyzed using gene frequencies obtained by simple gene counting and the chi-square test with Yates' correction for comparing observed and expected values.

Immunohistochemistory of the *HK2* and *NCK2*

Murine retinas were fixed with 4% PFA at 4°C overnight and then cryoprotected in phosphate buffered saline (PBS) with 20% sucrose. Cryosections (thickness 10 μm) were mounted on the slides and incubated with blocking buffer (10% goat serum, 0.5% gelatin, 3% BSA and 0.2% Tween 20 in PBS). Next, they were incubated with primary antibodies at 4°C overnight. Primary

Table 9. Clinical Characteristics of Subjects studied in Stage One and Two Screening.

Endophenotype		Age at diagnosis (y.o.)	Maximum IOP* (mmHg)	The Visual Field Score**
Stage One	POAG	56.9±11.4	25.3±5.6	2.8±1.0
	NTG	54.0±12.2	16.0±2.3	2.7±0.9
	Control	70.3±10.2	13.9±2.2	
Stage Two	POAG	57.8±12.0	23.5±5.3	−15.0±9.0 (dB)
	NTG	56.4±13.3	16.8±2.4	−11.0±7.1 (dB)
	Control	69.7±9.3	13.9±2.2	

*IOP; intra ocular pressure (under medication).
**The Visual Field Score was evaluated by Humphrey MD value or Goldmann perimetry (Stage One) and Humphrey MD value (Stage Two).
In Stage One, the severity of the visual field defects was scored from 1 to 5 according to previously reported criteria. The data obtained by two types of perimetry were combined using a five-point scale: 1, no alterations; 2, early defects; 3, moderate defects; 4, severe defects; and 5, light perception only or no light perception. The first four groups on this severity scale followed Kozaki's classification based on Goldmann perimetry or the classification was based on results of visual field perimetry (Humphrey Field Analyzer; Carl Zeiss Meditec, Dublin, CA). Kozaki's classification is widely used in Japan.

antibodies used were Mouse anti-Glial Fibrillary Acidic Protein (GFAP) (1:200; MAB360; Chemicon, Millipore, MA, USA), mouse anti-C38 (1:200; provided by Dr. Jun Kosaka), rabbit anti-NCK2 (1:200; ab14590; Abcam), or rabbit anti-HK2 (1:200; 2867S; Cell Signaling Technology, MA, USA). The sections were washed three times with PBST (PBS containing 0.2% Tween 20) and then incubated with secondary goat anti-rabbit IgG antibody (1:200; A11008 Invitrogen, Carlsbad, CA, USA) tagged with Alexa 488 or goat anti-mouse IgG A11030; Invitrogen, Carlsbad, CA, USA) tagged with Alexa 546 for 1 hour. The slides were washed three times and mounted with Vectashield mounting medium (H1000; Vector, Burlingame, CA).

Acknowledgments

The authors thank Dr. Duco I. Hamasaki for editing the manuscript, and thank Dr. Nariyuki Yamada and Prof. Makoto Tamai for experimental suggestions and support. We are grateful to Dr. Jun Kosaka for providing antibody mouse anti-C38.

Author Contributions

Conceived and designed the experiments: T. Funayama YM KN NF. Performed the experiments: DS T. Funayama YT AS KY MM AM TN NF. Analyzed the data: DS T. Funayama YM JER NF. Contributed reagents/materials/analysis tools: T. Funayama YT AS NY T. Fukuchi HA HI TN. Wrote the paper: DS KY JER NF.

References

1. Quigley H (1996) Number of people with glaucoma worldwide. Br J Ophthalmol 80: 389–393.
2. Quigley H (1993) Open-angle glaucoma. N Engl J Med 328: 1097–1106.
3. Hitchings RA, Anderton SA (1983) A comparative study of visual field defects seen in patients with low-tension glaucoma and chronic simple glaucoma. Br J Ophthalmol 67: 818–821.
4. Hitchings R (1992) Low tension glaucoma–its place in modern glaucoma practice. Br J Ophthalmol 76: 494–496.
5. Werner E (1996) Normal-tension glaucoma.; Ritch R SM, Krupin T, eds., editor. St.Louis: Mosby. 769–797 p.
6. Shiose Y, Kitazawa Y, Tsukahara S, Akamatsu T, Mizokami K, et al. (1991) Epidemiology of glaucoma in Japan–a nationwide glaucoma survey. Jpn J Ophthalmol 35: 133–155.
7. Iwase A, Suzuki Y, Araie M, Yamamoto T, Abe H, et al. (2004) The prevalence of primary open-angle glaucoma in Japanese: the Tajimi Study. Ophthalmology 111: 1641–1648.
8. Raymond V (1997) Molecular genetics of the glaucomas: mapping of the first five "GLC" loci. Am J Hum Genet 60: 272–277.
9. Sarfarazi M (1997) Recent advances in molecular genetics of glaucomas. Hum Mol Genet 6: 1667–1677.
10. Liu Y, Allingham RR (2011) Molecular genetics in glaucoma. Exp Eye Res 93: 331–339.
11. Pasutto F, Keller KE, Weisschuh N, Sticht H, Samples JR, et al. (2012) Variants in ASB10 are associated with open-angle glaucoma. Hum Mol Genet 21: 1336–1349.
12. Burdon KP, Macgregor S, Hewitt AW, Sharma S, Chidlow G, et al. (2011) Genome-wide association study identifies susceptibility loci for open angle glaucoma at TMCO1 and CDKN2B-AS1. Nat Genet 43: 574–578.
13. Ramdas WD, van Koolwijk LM, Lemij HG, Pasutto F, Cree AJ, et al. (2011) Common genetic variants associated with open-angle glaucoma. Hum Mol Genet 20: 2464–2471.
14. Wiggs JL, Yaspan BL, Hauser MA, Kang JH, Allingham RR, et al. (2012) Common variants at 9p21 and 8q22 are associated with increased susceptibility to optic nerve degeneration in glaucoma. PLoS Genet 8: e1002654.
15. Stoilova D, Child A, Trifan OC, Crick RP, Coakes RL, et al. (1996) Localization of a locus (GLC1B) for adult-onset primary open angle glaucoma to the 2cen-q13 region. Genomics 36: 142–150.
16. Akiyama M, Yatsu K, Ota M, Katsuyama Y, Kashiwagi K, et al. (2008) Microsatellite analysis of the GLC1B locus on chromosome 2 points to NCK2 as a new candidate gene for normal tension glaucoma. Br J Ophthalmol 92: 1293–1296.
17. Laakso M, Malkki M, Deeb SS (1995) Amino acid substitutions in hexokinase II among patients with NIDDM. Diabetes 44: 330–334.
18. Laakso M, Malkki M, Kekalainen P, Kuusisto J, Deeb SS (1995) Polymorphisms of the human hexokinase II gene: lack of association with NIDDM and insulin resistance. Diabetologia 38: 617–622.
19. Vidal-Puig A, Printz RL, Stratton IM, Granner DK, Moller DE (1995) Analysis of the hexokinase II gene in subjects with insulin resistance and NIDDM and detection of a Gln142->His substitution. Diabetes 44: 340–346.
20. Echwald SM, Bjorbaek C, Hansen T, Clausen JO, Vestergaard H, et al. (1995) Identification of four amino acid substitutions in hexokinase II and studies of relationships to NIDDM, glucose effectiveness, and insulin sensitivity. Diabetes 44: 347–353.
21. da-Silva WS, Gomez-Puyou A, de Gomez-Puyou MT, Moreno-Sanchez R, De Felice FG, et al. (2004) Mitochondrial bound hexokinase activity as a preventive antioxidant defense: steady-state ADP formation as a regulatory mechanism of membrane potential and reactive oxygen species generation in mitochondria. J Biol Chem 279: 39846–39855.
22. Santiago AP, Chaves EA, Oliveira MF, Galina A (2008) Reactive oxygen species generation is modulated by mitochondrial kinases: correlation with mitochondrial antioxidant peroxidases in rat tissues. Biochimie 90: 1566–1577.
23. Majewski N, Nogueira V, Bhaskar P, Coy PE, Skeen JE, et al. (2004) Hexokinase-mitochondria interaction mediated by Akt is required to inhibit apoptosis in the presence or absence of Bax and Bak. Mol Cell 16: 819–830.
24. Inagaki Y, Mashima Y, Fuse N, Ohtake Y, Fujimaki T, et al. (2006) Mitochondrial DNA mutations with Leber's hereditary optic neuropathy in Japanese patients with open-angle glaucoma. Jpn J Ophthalmol 50: 128–134.
25. Buday L, Wunderlich L, Tamas P (2002) The Nck family of adapter proteins: regulators of actin cytoskeleton. Cell Signal 14: 723–731.
26. Suzuki S, Mizutani M, Suzuki K, Yamada M, Kojima M, et al. (2002) Brain-derived neurotrophic factor promotes interaction of the Nck2 adaptor protein with the TrkB tyrosine kinase receptor. Biochem Biophys Res Commun 294: 1087–1092.
27. Harada C, Guo X, Namekata K, Kimura A, Nakamura K, et al. (2011) Glia- and neuron-specific functions of TrkB signalling during retinal degeneration and regeneration. Nat Commun 2: 189.
28. Wu Y, Smas CM (2008) Expression and regulation of transcript for the novel transmembrane protein Tmem182 in the adipocyte and muscle lineage. BMC Res Notes 1: 85.
29. Nakano M, Ikeda Y, Taniguchi T, Yagi T, Fuwa M, et al. (2009) Three susceptible loci associated with primary open-angle glaucoma identified by genome-wide association study in a Japanese population. Proc Natl Acad Sci U S A 106: 12838–12842.
30. Anderson DR, VM P (1999) Automated Static Perimetry. 2nd edition. St.Louis: Mosby.
31. Funayama T, Ishikawa K, Ohtake Y, Tanino T, Kurosaka D, et al. (2004) Variants in optineurin gene and their association with tumor necrosis factor-alpha polymorphisms in Japanese patients with glaucoma. Invest Ophthalmol Vis Sci 45: 4359–4367.

13

Common Variants in *CDKN2B-AS1* Associated with Optic-Nerve Vulnerability of Glaucoma Identified by Genome-Wide Association Studies in Japanese

Masakazu Nakano[1¶], Yoko Ikeda[2¶], Yuichi Tokuda[1¶], Masahiro Fuwa[1,3], Natsue Omi[1], Morio Ueno[2], Kojiro Imai[2], Hiroko Adachi[1], Masaaki Kageyama[3], Kazuhiko Mori[2], Shigeru Kinoshita[2*], Kei Tashiro[1*]

1 Department of Genomic Medical Sciences, Kyoto Prefectural University of Medicine, Kyoto, Japan, **2** Department of Ophthalmology, Kyoto Prefectural University of Medicine, Kyoto, Japan, **3** Research and Development Center, Santen Pharmaceutical Co. Ltd., Nara, Japan

Abstract

Background: To date, only a small portion of the genetic variation for primary open-angle glaucoma (POAG), the major type of glaucoma, has been elucidated.

Methods and Principal Findings: We examined our two data sets of the genome-wide association studies (GWAS) derived from a total of 2,219 Japanese subjects. First, we performed a GWAS by analyzing 653,519 autosomal common single-nucleotide polymorphisms (SNPs) in 833 POAG patients and 686 controls. As a result, five variants that passed the Bonferroni correction were identified in *CDKN2B-AS1* on chromosome 9p21.3, which was already reported to be a significant locus in the Caucasian population. Moreover, we combined the data set with our previous GWAS data set derived from 411 POAG patients and 289 controls by the Mantel-Haenszel test, and all of the combined variants showed stronger association with POAG ($P<5.8\times10^{-10}$). We then subdivided the case groups into two subtypes based on the value of intraocular pressure (IOP)—POAG with high IOP (high pressure glaucoma, HPG) and that with normal IOP (normal pressure glaucoma, NPG)—and performed the GWAS using the two data sets, as the prevalence of NPG in Japanese is much higher than in Caucasians. The results suggested that the variants from the same *CDKN2B-AS1* locus were likely to be significant for NPG patients.

Conclusions and Significance: In this study, we successfully identified POAG-associated variants in the *CDKN2B-AS1* locus using a Japanese population, i.e., variants originally reported as being associated with the Caucasian population. Although we cannot rule out that the significance could be due to the differences in sample size between HPG and NPG, the variants could be associated specifically with the vulnerability of the optic nerve to IOP, which is useful for investigating the etiology of glaucoma.

Editor: John R. B. Perry, Peninsula College of Medicine and Dentistry, United Kingdom

Funding: This work was supported by the grants from the Collaborative Development of Innovative Seeds of Japan Science and Technology Agency (JST) to MK and KT, from the Ministry of Health, Labor and Welfare of Japan to KM, SK and KT, and from Santen Pharmaceutical Co. Ltd. to SK and KT. The funders had no role in study design, data collection and analysis, decision to publish, or preparation of the manuscript.

Competing Interests: This study has been completed under the Collaborative Research Agreement executed by Kyoto Prefectural University of Medicine and Santen Pharmaceutical Co., Ltd. All materials and information produced throughout this study are parts of co-owned intellectual properties. MF and MK are employees of Santen Pharmaceutical Co., Ltd. This does not alter the authors' adherence to all the PLoS ONE policies on sharing data and materials.

* E-mail: tashiro@koto.kpu-m.ac.jp (KT); shigeruk@koto.kpu-m.ac.jp (SK)

¶ These authors contributed equally to this work.

Introduction

Glaucoma is a neurodegenerative ocular disease and one of the leading causes of irreversible blindness worldwide [1]. It is characterized by the progressive loss of retinal ganglion cells and optic nerve axons, resulting in visual field defects [2]. One of the well-known major risk factors for glaucoma is elevated intraocular pressure (IOP) [2]. Thus, the measurement of IOP is routinely involved in the diagnosis of glaucoma. In fact, the IOP level has been applied to subdivide the most common form of glaucoma, primary open-angle glaucoma (POAG), into two subtypes [3]: POAG with high (≥22 mmHg) IOP (POAG/HPG, high pressure glaucoma; hereafter referred to as "HPG") and with normal (<22 mmHg) IOP (POAG/NPG, normal pressure glaucoma; hereafter referred to as "NPG"). Interestingly, ~92% of the Japanese POAG patients are categorized into the NPG subtype [4], whereas ~41% of Caucasian POAG patients are categorized as NPG [5], thus showing a unique epidemiological distribution of Japanese patients compared with other ethnic groups.

Aside from IOP measurements, the diagnosis of glaucoma is commonly made by observing optic nerve degeneration and visual field defects by means of fundus examinations and visual field tests, respectively. In the case of HPG, early drug treatment to lower IOP immediately following the onset of visual field damage has been shown to be quite effective in slowing the irreversible progression toward blindness [6,7]. In contrast, since NPG patients show normal IOP, they are often misdiagnosed. Therefore, both fundus examinations of the optic nerve and visual field tests are critical for the proper diagnosis of NPG patients. However, due to the restriction of the healthcare expenditure to include those examinations into a person's regular medical checkup, especially in the preclinical state of glaucoma, it would be of great benefit if the risk of developing glaucoma could be ascertained based on a simple blood test to assess the genetic markers for the disease.

Since glaucoma shows familial aggregation and its prevalence varies between individuals of different ethnicities, it has been theorized that genetic factors play a significant role in the pathogenesis of glaucoma [8,9]. Therefore, several institutions are making profound efforts to discover single-nucleotide variants for glaucoma by conducting a genome-wide association study (GWAS) [10–14], and there are a few published reports of the association of particular loci, such as the *CAV1/CAV2* locus (7q31.1) [13] and the *TMCO1* or *CDKN2B-AS1* loci (1q24.1 or 9p21.3, respectively) [14], with POAG using Caucasian subjects. However, it appears that a controversy still exists as to determining the authentic variants associating with POAG, even within the same ethnicity of European descent [14,15]. We previously reported a GWAS and the subsequent follow-up study focused on the high-ranked variants identified in the initial population using in total of 1,575 Japanese subjects [10]. We identified six variants located in three loci, 1q43, 10p12.31, and 12q21.31, on the chromosome which were modestly associated with POAG, although the association results were not reproducible with a different population of different ethnicities [13,16,17]. In that previous study, we combined the patients from both HPG and NPG subtypes as a single case group in order to increase the statistical power [10]. Therefore, the genetic loci that were identified are most likely to be components of the molecular mechanism shared by both subtypes. Another Japanese group performed a GWAS [12] and discovered variants in *SRBD1* on 2p21 and *ELOVL5* on 6p12.1 that were associated with NPG (in that study, NPG was referred to as "normal tension glaucoma") [18]. However, since the findings in that study were derived from a single population, replication studies to support those findings still need to be conducted.

In this present study, we examined two independent GWAS data sets, and then performed a meta-analysis by combining the data sets in order to discover authentic genetic markers for POAG, HPG, or NPG. We succeeded in identifying some significant variants in the *CDKN2B-AS1* locus using a Japanese population, as that locus has also been shown to be significantly associated with POAG in Caucasians [14]. Moreover, the variants that passed the Bonferroni correction seemed to be associated with POAG and POAG/NPG, thus suggesting that the locus potentially affects the NPG, rather than the HPG, subtype of POAG. Although we still need to confirm our findings by use of a larger HPG cohort in order to increase the statistical power, the variants identified in this study could be associated specifically with the vulnerability of the optic nerve to IOP, thus enabling us to investigate the etiology of glaucoma.

Results

We first performed a GWAS in 833 POAG patients and 686 control subjects (hereafter referred to as "Present GWAS"; Figure 1A) who were selected and divided into case and control groups based on our strict diagnosis criteria. After genotyping, 653,519 SNPs passed the quality controls and were used for the association study (Figure 1A). In a quantile-quantile (Q-Q) plot

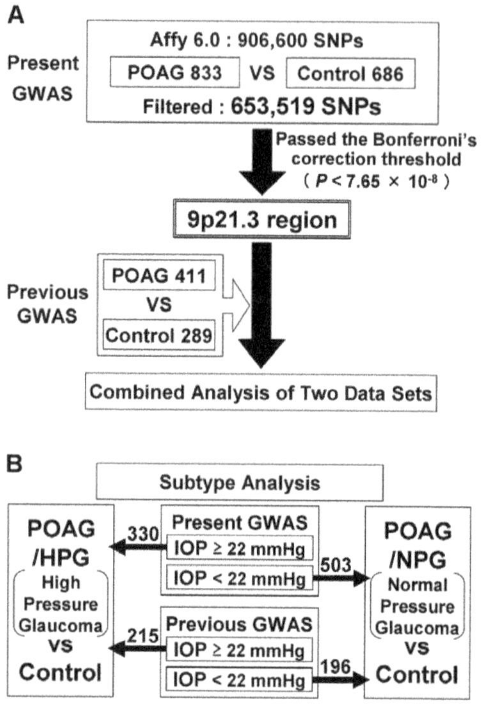

Figure 1. Study design. (A) We first performed the "Present GWAS" for POAG and identified the 9p21.3 locus. This result was confirmed by the combined analysis with the "Previous GWAS". (B) We then subdivided the POAG subjects into two subtypes, POAG/HPG and POAG/NPG, and each group was analyzed by combining the two data sets in order to investigate the differences of statistical significance in the 9p21.3 locus.

(Figure S1A), the genomic inflation factor (λ) showed 1.021, suggesting that the population substructure should not have any substantial effects on the association analysis. Under these conditions, we obtained 8 genome-wide significant SNPs (Table S1) that passed the Bonferroni correction threshold ($0.05/653{,}519 = 7.65 \times 10^{-8}$), of which 5 SNPs were located in *CDKN2B-AS1* on chromosome 9p21.3 (Figure 2). A few SNPs that showed modest to strong association were distributed across a single linkage disequilibrium (LD) block located in the locus (Figure S2). The remaining genome-wide significant SNPs identified from different chromosomes turned out to be genotyping errors due to the poor 2D clusters (Figure S3B–D).

Next, we updated the case and control groups of the previous GWAS population [10] with the latest clinical information and ended up with 411 POAG patients and 289 controls (hereafter referred to as "Previous GWAS"; Figure 1A). One SNP (rs8181047) of 5 genome-wide significant SNPs in *CDKN2B-AS1* identified from the Present GWAS was not able to be assessed in the Previous GWAS because a DNA probe of that particular SNP was not designed for the Affymetrix 500 K platform. Consequently, we combined the two sets of GWAS genotype data for the remaining 4 SNPs by use of the Mantel-Haenszel test [19], and the level of significance of all 4 SNPs increased from $P<5.2\times10^{-9}$ to $P<5.8\times10^{-10}$ (Table 1). These 4 SNPs were highly correlated with one another ($r^2>0.98$), and were considered to have a similar effect for POAG based on the conditional analysis. These results suggested that it was effective to combine the data since the population stratification between the two data sets seemed to be ignorable, which was also supported by the results of the heterogeneity test. Moreover, we assessed the confounding effects

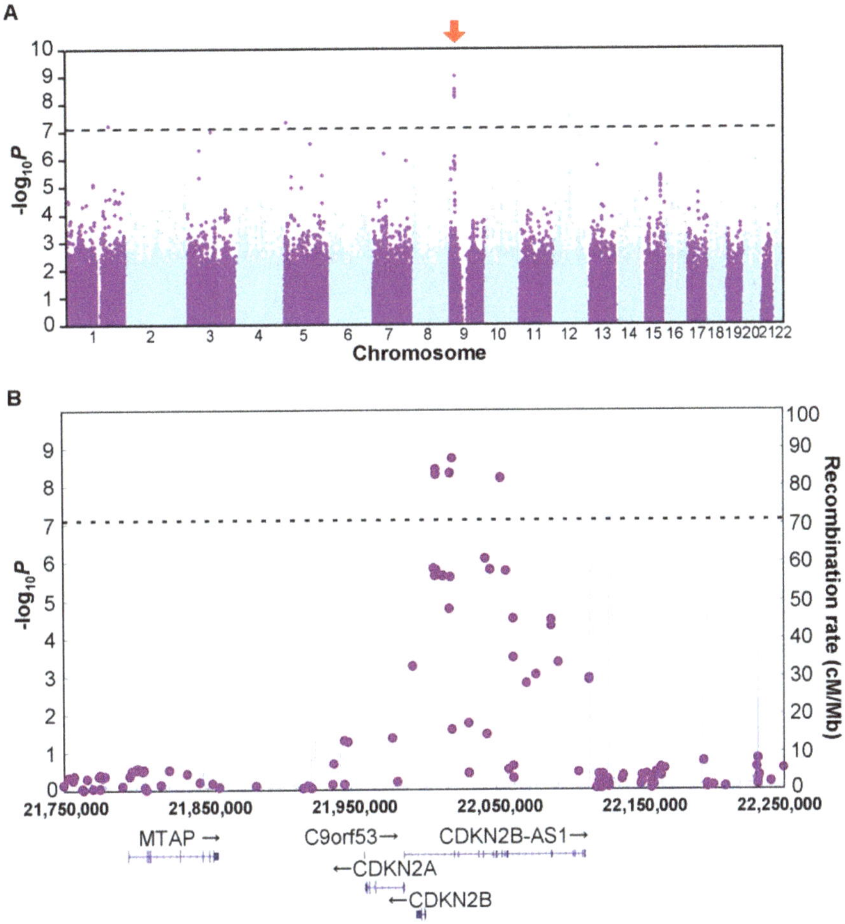

Figure 2. Association results of the Present GWAS. (A) The SNPs with a strong association appeared to exist in a cluster on chromosome 9 (red arrow). (B) The five significant SNPs that passed the Bonferroni correction threshold (horizontal dotted line) were identified in *CDKN2B-AS1* on the 9p21 locus. SNP positions followed the NCBI Build 36 coordinates. The genetic recombination rates (cM/Mb) estimated by HapMap Project [31] in Release 22 are indicated by the thin blue line.

for these SNPs with respect to age and gender, and none were found to be statistically significant (Table S2), thus suggesting that the obtained association results were specific to the case-control comparison. In addition, the two sets of GWAS data for 40 SNPs surrounding the significant 4 SNPs in the 9p21.3 locus were also combined and analyzed (Table S3, Table S4). Since these 44 SNPs, in total, were genotyped in both the Present and Previous GWAS, and all of the SNPs passed the genotyping quality controls, these SNPs should prove useful in providing a broader overview of the significance of the locus. The results showed that the significance of combined SNPs was generally high between 22.0–22.1 Mb (Figure 3A). Within the particular locus, there seemed to be two distinct LD blocks; one in the side including genome-wide significant SNPs ("LD Block 1" in Figure 3D) and one in the other side with modestly associated SNPs ("LD Block 2" in Figure 3D).

Table 1. Association results of genome-wide significant SNPs in the Present GWAS.

			Previous GWAS			Present GWAS			Previous & Present Combined		
SNP:risk allele	Chr.	Position	Frequency[a]	*P*	OR (95% CI)	Frequency[a]	*P*	OR (95% CI)	P^b	OR (95% CI)	Het-P^c
rs523096:A	9	22,009,129	0.89/0.84	6.0×10^{-3}	1.56 (1.13–2.14)	0.89/0.82	3.8×10^{-9}	1.86 (1.51–2.29)	1.6×10^{-10}	1.76 (1.48–2.10)	0.42
rs518394:C	9	22,009,673	0.89/0.85	1.5×10^{-2}	1.49 (1.08–2.07)	0.89/0.82	5.2×10^{-9}	1.85 (1.50–2.28)	5.8×10^{-10}	1.74 (1.46–2.07)	0.34
rs564398:A	9	22,019,547	0.90/0.85	4.7×10^{-3}	1.58 (1.15–2.18)	0.90/0.82	4.6×10^{-9}	1.86 (1.51–2.29)	1.4×10^{-10}	1.77 (1.49–2.11)	0.47
rs7865618:A	9	22,021,005	0.90/0.85	6.3×10^{-3}	1.56 (1.13–2.14)	0.90/0.82	2.0×10^{-9}	1.88 (1.53–2.32)	9.0×10^{-11}	1.78 (1.50–2.12)	0.39

[a]Risk allele frequency in POAG/controls.
[b]*P* value of combined 2 GWAS results by Mantel-Haenszel test.
[c]*P* value of Cochran's Q heterogeneity test between Previous and Present GWAS.

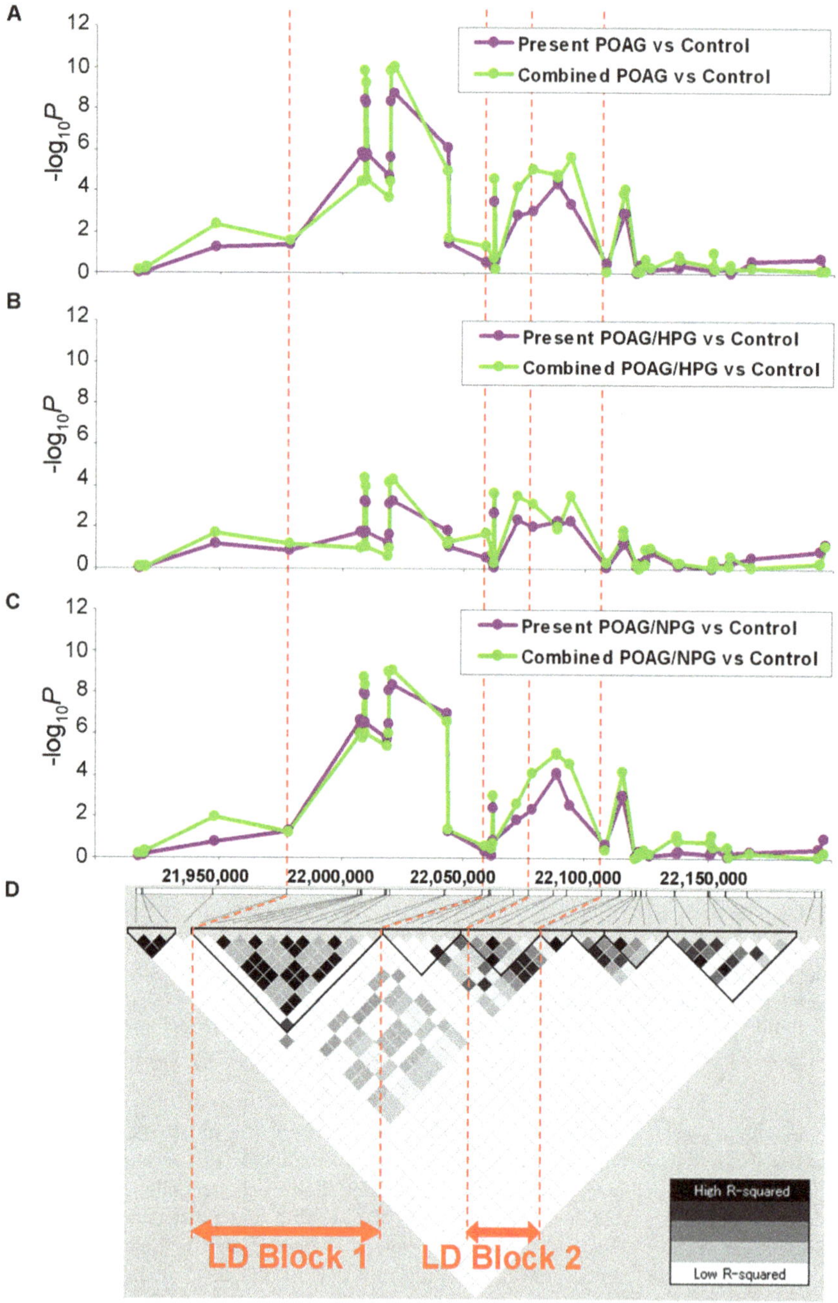

Figure 3. Combined analysis of the Present and Previous GWAS data in 9p21.3 locus. Three graphs representing the results of the association studies for POAG (A), HPG (B), and NPG (C) are shown in order from upper to lower, respectively. The results derived from the Present GWAS alone or the two combined GWAS data sets are indicated by the purple or green line graph plots, respectively. The lowest plot (D) shows an LD plot in the same region. All of the Present and Previous GWAS subject data was applied to draw the LD plot by Haploview v4.2. The color indicating pairwise r^2 and LD block were lined by using the confidence interval (95%) of pairwise D'. Vertical dashed redline indicates the same region between the upper graphs and LD Block 1 and 2 at the lowest.

For the subtype analyses (Figure 1B), the POAG patients from both the Present and Previous GWAS populations were divided into two subtypes based on the clinical record of IOP measurement: 1) POAG patients with HPG (IOP≥22 mmHg) and 2) those with NPG (i.e., patients who consistently showed an IOP of less than 22 mmHg) [3]. The number of subjects in each subtype was found to be 330 HPG and 503 NPG patients and 215 HPG and 196 NPG patients in the Present and Previous GWAS, respectively (Figure 1B). When we performed the analysis separately using the Present GWAS data set, the Q-Q plots of HPG vs control and NPG vs control appeared to be quite different from one another (Figure S1B, C). In particular, the HPG results indicated non-deviated Q-Q plots (Figure S1B). In fact, although none of the SNPs were genome-wide significant for HPG (Figure S4A), we obtained 4 genome-wide significant SNPs that passed the Bonferroni correction threshold for NPG (Table S1, Figure S4B). As for NPG, the significance level of all 4 SNPs also increased when the two data sets were combined (Figure 3C, Table S3,

Table S4), however, the significance was still far from the Bonferroni threshold of significance in relation to HPG (Figure 3B, Table S3, Table S4). Although the significance level of SNPs residing in LD Block 2 showed slight differences among the different subtypes, the level in LD Block 1 seemed to be determining the difference of significance between the two subtypes, thus suggesting that the variants on LD Block 1 are closely associated with the susceptibility to glaucoma in the 9p21.3 locus (Figure 3D). Surprisingly, all of the significant SNPs from NPG overlapped with those obtained from POAG (Table S1). However, when we performed the heterogeneity test between the HPG and NPG groups, the results were not significant ($P = 0.21$–0.25, Table S3), suggesting that the significant differences between the two subtypes could be due to the small sample size of the HPG group. Although we need to confirm the above results using a larger HPG cohort, these results suggested that the significant SNPs identified in *CDKN2B-AS1* on the 9p21.3 locus probably serve as genetic markers of glaucoma, which could be useful for investigating the etiology of glaucoma with respect to the vulnerability of the optic nerve to IOP.

Discussion

In this study, we successfully identified genetic markers in *CDKN2B-AS1* strongly associated with POAG and POAG/NPG, but not with HPG, by analyzing two GWAS data sets using independent study populations totaling 2,219 Japanese subjects. For the case-control study of the Present GWAS, we excluded the samples without hesitation that didn't meet our strict quality control (see Supporting Information S1). Since we succeeded in excluding the samples possessing a fair amount of no-call or missed-call genotype data, our more stringent filters certainly improved the actual genotyping results for the association studies performed later. Thus, we were able to obtain an increased level of significance without any substructure effects of the two populations based on the definite diagnosis when combining the genotyping results of the Present and Previous GWAS data sets (Figure 3).

Using our polished data sets derived from distinct case and control subjects (see Methods and Supporting Information S1), we succeeded in identifying a cluster of genome-wide significant SNPs associated with POAG in *CDKN2B-AS1*, a non-coding gene with an unknown function, on chromosome 9p21.3 (Figure 2A, B). Several variants in chromosome 9p21 have been found to be associated with a variety of common diseases, and 9p21 was initially identified as a locus for coronary artery disease (CAD) [20–23] and type-2 diabetes [24–26]. However, little is known about the biological meanings underlying the locus, as 9p21 is a "gene desert" locus and most of the variants identified were non-coding. Recently, Harismendy et al. [27] reported that they have identified 33 enhancers in 9p21, some of which being within *CDKN2B-AS1*, and it turned out to be the second densest gene desert for predicted enhancers, thus suggesting the regulatory role of sequences residing within non-coding loci. They finally determined a few adjacent, as well as distant (>45 kb), target gene regions relevant to CAD biology physically interacting with the enhancer by 3D-DSL (also known as "4C"), a chromatin conformation capture technology, in human vascular endothelial cells. Overall, their study has provided an excellent example of a solution to link the unknown meanings of statistical association to a biological function. Since the POAG variants were also identified in *CDKN2B-AS1*, the variants would probably affect the expression level of the downstream genes *CDKN2A* and *CDKN2B*. In fact, Burdon et al. reported up-regulated *CDKN2A* and *CDKN2B* expression in response to the elevated IOP [14], suggesting the involvement of the locus in molecular pathways leading to glaucoma development. Moreover, the possibility that the variants would also affect the distant unidentified target genes in the context of the complex etiology of glaucoma, as well as the nature of the identified locus [27], cannot be ruled out.

To date, several institutions have attempted to discover variants for glaucoma by conducting a GWAS, and a few published studies have reported the association of particular loci with POAG using Caucasian subjects (Table S5). Thorleifsson et al. reported the association of common variants near *CAV1/CAV2* on 7q31.1 using a population of European ancestry [13]. In contrast, Kuehn et al. reported that they failed to replicate their results in a United States cohort [15]. Moreover, meta-analysis of the association results derived from several institutions of Northern Europe, including the data from Thorleifsson et al. [13], identified a few new loci associated with POAG, including the *CDKN2B-AS1* locus on 9p21.3 [17]. Recently, the new loci at *TMCO1* on 1q24.1 and *CDKN2B-AS1* were reported to be associated with Australian populations [14]. Thus far, only the association of the *CDKN2B-AS1* locus was replicated, even within the same ethnicity of European descent. Interestingly, Thorleifsson et al. also showed a modest association with the *CAV1/CAV2* locus using Chinese subjects [13], although the allele frequency of the particular variant in Asian subjects was quite low when compared with that in Caucasians, suggesting etiological differences due to the genetic background. In fact, according to the results of our Present GWAS for POAG, we were unable to replicate the association with the *CAV1/CAV2* and *TMCO1* loci (Figure S5F, G, Table S5). Moreover, in the Present GWAS, we were unable to replicate the association results of the 6 SNPs identified in the previous study [10] (Table S5), even though the populations were of the same ethnic background, thus suggesting that we still need to discover authentic variants, irrespective of the difference in ethnicities, to elucidate the complex etiology of glaucoma. Consequently, it should be noted that the variants identified in the *CDKN2B-AS1* locus in this study using a Japanese population seemed to be shared with the Caucasian subjects (Table S5), thus showing that we have successfully obtained one of the authentic variants for POAG that is not ethnicity related.

In this study, we also subdivided the POAG subjects into two subtypes based on the IOP level measurements in an attempt to discover subtype-specific variants, which would be useful for investigating the different mechanism of each pathogenesis. Since the clinical states of both subtypes overlap almost completely, they are usually categorized as a single disease. However, as a unique epidemiological distribution compared with other ethnic groups, ~92% of the Japanese POAG patients fall into the NPG category, as determined by the Tajimi study [4], a robust epidemiology study. In fact, another Japanese group performed a GWAS focused on discovering NPG-specific variants [12]. They reported that the SNPs in *SRBD1* on 7q31.1 and *ELOVL5* on 6p12.1 were associated with NPG, although our group was unable to replicate those results (Figure S5D, E). On the contrary, we obtained an unexpected result that the variants associated with NPG were completely identical to those associated with POAG in *CDKN2B-AS1* identified in this study (Table S1). In contrast, none of the variants were significant for HPG (Figure 3B). Although we cannot rule out that the significance could be due to the differences in sample size between HPG and NPG cases according to the heterogeneity test ($P = 0.21$–0.25; Table S3), the results suggested that the genetic loci identified are most likely components of the molecular mechanism specific for NPG. It has been reported that there are differences in vulnerability of the optic nerve to IOP between HPG and NPG [18]. It has also been theorized that

CDKN2B-AS1 affects the susceptibility of the optic nerve [14,28]. Since the variants identified in this study seemed to be shared among different ethnicities in functional aspects as well, the other variants should be contributing to the unique epidemiology of NPG in Japanese. By continuing to build upon the detailed investigation, such as obtaining in-depth sequencing data of the non-coding 9p21 locus, it might be possible to reveal not only the molecular mechanism of glaucoma pathogenesis but also the genetic diversity that resides within the locus among different ethnic backgrounds.

Methods

Ethics statement

This study was approved by the Institutional Review Board of Kyoto Prefectural University of Medicine and all procedures were conducted in accordance with the Declaration of Helsinki. All participants provided written informed consent after an explanation of the nature and possible consequences of the study.

Case and control subjects for the Present GWAS

All participants were interviewed to determine their familial history of glaucoma and other ocular or general diseases. A total of 2,126 Japanese participants, including POAG patients, healthy volunteers, and patients with other ocular diseases, were recruited between March 2005 and December 2010 at the University Hospital of Kyoto Prefectural University of Medicine (Kyoto, Japan) to give peripheral blood samples for this study. A third person who was blind to both the blood sampling and genotyping assigned an anonymous code to each blood sample. Genomic DNA used for the genotyping experiments was isolated from the blood, and Epstein-Barr virus (EBV)-transformed lymphocytes were prepared from the remaining blood as previously described [29] to serve as the future resource of genomic DNA. POAG patients and controls suitable for this study were precisely selected based on the strict diagnosis as previously described [10]. In particular, subtype selection was performed by dividing POAG into two categories according to peak IOP without treatment; POAG/High Pressure Glaucoma (POAG/HPG, defined as ≥22 mmHg) and POAG/Normal Pressure Glaucoma (POAG/NPG) [3]. All of the diagnostic procedures, including case-control selection and subtype classification, were performed by three ophthalmologists (YI, MU, and KM) from a single institution. The age and female/male ratio of all of the subjects used in the Present and Previous GWAS are shown in Table S6. To examine the possible confounding effects of age and gender, we assessed the correlations between the values and the genotype data from the case and control samples by one-way ANOVA or chi-square test (Table S2).

SNP genotyping and quality control for the Present GWAS

First, 906,600 SNPs were genotyped for 2,126 Japanese subjects by Genome-Wide Human SNP Array 6.0 (Affymetrix, Santa Clara, CA) according to the manufacturer's instructions. As for the Present GWAS population, 839 POAG patients and 708 controls were selected after performing the quality control (QC) as described (Supporting Information S1). To exclude the potential inclusion of genetically related subjects into the population, identity-by-descent (IBD) estimates were performed for all possible combinations by PLINK v1.07 (http://pngu.mgh.harvard.edu/~purcell/plink/). In total, 6 POAG patients and 22 controls were assumed to be in first-degree relationships or in relationships with a few more-distant relatives, and were thus excluded from the Present GWAS population. Finally, the Present GWAS population ended up with 833 POAG patients, comprised of 330 HPG and 503 NPG patients, and 686 controls. Population stratification for the present GWAS population was examined by principal component analysis using EIGENSTRAT software v3.0 (http://genepath.med.harvard.edu/~reich/Software.htm). As for the reference genomic population, the four HapMap populations (CEU, YRI, JPT, and CHB) were simultaneously applied to EIGENSTRAT. The generated cluster plots indicated that our POAG and control population was genetically clustered within the JPT population, and there was no outlier sample (Figure S6). We performed SNP quality control for the population on the autosomal SNPs based on the following QC filters: (i) call rate per SNPs in case and control samples ≥95%, (ii) minor allele frequency (MAF) in case and control samples ≥1%, and (iii) Hardy-Weinberg equilibrium (HWE) in control samples P≥0.001. Consequently, we analyzed the remaining 653,519 SNPs for the Present GWAS population.

Population update for reanalyzing the Previous GWAS

Since 6 years had passed since the patients and healthy volunteers who participated in our Previous GWAS [10] were first recruited, we updated the case (n = 418) and control (n = 300) groups based on the latest clinical information. In total, 7 samples from the case group and 11 samples from the healthy control group were removed. The population for the reanalysis finally ended up with 411 POAG patients, comprised of 215 HPG and 196 NPG patients, and 289 controls. The Previous GWAS data was obtained by GeneChip® Human Mapping 500 K Array platform (Affymetrix) containing 500,568 SNPs. The quality control for the reanalysis was performed by using the same QC filters as used in the Present GWAS. Genotype data derived from the particular locus for combining with the Present GWAS data was extracted from these filtered SNPs.

Data management and statistical analysis

To manage and analyze all of the genotype data, we used our in-house Genoika Server System (SASA Plus Co., Ltd., Fukuoka, Japan), which was well improved from the system used in the Previous GWAS [10,30] by the same system engineers. In addition, to manage the Previous GWAS data effectively, the Labo Server System (World Fusion Co., Ltd.) was used simultaneously. The Genoika Server System comes with PLINK v1.07 (http://pngu.mgh.harvard.edu/~purcell/plink/), the R program v 2.9.2 and 2.10.1 (http://www.r-project.org/), EIGENSTRAT software v3.0 (http://genepath.med.harvard.edu/~reich/Software.htm), and Haploview 4.2 (http://www.broadinstitute.org/scientific-community/science/programs/medical-and-population-genetics/haploview/haploview) built in, and all the analyses were performed by use of this system. In addition, Microsoft Office Excel 2003 (Microsoft Corporation, Redmond, WA) was used for preparing the data sets and statistical analysis. The frequency of alleles in the case and control samples was compared by use of the basic allele test. The odds ratio (OR) and the upper and lower limit of the 95% confidence interval (CI) of each SNP were calculated for the allele possessing a higher frequency in the case samples than in the control samples. The HWE was evaluated by the chi-square test. Q-Q plots were generated by ranking the observed values from minimum to maximum and plotting them against their expected chi-square values using the "snpMatrix" package ver 1.14.6 in the R program (http://www.r-project.org/). We applied the Mantel-Haenszel test [19] to combine the data derived from the two data sets in order to reduce potential negative effects arising from the biases in age and female/male ratio among the populations (Table S6).

Supporting Information

Figure S1 Q-Q plots for the Present GWAS. Quantile-quantile (Q-Q) plots for the Present GWAS of POAG (A), HPG (B), and NPG (C) were generated by ranking the observed chi-square values from minimum to maximum and plotting them against their expected values. Genomic inflation factors (λ) are also shown. These plots were created using the R-package snpMatrix.

Figure S2 LD plots in the 9p21 locus. LD plots were generated from the Present GWAS data. The SNPs applied to these plots and the span of the region are the same as shown in Figure 2B. Upper and lower plots indicate the value of pairwise D′ and r2, respectively. The positions of 5 SNPs, which passed the Bonferroni correction threshold in the Present GWAS, are drawn in vertical dashed lines. These LD plots were generated using Haploview v4.2.

Figure S3 Genotyping error check. 2D-cluster plots for the representative SNPs obtained from chromosome 9 (A), chromosome 1 (B), chromosome 5 (C), and chromosome 12 (D) that showed genome-wide significance. These 2D cluster plots were drawn by Genotyping Console 4.1 software (Affymetrix).

Figure S4 GWAS results of two subtypes. Association results of the Present GWAS for the two subtypes of POAG, HPG (A) and NPG (B). The horizontal dashed line in each plot indicates the Bonferroni correction threshold for each study.

Figure S5 Evaluation of previously reported loci/genes. Evaluation of the POAG-associated loci/genes reported previously using our Present GWAS data. The genes located in the loci are as the follows: (A) ZP4, (B) PLXDC2, (C) TMTC2, (D) SRBD1, (E) ELOVL5, (F) CAV1/CAV2, and (G) TMCO1. Each locus was evaluated by the results of POAG vs control, POAG/HPG vs control, and POAG/NPG vs control. The plotted SNPs were selected from QC filtered SNPs. Target genes are placed in the center of the 500-kb spanned region. Plots are shown with genomic annotation and HapMap LD (JPT+CHB) made by the UCSC Genome Browser (Human Mar. 2006).

Figure S6 Population stratification analysis. Population stratification analysis by EIGENSTRAT in the Present GWAS data set. POAG samples separated with HPG and NPG groups were applied. The version of HapMap reference data is release22 (Build36). Since Control, NPG, HPG, and HapMap JPT samples were tightly overlapped, only the plots for NPG (yellow cross) are visible.

Table S1 Genome-wide significant SNPs that passed the Bonferroni correction threshold in the Present GWAS.

Table S2 Analysis of confounding effects of age and sex for the candidate SNPs.

Table S3 Present GWAS results in 9p21.3 locus.

Table S4 Combined GWAS results in 9p21.3 locus.

Table S5 Association results of Present GWAS for previously reported SNPs.

Table S6 Characteristics of the samples.

Supporting Information S1 Quality control for genotyping.

Acknowledgments

The authors wish to thank all the patients and volunteers who enrolled in the study. We also thank Professor T. Miki for managing the anonymous code-assignment process; M. Yamashita, S. Ohashi, and N. Saito for processing blood samples and performing genotyping; H. Yamada for the assistance in clinical information analysis; R. Sato and F. Sato (SASA Plus Co., Ltd., Fukuoka, Japan) for the management of genotype data and building the analyzing system; T. Ichikawa for excellent secretarial assistance; and J. Bush for reviewing the manuscript.

Author Contributions

Conceived and designed the experiments: SK KT. Performed the experiments: MN YI NO MU KI HA KM. Analyzed the data: MN YT SK KT. Contributed reagents/materials/analysis tools: YI MF MU KI MK KM SK. Wrote the paper: MN YI YT KM SK KT.

References

1. Quigley HA, Broman AT (2006) The number of people with glaucoma worldwide in 2010 and 2020. Br J Ophthalmol 90: 262–267.
2. Kwon YH, Fingert JH, Kuehn MH, Alward WL (2009) Primary open-angle glaucoma. N Engl J Med 360: 1113–1124.
3. European Glaucoma Society (2008) Terminology and guidelines for glaucoma, 3rd edition (Editrice Dogma, Savona, Italy).
4. Iwase A, Suzuki Y, Araie M, Yamamoto T, Abe H, et al. (2004) The prevalence of primary open-angle glaucoma in Japanese: the Tajimi Study. Ophthalmology 111: 1641–1648.
5. Klein BE, Klein R, Sponsel WE, Franke T, Cantor LB, et al. (1992) Prevalence of glaucoma. The Beaver Dam Eye Study. Ophthalmology 99: 1499–1504.
6. Heijl A, Leske MC, Bengtsson B, Hyman L, Bengtsson B, et al. (2002) Reduction of intraocular pressure and glaucoma progression: results from the Early Manifest Glaucoma Trial. Arch Ophthalmol 120: 1268–1279.
7. Leskea MC, Heijl A, Hyman L, Bengtsson B, Komaroff E (2004) Factors for progression and glaucoma treatment: the Early Manifest Glaucoma Trial. Curr Opin Ophthalmol 15: 102–106.
8. Hewitt AW, Craig JE, Mackey DA (2006) Complex genetics of complex traits: the case of primary open-angle glaucoma. Clin Experiment Ophthalmol 34: 472–484.
9. Fan BJ, Wiggs JL (2010) Glaucoma: genes, phenotypes, and new directions for therapy. J Clin Invest 120: 3064–3072.
10. Nakano M, Ikeda Y, Taniguchi T, Yagi T, Fuwa M, et al. (2009) Three susceptible loci associated with primary open-angle glaucoma identified by genome-wide association study in a Japanese population. Proc Natl Acad Sci U S A 106: 12838–12842.
11. Jiao X, Yang Z, Yang X, Chen Y, Tong Z, et al. (2009) Common variants on chromosome 2 and risk of primary open-angle glaucoma in the Afro-Caribbean population of Barbados. Proc Natl Acad Sci U S A 106: 17105–17110.
12. Meguro A, Inoko H, Ota M, Mizuki N, Bahram S (2010) Genome-wide association study of normal tension glaucoma: common variants in SRBD1 and ELOVL5 contribute to disease susceptibility. Ophthalmology 117: 1331–1338 e1335.
13. Thorleifsson G, Walters GB, Hewitt AW, Masson G, Helgason A, et al. (2010) Common variants near CAV1 and CAV2 are associated with primary open-angle glaucoma. Nat Genet 42: 906–909.
14. Burdon KP, Macgregor S, Hewitt AW, Sharma S, Chidlow G, et al. (2011) Genome-wide association study identifies susceptibility loci for open angle glaucoma at TMCO1 and CDKN2B-AS1. Nat Genet 43: 574–578.
15. Kuehn MH, Wang K, Roos B, Stone EM, Kwon YH, et al. (2011) Chromosome 7q31 POAG locus: ocular expression of caveolins and lack of association with POAG in a US cohort. Mol Vis 17: 430–435.

16. Rao KN, Kaur I, Chakrabarti S (2009) Lack of association of three primary open-angle glaucoma-susceptible loci with primary glaucomas in an Indian population. Proc Natl Acad Sci U S A 106: E125–126; author reply E127.
17. Ramdas WD, van Koolwijk LM, Lemij HG, Pasutto F, Cree AJ, et al. (2011) Common genetic variants associated with open-angle glaucoma. Hum Mol Genet 20: 2464–2471.
18. Japan Glaucoma Society (2006) Guidelines for glaucoma, 2nd edition.
19. Mantel N, Haenszel W (1959) Statistical aspects of the analysis of data from retrospective studies of disease. J Natl Cancer Inst 22: 719–748.
20. McPherson R, Pertsemlidis A, Kavaslar N, Stewart A, Roberts R, et al. (2007) A common allele on chromosome 9 associated with coronary heart disease. Science 316: 1488–1491.
21. Helgadottir A, Thorleifsson G, Manolescu A, Gretarsdottir S, Blondal T, et al. (2007) A common variant on chromosome 9p21 affects the risk of myocardial infarction. Science 316: 1491–1493.
22. Samani NJ, Erdmann J, Hall AS, Hengstenberg C, Mangino M, et al. (2007) Genomewide association analysis of coronary artery disease. N Engl J Med 357: 443–453.
23. Wellcome Trust Case Control Consortium (2007) Genome-wide association study of 14,000 cases of seven common diseases and 3,000 shared controls. Nature 447: 661–678.
24. Scott LJ, Mohlke KL, Bonnycastle LL, Willer CJ, Li Y, et al. (2007) A genome-wide association study of type 2 diabetes in Finns detects multiple susceptibility variants. Science 316: 1341–1345.
25. Saxena R, Voight BF, Lyssenko V, Burtt NP, de Bakker PI, et al. (2007) Genome-wide association analysis identifies loci for type 2 diabetes and triglyceride levels. Science 316: 1331–1336.
26. Zeggini E, Scott LJ, Saxena R, Voight BF, Marchini JL, et al. (2008) Meta-analysis of genome-wide association data and large-scale replication identifies additional susceptibility loci for type 2 diabetes. Nat Genet 40: 638–645.
27. Harismendy O, Notani D, Song X, Rahim NG, Tanasa B, et al. (2011) 9p21 DNA variants associated with coronary artery disease impair interferon-gamma signalling response. Nature 470: 264–268.
28. Ramdas WD, van Koolwijk LM, Ikram MK, Jansonius NM, de Jong PT, et al. (2010) A genome-wide association study of optic disc parameters. PLoS Genet 6: e1000978.
29. Traggiai E, Becker S, Subbarao K, Kolesnikova L, Uematsu Y, et al. (2004) An efficient method to make human monoclonal antibodies from memory B cells: potent neutralization of SARS coronavirus. Nat Med 10: 871–875.
30. Ueta M, Sotozono C, Nakano M, Taniguchi T, Yagi T, et al. (2010) Association between prostaglandin E receptor 3 polymorphisms and Stevens-Johnson syndrome identified by means of a genome-wide association study. J Allergy Clin Immunol 126: 1218–1225 e1210.
31. Frazer KA, Ballinger DG, Cox DR, Hinds DA, Stuve LL, et al. (2007) A second generation human haplotype map of over 3.1 million SNPs. Nature 449: 851–861.

14

Genome-Wide Linkage Scan for Primary Open Angle Glaucoma: Influences of Ancestry and Age at Diagnosis

Kristy R. Crooks[1]⁹, R. Rand Allingham[1,2]⁹, Xuejun Qin[1], Yutao Liu[1], Jason R. Gibson[1], Cecilia Santiago-Turla[2], Karen R. Larocque-Abramson[1], Elizabeth Del Bono[3], Pratap Challa[2], Leon W. Herndon[2], Stephen Akafo[4], Janey L. Wiggs[3], Silke Schmidt[1], Michael A. Hauser[1,2]*

1 Center for Human Genetics, Duke University Medical Center, Durham, North Carolina, United States of America, **2** Department of Ophthalmology, Duke University Eye Center, Duke University Medical Center, Durham, North Carolina, United States of America, **3** Department of Ophthalmology, Harvard Medical School and Massachusetts Eye and Ear Infirmary, Boston, Massachusetts, United States of America, **4** Unit of Ophthalmology, Department of Surgery, University of Ghana Medical School, Accra, Ghana

Abstract

Primary open-angle glaucoma (POAG) is the most common form of glaucoma and one of the leading causes of vision loss worldwide. The genetic etiology of POAG is complex and poorly understood. The purpose of this work is to identify genomic regions of interest linked to POAG. This study is the largest genetic linkage study of POAG performed to date: genomic DNA samples from 786 subjects (538 Caucasian ancestry, 248 African ancestry) were genotyped using either the Illumina GoldenGate Linkage 4 Panel or the Illumina Infinium Human Linkage-12 Panel. A total of 5233 SNPs was analyzed in 134 multiplex POAG families (89 Caucasian ancestry, 45 African ancestry). Parametric and non-parametric linkage analyses were performed on the overall dataset and within race-specific datasets (Caucasian ancestry and African ancestry). Ordered subset analysis was used to stratify the data on the basis of age of glaucoma diagnosis. Novel linkage regions were identified on chromosomes 1 and 20, and two previously described loci—GLC1D on chromosome 8 and GLC1I on chromosome 15—were replicated. These data will prove valuable in the context of interpreting results from genome-wide association studies for POAG.

Editor: Amanda Ewart Toland, Ohio State University Medical Center, United States of America

Funding: The funders had no role in study design, data collection and analysis, decision to publish, or preparation of the manuscript. This work was supported in part by a generous donation by Roger Milliken, Spartanburg, South Carolina and by the research infrastructure of the Duke Center for Human Genetics. This work was also supported by CTSA grant 1 UL1 RR024128-01 from NCRR/NIH, NIH grants R01EY013315 (MAH), R01EY019126 (MAH), RO1EY015543 (RRA), R01EY015872 (JLW), and P30EY014104 (Core support at the Massachusetts Eye and Ear Infirmary).

Competing Interests: The authors have declared that no competing interests exist.

* E-mail: mike.hauser@duke.edu

⁹ These authors contributed equally to this work.

Introduction

Glaucoma comprises a group of disorders that are characterized by retinal ganglion cell death and a characteristic pattern of progressive vision loss. POAG is the most common type of glaucoma globally [1], and it is estimated that by 2020 the number of people diagnosed with POAG in the United States alone will total more than 3 million [2]. It has long been recognized that there is a heterogeneous genetic component to POAG. Genome-wide linkage analyses have identified 14 loci, designated GLC1A-N, which are thought to contribute to POAG risk [2–18]. Causative mutations have been identified in genes within three of these loci: Myocilin (MYOC) on 1q24.3 (GLC1A) [12], optineurin (OPTN) on 10p15-14 (GLC1E) [8], and WD40-repeat 36 on 5q22.1 (GLC1G) [6]. Together, mutations in these three genes account for less than 10% of POAG cases [19]. Thus, the majority of the genetic etiology of POAG remains to be discovered.

Among the challenges in the study of POAG is genetic and phenotypic heterogeneity of study subjects. For example, while mutations in OPTN or MYOC both result in POAG, a missense change in OPTN (E50K) causes an adult-onset form of POAG that is characterized by normal intraocular pressures [8], whereas MYOC mutations can cause either adult-onset or juvenile-onset disease with highly elevated intraocular pressures [20]. Reducing this genetic variability in the study population is essential for identifying variants that contribute to POAG risk, and it can be achieved by phenotypic stratification. In the study of POAG and other complex diseases, phenotypic stratification by ordered subset analysis (OSA) [21] has been particularly successful in identifying genetically homogeneous subsets of families with increased evidence for linkage and in reducing linkage intervals for follow-up analysis. In OSA, families are ranked according to a phenotypic variable. In this study, families were sorted from lowest to highest average age at diagnosis (AAD, see Methods) of POAG in affected relatives. We chose this variable based on previous linkage analyses by our group [3] and others [22] that established AAD as an important source of genetic heterogeneity.

In this study we report the results of the largest SNP-based genome-wide POAG linkage study performed to date. Using both standard linkage methodology and OSA to account for genetic heterogeneity, our study identified global as well as ancestry-specific and phenotype-specific genomic regions that may harbor POAG susceptibility variants.

Results

Clinical data summary

Table 1 summarizes sample size and clinical characteristics of the study population. After exclusion of families segregating MYOC mutations, 786 sampled subjects from 134 multiplex families were analyzed. Clinical characteristics were similar among subjects of African ancestry and Caucasian ancestry. As expected, intraocular pressure (IOP) was clinically elevated in affected members of both ancestry groups, and pressures in those of African ancestry were significantly higher than those of Caucasian ancestry (31.5±1.0 versus 28.0±0.4 mmHg, $p \leq 0.003$). Both groups had an age at diagnosis (AAD, see Methods) that averaged in the 50 s and ranged from the 20 s to the 80 s. Slightly more than half the affected study subjects were female in both groups.

Whole genome linkage analysis

Figure 1 shows results of the multipoint linkage analyses for the overall dataset, based on 5,233 SNPs with an average intermarker distance of 0.68 cM. Parametric linkage analyses were performed using both dominant and recessive models. We found the strongest evidence for linkage at 20q13.12–13.13, with the peak marker rs911411 (multipoint HLOD = 2.3, 75.8 cM, dominant model). The one-lod unit support interval comprises the region between the markers rs765147 and rs718630.

Results of the two-point and multipoint linkage analyses for the Caucasian ancestry dataset and African ancestry dataset are shown in Figures 2 and 3, respectively. Among families of Caucasian ancestry, the best evidence for linkage was identified at 1q22–23.3, with the peak marker rs876537 (multipoint HLOD = 2.03, 154.5 cM, recessive model), and the one-lod unit support interval between markers rs2066981 and rs836. Among families of African ancestry, the strongest linkage was found at 20ptel-13, with the peak marker rs1342137 (multipoint HLOD = 2.09, 0.3 cM, dominant model), and the centromeric one-lod unit support boundary at rs600832.

The most notable linked regions for each dataset are shown in Table 2. In the combined dataset, there were four regions with multipoint lod scores >1.5. For the ancestry-specific datasets, all linked regions with both a multipoint lod score >1.5 and at least one two-point lod >1.5 within the one-lod support interval are shown. There were four such regions of interest in the Caucasian ancestry dataset, and two in the African ancestry dataset.

Ordered subset analysis

To examine whether AAD was a significant modifier of POAG linkage evidence, we performed OSA on the overall dataset, using ascending family mean AAD (lowest to highest age at diagnosis) as the covariate. We found significantly increased evidence for linkage to chromosomes 8 and 15 (empirical $p \leq 0.05$, with 10,000 permutations, Figure 4).

On chromosome 8 (Figure 4, left panel), the one-lod unit support interval comprised 22.1 cM with a maximum multipoint lod score of 2.03 at 117.2 cM (empirical $p = 0.04$). This region includes the previously reported POAG locus GLC1D [14]. All 26 families (13 Caucasian ancestry, 13 African ancestry) in the OSA subset had an average AAD below 50 years (mean 41, range: 28 to 49). In the complementary subset of 102 families (78 Caucasian ancestry, 34 African ancestry), the mean AAD was 62 years (range: 49 to 78).

The linkage region on chromosome 15 was found in the Caucasian early-onset dataset at 15q11–12 (Figure 4, right panel), comprising 13.6 cM with a maximum lod score of 3.17 at 3.2 cM (empirical $p = 7 \times 10^{-5}$), replicating our previously described GLC1I locus [3]. There were 19 families in this OSA subset, including the previously screened 11 families, all of which had an AAD below 53 years (mean: 45 years, range: 30 to 52 years). The complementary group of 68 families had an average age of onset of 63 years (range 52–78 years).

Discussion

We have conducted family-based linkage analysis to identify regions of the genome that may harbor POAG susceptibility variants. These linkage regions provide distinct and complementary data that can assist in the interpretation of genome-wide association studies. The overall dataset and the African ancestry dataset linked POAG to non-overlapping intervals on chromosome 20. As these regions appear to be distinct from the JOAG-linked locus GLC1K, located between D20S846 and rs6081603 [23], there may now be as many as three discrete regions of interest on this chromosome alone. The Caucasian ancestry dataset linked POAG to a novel locus on chromosome 1.

Two of the regions with evidence for linkage, 14q11.2 in the combined and Caucasian ancestry datasets and 20p13 in the

Table 1. Clinical characteristics of study populations.

		Caucasian ancestry	African ancestry	Total
Families	N	89	45	134
Individuals	N	538	248	786
Affected	N	278	123	401
	Mean age-of-onset in years (range)	59 (28–84)	54 (26–81)	58 (26–84)
	% female	54	56	54
	Mean maximum IOP	28.1	31.5	29.0
	Affected sibling pairs (N)	180	68	248
	Affected non-sib relative pairs (N)*	58	35	93
Unaffected	N	260	125	385
	Mean age-at-exam in years (range)	68 (50–83)	64 (45–76)	67 (45–83)
	% female	51	49	50

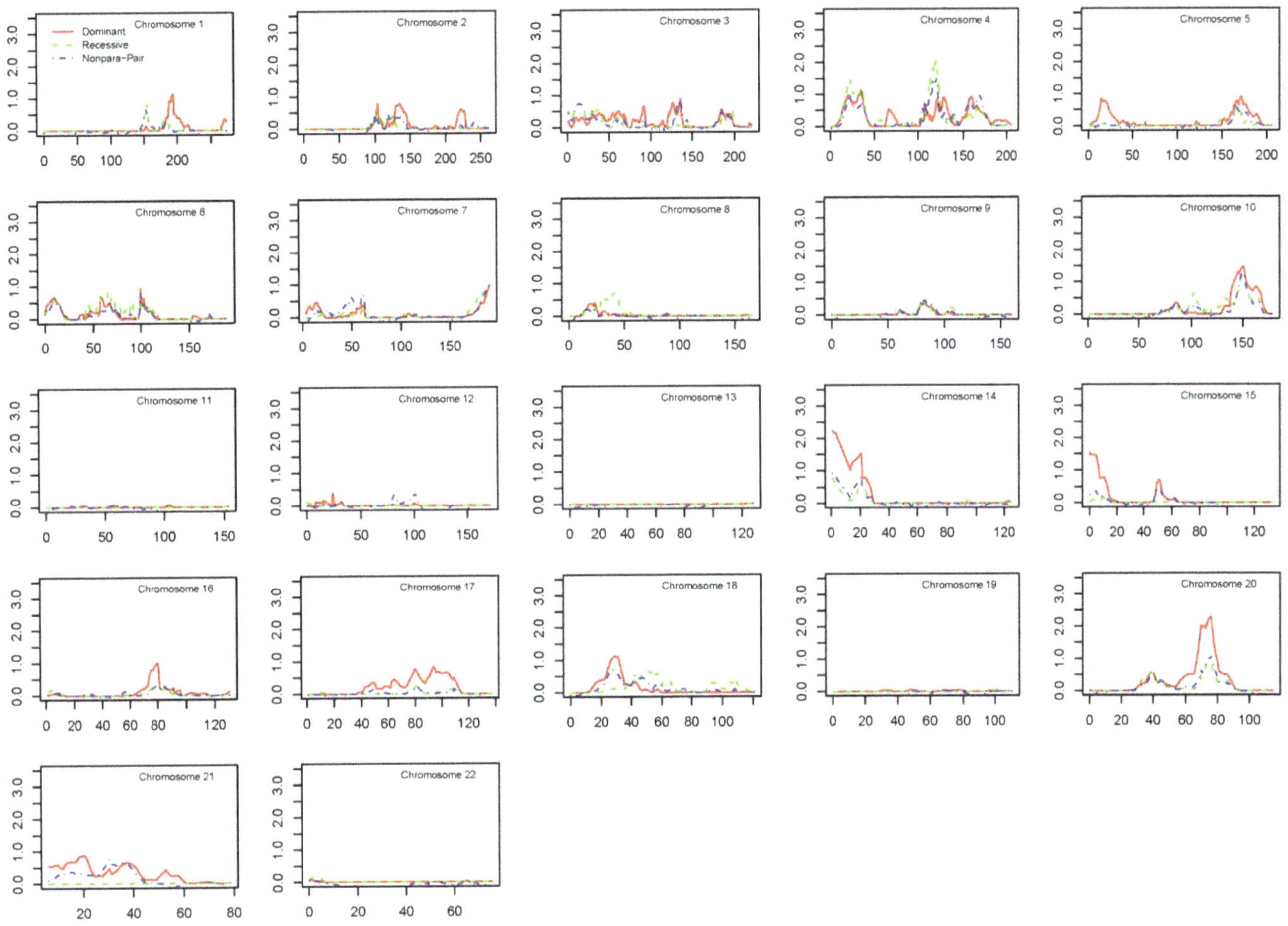

Figure 1. Linkage results for the combined dataset. Multipoint linkage scores for parametric dominant (red), parametric recessive (green), and nonparametric (blue) models are plotted for the combined dataset. Symbols indicate two-point lod scores ≥1.5 in the parametric dominant (red) and recessive (green) models.

African ancestry dataset, are telomeric. It is generally accepted that telomeric regions may give rise to false positive linkage peaks at a higher frequency than other regions of the chromosome. In the absence of confirmation, these regions of interest should be considered with caution and follow-up analysis should be delayed until the findings are replicated.

Using OSA, we found increased evidence for linkage in families with adult early-onset on chromosomes 8 and 15, replicating previous findings. The linkage region on chromosome 8 includes the GLC1D locus, which was first reported in a single family with an apparently Mendelian form of glaucoma [14]. It is not surprising that the one-lod unit support interval calculated here is somewhat larger than the reported GLC1D locus, considering the differences between a nonparametric linkage analysis of a complex phenotype in a larger family collection, compared to recombination-based linkage mapping within a single large pedigree. Interestingly, the age-at-onset of glaucoma in that pedigree is reported as "within the third to fourth decade of life" which is consistent with the AAD of the OSA-identified subset of families reported here. Our finding suggests the possibility that one or more variants in the GLC1D region may give rise to both rare Mendelian and more common non-Mendelian forms of early-onset POAG.

We have previously reported microsatellite linkage to proximal 15q in a collection of 15 (11 Caucasian and 4 African American) early onset families [3]. Our current dataset comprises 34 early-onset families (19 Caucasian ancestry, 15 African ancestry). With the additional families, we were able to divide the dataset based on ancestry and analyze the two groups separately. We replicated linkage to GLC1I in the Caucasian dataset (19 families, including the 11 families reported earlier). In the current report, the one-lod unit support interval is larger and the peak lod score marginally lower than in the previous report. This likely reflects the nature of the individually more informative microsatellite markers compared to SNPs, rather than different underlying genes in the two OSA subsets. There was no evidence for linkage to POAG in the African ancestry early-onset dataset.

In conclusion, we have reported results of the first SNP-based genome-wide linkage analysis of POAG. We identified regions of interest for further investigation in a dataset of African ancestry, a dataset of Caucasian ancestry, and in the combined dataset. We also replicated two previously-reported early-onset POAG loci, strengthening the case that these regions may harbor one or more genes that are either causative for early-onset glaucoma or that modulate the age at which symptoms are first evident. We expect that the results reported here will prove useful in the context of interpreting and strengthening results from genome-wide association studies and will complement efforts to better understand the complex genetic etiology of glaucoma.

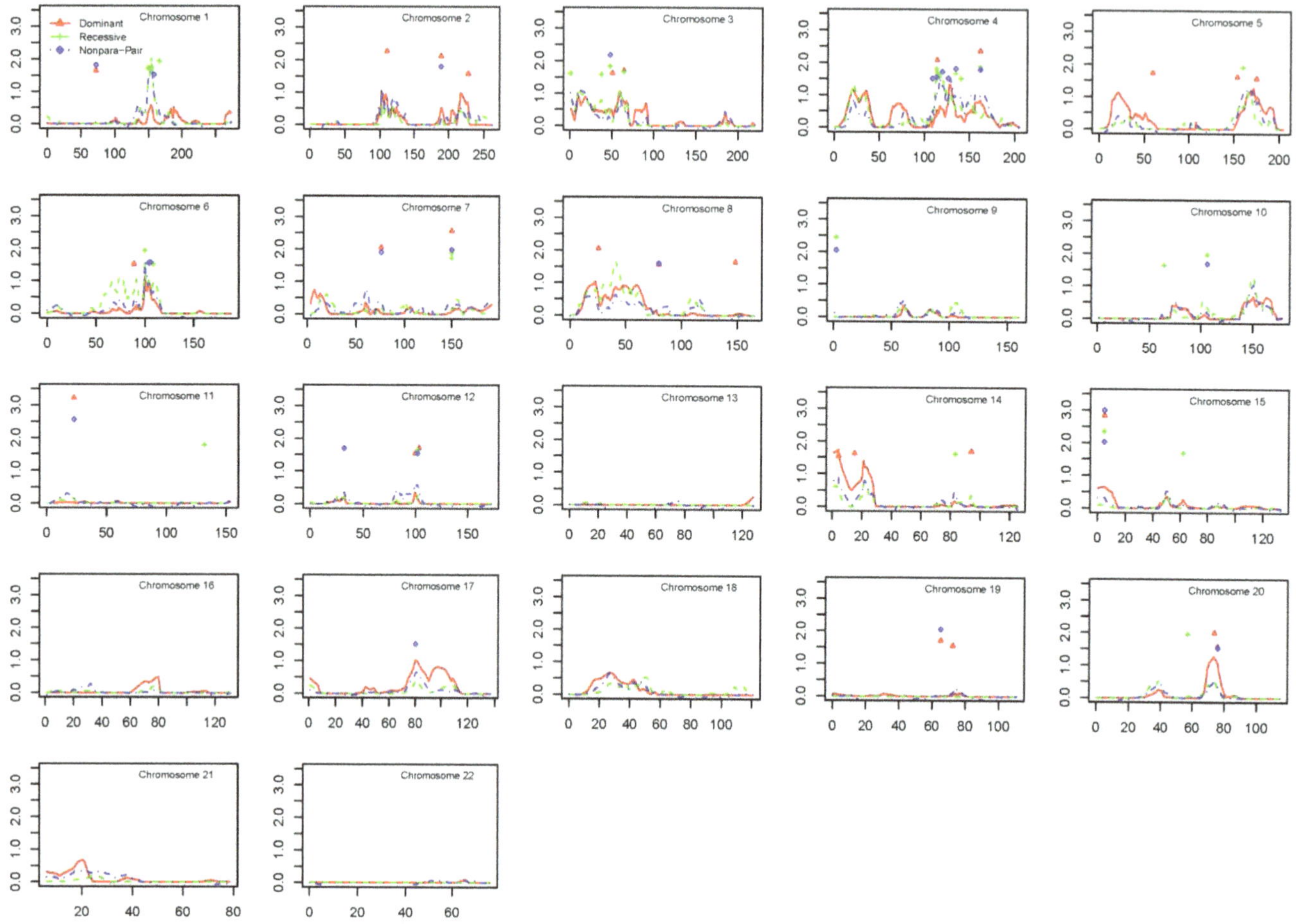

Figure 2. Linkage results for the Caucasian ancestry dataset. Multipoint linkage scores for parametric dominant (red), parametric recessive (green), and nonparametric (blue) models are plotted for the Caucasian ancestry dataset. Symbols indicate two-point lod scores ≥1.5 in the parametric dominant (red) and recessive (green) models.

Materials and Methods

Subjects

This study adhered to the tenets of the Declaration of Helsinki. Written informed consent was obtained from all participating individuals. Caucasian and African-American subjects were recruited at the Duke Eye Center (Durham, NC). Caucasian subjects were also enrolled at the Massachusetts Eye and Ear Infirmary (Boston, MA). African subjects were enrolled at the University of Ghana. The research was reviewed and approved by the Institutional Review Board from all participating institutions, including Duke University Medical Center, the Massachusetts Eye and Ear Infirmary and the Noguchi Memorial Institute of Medical Research of the College of Health Sciences, University of Ghana.

POAG probands were unrelated and met the following three inclusion criteria: (1) intraocular pressure greater than 22 mm Hg in both eyes without medications or greater than 19 mm Hg with two or more medications; (2) glaucomatous optic neuropathy in both eyes; and (3) visual field loss consistent with optic nerve damage in at least one eye. Other affected members met at least 2 of these criteria. Glaucomatous optic neuropathy was defined as cup-to-disc ratio higher than 0.7 or focal loss of the nerve fiber layer (notch). Visual fields were performed by using standard automated perimetry. Exclusion criteria included the presence of any secondary form of glaucoma. Consenting family members who did not meet the above criteria were enrolled, but their genotypes were used only to establish linkage phase. The MYOC gene was sequenced in all probands. Families with disease-associated MYOC mutations were excluded from analysis. Age at diagnosis (AAD) was self-reported by POAG cases as the age at which they were first told by an eye specialist that they 1) had elevated intraocular pressure, 2) were prescribed IOP-lowering eye medications, or 3) had glaucoma.

Sample preparation and genotyping

To conduct the genome screen, samples were genotyped using the Illumina GoldenGate Linkage 4 Panel or the Illumina Infinium Human Linkage-12 Panel. DNA from two CEPH individuals and two quality control samples were included in each 96-well plate used for genotyping, and a 100% match of these samples was required for inclusion of a marker in the analysis. A minimum genotyping efficiency of 95% was required for each marker.

Pedigree relationships were tested with RELPAIR [24], which uses identity-by-descent allele sharing estimates for statistical inference of biological relationships within and across the specified family structures. Discrepancies between specified and inferred relationships, typically due to sample switches, were addressed by removing four unresolved individuals and two families from the analysis. Genotypes that were inconsistent with Mendelian

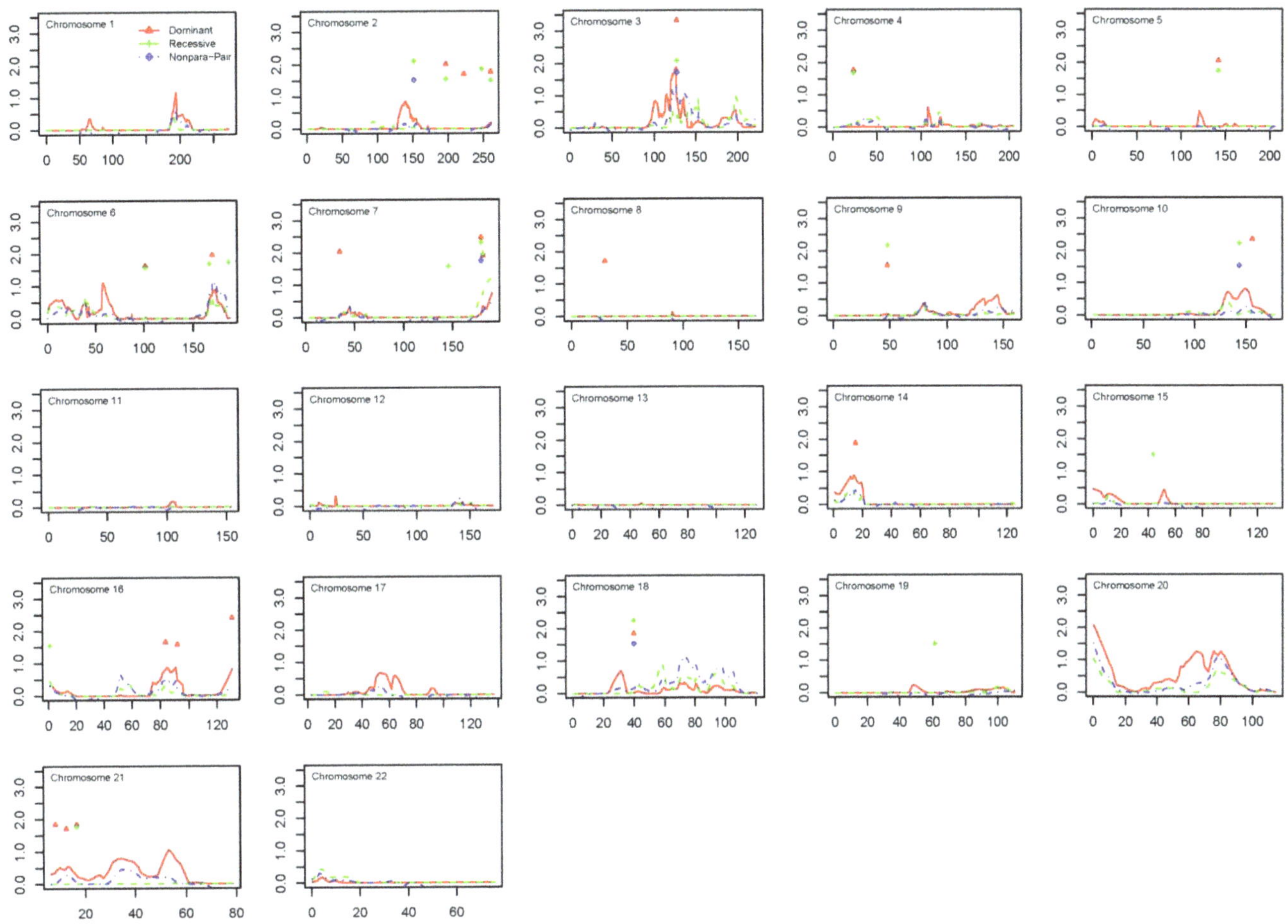

Figure 3. Linkage results for the African ancestry dataset. Multipoint linkage scores for parametric dominant (red), parametric recessive (green), and nonparametric (blue) models are plotted for the African ancestry dataset. Symbols indicate two-point lod scores ≥1.5 in the parametric dominant (red) and recessive (green) models.

Table 2. Linkage analysis results.

Dataset	Chromosome	Location (cM)	SNP	peak multipoint lod (model)	peak 2-point lod
Combined	20q13.13	67–78	rs911411	2.3 (dom)	N/A
	14q11.2	0–12	rs1959344	2.2 (dom)	N/A
	4q26	111–124	rs814397	2.0 (rec)	N/A
	15q11.2	0–14	rs1722791	1.5 (dom)	N/A
Caucasian ancestry	1q23.2	148–158	rs876537	2.0 (rec)	1.8
	4q25	111-126	rs701760	1.9 (rec)	1.8
	14q11.2	0–28	rs1713423	1.8 (dom)	1.6
	6q15	98–114	rs1979797	1.6 (rec)	1.9
African ancestry	20p13	0–10	rs1774116	2.1	1.5
	3q13.32	119–130	rs1348969	1.8 (dom)	3.3

For the combined dataset, all linked regions with a peak multipoint lod >1.5 are shown. For the ancestry-specific datasets, all linked regions with both a multipoint lod >1.5 and at least one two-point lod ≥1.5 within the one-lod support interval are shown.

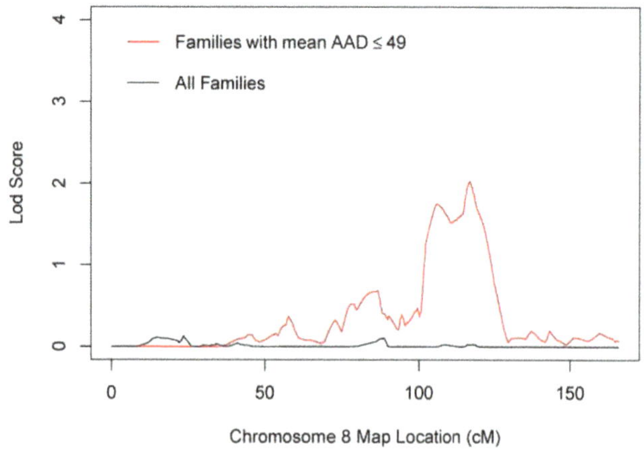

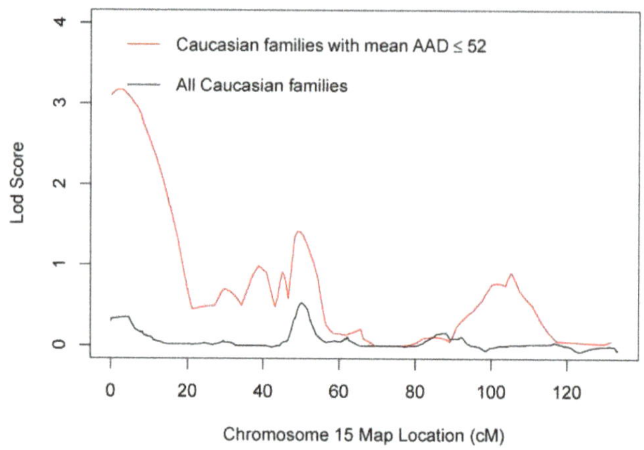

Figure 4. OSA results for chromosomes 8 and 15. Ordered subset analysis (red line) indicates improved evidence for linkage to chromosome 8 (left panel) among families with a mean age of onset ≤49 years. The black line plots non-parametric linkage analysis in all families in the combined dataset. Improved evidence for linkage to chromosome 15 (right panel) was demonstrated among Caucasian families with a mean age of onset ≤52 years. The black line plots non-parametric linkage analysis in all Caucasian families.

inheritance were identified with the program PEDCHECK [25] and removed prior to the linkage analysis.

Whole genome linkage analysis

The final linkage analysis included 5233 single nucleotide polymorphisms (SNPs). Marker order and intermarker distances (in cM) were derived from the Decode linkage maps [26]. For markers not included in that panel, genetic distances were interpolated based on physical distances (1 cM~1 Mb). The software MERLIN [27] was used to calculate nonparametric two-point and multipoint lod scores, using the exponential model and Spairs allele sharing statistic [28]. Parametric affecteds-only heterogeneity lod scores (HLODs) assuming a dominant (disease allele frequency 0.01) or recessive (disease allele frequency 0.2) model were also computed with MERLIN. For the separate analysis of Caucasian and African ancestry datasets, ethnicity-specific marker allele frequencies were estimated from all genotyped individuals [29]. To avoid an inflation of lod scores due to misspecified allele frequencies, particularly for markers with rare minor alleles in one of the two ethnicities, we also used these ethnicity-specific marker allele frequencies in the overall analysis. This was done by modifying the analysis files to include two "dummy markers" at the same map position as the real marker. The dummy markers had ethnicity-specific allele frequencies, with observed genotypes for samples of one ethnicity, but missing genotypes for the other. This computational approach allowed for the appropriate calculation of joint multipoint lod scores, which combine linkage information across map positions (i.e., at and in-between genotyped markers); joint two-point lod scores could not be calculated. To avoid an inflation of linkage evidence due to inter-marker LD in the absence of parental genotypes, we estimated haplotype frequencies of SNP clusters in high pairwise LD, using a threshold of $r^2 = 0.16$ to define these clusters [30,31].

Ordered subset analysis (OSA)

Based on previous POAG linkage analyses [3,22], we used OSA [21] to test whether AAD was a significant source of linkage heterogeneity in our dataset. Families were sorted by increasing average AAD in affected relatives and nonparametric linkage analysis was performed one family at a time in the AAD-based order until the family subset generating the maximum lod score anywhere on the given chromosome was identified. This maximum could occur at different map positions for different family subsets. Permutation testing was employed to test whether the observed increase in linkage evidence in this family subset was greater than expected by chance. To this end, families were randomly ordered and the lod score maximization procedure was repeated 10,000 times to calculate the proportion of random permutations with a maximum subset-based lod score at least as large as the observed one (empirical p-value). The OSA null hypothesis specifies no relationship between family-specific covariate and family-specific linkage evidence. Rejection of this null hypothesis suggests that the covariate, here AAD, is a statistically significant (empirical p-value≤0.05) source of linkage heterogeneity.

Acknowledgments

We would like to extend special thanks to Daniel Weeks for statistical assistance in calculating joint multipoint lod scores using multiple ethnicities.

Author Contributions

Conceived and designed the experiments: MAH SS RRA JRG. Performed the experiments: KRL-A YL JRG. Analyzed the data: XQ SS JRG. Contributed reagents/materials/analysis tools: JLW PC LWH SA CS-T EDB JRG. Wrote the paper: KRC RRA MAH SS JRG.

References

1. Quigley HA (1996) Number of people with glaucoma worldwide. Br J Ophthalmol 80: 389–393.
2. Friedman DS, Wolfs RC, O'Colmain BJ, Klein BE, Taylor HR, et al. (2004) Prevalence of open-angle glaucoma among adults in the United States. Arch Ophthalmol 122: 532–538.
3. Allingham RR, Wiggs JL, Hauser ER, Larocque-Abramson KR, Santiago-Turla C, et al. (2005) Early Adult-Onset POAG Linked to 15q11–13 Using Ordered Subset Analysis. Invest Ophthalmol Vis Sci 46: 2002–2005.
4. Baird PN, Foote SJ, Mackey DA, Craig J, Speed TP, et al. (2005) Evidence for a novel glaucoma locus at chromosome 3p21–22. Hum Genet 117: 249–257.
5. Lin Y, Liu T, Li J, Yang J, Du Q, et al. (2008) A genome-wide scan maps a novel autosomal dominant juvenile-onset open-angle glaucoma locus to 2p15–16. Mol Vis 14: 739–744.
6. Monemi S, Spaeth G, Dasilva A, Popinchalk S, Ilitchev E, et al. (2005) Identification of a novel adult-onset primary open-angle glaucoma (POAG) gene on 5q22.1. Hum Mol Genet 14: 725–733.

7. Pang CP, Fan BJ, Canlas O, Wang DY, Dubois S, et al. (2006) A genome-wide scan maps a novel juvenile-onset primary open angle glaucoma locus to chromosome 5q. Mol Vis 12: 85–92.
8. Rezaie T, Child A, Hitchings R, Brice G, Miller L, et al. (2002) Adult-onset primary open-angle glaucoma caused by mutations in optineurin. Science 295: 1077–1079.
9. Sarfarazi M, Child A, Stoilova D, Brice G, Desai T, et al. (1998) Localization of the fourth locus (GLC1E) for adult-onset primary open-angle glaucoma to the 10p15-p14 region. Am J Hum Genet 62: 641–652.
10. Sheffield VC, Stone EM, Alward WL, Drack AV, Johnson AT, et al. (1993) Genetic linkage of familial open angle glaucoma to chromosome 1q21–q31. Nat Genet 4: 47–50.
11. Stoilova D, Child A, Trifan OC, Crick RP, Coakes RL, et al. (1996) Localization of a locus (GLC1B) for adult-onset primary open angle glaucoma to the 2cen-q13 region. Genomics 36: 142–150.
12. Stone EM, Fingert JH, Alward WLM, Nguyen TD, Polansky JR, et al. (1997) Identification of a gene that causes primary open angle glaucoma. Science 275: 668–670.
13. Suriyapperuma SP, Child A, Desai T, Brice G, Kerr A, et al. (2007) A new locus (GLC1H) for adult-onset primary open-angle glaucoma maps to the 2p15–p16 region. Arch Ophthalmol 125: 86–92.
14. Trifan OC, Traboulsi EI, Stoilova D, Alozie I, Nguyen R, et al. (1998) A third locus (GLC1D) for adult-onset primary open-angle glaucoma maps to the 8q23 region. Am J Ophthalmol 126: 17–28.
15. Wang DY, Fan BJ, Chua JK, Tam PO, Leung CK, et al. (2006) A genome-wide scan maps a novel juvenile-onset primary open-angle glaucoma locus to 15q. Invest Ophthalmol Vis Sci 47: 5315–5321.
16. Wiggs JL, Lynch S, Ynagi G, Maselli M, Auguste J, et al. (2004) A genomewide scan identifies novel early-onset primary open-angle glaucoma loci on 9q22 and 20p12. Am J Hum Genet 74: 1314–1320.
17. Wirtz MK, Samples JR, Kramer PL, Rust K, Topinka JR, et al. (1997) Mapping a gene for adult-onset primary open-angle glaucoma to chromosome 3q. Am J Hum Genet 60: 296–304.
18. Wirtz MK, Samples JR, Rust K, Lie J, Nordling L, et al. (1999) GLC1F, a new primary open-angle glaucoma locus, maps to 7q35–q36. Arch Ophthalmol 117: 237–241.
19. Allingham RR, Liu Y, Rhee DJ (2009) The genetics of primary open-angle glaucoma: a review. Exp Eye Res 88: 837–844.
20. Alward WL, Fingert JH, Coote MA, Johnson AT, Lerner SF, et al. (1998) Clinical features associated with mutations in the chromosome 1 open-angle glaucoma gene (GLC1A). N Engl J Med 338: 1022–1027.
21. Hauser ER, Watanabe RM, Duren WL, Bass MP, Langefeld CD, et al. (2004) Ordered subset analysis in genetic linkage mapping of complex traits. Genet Epidemiol 27: 53–63.
22. Woodroffe A, Krafchak CM, Fuse N, Lichter PR, Moroi SE, et al. (2006) Ordered subset analysis supports a glaucoma locus at GLC1I on chromosome 15 in families with earlier adult age at diagnosis. Exp Eye Res 82: 1068–1074.
23. Sud A, Del Bono EA, Haines JL, Wiggs JL (2008) Fine mapping of the GLC1K juvenile primary open-angle glaucoma locus and exclusion of candidate genes. Mol Vis 14: 1319–1326.
24. Epstein MP, Duren WL, Boehnke M (2000) Improved inference of relationship for pairs of individuals. Am J Hum Genet 67: 1219–1231.
25. O'Connell JR, Weeks DE (1998) PedCheck: a program for identification of genotype incompatibilities in linkage analysis. Am J Hum Genet 63: 259–266.
26. Kong X, Murphy K, Raj T, He C, White PS, et al. (2004) A combined linkage-physical map of the human genome. Am J Hum Genet 75: 1143–1148.
27. Abecasis GR, Cherny SS, Cookson WO, Cardon LR (2002) Merlin–rapid analysis of dense genetic maps using sparse gene flow trees. Nat Genet 30: 97–101.
28. Kong A, Cox NJ (1997) Allele-sharing models: LOD scores and accurate linkage tests. Am J Hum Genet 61: 1179–1188.
29. Broman KW (2001) Estimation of allele frequencies with data on sibships. Genet Epidemiol 20: 307–315.
30. Abecasis GR, Wigginton JE (2005) Handling marker-marker linkage disequilibrium: pedigree analysis with clustered markers. Am J Hum Genet 77: 754–767.
31. Boyles AL, Scott WK, Martin ER, Schmidt S, Li YJ, et al. (2005) Linkage disequilibrium inflates type I error rates in multipoint linkage analysis when parental genotypes are missing. Hum Hered 59: 220–227.

15

Early Reduction of Microglia Activation by Irradiation in a Model of Chronic Glaucoma

Alejandra Bosco[1], Samuel D. Crish[2¤], Michael R. Steele[1], Cesar O. Romero[1], Denise M. Inman[3¤], Philip J. Horner[3], David J. Calkins[2], Monica L. Vetter[1]*

1 Department of Neurobiology and Anatomy, University of Utah, Salt Lake City, Utah, United States of America, 2 Department of Ophthalmology and Visual Sciences, Vanderbilt University, Nashville, Tennessee, United States of America, 3 Department of Neurosurgery, University of Washington, Seattle, Washington, United States of America

Abstract

Glaucoma is a neurodegenerative disease that results in the progressive decline and ultimate death of retinal ganglion cells (RGCs). While multiple risk factors are associated with glaucoma, the mechanisms leading to onset and progression of the disease remain unknown. Molecular analysis in various glaucoma models has revealed involvement of non-neuronal cell populations, including astrocytes, Mueller glia and microglia, at early stages of glaucoma. High-dose irradiation was reported to have a significant long-term protective effect in the DBA/2J (D2) mouse model of glaucoma, although the cellular and molecular basis for this effect remains unclear. In particular, the acute effects of irradiation on specific cell populations, including non-neuronal cells, in the D2 retina and nerve have not been assessed. Here we report that irradiation induces transient reduction in proliferating microglia within the optic nerve head and glial lamina within the first week post-irradiation. This was accompanied by reduced microglial activation, with no effect on astrocyte gliosis in those regions. At later stages we confirm that early high-dose irradiation of the mouse head results in improvement of axonal structural integrity and anterograde transport function, without reduction of intraocular pressure. Thus reduced microglial activation induced by irradiation at early stages is associated with reduced optic nerve and retinal neurodegeneration in the D2 mouse model of glaucoma.

Editor: Andreas Ohlmann, University of Regensburg, Germany

Funding: Funded by a generous grant from the Melza M. and Frank Theodore Barr Foundation through the Glaucoma Research Foundation (www.glaucoma.org/) (Catalyst for a Cure to MLV, PJH and DJC) and NIH grant # R01EY02878 to MLV. The funders had no role in study design, data collection and analysis, decision to publish, or preparation of the manuscript.

Competing Interests: The authors have declared that no competing interests exist.

* E-mail: monica@neuro.utah.edu

¤ Current address: Northeast Ohio Medical University, Rootstown, Ohio, United States of America

Introduction

Glaucoma is a neurodegenerative disease that destroys vision through progressive degeneration of the optic nerve and decline and death of retinal ganglion cells (RGCs). This disease affects roughly 70 million people, and is a leading cause of non-curable vision loss [1]. Multiple risk factors contribute to glaucoma, including race, age and elevated intraocular pressure [2,3]. However, how these factors influence neuronal loss in glaucoma is complex. In human patients, as well as in experimental animal models, there is evidence that age- and IOP-related RGC axon damage first occurs in the optic nerve head (ONH), where optic axons exit the eye [4]. But degenerative changes also affect other RGC compartments, localized to the retina, nerve and brain, in an asynchronous manner, impacting cell somata, dendrites and their synapses, myelinated axons, and axonal terminations [5,6,7].

Analysis of molecular and cellular changes in various animal models of glaucoma have suggested involvement of diverse non-neuronal cell populations, including astrocytes, Mueller glia and microglia, although the relative contributions of these glial cells to RGC degeneration or protection remain unclear [8]. Microglia are resident immune cells of the central nervous system that have been implicated in neurodegenerative diseases, including glaucoma [8,9]. These glial cells respond to neuronal stress or injury with changes in distribution and cell activation, which involves simplification of cell morphology, expression of various growth factors and cytokines, and in some cases migration, proliferation or phagocytic activity [9,10]. Notably, microglia reside in proximity to all RGC compartments impacted in glaucoma including dendrites and synapses, cell somata, and axons [11]. In human glaucoma, activated microglia have been found clustered in the region of the ONH, which is the site of initial axonal injury [12].

In the DBA/2J mouse (D2), which is an established model of inherited pigmentary glaucoma [13], microglia become activated prior to evidence of RGC structural decline [11]. Spatially, activated microglia first localize to the ONH and lamina around unmyelinated optic axons [11], the presumed sites of initiation of optic neuropathy in D2 mice [14,15]. At later stages microglia activation spreads to the peripheral inner retina [11], and this is associated with slow microglial proliferation that doubles retinal microglia numbers from 4 to 10 months of age [16]. Consistent with involvement of microglia in glaucoma, microarray analysis of the D2 mouse has shown that there are changes in gene expression within the retina as well as the ONH that suggest an innate immune response [17,18,19]. Similar changes in gene expression have been reported in microarray studies of the retina following acute IOP elevation in various species [20,21,22,23]. Furthermore, early and chronic deactivation of microglia by administration of minocycline results in improved RGC axonal integrity and transport function [24]. Thus microglia activation represents a significant and early component of pathology in glaucoma.

High-dose radiation treatment of the entire animal with syngeneic bone marrow transfer (BMT) had an unexpected and remarkably profound protective effect on glaucomatous damage in the D2 mouse [25]. Neither iris disease nor IOP elevation were affected by treatment, but there was dramatic improvement in axon preservation out to 14 months of age, when most D2 mice normally show severe optic nerve pathology. In addition, there was protection against RGC somal loss and excavation of the ONH. The protective effect was also observed with irradiation of the head or eye without BMT [26]. In these studies irradiation was performed from 5 to 8 weeks of age, which is just prior to significant microglial activation in the D2 mouse [11]. Thus, it is possible that treatment had an effect on microglia with the potential to impact the subsequent course of degeneration.

Here we tested the effects of high-dose irradiation of the head region alone on D2 mice and found transient reduction in proliferating microglia within the ONH and glial lamina, with maximal effect within the first week post-irradiation. This was accompanied by reduced microglial activation within the central retina and proximal optic nerve compartments, with no effect on astrocyte gliosis in those regions. We also found significant improvement in axonal survival and anterograde transport without reduction of IOP, confirming that bone marrow transfer is not required to abate degeneration. Thus, one consequence of high-dose irradiation is to acutely reduce the levels of microglia activation in this glaucoma model.

Materials and Methods

Ethics Statement

This study was performed in strict accordance with the recommendations in the Guide for the Care and Use of Laboratory Animals of the National Institutes of Health. The protocol was approved by the Institutional Animal Care and Use Committee of the University of Utah (Animal Welfare Assurance Number: A3031-01). All procedures were performed under avertin anesthesia, and every effort was made to minimize suffering.

Animals

Adult DBA/2J mice (Jackson Laboratory (JAX), Bar Harbor, ME; stock # 000671) served as an experimental model of inherited pigmentary glaucoma, and its DBA/2J-Gpnmb+/Sj substrain (stock # 007048) as non-glaucoma control [27,28]. These strains are referred to as D2 and D2G mice, respectively. Mice were bred and aged at the University of Utah in a pathogen-free barrier facility under a 12 hr light/dark cycle, and every 4 generations breeders purchased from JAX were introduced to avoid genetic drift. Mice under anesthesia were identified with ear tattoos (Harvard Apparatus, Holliston, MA). D2.CX3CR1$^{gfp/+}$ mice, where microglia (and other myeloid cells) specifically express GFP under the control of fractalkine receptor locus [29], were generated after backcrossing B6.129P-*CX3CR1*^{tm1Litt}/J mice (JAX stock #005582) onto the D2 background for over 10 generations. All animal maintenance and procedures were approved by the University of Utah Institutional Animal Care and Use Committee, and followed the Statement for the Use of Animals in Ophthalmic and Vision Research from the Association for Research in Vision and Ophthalmology (ARVO).

Head irradiation

Four to six week-old female and male D2 mice had the rostral half of their heads exposed to a single high dose of electromagnetic radiation (8 Gy or 800 rads, 1 Gy/min) delivered by a biological X-ray generator (X-Rad 320, Precision X-Ray, North Branford, CT). To restrict irradiation to the eyes and visual pathways, each mouse was positioned inside a 50 mL conical tube with its muzzle exposed through the truncated end of the tube, while the rest of the body was shielded with two 6 mm-thick lead plates. Irradiation targeted an area delimited by the base of the ears and the beginning of the eyes, sparing the nose. The head region and the depths targeted were maintained constant across animals with the aid of reference collimated light and focusing LEDs. During the procedure, mice were anesthetized via intraperitoneal Avertin injection, and kept warm over isothermal pads (Braintree Scientific, Braintree, MA).

Intraocular pressure (IOP) measurement

IOP was measured monthly from 2 to 8 months of age in both irradiated and untreated D2 mice using the TonoLab (Colonial Medical Supply, Franconia, NH), as previously described [11]. Each data point represents individual (per eye) monthly, mean IOP values (20 readings). Mean value per age and experimental group were tabulated, as well as sample size.

Optic nerve histology and analysis

Axon counts were obtained in optic nerve cross-sections (2 μm-thick) from 9–12 month-old irradiated and control D2 mice. Optic nerves 2 mm proximal to the globe were stained with paraphenylenediamine (PPD) and counterstained with toluidine blue then prepared for plastic embedding and semithin sectioning, as previously described [30,31,32]. Using differential interference contrast optics at 100× magnification, cross-sections of optic nerve were photographed en montage using an Olympus Provis AX70 microscope. Custom algorithms were used to identify and count axons across the entire cross-section, as previously described [33].

Anterograde transport analysis

To measure the preservation of RGC axonal transport from the retina to the superior colliculus (SC), cholera toxin β-subunit (CTB) transport was assayed in 10–12 month-old irradiated and non-irradiated mice as recently described [31]. Briefly, 1 μL of 1% CTB conjugated to Alexa Fluor 488 nm (Molecular Probes, Eugene, OR) in sterile PBS was injected intravitreally, using a 33 G needle attached to a 25 μL Hamilton syringe (Hamilton Co., Reno, NV). After 2 days, serial coronal brain sections (50 μm) were collected from mice prepared by transcardial perfusion with 4% paraformaldehyde in PBS. CTB signal was imaged throughout alternate SC sections to reconstruct the total retinotopic map in the superficial layers. CTB signal was normalized to the background of the deeper, non-retinorecipient layers and label and density was calculated and plotted across the total SC. CTB density is represented colorimetrically, and the fraction of intact transport map is defined as the percent area with CTB signal ≥70%.

Retrograde Transport Analysis

To measure retrograde transport of cargo from superior colliculus to retina within the retinal ganglion cell axons, a small burr hole was drilled through the skull above the superior colliculus in anesthetized mice; FluoroGold was injected (1 µL, bilaterally) as described (Buckingham, et al., 2008). The holes were plugged with Gelfoam (Pfizer) soaked in 5% FluoroGold. Three days later, retinas were collected from mice after transcardial perfusion with 0.1M PBS followed by 4% paraformaldehyde in PBS, dissected out, immunolabeled with NeuN (1:500, Millipore, Temecula, CA) and FluoroGold (1:500, Millipore), mounted flat with gelvitol, then coverslipped. Unbiased stereological analysis of NeuN and FG-positive cell number was undertaken in whole-mount retinas using the optical fractionator module within StereoInvestigator software (MicroBrightfield, Middlebury, VT).

Retinal immunofluorescence, microscopy and analysis

Processing, immunostaining and imaging of retinal whole-mounts and cryosections (30 µm-thick) including the ONH, OL and proximal ON regions were performed as previously described [11]. We used polyclonal antibodies against Brn3 to identify RGCs, which recognize its three isoforms, (1:50, C-13; Santa Cruz, Santa Cruz, CA), Iba1 to identify microglia (1:1,000; Wako, Richmond, VA), and monoclonal antibodies against GFAP to label astrocytes (1:1,000; Sigma, St. Louis, MO), and against the 68 and 200 kDa isoforms of phosphorylated neurofilament to identify optic axons (1:50, clone 2f11; Dako, Carpinteria, CA). An antibody recognizing PCNA was used to identify mitotic cells (1:500, clone PC10; Dako, Carpinteria, CA), which required prior antigen unmasking with a solution of 0.18 mM citric acid, 77 µM sodium citrate, pH 6 for 15 min at 90°C. Immunostaining of retinal wholemounts and sections consisted of a 3-day incubation of three different primary antibodies at 4°C, followed by 2 hr incubation in Alexa Fluor-conjugated secondary antibodies (1:400, Molecular Probes). Confocal images were acquired with identical settings for each marker to allow comparison across samples (A1 and NIS-Elements 3.1, Nikon, Melville, NY), and are published with minimal adjustment of brightness (Photoshop CS3, Adobe Systems, San Jose, CA). Each flat mounted retina was imaged by acquiring 625 XY images throughout inner 25–35 µm of the retina (0.7 µm-step). For analysis, these images were stitched to produce a high-resolution image (0.41 µm/pixel) of the retinal surface, and published as maximal intensity projections that span the nerve fiber layer (NFL) and ganglion cell layer (GCL). To represent variations in relative intensity of protein levels, some published images were pseudocolored as indicated by a color code bar. Confocal images of cryosections of the central retina and proximal optic nerve regions show 20-µm thick maximal intensity projections.

Microglia cell counting

Total and proliferating microglial cells were counted in images of radial sections along the central retina and proximal optic nerve from irradiated D2 mice (1, 7 and 30 days post-treatment) and aged-matched untreated D2 mice. Cells were counted within areas localized to the head, laminar and myelinated optic nerve regions, defined as ONH (150 µm below NFL-plane), OL (100 µm from choroidal plane), and ON (250 µm from OL). Briefly, total microglia numbers were obtained from counting Iba1-positive cells with an identifiable Hoechst-stained nucleus (total microglia) within each nerve region. Proliferating microglia were recognized as cells with cytosolic Iba1 and nuclear PCNA, unambiguously identified by tracing their linear density profile across the cell soma, in single optical slice views. Cell counts in each compartment were normalized to represent percentage of proliferating cells and cells per mm^2.

Detection of apoptotic microglia

To detect apoptosis in microglial cells, avoiding artifacts derived from euthanasia and histology, we used D2.CX3CR1$^{gfp/+}$ mice, in which microglia express GFP, and delivered SR-FLIVO, a red-fluorescent tracer that selectively forms covalent bonds with active caspases *in vivo* (Immunochemistry Technologies LLC, Bloomington, MN). Following manufacturer's protocol, 100 µL FLIVO was administered to 2–3 month-old mice via tail vein injection 8 hr after irradiation and 8 hr before sacrifice, which was replicated in non-irradiated control mice. Retinas were dissected and flat mounted fresh, then fixed for 30 min and counterstained with Hoechst 33258 (Invitrogen, Carlsbad, CA). Confocal images were collected for each entire retina as described above.

Quantitative real time PCR analysis

Levels of Iba1 mRNA expression were measured in a sample that included the central 1-mm of retina, with its ONH and OL, using techniques and primers previously described [11]. Iba1 expression was assessed 1 week and 4 to 6 weeks after irradiation, and compared to untreated age-matched D2 and D2G samples (n = 10 per timepoint and strain). Data is presented as mean fold change normalized to β-actin expression within each sample.

Statistical analysis

Statistical significance was determined using two-way analysis of variance, followed by two-tailed Student's t-test (GraphPad, La Jolla, CA). Statistical significance is indicated by asterisks, $p<0.05$ (*) and $p<0.01$ (**). Sample sizes are also reported in Figure legends.

Results

High dose head irradiation alters early microgliosis

One effect of high-dose irradiation is to kill dividing cells, so we hypothesized that irradiation may be affecting a proliferative glial cell population in the retina, optic nerve head (ONH), optic lamina (OL), or optic nerve (ON). Previous analysis has shown that microglia represent the only significant dividing cell population in the D2 retina, doubling their numbers from 4 to 10 months of age [16]. Furthermore, we previously showed that microglial cell density increased in the central inner retina and ONH in D2 mice by 3 months of age versus D2G controls, suggesting increased proliferation [11]. To directly assess whether microglia are proliferating at 4 to 6 weeks of age (the time of irradiation) in the central retina, ONH, OL and/or proximal ON, radial retinal sections were double-immunostained for Iba1 and PCNA to identify and quantify dividing microglial cells within each region (Fig. 1A, B). Numerous PCNA+/Iba1+ cells were detected in the ONH, OL and ON from non-irradiated D2 animals, suggesting the presence of proliferating microglia (Fig. 1C, E). Few PCNA+/Iba1+ cells localized to the peripheral retina (data not shown), consistent with previous analysis [16].

To assess the effects of irradiation on microglia in the eye, we selected mice from 4 to 6 weeks of age, shielded the body with lead plates, and delivered a single high dose of X-irradiation (8 Gy) to the rostral half of the head spanning the eye region and visual pathway (see Methods and Fig. S1). IOP was measured monthly from 2 to 8 months of age in both non-irradiated and irradiated mice. The irradiated cohort of D2 mice still showed the expected IOP elevation (>20 mm Hg) by 7–8 months (Fig. S2), consistent with previous reports [25,26]. We then assessed the effects of irradiation on proliferating microglia and found that in irradiated D2 mice, the presence of PCNA+/Iba1+ cells was dramatically reduced one week post-irradiation (Fig. 1D, F). To determine

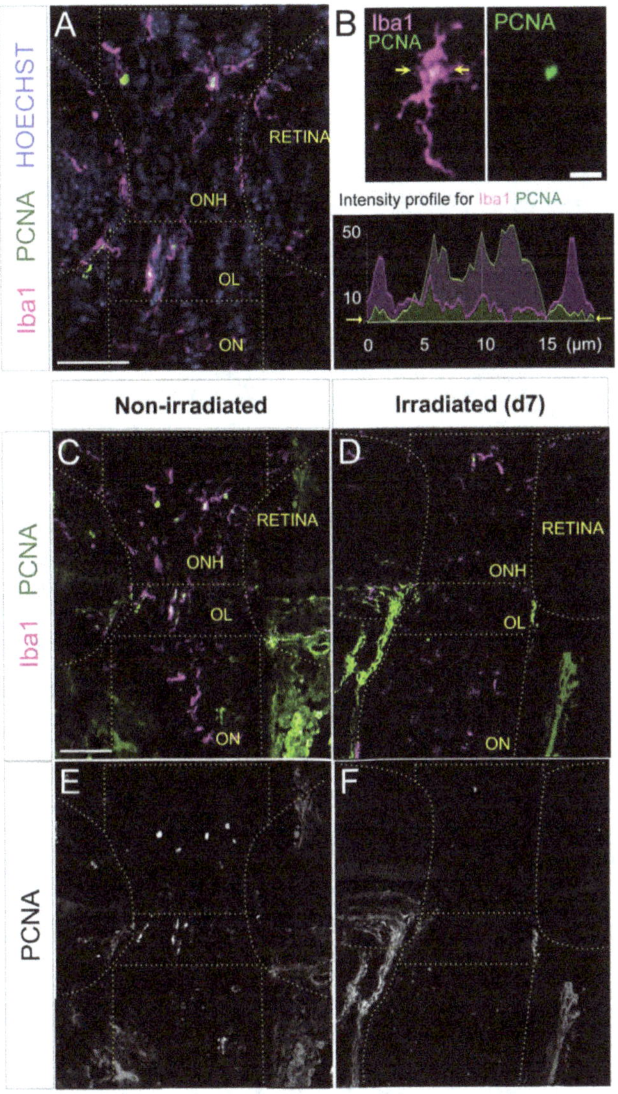

Figure 1. Irradiation results in depletion of proliferative microglia within the proximal optic nerve regions. *(A)* Iba1-positive cells with and without nuclear expression of the proliferative marker (PCNA) were detected in radial sections along the ONH, OL and proximal ON (delineated) shown in a single 1 μm optical slice. *(B)* Overlay of Iba1 and PCNA, plus single-channel view for PCNA. Scale bar represents 10 μm. The colocalization of Iba1 and PCNA to individual cells was confirmed by tracing their linear intensity profiles in single optical slices (between the arrows). Cycling microglial cells were positively identified by the nuclear localization of PCNA expression within the cytoplasmic Iba1 expression (graph). *(C, E)* Non-irradiated D2 mice show concentration of proliferating microglia within the unmyelinated ONH and OL, shown in a maximal Z-projection. Cycling microglia have a green or white nucleus in the overlay view of Iba1 and PCNA stainings, which is shown as single PCNA-channel for clarity. *(D, F)* 7 days (d7) after irradiation microglia proliferation appears negligible along the proximal nerve, as shown in a maximal Z-projection. Scale bars, 100 μm.

whether this was due to induction of apoptosis we delivered SR-FLIVO probe to 2–3 month-old D2.CX3CR1$^{gfp/+}$ mice by tail vein injection 8 hours post-irradiation, then sacrificed animals 8 hours later for retina dissection and analysis. We detected apoptotic microglia in irradiated mice, which were mostly concentrated in the central retina, while apoptotic microglia were absent in non-irradiated controls (Fig. S3).

To quantify the effect of radiation on proliferating microglia, we counted the percent of Iba1+ PCNA+ microglia localized to the ONH, OL and proximal ON in untreated D2 animals, and at 1, 7 and 30 days post-irradiation. In non-irradiated 4 to 6 week-old D2 mice we found proliferating microglia in all three regions, but detect the highest proportion in the lamina (OL), representing half of the microglia population in this region (Fig. 2A). At both 1 and 7 days post-irradiation, proliferating microglia were dramatically reduced in the ONH, OL and ON, with some recovery in the ONH by 7 days. By 30 days post-irradiation the proportion of cycling microglia within both the ONH and OL had recovered to nearly half of their original numbers, while the repopulation within the first 250 μm of ON was complete (Fig. 2A). When we assessed changes in overall density of microglia, we found a general reduction in all compartments at 1 day post-irradiation, but most significantly in the OL, consistent with the high proportion of proliferating microglia in that region (Fig. 2B). Microglial cell density was restored to levels approaching non-irradiated D2 mice by 7 days post-irradiation and was maintained out through 30 days. Thus, we conclude that irradiation has an acute and significant effect by reducing the presence of proliferating microglia.

Irradiation results in reduced levels of microglia activation

Since the numbers of proliferating microglia were acutely reduced by high dose irradiation, we sought to investigate whether irradiation also had an acute effect on the level of microglial activation, as well as an impact on the peak activation detectable by 3 months of age in the central retina and ONH of D2 mice [11]. To quantify changes in Iba1 mRNA expression 7 days and 30 to 45 days post-irradiation, we performed quantitative RT-PCR on mRNA isolated from microdissected samples that included the central 100 μm of central retina, the unmyelinated optic nerve regions and the first ~200 μm of myelinated optic nerve. We compared these samples to age-matched control samples from non-irradiated D2 and D2G retinas. After 7 days, irradiation did not alter the levels of Iba1 expression, which are low at this age and were comparable between the three groups analyzed. Normally there is an increase in microglia activation in the central retina and proximal nerve region by 3 months of age [11], which is also observed here as indicated by an elevation of Iba1 expression (Fig. 3A). In irradiated D2 tissue at this age, which is 30 to 45 days after irradiation, we found a significant reduction in Iba1 expression down to levels corresponding to those in tissue from non-glaucoma D2G mice (Fig. 3A), suggesting that irradiation prevents the increase in microglia activation. We conclude that, after high dose irradiation, the microglia localized to the central retina and proximal nerve region show sustained reduced levels of activation, comparable to non-glaucoma controls.

The striking finding that irradiation lowers the levels of Iba1 mRNA expression to control levels by 3 months of age was confirmed by immunostaining retinal wholemounts from non-irradiated and irradiated D2 mice for Iba1. To assess microglia activation, microglia localized to the central retina and optic disc were imaged at high resolution. We found that non-irradiated D2 retinas show clustering of microglia with large soma size and reduced branching within the central retina, demonstrating cell activation (Fig. 3B, B'). In contrast, irradiated retinas show microglia with small somata and thinner branches, and therefore with reduced levels of activation (Fig. 3D, D'). High levels of Iba1

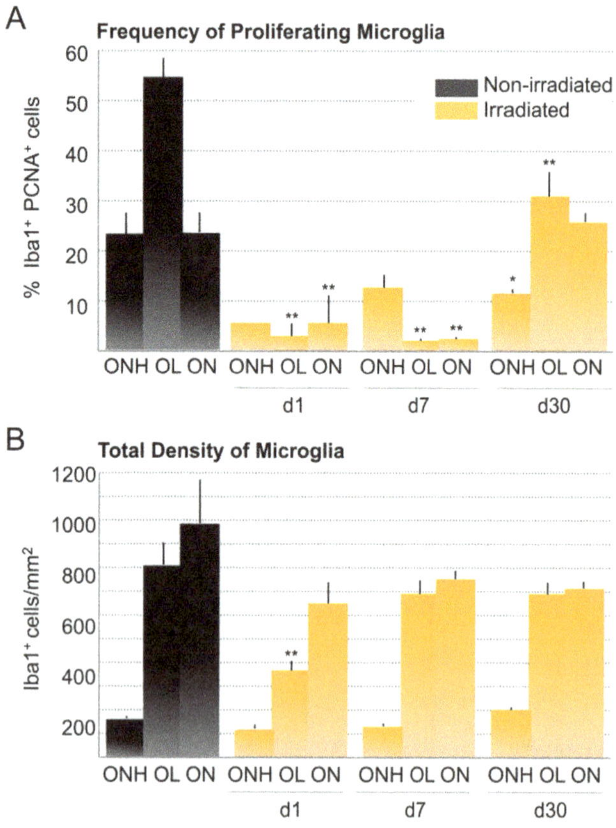

Figure 2. Irradiation reduces microgliosis in the unmyelinated optic nerve. Quantification of the proportion of cycling microglial cells (PCNA and Iba1-positive) per optic nerve compartment in non-irradiated and irradiated D2 mice (n=6 samples per timepoint and experimental group). The statistical significance indicated for each compartment and timepoint is relative to non-irradiated controls. *(A)* In non-irradiated D2 mice aged 4 to 6 weeks, the proportion of proliferating microglia is ~50% within the OL, and ~25% within the ONH and ON. At 1 day and 7 days after irradiation, numbers of cycling microglia are reduced in all optic nerve portions, with maximal reduction within the OL ($p<0.001$), and with significant effect in the ONH and proximal ON ($p<0.01$). 30 days post-treatment the unmyelinated ONH and OL compartments have recovered only half of its original proliferating microglia, whereas the proximal ON has been repopulated. *(B)* Total number of Iba1-positive microglia (per area) within each optic nerve compartment. The density of total microglia demonstrates that irradiation has an acute and specific effect on cycling microglia resident within the OL ($p<0.01$).

expression was observed in numerous microglial cells in non-irradiated D2 retinas (Fig. 3C, C'; pseudocolored, with red representing the highest levels of expression), and this is clearly reduced in age-matched tissue after irradiation (Fig. 3D, E; pseudocolored). Our findings indicate that irradiation suppresses the intense microglia activation, characteristic of the early D2 retina.

Irradiation did not induce early gliosis

Glaucoma-like pathology in the D2 retina is also associated with significant astrocyte and Mueller cell reactive gliosis, which is evident by upregulation of GFAP expression [16]. To assess whether irradiation induces gliosis at 3 months of age, we generated radial sections through the central retina and its proximal optic nerve regions and immunostained them for GFAP. Non-irradiated and irradiated D2 mice showed similar levels and

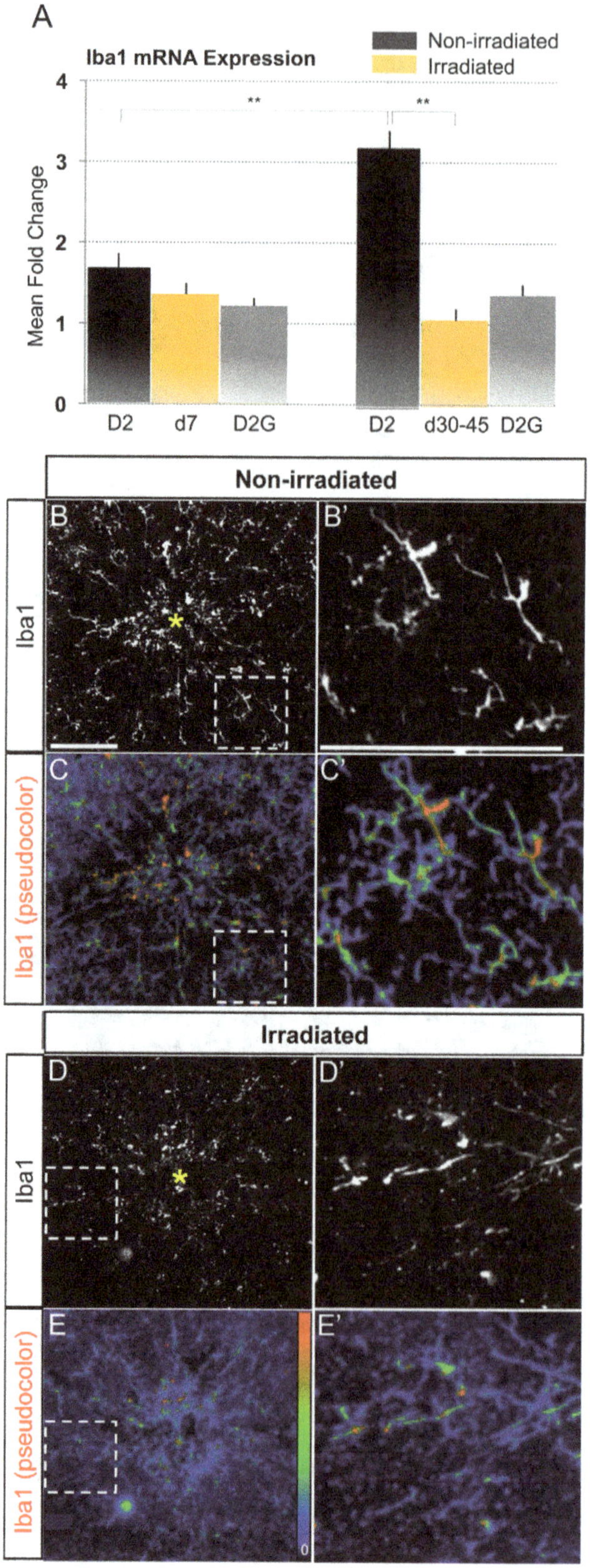

Figure 3. Irradiation reduced early microglia activation within the central retina and proximal optic nerve compartments. *(A)* Quantitative RT-PCR analysis of Iba1 transcript in a sample including the central 100 μm of retina, ONH, OL and proximal 200 μm of myelinated optic nerve, collected from non-irradiated D2 and non-glaucoma D2G, and irradiated D2 mice (n=10 per group and age). 7 days post-

irradiation there are comparable levels of Iba1 expression as in age-matched non-irradiated D2 or D2G samples. 30 to 45 days after irradiation Iba1 expression is significantly lower than the elevated levels of expression seen in non-irradiated D2 tissue at this age ($p<0.01$), and is comparable to levels of Iba1 expression in age-matched non-glaucoma D2G mice. *(B, C)* Representative retinal wholemounts from non-irradiated and irradiated D2 mice at 3 months of age show clustering of large, activated microglia with high Iba1 expression within the central retina and optic disc (yellow asterisk) in non-irradiated conditions. In age-matched irradiated mice few high-Iba1 expressing microglia are detectable, and display little clustering. *(D, E)* In non-irradiated D2 retinas, Iba1 expression (pseudocolor code indicated as inset bar) is highly upregulated in the microglial cells concentrated at the optic disc, while only few cells show high expression levels in untreated D2. (B′–E′) High magnification views of framed areas shown in B–E. Scale bars, 100 μm.

patterns of GFAP expression, confined in the retina to the NFL where astrocytes reside, and spanning the proximal optic nerve segments (Fig. S4).

Irradiation reduces RGC axon degeneration

After 9 months of age, optic nerves from non-irradiated D2 mice showed significant structural degeneration, including an abundance of dystrophic axons with expanded diameters and compacted myelin sheaths, dense and dark axonal profiles with multilayered myelin sheaths, and enlarged glial cell somata, indicative of gliosis (Fig. 4A, C), consistent with previous reports [32]. In contrast, irradiated mice showed relatively normal optic nerves with few degenerating axonal profiles and generally intact myelin sheaths (Fig. 4B, D). Since D2 mice typically show significant axon loss by 10 to 12 months of age we quantified axons to assess whether irradiation had a protective effect. We found that irradiated D2 mice had significantly larger axon numbers as compared to untreated D2 mice, indicating reduction of RGC axonal degeneration (Fig. 4E).

Another feature of axonal decline in the D2 mouse is progressive loss of anterograde axonal transport from the retina to the superior colliculus (SC), which is severely compromised by 11–12 months of age [31]. To assess whether this is improved by irradiation, we performed intravitreal injection of cholera toxin β-subunit (CTB) in live mice, which is actively taken up by RGCs and transported by their axons to the superficial layers of the SC. Coronal sections of 11-month old SC of non-irradiated D2 mice reveal almost complete loss of CTB label along the medial-lateral extent of the SC, throughout its entire length (Fig. 4F, H). In contrast, irradiated 12-month old mice showed persistent CTB label throughout the entire SC (Fig. 4G, I). We quantified this effect across multiple animals by calculating the percentage of animals with intact anterograde axonal transport, as defined by ≥70% CTB signal density, and found a significant increase in irradiated D2 mice compared to untreated animals (Fig. 4J). Thus, axonal transport function is also robustly preserved in D2 mice by high-dose head irradiation.

Previous reports have demonstrated significant decline in retrograde transport of FluoroGold tracer in advance of significant RGC death (Buckingham, et al., 2008). Significantly, irradiation did not have a direct toxic effect on cells in the ganglion cell layer since the NeuN+ cell numbers did not differ between irradiated and non-irradiated control (Fig. 4M). Irradiated mice injected with FluoroGold demonstrated no significant improvement of retrograde transport of the tracer as compared to non-irradiated mice, although there was a trend towards increased transport (Fig. 4M).

Irradiation improves retinal ganglion cell integrity. Since RGC optic axon structure and transport

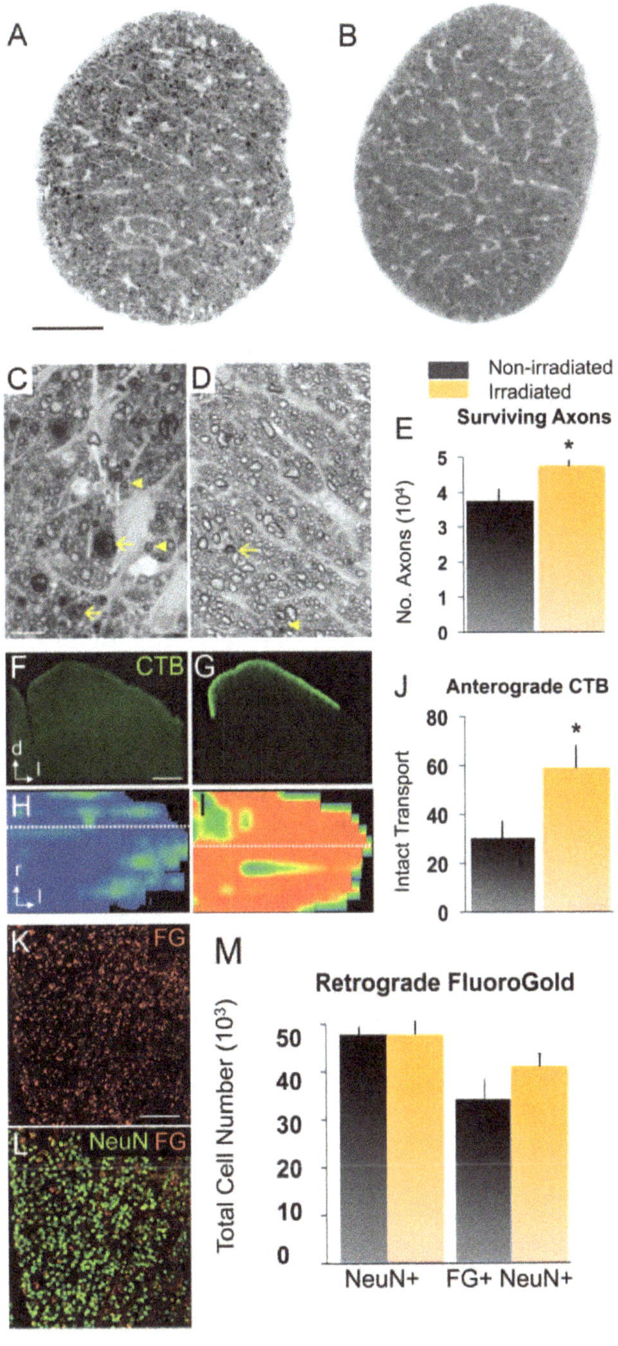

Figure 4. Head irradiation protects D2 mice from optic nerve degeneration. *(A, B)* Optic nerve cross-sections stained with PPD, from naïve (11 mo old) and irradiated (12 mo old) D2 mice. Scale bar, 250 μm. (C, D) Higher magnification view of the same nerves. Scale bar, 10 μm. *(C)* Non-irradiated D2 nerves show abundant degenerating axon profiles with dark, condensed axoplasm (arrowheads) and disorganized myelin sheaths (arrows), as well as extensive gliosis. *(D)* Irradiated D2 nerves mostly show healthy axons with clear axoplasm and uniform myelin sheaths, and rare degenerating profiles (arrows). *(E)* Total optic axon counts from irradiated D2 nerves ($n=29$; 12 mo old) show a significant increase in mean axon number compared to non-irradiated D2 mice ($n=16$; 10 and 11 mo old; $p<0.01$). *(F–J)* The anterograde transport of CTB by RGC axons from the retina to the superior colliculus (SC) was measured in non-irradiated ($n=16$; 10 and 11 mo old) and irradiated D2 mice ($n=17$; 12 mo old). *(F)* Non-irradiated D2 mice (11 mo old) showed severe loss of CTB signal, as seen in coronal section of the SC (dorsal, d; lateral, l). Scale bar, 500 μm. *(G)* Irradiated D2 mice (12 mo old) showed persistent CTB transport to the superficial layers of

the SC. *(H, I)* Reconstruction of the retinotopic SC map, showing the density of CTB signal (red, green and blue indicate 100, 50 and 0% density, respectively). Dotted lines indicate location of sections shown in F and G; rostral, r; lateral, l. *(H)* Non-irradiated D2 mice showed near total CTB depletion. *(I)* Irradiated D2 mice showed almost complete CTB label and a normal retinotopic pattern. *(J)* Irradiation significantly protected axonal anterograde transport in D2 optic nerves ($p<0.05$). K) Flat-mount of an irradiated D2 retina at 9 mo of age showing FG labeled cells (red). L) Most NeuN+ RGCs (green) in this retina are retrogradely labeled with FG (red). Scale bar, 100 μm. M) Quantitative stereology of both NeuN+ RGCs and FG+/NeuN+ RGCs in flat-mounted retinas. Non-irradiated retinas (dark bars, n = 8; 9–10 mo old) and irradiated retinas (yellow bars, n = 8; 9–10 mo old) showed no differences in the total number of NeuN+ RGCs per retina between treatments, but slightly more retrogradely labeled FG+ RGCs in the irradiated retinas. Error bars = SEM.

function were preserved by irradiation, we investigated whether there is also preservation of intraretinal RGC compartments. To identify and assess the health status of RGCs, we collected retinas from 12 month-old mice that had received high-dose head irradiation at 4 to 6 weeks of age and, and compared these to non-irradiated D2 controls. We performed immunostaining in whole retinas with a Brn3 antibody that recognizes all isoforms of Brn3, a POU homeodomain transcription factor that identifies the majority of adult mouse RGCs. Brn3 expression is known to downregulate in aged D2 retinas prior to RGC loss (Buckingham et al., 2008; Soto et al., 2008). Confocal images of retinal flat-mounts showed that irradiated mice displayed a higher density of RGC somata expressing Brn3 compared to non-irradiated mice, as well as relatively more intense levels of Brn3 expression (Fig. 5A, B). Half of the non-irradiated D2 retinas analyzed (4/8 retinas) showed almost complete or severe loss of Brn3 immunostaining throughout the entire GCL, while only one irradiated retina (1/8 retinas) showed a significant portion of the retina with reduced Brn3, with none showing the most severe loss.

In the same tissue we performed co-immunostaining for phosphorylated neurofilament (pNF), which is normally localized to optic axons, but aberrantly accumulates within the somata, dendrites and intraretinal axon segment of declining RGCs in D2 mice [15]. We found that in non-irradiated D2 retinas, there were reduced numbers of pNF-labeled axons overall, as well as beading or fragmentation of the remaining axons (Fig. 5C). In contrast, RGCs in irradiated mice showed uniform levels of pNF expression along their intraretinal axons, although axonal beading was present in the far peripheral retina (Fig. 5D). Somal and dendrite accumulation of pNF immunostaining was detected in most non-irradiated D2 retinas, particularly in RGCs localized to the mid- and far-peripheral retina (Fig. 5C, arrowheads), and in some cases somal pNF was observed within every declining RGC in the far-periphery (4/8 retinas). However, irradiated retinas had very few RGCs with somal pNF build up, with only low levels of accumulation (Fig. 5D, arrowhead; 7/8 retinas). The merged view of the Brn3 and pNF immunostainings reveals that in the non-irradiated retina there is colocalization of dystrophic axons to areas with reduced density of Brn3-positive cells, while these areas are reduced, but not completely absent, in retinas from irradiated mice (Fig. 5E, F).

Since microglia activation is associated with neuron decline and degeneration in glaucoma and other neurodegenerative conditions, we immunostained the same tissue for Iba1 to assess the distribution and presence of activated microglia, identifiable by enlarged somata, thick processes and upregulation of Iba1 expression. We observed higher density of Iba1-positive microglia in non-irradiated D2 retinas (Fig. 5G), in comparison to irradiated ones (Fig. 5H). Moreover, non-irradiated retinas showed a more irregular tiling of microglia resident in the NFL and GCL (Fig. 5G, H). The presence of activated microglia was noticeably reduced in irradiated retinas, presumably due to reduced RGC decline and degeneration. Most cells showed complex, slender processes and small somata (Fig. 5H, H'), versus the conspicuous soma and processes of activated microglia in non-irradiated retinas (Fig. 5G, G'). Thus, head irradiation results in overall improvement of RGC integrity at 12 months of age, when the RGC somal loss by apoptosis is quite apparent in a majority of D2 mice [13,34,35,36]. The late effect includes preservation of Brn3 expression and reduction of pNF buildup, in conjunction with reduced microglia activation.

Discussion

Here we examined the acute effects of high-dose irradiation on microglia in the D2 mouse glaucoma model. We found that irradiation causes an immediate reduction in proliferating microglia in the optic nerve head and glial lamina region, as well as a sustained reduction in the levels of microglia activation in the central retina, optic nerve head and laminar region. We also confirmed that irradiation of the head alone reduces RGC degeneration, improving both the structural integrity of the axons as well as anterograde axonal transport at later stages. While the effects of high dose irradiation on neuronal tissue are complex, these findings suggest that a component of the response to irradiation involves changes in microglia.

High-dose irradiation has previously been shown to have significant effects on microglia, particularly in the young brain where proliferating microglia are more abundant than in the adult. For example, following high-dose irradiation of rats at P9 or P21, apoptotic microglia were evident by six hours, with a significant decrease in microglia cell numbers seven days later [37]. In the D2 retina, it has previously been shown that the major proliferating cell population is microglia [16], consistent with our observation that these cells are vulnerable to irradiation. Previously we reported microgliosis, as well as clustering and activation of microglial cells in the inner central retina and unmyelinated optic nerve regions (ONH and OL) in D2 mice at early ages [11]. In this study we found evidence for proliferating microglia concentrated in the OL by 1 mo of age, which were depleted by high-dose irradiation. In some cases, whole brain irradiation has been associated with increased microglia activation coupled with secondary astrocyte gliosis [38], although this was not observed here. In the D2 retina, the effect may target proliferating microglia, which are selectively increased in this disease model.

In this study, irradiation was performed in young D2 animals, from 4 to 6 weeks of age, which is prior to the onset of detectable neurodegeneration of RGCs. Since microglia activation can be detrimental to neurons [9], it is possible that the protective effect of irradiation is due to selective depletion of an activated, proliferating population of microglia, resulting in less neuronal damage. In support of this idea we have found that other interventions that reduce the levels of microglia activation, such as long-term minocycline treatment, can improve RGC axon integrity and axon transport function [24]. High dose irradiation with bone marrow transfer has also been shown to be neuroprotective in another neurodegenerative disease, Sandhoff's disease, which is an inherited lysosomal storage disorder causing acute and rapid neuronal decline usually leading to early childhood death [39]. Interestingly, neurodegeneration in this disease is preceded by extensive microglia activation in both human cases as well as in a mouse model of the disease, which was prevented by the

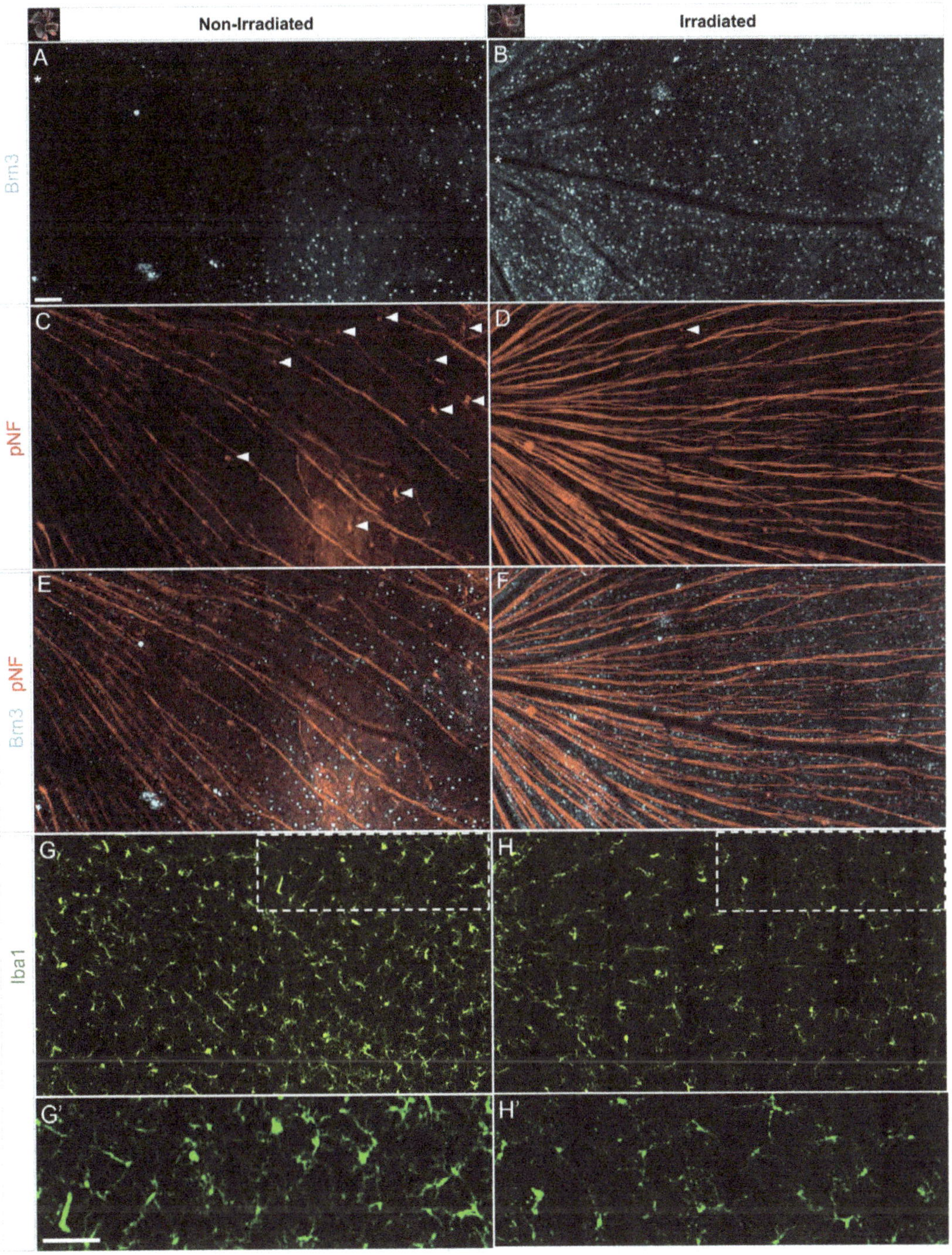

Figure 5. Irradiation reduces RGC decline and microglia activation within the retina. Confocal images of triple-immunostained (Brn3, pNF and Iba1) flat-mounted retinas from non-irradiated (11 mo old) and irradiated (12 mo old) D2 mice (n = 8 retinas per group). Representative fields (~1.6×0.9 mm^2) show matching position (optic disc at left of asterisks) and a projection of the NFL and GCL, from central to peripheral eccentricities. *(A–B)* Most of the non-irradiated retina displays low numbers of RGCs expressing Brn3, whereas irradiated mice maintain a higher density of brightly labeled RGCs. *(C, D)* Co-immunostaining for pNF in the same non-irradiated retina shows a reduced number of optic axons, thinner axonal bundles and defasciculated axons that show beaded profiles in their entire length. In the irradiated retina, RGC axons are organized in bundles that show a higher and uniform pNF content, and some fragmentation mostly limited to the peripheral area. Only non-irradiated retinas show abundant RGCs with somadendritic accumulation of pNF (arrowheads). *(E, F)* Overlay of Brn3 and pNF staining reveals the colocalization of declining axons and sparse Brn3-positive RGCs in the non-irradiated D2 retina, in contrast to healthier, fasciculated axons in the irradiated mice. *(G, H)* Reflecting the abnormalities shown by the RGC markers, microglia (Iba1) had altered tiling around RGC axons and variable, increased density in non-irradiated retinas. Activated microglia, recognizable by their enlarged somata and reduced branching, were abundant in the non-irradiated retina, and infrequent in the irradiated ones. (G', H') High magnification views of framed areas shown in G, H. Scale bars, 100 μm.

irradiation and bone marrow transfer procedure in mice [39]. In this case, the effects of irradiation versus bone marrow transplantation were not tested. Nevertheless, it raises the possibility that irradiation may have similar neuroprotective effects in other disease models since early microglial activation has been reported for a number of neurodegenerative diseases [40]. However caution is warranted, since radiation retinopathy associated with adverse effects on retinal vasculature can be a significant complication of irradiating the retina, with few therapeutic options [41,42,43].

It is also possible that irradiation has a direct effect on other retinal cell populations, since there is precedence for irradiation impacting neural tissue. For example, therapeutic irradiation of the brain is used for treating brain tumors, but is known to induce cognitive deficits [44,45]. Some of this may be due to the depletion of dividing neural stem cells and neural precursors in the ventricular zone of some brain regions [44]. This is unlikely to be a factor in this study since there are no dividing neural precursors or stem cells within the retina at this stage, with only microglia and pericytes dividing in the D2 retina [16]. In addition, postmitotic neurons are generally thought to be more radio-resistant [46]. We did not observe any significant acute effects of irradiation on RGC structural integrity (data not shown), suggesting that RGCs are relatively resistant to radiation-induced damage.

More subtle effects on neurons have been associated with irradiation. For example in hippocampal pyramidal neurons irradiation caused a loss of expression of some neuronal genes, such as NeuN, within 7 days [47]. In addition, irradiation has been shown to affect behaviorally induced expression of the immediate-early gene *Arc* (activity-regulated cytoskeleton-associated protein), suggesting alteration of neuronal function [48]. However, we observed normal expression of Brn3 and NeuN, suggesting that RGC gene expression is not negatively affected by irradiation. While these other studies suggest that irradiation causes reduction of neuronal integrity and function, it remains possible that exposure of the retina to high-dose irradiation alters neuronal gene expression, potentially rendering RGCs resistant to subsequent insult in this glaucoma model.

Retinal pericytes, which are associated with the retinal vasculature, also proliferate in the D2 retina [16], so these cells may also be impacted by high-dose irradiation, as suggested by our detection of activated caspases in diminutive cells along vessel walls. In fact, in other studies irradiation has been shown to acutely affect the integrity of the blood–brain barrier and blood-retinal barrier and promote the influx of bone-marrow-derived cells [49,50,51,52], while under normal conditions, bone marrow-derived myeloid cells rarely infiltrate the CNS [53]. Consistent with this, it has been clearly demonstrated in the retina that irradiation triggers recruitment of blood-derived monocytes, as detected by transplantation of GFP-labeled bone marrow cells into mice following whole body irradiation [51,52,54]. This influx of GFP+ cells into the retina was prevented by shielding of the head, demonstrating that irradiation of the retina is required and that normal microglial cell turnover from circulating monocytes is low [52,55].

In contrast, Howell et al. report that irradiation of the head or eyes of the D2 mouse at 2 months of age prevents proinflammatory monocytes from entering the optic nerve when analyzed at 10.5 months of age, but prior to detectable neuronal damage, and they provide evidence that these infiltrating monocytes contribute to neuronal decline in D2 glaucoma [26]. Thus, monocyte infiltration may be a critical component of disease in this model. However, it remains to be determined how early irradiation inhibits the invasion of monocytes at much later ages, especially when in other models irradiation promotes monocyte invasion [52]. Importantly, bone marrow-derived myeloid cells may have functions or responses that are distinct from those of resident microglia [53,56,57], potentially impacting the course of disease. In our study, Iba1 does not distinguish macrophages from microglia, so it is possible that macrophages are recruited at early stages as well. It remains to be determined whether this contributes to the effects of irradiation in the D2 model of glaucoma.

Supporting Information

Figure S1 Experimental design. *(A)* D2 mice received a single high-dose of X-irradiation targeting their eyes and visual pathways at a prepathological age of 4 to 6 weeks of age. Microglial changes following irradiation were examined in a cohort of young mice, while optic neuropathy was measured in aged mice. Identical analysis was performed in age-matched non-irradiated D2 mice as well as non-glaucoma D2G mice. *(B)* Radiation was confined to the rostral half of the head targeting eyes and visual pathways (orange rectangle). This area was consistently positioned with reference collimated light (white rectangle) and focusing LEDs. The nose and regions behind the ears (5-mm post-lambda, λ) were spared, as was the body by shielding with lead plates.

Figure S2 Intraocular pressure (IOP) elevated with similar patterns in D2 mice from 2 to 8 months of age, regardless of irradiation. A summary of mean IOP per month (and sample size) shows that irradiation did not prevent IOP elevation.

Figure S3 Irradiation selectively induces apoptosis in retinal microglia. Representative retinal wholemounts from non-irradiated and irradiated D2.CX3CR1$^{gfp/+}$ mice, where microglia expresses GFP under the control of fractalkine-receptor locus (optic disc position indicated by asterisk). Apoptotic cells were detected with SR-FLIVO, which selectively binds cleaved caspases and emits at 600 nm. *(A)* Non-irradiated retinas show only very small apoptotic cells positioned along large blood vessels, probably corresponding to pericytes. *(B)* Irradiated retinas, instead, show numerous and conspicuous apoptotic microglia mostly localized to the optic disc and central retina. Some microglial cells are detectable in the mid-peripheral retina (arrowheads). Notice that, relative to non-irradiated mice, the regularity of microglial cell tiling is lost, and fewer cells with complex branching are present in the central retina. *(C, D)* Detailed view of the optic disc area (inset in A, B) showing the overlay of FLIVO and GFP highlights the virtual absence of apoptosis in the non-irradiated retina, and the clear overlap of both stainings to cells with activated shape. n = 3 per group. Scale bars, 100 μm *(A, B)*, 10 μm *(C, D)*.

Figure S4 Irradiation does not induce early gliosis. *(A, B)* Images of representative radial sections through the central retina and proximal optic nerve from 3 month-old D2 mice detects comparable GFAP expression in astrocytes, but not in Mueller cells, regardless of treatment. Co-immunostaining for Iba1 shows the relative reduction of microglial cells in the irradiated ONH and OL, relative to the non-irradiated sample. *(C, D)* High-magnification view of astrocytes localized to the OL (insets in A, B) show similar cell size and shape under both experimental conditions, while microglia display morphological signs of activation in the non-irradiated tissue. Scale bar, 100 μm (A, B), 10 μm (C, D).

Acknowledgments

We thank N. Marsh-Armstrong for comments on the manuscript.

Author Contributions

Conceived and designed the experiments: AB MLV. Performed the experiments: AB SDC MRS COR DMI. Analyzed the data: AB MRS DMI DJC. Contributed reagents/materials/analysis tools: MLV PJH DJC. Wrote the paper: MLV. Edited the manuscript: AB SDC DMI PJH DJC MLV.

References

1. Quigley HA, Broman AT (2006) The number of people with glaucoma worldwide in 2010 and 2020. Br J Ophthalmol 90: 262–267.
2. Sommer A (1996) Glaucoma risk factors observed in the Baltimore Eye Survey. Current opinion in ophthalmology 7: 93–98.
3. Gupta N, Yucel YH (2007) Glaucoma as a neurodegenerative disease. Curr Opin Ophthalmol 18: 110–114.
4. Burgoyne CF (2011) A biomechanical paradigm for axonal insult within the optic nerve head in aging and glaucoma. Experimental eye research 93: 120–132.
5. Crish SD, Calkins DJ (2011) Neurodegeneration in glaucoma: progression and calcium-dependent intracellular mechanisms. Neuroscience 176: 1–11.
6. Stevens B, Allen NJ, Vazquez LE, Howell GR, Christopherson KS, et al. (2007) The classical complement cascade mediates CNS synapse elimination. Cell 131: 1164–1178.
7. Whitmore AV, Libby RT, John SW (2005) Glaucoma: thinking in new ways-a role for autonomous axonal self-destruction and other compartmentalised processes? Prog Retin Eye Res 24: 639–662.
8. Johnson EC, Morrison JC (2009) Friend or foe? Resolving the impact of glial responses in glaucoma. J Glaucoma 18: 341–353.
9. Hanisch UK, Kettenmann H (2007) Microglia: active sensor and versatile effector cells in the normal and pathologic brain. Nat Neurosci 10: 1387–1394.
10. Block ML, Zecca L, Hong JS (2007) Microglia-mediated neurotoxicity: uncovering the molecular mechanisms. Nat Rev Neurosci 8: 57–69.
11. Bosco A, Steele MR, Vetter ML (2011) Early microglia activation in a mouse model of chronic glaucoma. J Comp Neurol 519: 599–620.
12. Neufeld AH (1999) Microglia in the optic nerve head and the region of parapapillary chorioretinal atrophy in glaucoma. Arch Ophthalmol 117: 1050–1056.
13. Libby RT, Anderson MG, Pang IH, Robinson ZH, Savinova OV, et al. (2005) Inherited glaucoma in DBA/2J mice: pertinent disease features for studying the neurodegeneration. Vis Neurosci 22: 637–648.
14. Howell GR, Libby RT, Jakobs TC, Smith RS, Phalan FC, et al. (2007) Axons of retinal ganglion cells are insulted in the optic nerve early in DBA/2J glaucoma. J Cell Biol 179: 1523–1537.
15. Soto I, Oglesby E, Buckingham BP, Son JL, Roberson ED, et al. (2008) Retinal ganglion cells downregulate gene expression and lose their axons within the optic nerve head in a mouse glaucoma model. J Neurosci 28: 548–561.
16. Inman DM, Horner PJ (2007) Reactive nonproliferative gliosis predominates in a chronic mouse model of glaucoma. Glia 55: 942–953.
17. Steele MR, Inman DM, Calkins DJ, Horner PJ, Vetter ML (2006) Microarray analysis of retinal gene expression in the DBA/2J model of glaucoma. Invest Ophthalmol Vis Sci 47: 977–985.
18. Fan W, Li X, Wang W, Mo JS, Kaplan H, et al. (2010) Early Involvement of Immune/Inflammatory Response Genes in Retinal Degeneration in DBA/2J Mice. Ophthalmology and eye diseases 1: 23–41.
19. Howell GR, Macalinao DG, Sousa GL, Walden M, Soto I, et al. (2011) Molecular clustering identifies complement and endothelin induction as early events in a mouse model of glaucoma. The Journal of clinical investigation 121: 1429–1444.
20. Ahmed F, Brown KM, Stephan DA, Morrison JC, Johnson EC, et al. (2004) Microarray analysis of changes in mRNA levels in the rat retina after experimental elevation of intraocular pressure. Invest Ophthalmol Vis Sci 45: 1247–1258.
21. Johnson EC, Jia L, Cepurna WO, Doser TA, Morrison JC (2007) Global changes in optic nerve head gene expression after exposure to elevated intraocular pressure in a rat glaucoma model. Invest Ophthalmol Vis Sci 48: 3161–3177.
22. Lam TT, Kwong JM, Tso MO (2003) Early glial responses after acute elevated intraocular pressure in rats. Invest Ophthalmol Vis Sci 44: 638–645.
23. Miyahara T, Kikuchi T, Akimoto M, Kurokawa T, Shibuki H, et al. (2003) Gene microarray analysis of experimental glaucomatous retina from cynomologous monkey. Invest Ophthalmol Vis Sci 44: 4347–4356.
24. Bosco A, Inman DM, Steele MR, Wu G, Soto I, et al. (2008) Reduced retina microglial activation and improved optic nerve integrity with minocycline treatment in the DBA/2J mouse model of glaucoma. Invest Ophthalmol Vis Sci 49: 1437–1446.
25. Anderson MG, Libby RT, Gould DB, Smith RS, John SW (2005) High-dose radiation with bone marrow transfer prevents neurodegeneration in an inherited glaucoma. Proc Natl Acad Sci U S A 102: 4566–4571.
26. Howell GR, Soto I, Zhu X, Ryan M, Macalinao DG, et al. (2012) Radiation treatment inhibits monocyte entry into the optic nerve head and prevents neuronal damage in a mouse model of glaucoma. The Journal of clinical investigation.
27. Howell GR, Libby RT, Marchant JK, Wilson LA, Cosma IM, et al. (2007) Absence of glaucoma in DBA/2J mice homozygous for wild-type versions of Gpnmb and Tyrp1. BMC Genet 8: 45.
28. John SW, Smith RS, Savinova OV, Hawes NL, Chang B, et al. (1998) Essential iris atrophy, pigment dispersion, and glaucoma in DBA/2J mice. Invest Ophthalmol Vis Sci 39: 951–962.
29. Jung S, Aliberti J, Graemmel P, Sunshine MJ, Kreutzberg GW, et al. (2000) Analysis of fractalkine receptor CX(3)CR1 function by targeted deletion and green fluorescent protein reporter gene insertion. Mol Cell Biol 20: 4106–4114.
30. Buckingham BP, Inman DM, Lambert W, Oglesby E, Calkins DJ, et al. (2008) Progressive ganglion cell degeneration precedes neuronal loss in a mouse model of glaucoma. J Neurosci 28: 2735–2744.
31. Crish SD, Sappington RM, Inman DM, Horner PJ, Calkins DJ (2010) Distal axonopathy with structural persistence in glaucomatous neurodegeneration. Proceedings of the National Academy of Sciences of the United States of America 107: 5196–5201.
32. Inman DM, Sappington RM, Horner PJ, Calkins DJ (2006) Quantitative correlation of optic nerve pathology with ocular pressure and corneal thickness in the DBA/2 mouse model of glaucoma. Invest Ophthalmol Vis Sci 47: 986–996.
33. Sappington RM, Carlson BJ, Crish SD, Calkins DJ (2010) The microbead occlusion model: a paradigm for induced ocular hypertension in rats and mice. Investigative ophthalmology & visual science 51: 207–216.
34. Libby RT, Li Y, Savinova OV, Barter J, Smith RS, et al. (2005) Susceptibility to neurodegeneration in a glaucoma is modified by Bax gene dosage. PLoS Genet 1: 17–26.
35. Reichstein D, Ren L, Filippopoulos T, Mittag T, Danias J (2007) Apoptotic retinal ganglion cell death in the DBA/2 mouse model of glaucoma. Experimental eye research 84: 13–21.
36. Schlamp CL, Li Y, Dietz JA, Janssen KT, Nickells RW (2006) Progressive ganglion cell loss and optic nerve degeneration in DBA/2J mice is variable and asymmetric. BMC Neurosci 7: 66.
37. Kalm M, Lannering B, Bjork-Eriksson T, Blomgren K (2009) Irradiation-induced loss of microglia in the young brain. Journal of neuroimmunology 206: 70–75.
38. Hwang SY, Jung JS, Kim TH, Lim SJ, Oh ES, et al. (2006) Ionizing radiation induces astrocyte gliosis through microglia activation. Neurobiology of disease 21: 457–467.
39. Wada R, Tifft CJ, Proia RL (2000) Microglial activation precedes acute neurodegeneration in Sandhoff disease and is suppressed by bone marrow transplantation. Proceedings of the National Academy of Sciences of the United States of America 97: 10954–10959.
40. Yoshiyama Y, Higuchi M, Zhang B, Huang SM, Iwata N, et al. (2007) Synapse loss and microglial activation precede tangles in a P301S tauopathy mouse model. Neuron 53: 337–351.
41. Giuliari GP, Sadaka A, Hinkle DM, Simpson ER (2011) Current treatments for radiation retinopathy. Acta oncologica 50: 6–13.
42. Gupta A, Dhawahir-Scala F, Smith A, Young L, Charles S (2007) Radiation retinopathy: case report and review. BMC ophthalmology 7: 6.
43. Horgan N, Shields CL, Mashayekhi A, Shields JA (2010) Classification and treatment of radiation maculopathy. Current opinion in ophthalmology 21: 233–238.
44. Fike JR (2011) Physiopathology of radiation-induced neurotoxicity. Revue neurologique 167: 746–750.
45. Sarkissian V (2005) The sequelae of cranial irradiation on human cognition. Neuroscience letters 382: 118–123.
46. Ben Abdallah NM, Slomianka L, Lipp HP (2007) Reversible effect of X-irradiation on proliferation, neurogenesis, and cell death in the dentate gyrus of adult mice. Hippocampus 17: 1230–1240.
47. Wu KL, Li YQ, Tabassum A, Lu WY, Aubert I, et al. (2010) Loss of neuronal protein expression in mouse hippocampus after irradiation. Journal of neuropathology and experimental neurology 69: 272–280.
48. Rosi S, Andres-Mach M, Fishman KM, Levy W, Ferguson RA, et al. (2008) Cranial irradiation alters the behaviorally induced immediate-early gene arc (activity-regulated cytoskeleton-associated protein). Cancer research 68: 9763–9770.
49. Ajami B, Bennett JL, Krieger C, Tetzlaff W, Rossi FM (2007) Local self-renewal can sustain CNS microglia maintenance and function throughout adult life. Nat Neurosci 10: 1538–1543.

50. Mildner A, Schmidt H, Nitsche M, Merkler D, Hanisch UK, et al. (2007) Microglia in the adult brain arise from Ly-6ChiCCR2+ monocytes only under defined host conditions. Nature neuroscience 10: 1544–1553.

51. Xu H, Chen M, Mayer EJ, Forrester JV, Dick AD (2007) Turnover of resident retinal microglia in the normal adult mouse. Glia 55: 1189–1198.

52. Muther PS, Semkova I, Schmidt K, Abari E, Kuebbeler M, et al. (2010) Conditions of retinal glial and inflammatory cell activation after irradiation in a GFP-chimeric mouse model. Investigative ophthalmology & visual science 51: 4831–4839.

53. Prinz M, Mildner A (2011) Microglia in the CNS: immigrants from another world. Glia 59: 177–187.

54. Chen M, Zhao J, Luo C, Pandi SP, Penalva RG, et al. (2012) Para-inflammation-mediated retinal recruitment of bone marrow-derived myeloid cells following whole-body irradiation is CCL2 dependent. Glia 60: 833–842.

55. Kaneko H, Nishiguchi KM, Nakamura M, Kachi S, Terasaki H (2008) Characteristics of bone marrow-derived microglia in the normal and injured retina. Invest Ophthalmol Vis Sci 49: 4162–4168.

56. Mildner A, Schlevogt B, Kierdorf K, Bottcher C, Erny D, et al. (2011) Distinct and non-redundant roles of microglia and myeloid subsets in mouse models of Alzheimer's disease. The Journal of neuroscience : the official journal of the Society for Neuroscience 31: 11159–11171.

57. Prinz M, Priller J, Sisodia SS, Ransohoff RM (2011) Heterogeneity of CNS myeloid cells and their roles in neurodegeneration. Nature neuroscience 14: 1227–1235.

16

GALC Deletions Increase the Risk of Primary Open-Angle Glaucoma: The Role of Mendelian Variants in Complex Disease

Yutao Liu[1,2]*, Jason Gibson[1,2], Joshua Wheeler[1,2], Lydia Coulter Kwee[1,2], Cecile M. Santiago-Turla[3], Stephen K. Akafo[4], Paul R. Lichter[5], Douglas E. Gaasterland[7], Sayoko E. Moroi[5], Pratap Challa[3], Leon W. Herndon[3], Christopher A. Girkin[8], Donald L. Budenz[9], Julia E. Richards[5,6], R. Rand Allingham[3], Michael A. Hauser[1,2,3]

1 Center for Human Genetics, Duke University Medical Center, Durham, North Carolina, United States of America, **2** Department of Medicine, Duke University Medical Center, Durham, North Carolina, United States of America, **3** Duke University Eye Center, Duke University Medical Center, Durham, North Carolina, United States of America, **4** Unit of Ophthalmology, Department of Surgery, University of Ghana Medical School, Korle Bu, Ghana, **5** Department of Ophthalmology and Visual Sciences, University of Michigan, Ann Arbor, Michigan, United States of America, **6** Department of Epidemiology, University of Michigan, Ann Arbor, Michigan, United States of America, **7** Eye Doctors of Washington, Chevy Chase, Maryland, United States of America, **8** Department of Ophthalmology, University of Alabama at Birmingham, Birmingham, Alabama, United States of America, **9** Department of Ophthalmology, Bascom Palmer Eye Institute, Miami, Florida, United States of America

Abstract

DNA copy number variants (CNVs) have been reported in many human diseases including autism and schizophrenia. Primary Open Angle Glaucoma (POAG) is a complex adult-onset disorder characterized by progressive optic neuropathy and vision loss. Previous studies have identified rare CNVs in POAG; however, their low frequencies prevented formal association testing. We present here the association between POAG risk and a heterozygous deletion in the galactosylceramidase gene (*GALC*). This CNV was initially identified in a dataset containing 71 Caucasian POAG cases and 478 ethnically matched controls obtained from dbGAP (study accession phs000126.v1.p1.) ($p = 0.017$, fisher's exact test). It was validated with array comparative genomic hybridization (arrayCGH) and realtime PCR, and replicated in an independent POAG dataset containing 959 cases and 1852 controls ($p = 0.021$, OR (odds ratio) $= 3.5$, 95% CI −1.1–12.0). Evidence for association was strengthened when the discovery and replication datasets were combined ($p = 0.002$; $OR = 5.0$, 95% CI 1.6–16.4). Several deletions with different endpoints were identified by array CGH of POAG patients. Homozygous deletions that eliminate GALC enzymatic activity cause Krabbe disease, a recessive Mendelian disorder of childhood displaying bilateral optic neuropathy and vision loss. Our findings suggest that heterozygous deletions that reduce GALC activity are a novel mechanism increasing risk of POAG. This is the first report of a statistically-significant association of a CNV with POAG risk, contributing to a growing body of evidence that CNVs play an important role in complex, inherited disorders. Our findings suggest an attractive biomarker and potential therapeutic target for patients with this form of POAG.

Editor: Reiner Albert Veitia, Institut Jacques Monod, France

Funding: This work is supported by National Institutes of Health (NIH) grants R01EY013315 (MAH), R01EY019126 (MAH), R03EY014939 (RRA), R01EY015543 (RRA), R01EY011671 (JER), R01EY09580 (JER), the Glaucoma Research Foundation (YL), National Glaucoma Research of American Health Assistance Foundation (YL), Research to Prevent Blindness (JER) and The Glaucoma Foundation (YL). This study was also supported in part by Duke University's CTSA grant 1 UL1 RR024128-01 from NCRR/NIH, as well as the research infrastructure of the Duke Center for Human Genetics. The funders had no role in study design, data collection and analysis, decision to publish, or preparation of the manuscript.

Competing Interests: The authors have declared that no competing interests exist.

* E-mail: yutao.liu@duke.edu

Introduction

Glaucoma is the leading cause of irreversible blindness worldwide [1]. As a heterogeneous group of disorders, glaucoma is a pathologic condition characterized by progressive loss of retinal ganglion cells with corresponding loss of the visual field. Primary open-angle glaucoma (POAG, OMIM #137760) is the most common form of glaucoma [2]. POAG is characterized by typical glaucomatous changes of the optic nerve and vision loss in the absence of secondary causes. Well recognized risk factors for the development of POAG include elevated intraocular pressure (IOP), increasing age, African ancestry, and family history of glaucoma [3,4]. Genetics plays an important role in the pathogenesis of POAG [2,3,5]. Traditional linkage studies have identified many genomic regions (GLC1 loci) for familial cases [6]. Among these, mutations in several genes, such as myocilin, optineurin, *WDR36* (WD repeat domain 36) and *CYP1B1* (cytochrome P450 1B1), are causal or associated with increased risk of developing POAG in multiple populations [7,8,9,10,11]. Association studies have identified many variants that may contribute to POAG [6,12]. Recently, genome-wide association studies have been used to identify genetic risk factors for POAG or glaucoma-related ocular phenotypes [13,14,15,16,17,18,19]. These genes and regions include caveolin 1 and 2 (*CAV1/2*), transmembrane and coiled-coil domains 1 (*TMCO1*), SIX homeobox 1 (*SIX1*), and cyclin-dependent kinase inhibitor 2B (*CDKN2B*) [13,19,20].

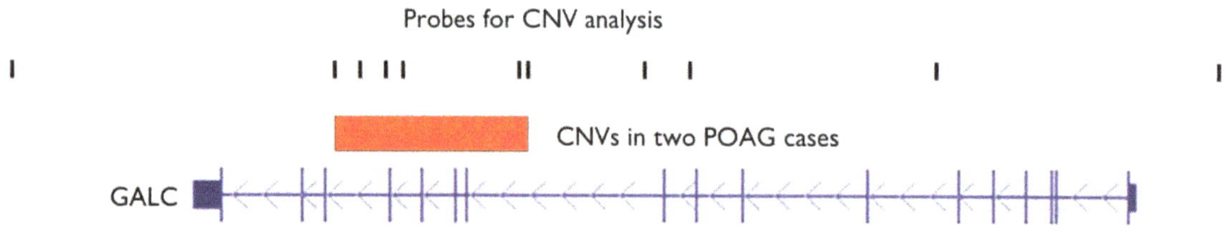

Figure 1. Heterozygous DNA deletion in the GALC gene. A heterozygous DNA deletion in the galactosylceramidase (*GALC*) gene present in 2 of 71 POAG cases and absent in 478 controls. The deletion was identified through six probes common to both the Illumina HumanCNV370-Duo and Human610-Quad BeadChips. The deletion indicated by the red-colored box includes five exons (exons 11–15) and abolishes enzymatic activity.

In addition to DNA sequence variation, DNA copy number variations (CNV) have been increasingly reported in human genetic disorders such as autism, HIV/AIDS, and cancer [21]. However, the role of CNV in POAG has been unclear. Abu-Amero et al. found no evidence of CNVs associated with POAG among 27 POAG cases and 12 controls using array comparative genomic hybridization (array CGH) [22]. However, in a larger dataset, Davis et al. using SNP genotyping arrays [23] studied 400 POAG cases and 500 non-glaucoma controls and found eleven rare CNVs that may be relevant to POAG. Fingert et al. recently identified a large duplication of *TBK1* (Tank-binding kinase 1) in patients with normal tension glaucoma [24]. Replications of these studies in larger datasets will help to clarify the importance of these CNVs in glaucoma risk.

In order to systematically examine the role of CNVs in POAG, we performed a discovery project using a genome-wide SNP genotyping array in a POAG case-control dataset. A set of candidate CNVs was selected for validation using realtime PCR. One specific CNV in the galactosylceramidase (*GALC*, OMIM *606890) gene was further examined in an independent case-control dataset. The heterozygous loss of the *GALC* gene was confirmed using three-primer PCR assays and array CGH.

Results

In the discovery phase of our study, we performed genome-wide DNA copy number variant analysis in 92 POAG cases genotyped on the Illumina HumanHap610 BeadChip. The CNV frequencies in our POAG patients were compared to publicly available controls genotyped on the Illumina HumanCNV370 BeadChip (dbGAP study accession phs000126.v1.p1.c1). The analysis was limited to the 363,185 markers shared between the two BeadChip platforms. After applying quality control protocols described in the methods section, 71 POAG samples and 478 dbGAP controls (greater than 40 years old) were analyzed using PennCNV software. Overall, 15,940 CNV calls were generated for a total of 549 DNA samples, with an average of 29 CNV events per sample. About one third of CNV calls overlapped with known coding genes. We performed a case-control comparison with all the identified CNVs. However, none of the CNVs reached genome-wide significance (p value$<5\times10^{-8}$). CNVs in five genomic regions were selected for further follow-up based on their potential functional annotation and relative frequency in cases versus controls. These five candidate regions were *RASA4* (RAS p21 protein activator 4), *EYA1* (eyes absent 1 homolog 1), *CROCC* (ciliary rootlet coiled-coil, rootletin), *ALDH1A2* (aldehyde dehydrogenase 1 family, member A2), and *GALC* (galactosylceramidase).

In order to validate the CNV calls generated from the SNP genotyping array, we used TaqMan-based realtime PCR on the 71 genotyped POAG cases using probes in these five selected regions. Realtime PCR validated the presence of the *GALC* deletion, but not the CNV calls in the regions of *RASA4*, *EYA1*, *CROCC*, or *ALDH1A2*. In the discovery dataset, 2/71 (2.8%) POAG cases were identified with heterozygous deletions in *GALC* while none were found in 478 age-matched US Caucasian controls (**Figure 1**). The difference in allele frequency between cases and controls was statistically significant (p = 0.017, Fisher's exact test). The *GALC* deletion was further validated in the POAG cases using a human chromosome 14-specific CGH array (Roche NimbleGen, Inc., Madison, WI) which demonstrated that it encompasses a 31 kb genomic region (**Figure 2**).

Association of the *GALC* CNV was replicated in a second Caucasian POAG case/control dataset. This dataset consisted of 959 cases and 1104 examined normal controls genotyped with realtime PCR that were augmented by an additional 748 publicly available population controls (greater than 40 years old) genotyped with the Affymetrix 6.0 array [25]. In this analysis, 9/959 POAG cases (0.94%) and 5/1852 controls (0.27%) carried the heterozygous DNA loss in *GALC* (P = 0.021, Fisher's exact test; OR = 3.5, 95%CI 1.1–12.0). After combining the discovery and replication datasets the strength of association was increased (p = 0.002, Fisher's exact test, OR = 5.0, 95% CI 1.6–16.4). The CNV deletion for *GALC* was found in 1.07% of POAG cases and 0.21% of the controls in the combined Caucasian dataset. There were no significant differences in age-at-diagnosis, maximum IOP, or visual acuity in POAG cases with the *GALC* deletion compared with POAG cases without the deletion. Realtime PCR-based screening was applied to African American (400 cases/290 controls) and West African (Ghana) (190 cases/500 controls) case-control datasets. No *GALC* CNV deletions were identified in either dataset (**Table 1**). This suggests that *GALC* deletions are either absent or extremely rare in individuals of West African ancestry. This finding is supported Shaikh *et al.* who report that *GALC* deletions were absent in 694 African American samples [25].

To further define the observed deletion, we used a 3-primer PCR assay (**Figure 3**) to examine our POAG cases and controls [26,27,28]. Three samples carry a previously reported 31 kb deletion (Human genome build 37, chromosome 14: 88,391,505–88,423,176) while the others have deletions with previously unreported and variable endpoints in our POAG cases. The heterogeneity of *GALC* CNV events was validated by array CGH (**Figure 4**). The 31 kb *GALC* deletion has been reported to carry a 4 bp direct repeat (TATC) at the deletion junction [26].

Discussion

We have identified CNV deletions of *GALC* that, when heterozygous, increase risk of POAG by four-fold in Caucasian

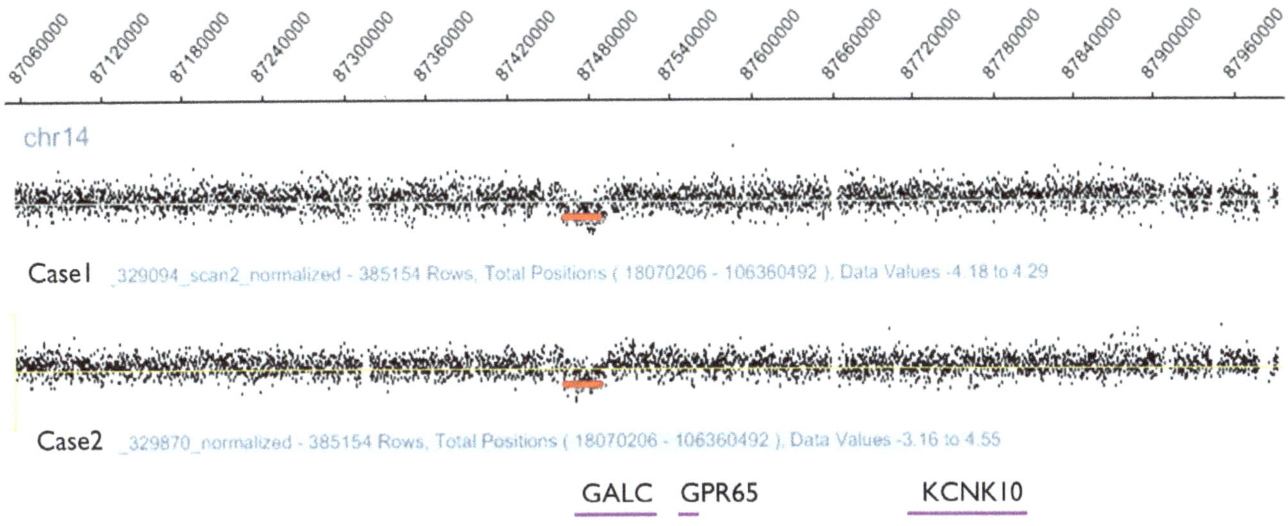

Figure 2. Validation of *GALC* deletion with array CGH. The *GALC* deletion from Figure 1 was validated with high resolution chromosome 14 specific CGH array. This figure showed a 31 kb deletion in the *GALC* gene, indicated by the red line.

individuals. CNV deletions were not found in subjects of African ancestry. The normal *GALC* mRNA encodes an 80 kDa precursor, which is processed into 50 and 30 kDa subunits to form an enzymatically active complex [26,29]. The 31 Kb *GALC* deletion abolishes production of the 30 kDa subunit and results in the production of a significantly shortened (15%) 50 kDa subunit [26]. *GALC* encodes the enzyme galactosylceramidase, which is required for the degradation of specific galactolipids in the white matter of the central and peripheral nervous system. These galactolipids include galactosylceramide, galactosylsphingosine (psychosine), lactosylceramide, and monogalactosyldiglyceride. GALC is critical in the maintenance of the myelin sheath, which functions as the protective covering around certain nerve cells to ensure the rapid transmission of nerve impulses. Psychosine forms during the production of myelin and is catabolized in part by GALC. Normally, only small amounts of psychosine are present in the brains of individuals with normal GALC enzymatic activity; however complete loss of activity leads to accumulation of psychosine and galactosylceramide, resulting in the development of Krabbe disease, a form of globoid cell leukodystrophy. Krabbe disease is a rare, autosomal recessive disorder of the central and peripheral nervous system [30] that is characterized by increased muscle tone, impaired motor control, seizures, hearing loss and vision loss.

Among all the *GALC* mutations causing Krabbe disease, the most common in Caucasian individuals (40–45%) is the large 31-kb deletion beginning in intron 10 and continuing past the end of *GALC* [29,30]. This deletion has not been reported in African American or African Krabbe disease patients. Based on the incidence of Krabbe disease in the United States (1 in 100,000 births) [29,30], the estimated combined frequency of all functionally-relevant *GALC* mutations is 0.003, implying a population frequency of the 30-kb deletion of approximately 0.0013, very similar to the frequency of 0.0011 we have detected in the present study (5 deletions in 4660 chromosomes of 2330 controls). This frequency match suggests that the controls included in our studies are appropriate and representative of the overall Caucasian population.

Although optic neuropathy with associated loss of vision is one of the most common clinical manifestations of Krabbe disease, poor patient prognosis has limited studies of the molecular mechanism of vision loss. In 1978, Brownstein et al. reported optic atrophy in an infant Krabbe disease patient [31]. Absence of GALC activity and accumulation of its substrates, galactosylcer-

Table 1. Summary of *GALC* deletion screening in all datasets.

Dataset	Ethnicity	Sample size (cases/controls)	Deletion events (cases/controls)	Fisher's exact p-value	Odds Ratio (95% CI)	Experimental Platform
Discovery	Caucasian	71/478	2 (2.8%)/0	0.017	Infinite	SNP-based array
Replication	Caucasian	959/1852	9 (0.94%)/5 (0.27%)	0.021	3.5 (1.1–12.0)	Realtime PCR+SNP-based array
Combined	Caucasian	1030/2330	11 (1.07%)/5 (0.21%)	0.002	5.0 (1.6–16.4)	Array & PCR
Duke	African American	400/290	0/0	1.000	N/A	Real time PCR
CHOP	African American	0/694	0/0	1.0	N/A	SNP-based array
Duke	Ghanaian	190/500	0/0	1.000	N/A	Real time PCR

The CHOP dataset was obtained from the Copy Number Variation project at the Children's Hospital of Philadelphia (CHOP) [25]; Fisher's exact p-value was based on one-tailed test, as we hypothesize that loss or decrease of GALC function results in POAG risk.

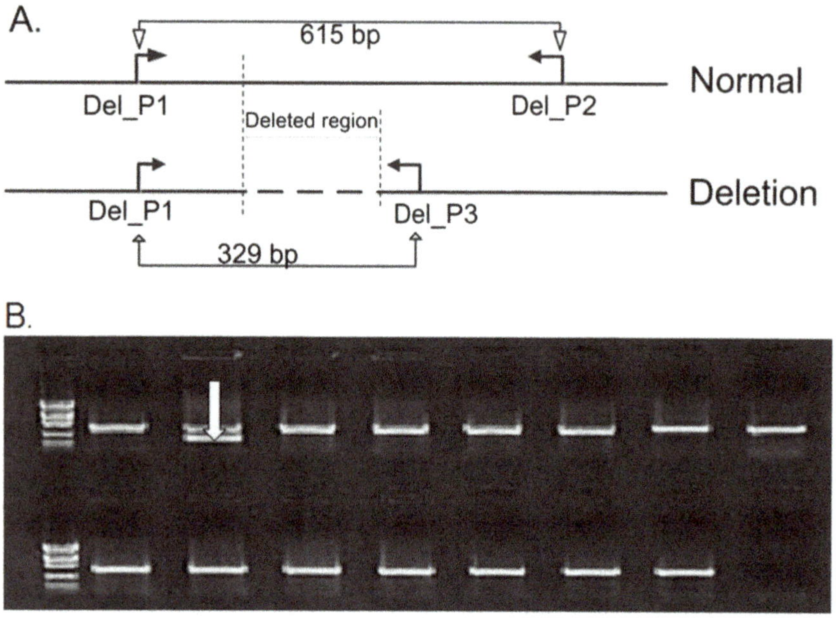

Figure 3. Three-Primer PCR assay for *GALC* deletion. (A) Schematic diagram of a portion of the *GALC* gene showing the region around the known GALC deletion. Both primers Del_P1 and Del_P3 are located outside of the deletion while primer Del_P2 is inside the deletion and close to the left breakpoint. (B) DNA samples with heterozygous deletion produced two DNA bands (329 bp and 615 bp in size) while DNA samples without GALC deletion generated one DNA band of 615 bp in size. The white arrow indicates the DNA sample with heterozygous deletion.

cbroside and psychosine, in the optic nerve caused optic nerve fiber and ganglion cell layer degeneration [31]. The carriers of *GALC* mutations are known to have reduced enzymatic activity [29,30], and we hypothesize that this reduced activity is the mechanism by which *GALC* deletions increase risk of POAG. Measurements of GALC enzymatic activity could be used to screen patients for risk of POAG. Currently it is estimated that there are hundreds of thousands of individuals who carry *GALC* deletions in the United States [29,30]. The findings reported here show that these carriers are at increased risk for glaucoma. In addition, the variability of GALC activity in the general population is broad. These estimates suggest that a substantial fraction of the population is expected to have as little as 20–30% of the normal GALC enzymatic activity levels [29,30]. It will be important to examine POAG-related phenotypes in the parents or grandparents of Krabbe disease patients, especially those GALC deletion carriers. This examination will provide direct evidence to the functional involvement of GALC in the pathogenesis of glaucoma. This work is currently underway.

McCarroll et al. and Redon et al. have reported two CEPH individuals (NA12716 and NA11840) with a heterozygous 24 kb deletion in the *GALC* gene using the Affymetrix 6.0 array [32,33]. Supplementary data from two genome-wide expression studies using HapMap samples [34,35], indicates that the *GALC* gene

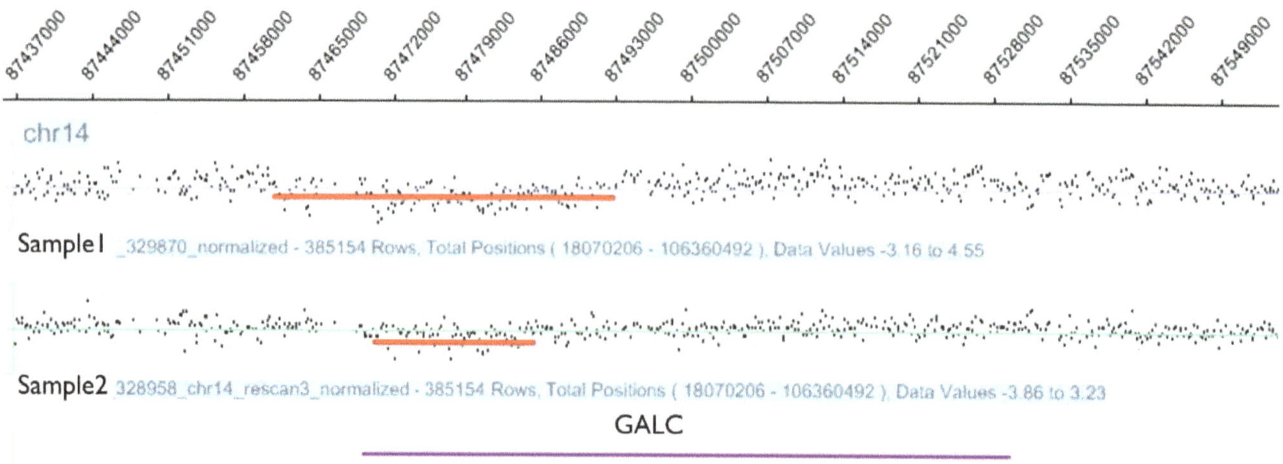

Figure 4. Heterogeneity of *GALC* deletions in different DNA samples. Two heterozygous *GALC* deletions with different end-points were identified by array CGH, indicated by the red line. The lower diagram shows the previously reported 31 kb *GALC* deletion while the upper diagram shows a smaller deletion of approximately 15 kb.

expression in these two CEPH individuals is the lowest in their respective families (pedigrees 1358 and 1349). Further, the GALC activity for these individuals is in the lowest 20th percentile compared to 90 other Caucasian subjects. These data suggest that GALC enzymatic activity may constitute a potential biomarker as well as therapeutic target for POAG.

In conclusion, this is the first study to report the role of heterozygous *GALC* deletions as a significant risk factor for POAG. We hypothesize that increased POAG risk is mediated through reduced gene expression and enzymatic activity that in turn leads to functional deficits in retinal ganglion cells. Further studies are warranted on the role of GALC in optic nerve function, the impact of *GALC* mutations in pathogenesis of glaucoma, and galactosylceramidase activity as a biomarker and a potential therapeutic target for POAG.

Materials and Methods

Ethics Statement

This study was reviewed and approved by the Institutional Review Board of Duke University Medical Center (Durham, NC) and adhered to the tenets of the Declaration of Helsinki. Written informed consent was obtained from all study participants.

Study Sample and Phenotype Description

Subjects with POAG were unrelated and met the following inclusion criteria [36] : 1) glaucomatous optic neuropathy in both eyes; 2) visual field loss consistent with optic nerve damage in at least one eye. Glaucomatous optic neuropathy was defined as a cup-to-disc ratio greater than 0.7 or focal loss of the nerve fiber layer resulting in a notch in the neuroretinal rim, associated with a glaucomatous visual field defect. Visual fields were performed using standard automated perimetry or frequency doubling test (FDT) [1]. IOP was not used as an inclusion criterion. The exclusion criteria for POAG subjects included the diagnosis or history of a secondary form of glaucoma or history of ocular trauma. Medical records for all POAG cases and control subjects were reviewed by professionally trained glaucoma subspecialists (RRA, SEM). The examined control subjects were unrelated and met the following criteria: 1) no self-report of a first-degree relative with glaucoma; 2) IOP less than 21 mmHg in both eyes without treatment; 3) no evidence of glaucomatous optic neuropathy in either eye; 4) normal visual field in both eyes.

We have used a two–stage study design: discovery and replication phases. The Caucasian POAG cases in the discovery phase were recruited at Duke University Eye Center. The Caucasian controls in the discovery phase were controls from a previous Parkinson's GWAS study (dbGAP study accession phs000126.v1.p1.c1). This study only uses those controls at least 40 years of age, with a total of 478 individuals. These controls are negative for neurologic disease and do not have a family history of any neurodegenerative disease. They are Caucasian and non-Hispanic subjects. They were enrolled at either Boston University or Indiana University and deposited into the NINDS Repository. The Caucasian POAG cases in the replication phase were enrolled at several sites: Duke University Eye Center, the University of Michigan Kellogg Eye Center, or Eye Doctors of Washington at Chevy Chase, MD. The examined control individuals in the replication phase were enrolled at either Duke University Eye Center or the University of Michigan Kellogg Eye Center. In the replication phase, we also included 748 US Caucasian controls from a previous Bipolar dbGAP GWAS study (phs000017.v2.p1) with an age cut-off at 40 years old. These controls will serve as non-examined population controls. These controls were genotyped using Affymetrix 6.0 array containing 1,800,000 probes for CNV analysis. All the African American POAG cases and controls were enrolled at Duke University Eye Center. The Ghanaian POAG cases and controls were collected in Ghana (West Africa).

CNV Calling

Extraction of genomic DNA by standard techniques (Gentra, Minneapolis, MN) was carried out for 1130 Caucasian POAG cases, 1350 Caucasian controls, 400 African American POAG cases, 300 African American controls, 190 Ghanaian POAG cases and 500 Ghanaian controls. Ninety-two POAG cases were subjected to genome-wide SNP genotyping with the Infinium II Human610-Quad BeadChip (Illumina, San Diego, CA, USA) at the Molecular Genetics Core of the Center for Human Genetics at Duke University. High quality genomic DNA (500 ng) was used to genotype each sample according to the manufacturer's guidelines [37]. BeadStudio software (Illumina) was used to analyze DNA genotype and intensity. For 943 controls we obtained the genotype and intensity files from dbGAP (study accession phs000126.v1.p1). These samples were genotyped using Illumina HumanCNV370-Duo BeadChip. For CNV analysis, samples were required to have the following criteria: First, only samples with call rates >98% were included. Second, only samples with the standard deviation of normalized intensity (Log R Ratio, LRR) ≤0.35 were included. Third, only samples where the correlation of LRR to wave model ranged between −0.2 and 0.4 were included. Finally, only samples with the initial CNV call count ≤40 were included in the analysis. A total of 71 POAG cases and 478 controls met all inclusion measures in the final CNV analysis. For those 748 GAIN controls genotyped with Affymetrix 6.0 array, we applied a similar quality control procedure: 1) standard deviation of LRR ≤0.35; 2) a minimum of 5 probes per CNV due to a much higher density of probes (a total of 1.8 million probes per sample); 3) ≤100 CNV calls per sample; 4) drift of B allele frequency (BAF) ≤0.01; and 5) wave factor ≤0.05.

To call CNVs, we used the PennCNV algorithm [38], which combines multiple sources of information, including LRR and BAF at each SNP marker. We required a minimum of 3 consecutive probes for a CNV call. Since POAG cases and controls were genotyped with different types of Illumina Beadchips, only SNPs and probes shared in common between these two Beadchips (approximately 370,000) were utilized to generate CNV calls. The differences in CNV frequency between POAG cases and controls were evaluated using Fisher's exact test. A list of specific CNVs was selected for further validation using realtime PCR in a large POAG case/control dataset.

CNV Validation and Screening by Realtime PCR

To validate the CNVs determined by PennCNV, we selected five candidate CNVs identified in the initial genome-wide screen. We used TaqMan® Copy Number Assays from ABI (Applied Biosystems Inc, Carlsbad, CA, USA) on the ABI Prism® 7900HT Sequence Detection System for validation and further screening in additional POAG cases and controls. A VIC-labeled Copy Number Assay for RNase P was selected to be an endogenous control as it performed in the same reaction with gene-specific assays. Only one probe was selected for each CNV region. Each sample was assayed with four replicates by using 10 ng DNA in each reaction in 384-well format. The CNV calls were generated with SDS software and CopyCaller™ from ABI (Applied Biosystems Inc, Carlsbad, CA, USA). A known CEPH sample was used as a reference for a copy number of 2. This CEPH sample was already examined by SNP microarray to contain two copies of candidate CNV regions. In order to make CNV calls in

CopyCaller^{TM} software, a confidence score of greater than 0.95 was required with four replicates.

The CNV assay for *EYA1* gene used Hs03668790 to target intron 7. The assay for the *CROCC* gene used Hs01817683 to target the boundary of exon 3 and intron 3. The assay for *ALDH1A2* gene used Hs02281830 to target the boundary of intron 7 and exon 8. The assay for *RASA4* was custom-designed to target the genomic region between exon 1 and exon 3. The specific CNV assay for the *GALC* gene used Hs00121467 to target exon 13. The assay for *GALC* was run with all Caucasian, African American, and Ghana case-control samples as well as a multiplex familial POAG cohort.

Three-primer PCR assay for *GALC* Deletion

We utilized a three-primer PCR assay that was developed previously [26] to examine a known deletion in the *GALC* gene. The primer sequences were Del_P1: 5′-CCTATATGGAAAA-CAATGTGG-3′, Del_P2: 5′-AAGGAGCTAACATTTCAGGC-3′; and Del_P3: 5′- AAGGAGCTAACATTTCAGGC-3′. Primers Del_P1 and Del_P3 were outside of the genomic deletion, while primer Del_P2 was inside of the deleted region and close to Del_P1 (**Figure 3**). Individuals with a homozygous deletion generate a 329 bp fragment with PCR primers Del_P1 and Del_P3 while subjects without deletion produce a 615 bp fragment with PCR primers Del_P1 and Del_P2. Individuals with a heterozygous deletion generate two PCR fragments of 329 and 615 bp in size. This three-primer PCR reaction was used to examine all POAG cases and controls.

Validation with Array CGH

Selected DNA samples were examined with CGH array experiments for CNV changes in *GALC*. A high-resolution chromosome 14 specific CGH array was used according to the standard protocols provided by the manufacturer (Roche-NimbleGen, Inc, Madison, WI, USA) [39]. For each sample, 1 µg high quality undegraded DNA was included with human reference DNA from HapMap. The human chromosome 14-specific CGH array provides measurements from 385,000 unique genomic loci on chromosome 14. The experimental sample was labeled with Cy3 and reference sample was with Cy5. The arrays were scanned on an Axon 4100A scanner (Molecular Devices, Sunnyvale, CA, USA). TIFF images were analyzed using NimbleScan 2.5 software to obtain fluorescent intensity and the copy number was further determined using the segMNT algorithm with a 10× averaging window and minimum difference in log ratio of 0.2. A minimum of 10 consecutive probes was required to make CNV calls. The copy number variation result was visualized using SignalMap 1.8 from Roche NimbleGen.

Acknowledgments

We are grateful to the study participants, without whom this work would not have been possible. We thank two previous genome-wide association studies in dbGAP: Whole Genome Association Study of Bipolar Disorder (phs000017.v2.p1) and CIDR: Genome Wide Association Study in Familial Parkinson Disease (PD) (phs000126.v1.p1).

Author Contributions

Conceived and designed the experiments: YL RRA JER PRL MAH. Performed the experiments: YL JG JW MAH RRA. Analyzed the data: YL RRA LCK CMST JG MAH. Contributed reagents/materials/analysis tools: YL JW RRA LCK CMST SKA CAG DLB JER SEM PRL DEG PC LWH MAH. Wrote the paper: YL RRA JG JER PRL CAG DEG DLB SEM PC LWH MAH.

References

1. Quigley HA, Broman AT (2006) The number of people with glaucoma worldwide in 2010 and 2020. Br J Ophthalmol 90: 262–267.
2. Liu Y, Allingham RR (2011) Molecular genetics in glaucoma. Exp Eye Res.
3. Libby RT, Gould DB, Anderson MG, John SW (2005) Complex genetics of glaucoma susceptibility. Annu Rev Genomics Hum Genet 6: 15–44.
4. Manni G, Oddone F, Parisi V, Tosto A, Centofanti M (2008) Intraocular pressure and central corneal thickness. Prog Brain Res 173: 25–30.
5. Kwon YH, Fingert JH, Kuehn MH, Alward WL (2009) Primary open-angle glaucoma. N Engl J Med 360: 1113–1124.
6. Allingham RR, Liu Y, Rhee DJ (2009) The genetics of primary open-angle glaucoma: a review. Exp Eye Res 88: 837–844.
7. Rezaie T, Child A, Hitchings R, Brice G, Miller L, et al. (2002) Adult-onset primary open-angle glaucoma caused by mutations in optineurin. Science 295: 1077–1079.
8. Stone EM, Fingert JH, Alward WL, Nguyen TD, Polansky JR, et al. (1997) Identification of a gene that causes primary open angle glaucoma. Science 275: 668–670.
9. Monemi S, Spaeth G, DaSilva A, Popinchalk S, Ilitchev E, et al. (2005) Identification of a novel adult-onset primary open-angle glaucoma (POAG) gene on 5q22.1. Hum Mol Genet 14: 725–733.
10. Stoilov I, Akarsu AN, Sarfarazi M (1997) Identification of three different truncating mutations in cytochrome P4501B1 (CYP1B1) as the principal cause of primary congenital glaucoma (Buphthalmos) in families linked to the GLC3A locus on chromosome 2p21. Hum Mol Genet 6: 641–647.
11. Vasiliou V, Gonzalez FJ (2008) Role of CYP1B1 in glaucoma. Annu Rev Pharmacol Toxicol 48: 333–358.
12. Fuse N (2010) Genetic bases for glaucoma. Tohoku J Exp Med 221: 1–10.
13. Burdon KP, Macgregor S, Hewitt AW, Sharma S, Chidlow G, et al. (2011) Genome-wide association study identifies susceptibility loci for open angle glaucoma at TMCO1 and CDKN2B-AS1. Nat Genet 43: 574–578.
14. Cornelis MC, Agrawal A, Cole JW, Hansel NN, Barnes KC, et al. (2010) The Gene, Environment Association Studies consortium (GENEVA): maximizing the knowledge obtained from GWAS by collaboration across studies of multiple conditions. Genet Epidemiol 34: 364–372.
15. Lu Y, Dimasi DP, Hysi PG, Hewitt AW, Burdon KP, et al. (2010) Common genetic variants near the Brittle Cornea Syndrome locus ZNF469 influence the blinding disease risk factor central corneal thickness. PLoS Genet 6: e1000947.
16. Macgregor S, Hewitt AW, Hysi PG, Ruddle JB, Medland SE, et al. (2010) Genome-wide association identifies ATOH7 as a major gene determining human optic disc size. Hum Mol Genet 19: 2716–2724.
17. Meguro A, Inoko H, Ota M, Mizuki N, Bahram S (2010) Genome-wide association study of normal tension glaucoma: common variants in SRBD1 and ELOVL5 contribute to disease susceptibility. Ophthalmology 117: 1331–1338 e1335.
18. Ramdas WD, van Koolwijk LM, Ikram MK, Jansonius NM, de Jong PT, et al. (2010) A genome-wide association study of optic disc parameters. PLoS Genet 6: e1000978.
19. Thorleifsson G, Walters GB, Hewitt AW, Masson G, Helgason A, et al. (2010) Common variants near CAV1 and CAV2 are associated with primary open-angle glaucoma. Nat Genet 42: 906–909.
20. Ramdas WD, van Koolwijk LM, Lemij HG, Pasutto F, Cree AJ, et al. (2011) Common genetic variants associated with open-angle glaucoma. Hum Mol Genet 20: 2464–2471.
21. Zhang F, Gu W, Hurles ME, Lupski JR (2009) Copy number variation in human health, disease, and evolution. Annu Rev Genomics Hum Genet 10: 451–481.
22. Abu-Amero KK, Hellani A, Bender P, Spaeth GL, Myers J, et al. (2009) High-resolution analysis of DNA copy number alterations in patients with primary open-angle glaucoma. Mol Vis 15: 1594–1598.
23. Davis L, Meyer K, Schindler E, Beck J, Rudd D, et al. (2011) Copy Number Variations (CNVs) and Primary Open Angle Glaucoma (POAG). Invest Ophthalmol Vis Sci.
24. Fingert JH, Robin AL, Stone JL, Roos BR, Davis LK, et al. (2011) Copy number variations on chromosome 12q14 in patients with normal tension glaucoma. Hum Mol Genet 20: 2482–2494.
25. Shaikh TH, Gai X, Perin JC, Glessner JT, Xie H, et al. (2009) High-resolution mapping and analysis of copy number variations in the human genome: a data resource for clinical and research applications. Genome Res 19: 1682–1690.
26. Luzi P, Rafi MA, Wenger DA (1995) Characterization of the large deletion in the GALC gene found in patients with Krabbe disease. Hum Mol Genet 4: 2335–2338.
27. Rafi MA, Luzi P, Chen YQ, Wenger DA (1995) A large deletion together with a point mutation in the GALC gene is a common mutant allele in patients with infantile Krabbe disease. Hum Mol Genet 4: 1285–1289.

28. Luzi P, Rafi MA, Wenger DA (1995) Structure and organization of the human galactocerebrosidase (GALC) gene. Genomics 26: 407–409.
29. Wenger DA, Rafi MA, Luzi P (1997) Molecular genetics of Krabbe disease (globoid cell leukodystrophy): diagnostic and clinical implications. Hum Mutat 10: 268–279.
30. Wenger DA, Rafi MA, Luzi P, Datto J, Costantino-Ceccarini E (2000) Krabbe disease: genetic aspects and progress toward therapy. Mol Genet Metab 70: 1–9.
31. Brownstein S, Meagher-Villemure K, Polomeno RC, Little JM (1978) Optic nerve in globoid leukodystrophy (Krabbe's disease). Ultrastructural changes. Arch Ophthalmol 96: 864–870.
32. McCarroll SA, Kuruvilla FG, Korn JM, Cawley S, Nemesh J, et al. (2008) Integrated detection and population-genetic analysis of SNPs and copy number variation. Nat Genet 40: 1166–1174.
33. Redon R, Ishikawa S, Fitch KR, Feuk L, Perry GH, et al. (2006) Global variation in copy number in the human genome. Nature 444: 444–454.
34. Zhang W, Duan S, Bleibel WK, Wisel SA, Huang RS, et al. (2009) Identification of common genetic variants that account for transcript isoform variation between human populations. Hum Genet 125: 81–93.
35. Spielman RS, Bastone LA, Burdick JT, Morley M, Ewens WJ, et al. (2007) Common genetic variants account for differences in gene expression among ethnic groups. Nat Genet 39: 226–231.
36. Liu Y, Schmidt S, Qin X, Gibson J, Hutchins K, et al. (2008) Lack of association between LOXL1 variants and primary open-angle glaucoma in three different populations. Invest Ophthalmol Vis Sci 49: 3465–3468.
37. Glessner JT, Wang K, Cai G, Korvatska O, Kim CE, et al. (2009) Autism genome-wide copy number variation reveals ubiquitin and neuronal genes. Nature 459: 569–573.
38. Wang K, Li M, Hadley D, Liu R, Glessner J, et al. (2007) PennCNV: an integrated hidden Markov model designed for high-resolution copy number variation detection in whole-genome SNP genotyping data. Genome Res 17: 1665–1674.
39. Fraser CR, Wang W, Gomez M, Zhang T, Mathew S, et al. (2009) Transformation of chronic lymphocytic leukemia/small lymphocytic lymphoma to interdigitating dendritic cell sarcoma: evidence for transdifferentiation of the lymphoma clone. Am J Clin Pathol 132: 928–939.

17

Analysis of Pulsatile Retinal Movements by Spectral-Domain Low-Coherence Interferometry: Influence of Age and Glaucoma on the Pulse Wave

Carolyne Dion[1,2†], Kanwarpal Singh[1,2], Tsuneyuki Ozaki[1,2], Mark R. Lesk[2,3], Santiago Costantino[2,3,4*]

1 Institut National de la Recherche Scientifique - Énergie, Matériaux et Télécommunications, Varennes, Québec, Canada, **2** Centre de Recherche de l'Hôpital Maisonneuve-Rosemont, Montréal, Québec, Canada, **3** Department of Ophthalmology, Faculty of Medicine, Université de Montréal, Montréal, Québec, Canada, **4** Biomedical Engineering Institute, Université de Montréal, Montréal, Québec, Canada

Abstract

Recent studies have shown that ocular hemodynamics and eye tissue biomechanical properties play an important role in the pathophysiology of glaucoma. Nevertheless, better, non-invasive methods to assess these characteristics *in vivo* are essential for a thorough understanding of degenerative mechanisms. Here, we propose to measure ocular tissue movements induced by cardiac pulsations and study the ocular pulse waveform as an indicator of tissue compliance. Using a novel, low-cost and non-invasive device based on spectral-domain low coherence interferometry (SD-LCI), we demonstrate the potential of this technique to differentiate ocular hemodynamic and biomechanical properties. We measured the axial movement of the retina driven by the pulsatile ocular blood flow in 11 young healthy individuals, 12 older healthy individuals and 15 older treated glaucoma patients using our custom-made SD-OCT apparatus. The cardiac pulse was simultaneously measured through the use of an oximeter to allow comparison. Spectral components up to the second harmonic were obtained and analyzed. For the different cohorts, we computed a few parameters that characterize the three groups of individuals by analyzing the movement of the retinal tissue at two locations, using this simple, low-cost interferometric device. Our pilot study indicates that spectral analysis of the fundus pulsation has potential for the study of ocular biomechanical and vascular properties, as well as for the study of ocular disease.

Editor: Bang V. Bui, Univeristy of Melbourne, Australia

Funding: The study was supported by the Ministère du Développement Économique de l'Innovation et de l'Exportation du Québec, the Fonds Québécois de la Recherchesur la Nature et les Technologies, the Canadian Institutes of Health Research, the Fonds de la Recherche en Santé du Québec, le Fonds de Recherche en Ophthalmologie de Universite de Montreal and the Natural Sciences and Engineering Research Council of Canada. The funders had no role in study design, data collection and analysis, decision to publish, or preparation of the manuscript.

Competing Interests: The authors have declared that no competing interests exist.

* E-mail: santiago.costantino@umontreal.ca

† Deceased.

Introduction

The pathophysiology of glaucoma, is still under debate: although elevated intraocular pressure (IOP) is the major risk factor [1], there is increasing evidence that the pathogenesis of glaucoma is also linked to the biomechanical properties of the eye [2–5] and to abnormal ocular blood flow (OBF) [6,7]. Both IOP and OBF are pulsatile by nature, being in close relationship with the cardiovascular system activity. [8] Numerous studies have demonstrated reduced IOP pulse amplitudes and reduced pulsatile ocular blood flow in glaucoma patients compared with control subjects[9–11]. However, to our knowledge, very little work has been devoted to the analysis of the pulse waveform itself to determine whether it can be used for differentiating diseased from healthy individuals. For instance, Evans *et al.* [12] have shown that the spectral power of the second, third and fourth harmonic components of the IOP pulse is significantly lower in glaucomatous groups compared to normal groups. Unfortunately, assessment of the IOP relies on the use of contact techniques such as pneumotonography [13] or variants of the Goldman's applanation tonometer [14]. Since Fourier analysis of the pulsatile IOP requires relatively long data acquisition time, which may lead to serious patient discomfort because of direct eye contact, such type of investigation for screening purposes remains unpopular in ophthalmology clinics and researches.

In systemic circulation, however, the use of Fourier analysis to study the pressure and blood flow waveforms has been a standard method of evaluating impedance of the arterial wall. [15,16] As an example, such analysis can be used to study the influence of vasodilator drugs on the vascular arterial compliance [17] or allow better insights into the vascular status of specific organs, such as in cerebral hemodynamics. [18,19] In ophthalmology, spectral analysis has been widely used for the study of ocular tremors, [20,21] pupil size fluctuation, [22,23] and corneal[24–26] and retinal [22,26,27] movements, providing better understanding of the ocular deformation in relation with the cardiopulmonary system. More recently, Plumb *et al.* [28] have shown that spectral analysis of the Doppler flow velocity waveform of the ophthalmic artery revealed significant differences in the percentage power of the first four lower frequency sinusoidal components between subjects with type 2 diabetes and healthy controls. Thus, a comprehensive assessment of waveforms can be a very powerful tool for studying pulsatile biomechanical systems.

On the other hand, tremendous efforts have been deployed over the years to elaborate non-invasive instruments to measure pulsatile ocular movements for assessing ocular hemodynamics and/or biomechanics.[4,22,24–26,29,30] We have recently demonstrated the capabilities of spectral-domain low coherence interferometry (SD-LCI) to extract displacement information from sequential axial scans of the eye. [26] This homemade system was successfully used to measure longitudinal retinal and corneal movements *in vivo* in healthy volunteers. [27] It was found that the movements of the cornea and the retina are highly correlated with each other, where the amplitude of both tissues is almost equal. In light of these results, the aim of this work is to demonstrate that the measurement of the longitudinal retinal displacements performed using SD-LCI, along with comprehensive Fourier analysis, can be used to differentiate individuals with different eye hemodynamic and biomechanical properties. Measurements can be achieved with a reliable device, whose principle components consist of a steady low-power broadband laser source, diffractive optics and a camera. We show that the ratio between the fundamental and second harmonic spectral components of the longitudinal retinal movement, the phase shift between these two harmonics, and the phase shift between the movement and the cardiac pulses showed distinctive signatures for the groups varying in age (35 vs 60 years old) and eye condition (normal vs glaucoma).

Methods

Experimental Set-up

Figure 1 shows a schematic diagram of the optical SD-LCI system. A fiber-based Michelson interferometer was built using a superluminescent diode (SLD, Superlum) with central wavelength of 844 nm and 46 nm bandwidth. The beam was split using a 2×2, 80:20 fiber coupler into the reference and sample arms terminated with fiber collimators. The collimated sample beam was focused by the eye on to the fundus. The sample arm was also coupled to a fundus camera (Topcon) equipped with an infrared CCD camera (Pulnix), which assured, along with a fixation point, proper positioning of the beam onto the fundus either at the macula or optic disk. The SLD power incident onto the eye was set constant to 700 μW, which is safe for continuous illumination of the human eye according to ANSI safety standards. [31] At the reference arm, the light was reflected by a broadband mirror placed on a motorized translation stage (Zaber Technology). The reference arm beam was attenuated by a neutral density filter (NDF) in order to keep its total intensity below the saturation level of the detector. The two reflected beams (one reflected from the eye layer of interest and the other from the reference mirror) were recombined in the fiber coupler, then dispersed using a diffraction grating (1200 lines/mm) and focused by an achromatic lens (f=200 mm) onto a linear CCD camera (Spyder 3, Dalsa Technology). The camera exposure time was set to 400 μs. The full SLD spectrum spanned 700 pixels on the linear CCD camera, which allowed a theoretical depth range of ~1.2 mm and longitudinal resolution of ~7 μm in air. The measured sensitivity close to the zero delay position was found to be 94 dB with a decay of 15 dB as one approached 80% of the maximal depth range. Calibration and dispersion compensation of the system were achieved by measuring the position of the peak in the axial scan as a function of the position of the translation stage, repeating this measurement at 100 μm intervals. [32] To establish a relationship between the eye movements and the cardiac pulsations, a custom-made oximeter was placed on the earlobe during measurements to record the pulse of the subjects using a data acquisition card (Labjack, Lakewood, CO). The signals from the linear CCD camera and the oximeter were processed using a dual core 2.0 GHz computer with custom software (LabView, National Instruments). Overall, the total data acquisition time of the CCD camera and oximeter signals provided a sampling rate of 100 Hz. Data was acquired for approximately 20 seconds and stored for later processing.

Data Analysis

Retinal axial scans (A-scans), or depth profiles, were obtained from the Fast Fourier Transform (FFT) of the SLD spectrum recorded by the CCD camera. A typical A-scan of the retinal layers at the macula region is shown in Fig. 2(a), where FFT peaks can be assigned to reflective interfaces in the sample, which in the present example, to the nerve fiber layer (NFL) and retinal pigment epithelium (RPE). In order to illustrate how the reflectivity profile of the tissues changes during the movements, two A-scans acquired at the retina and the optic disc are plotted simultaneously (Figure S2 and Figure S3 in supplementary information) at extreme time points of the cardiac cycle. For measuring at the optic disc, the probing beam was focused and its position was monitored using a fundus camera throughout the measurement. In order to minimize displacements off the optic disc, the subject was asked to fixate at an illuminated point. As described in a previous paper, [26] measurement of the movement relies on locating the centroid position of FFT peaks in sequential A-scans. An example of such displacement measurements obtained with this procedure is shown along with the oximeter signal in Fig. 2(b). Measurements in which patients blinked for a significant fraction of time were visually identified and discarded for analysis. In addition, frequencies lower than 0.5 Hz and higher than 7 Hz were removed by using a squared band pass filter. No special processing was applied to short blinks, since the frequency filter basically removed their potential contribution. Next, the effective movement amplitude of a given retinal layer was determined by calculating the root mean square of the axial position.

A simple way to inspect the pulse waveform characteristics is to perform Fast Fourier Transform on the pulsatile signal as a function of time. Figure 2(c) and (d) show typical spectral characteristics of the retinal movement and heart signal. The data shown in Fig. 2(c) illustrates that both, the movement and oximeter signals show matched fundamental frequencies (f_1) and second harmonics (f_2). In Fig. 2, for simplicity reasons, data with a narrow spread in the cardiac frequencies is shown, but in several cases the heart signal is non-stationary, which leads to spreading of the frequency components. Such an example is shown in Figure S1.

Although a novel concept in ophthalmology, harmonic components of tissue movements have been found in cardiovascular research to be associated with the vessel's vascular impedance and wave reflections from the distal arterial tree. [15,16] From the analysis of spectral power and phase data, additional parameters can also be extracted: (*i*) the ratio between the integrated signal under the second harmonic and fundamental frequency peaks of the movements ($R_{Mvt} = A_{2\text{-}Mvt}/A_{1\text{-}Mvt}$) and heart signal ($R_{Oxi} = A_{2\text{-}Oxi}/A_{1\text{-}Oxi}$); (*ii*) the phase shift between the fundamental frequency of the movement with respect to the oximeter fundamental frequency ($\Theta = \Phi_{1\text{-}Mvt}\text{-}\Phi_{1\text{-}Oxi}$), and (*iii*) the phase shift between the second harmonic with respect to fundamental frequency for both the movement ($\Pi_{Mvt} = \Phi_{2\text{-}Mvt}\text{-}\Phi_{1\text{-}Mvt}$) and the heart signal ($\Pi_{Oxi} = \Phi_{2\text{-}Oxi}\text{-}\Phi_{1\text{-}Oxi}$). Integrated signals were computed as the area under each frequency peak in the Fourier space, and phase

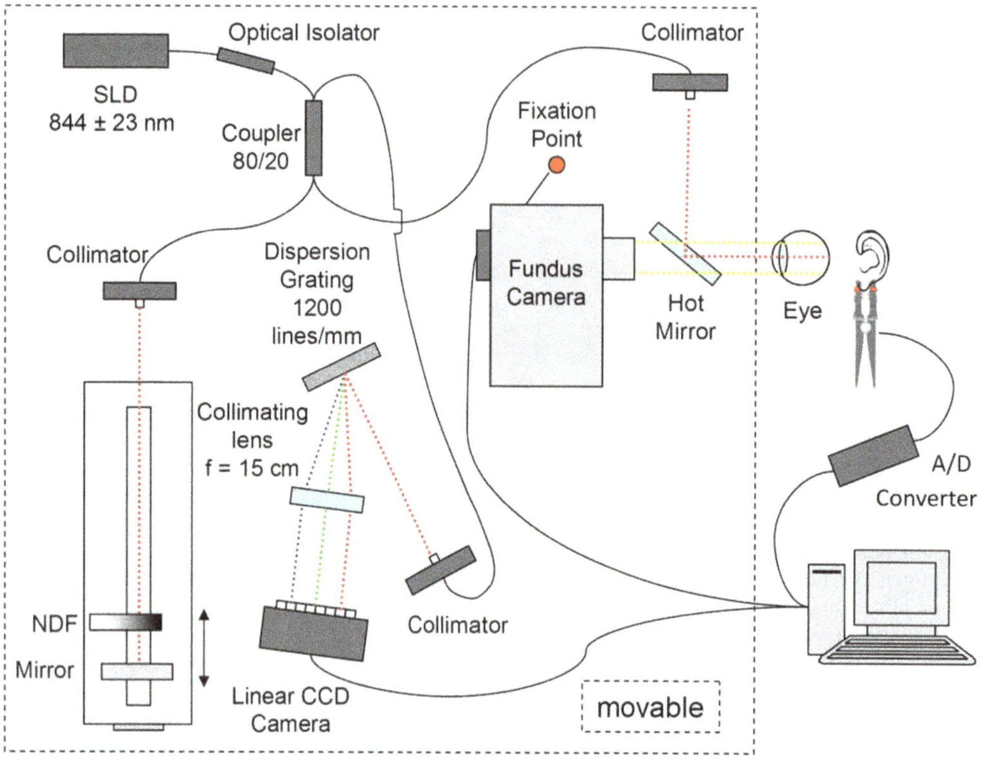

Figure 1. Schematic diagram of a FD-LCI system.

was also averaged for the same frequency ranges. These three parameters were evaluated and compared for different cohorts of individuals.

Clinical Subjects

Thirty-eight individuals were recruited from the Maisonneuve-Rosemont Ophthalmology Clinic and Research Center and all experiments were approved by the ethics committee of the Maisonneuve-Rosemont hospital. The procedure and the consequences were described to all the individuals and informed consent was obtained. The procedure adheres to the Declaration of Helsinki. Three cohorts were formed: 11 younger healthy individuals, 12 older healthy individuals, and 15 older treated glaucoma patients. The characteristics of these groups are shown in Table 1. Gender distribution among individuals was similar for the three groups, and age distribution was also similar for the old-healthy and old-glaucoma groups. It is worth mentioning that the three different cohorts were matched for heart rate. Heart rate has been shown to be significantly correlated to measures of the IOP pulse wave, *i.e.* the higher the heart rate, the lower the pulse amplitude, pulse volume and pulsatile ocular blood flow. With the groups matched for heart rate, this factor is eliminated. [12] Diagnosis of glaucoma was made on visual field analysis and optic disk appearance in accordance with established clinical parameters. [33] The average ± standard deviation of the mean defect was found to be 1.61±1.63 dB in glaucoma patients. At the time of study, glaucoma patients had already been treated for their disease with medication controlling increased IOP or laser surgery. The medication used to control the IOP was one of the following; Xalatan die HS, Lumigan HS, Cosopt Bid, Bitoptic Bid, Travatan die HS. For each patient, the eye with greatest optic disk cupping was selected for evaluation. Control healthy subjects had no history of ophthalmic disorders and the results of an ophthalmic examination were normal. The right eye of each individual in both healthy groups was used for evaluation. Neither pupil dilatation nor corneal anesthesia were required for SD-LCI measurements and proper positioning with infrared fundus camera. Axial movements of the retina at both the optic disk and the macula region were measured using the system described above, with participants properly positioned on a chin rest. Several series of twenty-second measurements separated by 1-minute pauses were recorded for each individual. For each patient, data analysis was performed for all series, while data with the best signal-to-noise ratio in the movement FFT spectral power was selected for further comparison. For comparison between different cohorts, data was checked for normality using the Shapiro–Wilk test and results are presented in Table S1. All data sets were found to be normal at a significance level lower than 0.01. Unpaired Student's *t*-tests were used to compare differences between groups at each eye position. Pearson's product moment correlation analysis was used to evaluate associations between variables, and p values lower than 0.05 were considered statistically significant.

Results

Ocular movements at the macula and optic disk regions were analyzed for the three groups. Comparison of the calculated parameters for each of these groups at both the macula and optic disk regions is shown as multiple boxplots in Fig. 3. In Fig. 3(a) the effective amplitude of the movements, which are approximately 50 μm is displayed. Overall, the effective amplitude of the movement seems to be greater at the optic disk than at the macula, but this difference does not reach significance in our small pilot test. In addition, no significant difference in effective amplitude between the three groups is observed. Finally, it should be noted here that this device measures overall changes in the

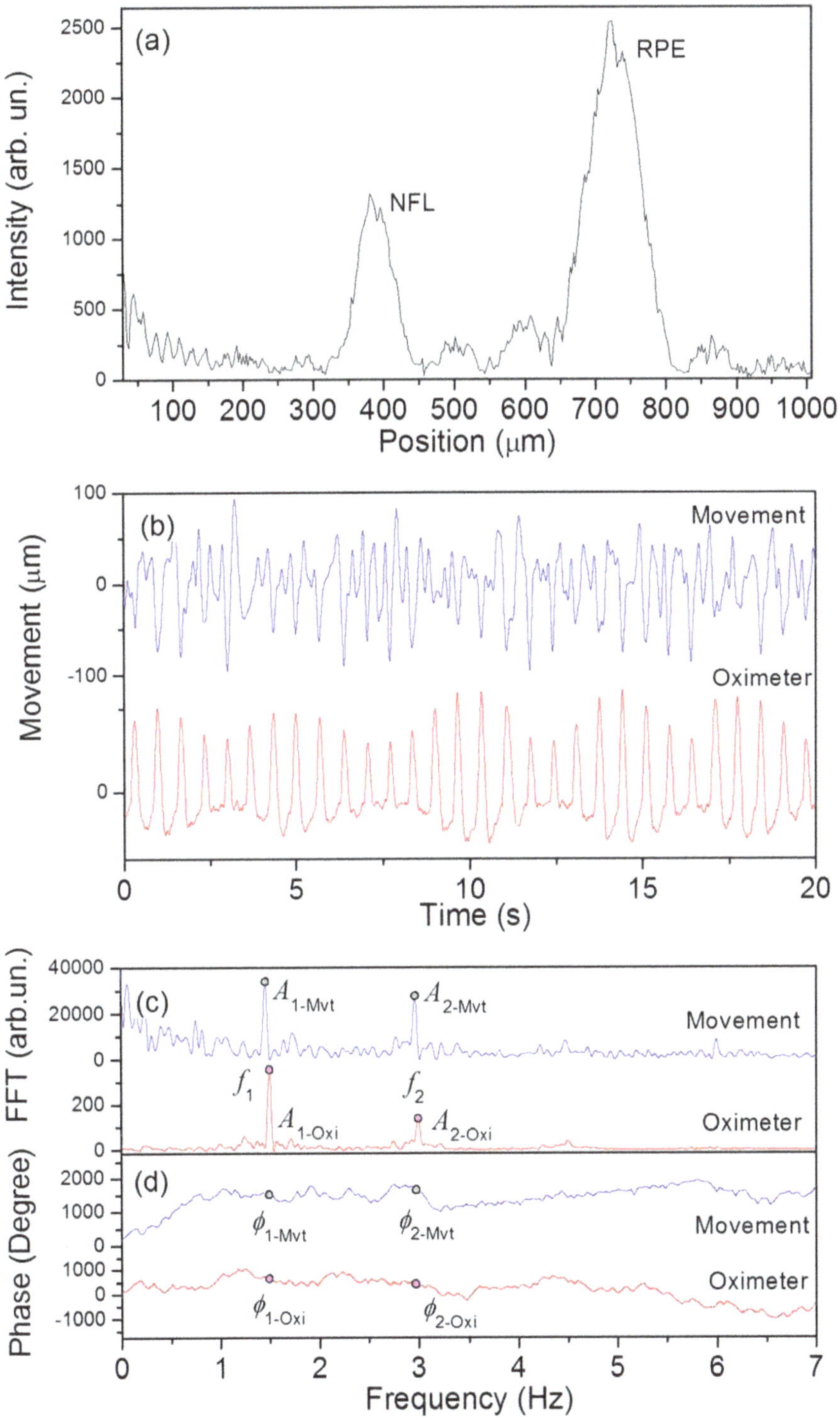

Figure 2. Representative data and movement analysis. (a) Typical A-scan produced by the retina where the nerve fiber layer (NFL) and retinal pigment epithelium (RPE) are clearly observed. (b) Position of the retina in the macula region as a function of time along with oximeter signal, as recorded by the SD-LCI for a 30-years-old normal female subject. Movement and oximeter signal FFT analysis are shown in (c) and (d).

optical path length, this includes not only the fundus pulse amplitude (FPA), but also full-eye displacements. FPA is a few microns (approximately 5 microns), which is one order of magnitude smaller than what we observed as effective amplitude of the retina in our study. This full movement can be measured using a very simple device, but a mechanical interpretation becomes more complicated.

We compared the amplitude of the two most important frequency components. Fig. 3 (b) shows the ratio between the integrated signal under the second harmonic and fundamental peaks of the movements (R_{Mvt}). Within a specific cohort, there is no significant difference of R_{Mvt} between the macula and the optic disk. In most cases, the fundamental frequency integrates the majority of the power as mean R_{Mvt} values are below unity.

Table 1. Characteristics of young healthy, old healthy and old glaucoma subjects.

Parameter	Younger Healthy	Older Healthy	Older Glaucoma
Age (years)	35±7	60±12	60±10
Sex (F/M)	5/6	7/5	9/6
Heart Rate (Hz)	1.19±0.16	1.19±0.12	1.14±0.13
Blood pressure (systolic)	115±10	125±9	118±13
Blood pressure (diastolic)	72±7	81±4	73±7

However, younger individual present mean R_{Mvt} values higher than one, which means that the second harmonic is the dominant frequency of the movement. Statistical analysis reveals that R_{Mvt} is definitely higher in younger healthy individuals than in older healthy subjects at both the macula ($p=0.042$) and the optic disk ($p=0.018$). This ratio is also higher for glaucoma patients in comparison to age-matched healthy individuals, though this difference is solely significant at the optic disk ($p=0.029$).

Next, we compared the temporal delays between the heart signal and the different frequency components. We present in Fig. 3 (c) these phase shifts between the movement fundamental frequency with respect to the oximeter signal fundamental frequency at the macula and the optic disk (Θ). Significant differences between the three groups are obtained at the macula, where both young healthy individuals ($p=0.041$) and glaucoma patients ($p=0.044$) present higher phase shift values than the ones obtained for older healthy people.

Finally, we present in Fig. 3 (d) the phase shifts between the second harmonic and the fundamental frequency component of the movement (Π_{Mvt}) at the macula and the optic disk. Non negligible differences between the three groups are obtained at the macula, where both young healthy subjects ($p=0.063$) and glaucoma patients ($p=0.059$) present lower phase shift values than the ones obtained for older healthy individuals, but these differences did not reach statistical significance.

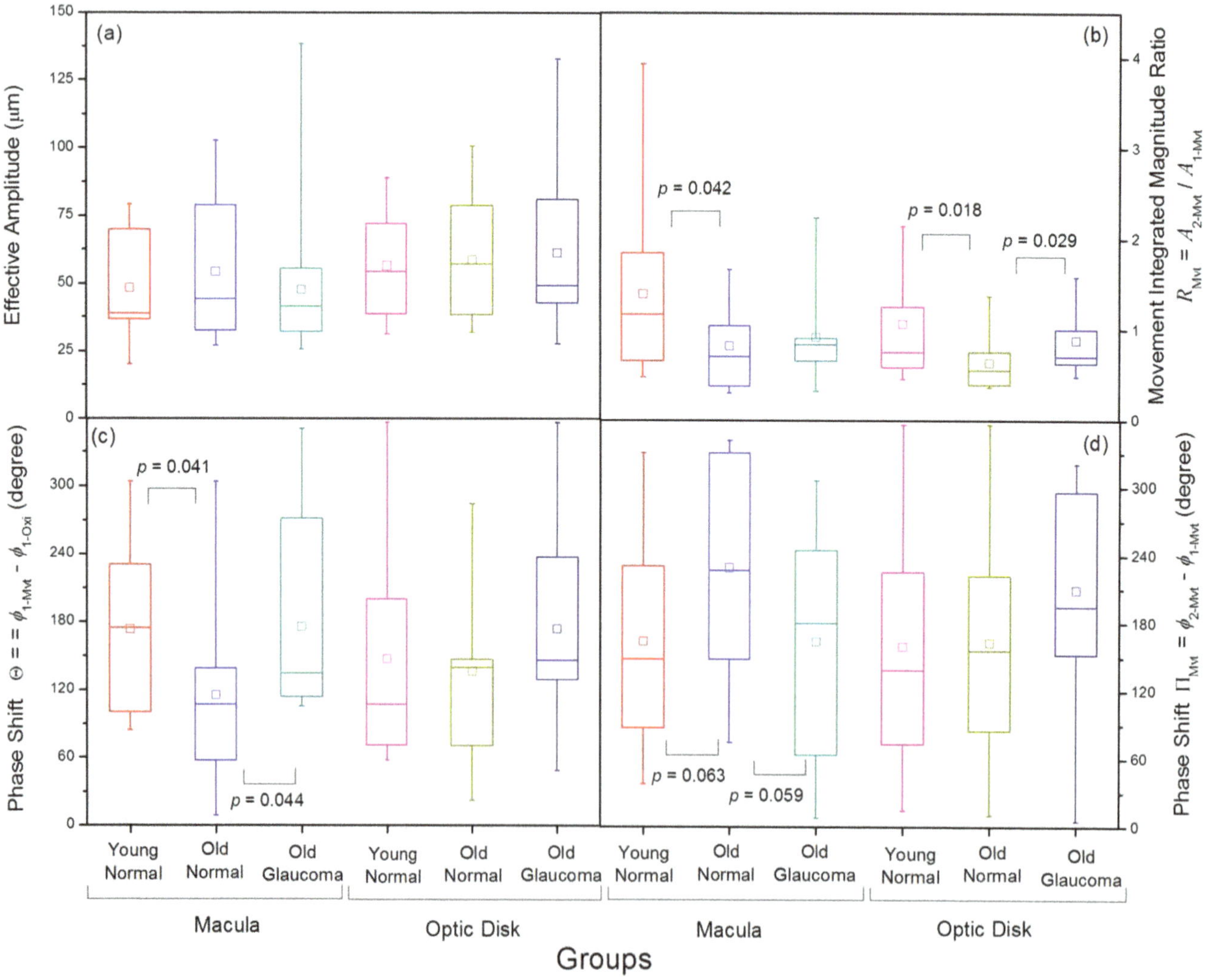

Figure 3. Eye movement at the macula and optic disk region was investigated for the three subject groups. In (a) are compared the effective amplitude of the movement, in (b) the FFT integrated amplitude ratio between the movement fundamental frequency and the movement second harmonic, in (c) the phase shift between the movement fundamental frequency with respect to the oximeter signal fundamental frequency, and in (d) the phase shift between the movement second harmonic with respect to movement fundamental frequency.

Discussion

The results displayed in Fig. 3 showed that the pulsatile eye movement could readily be described in the frequency domain. We found a few parameters that characterize the three groups of individuals by analyzing the movement of the retinal tissue at two locations, using a simple, low-cost interferometric device. Our analysis revealed that the power spectral ratio between the second harmonic and the fundamental frequency components of the movement (R_{Mvt}), the phase shift between the second harmonic and the fundamental frequency components of the movement (Θ), and the phase shift between the fundamental frequency of the movement with respect to the oximeter fundamental frequency (Π_{Mvt}) can be used as parameters to differentiate cohorts with respect to the individuals average age (35 vs 60 years old) and eye condition (normal vs glaucoma). Although, these parameters showed similar tendencies among the various groups, more distinctive differences (lower p values) were obtained at the macula. This is probably due to the lower tissue reflectivity at the optic disk compared to the macula, which considerably reduces the overall quality of the data.

An important feature that our study demonstrates is that all groups of subjects showed comparable effective amplitudes of the movement at both the macula and optic disk. This indicates that changes of the eye hemodynamic and biomechanical properties can be detected on the pulse waveform and phase with respect to the heart signal rather than simply the amplitude. The observed differences among different cohorts can be attributed to changes in the biomechanical properties such as stiffening of the eye with age or disease. These biomechanical changes are observed as different time delays between blood-flow-driven oscillations in separate regions of the eye. Nevertheless, it remains speculative to provide an insightful explanation or a mechanical model for this. Although it has been found previously that older eyes are more rigid than the younger eyes, the exact mechanism through which the biomechanical properties of the eye get modified with the progression of the age are not well understood.

Previous investigations of arterial blood pressure have associated higher harmonics in vessel displacement to vascular impedance, which depends on the dimension and viscoelastic properties of arteries, in addition to the viscoelastic properties of the blood. [16] Based on these results, we can postulate that the observed variations of R_{Mvt}, Θ and Π_{Mvt} are directly related to differences in the ocular vascular status. However, it is important to note that the eye movement from which our analysis is derived is not solely dependent on the eye's vasculature. Indeed, the retinal tissue kinematics is also likely to dependent on the impedance of scleral tissue. Therefore, even if SD-LCI along with exhaustive spectrum analysis could become a method to characterize ocular tissues, it is still premature to fully identify the hemodynamic status and the biomechanical properties from the eye kinematics.

Conclusion

Our study showed that spectral decomposition of the pulsatile retinal movements measured with a non-invasive SD-LCI system could be used to characterize the response of retinal and optic nerve head tissues to the cardiac pulsation. The power spectral ratio between the fundamental and second harmonic components of the movement, the phase shift between these two harmonics, and the phase shift between the movement and the cardiac pulses showed distinctive signatures between the groups we compared.

It is important to state that further studies with larger cohorts are required to determine whether our findings will have physiological and clinical utility in glaucoma diagnosis. Furthermore, a better physical description of the movement of the different eyes tissues will help us improve this description and the details of how these movements are described. Overall, this study seeks to show how axial retinal displacements measured with our SD-LCI could be a promising method to differentiate individuals with different ocular hemodynamic and/or biomechanical properties. As a first step towards a potential screening method for glaucoma, we succeeded in defining parameters to group the individuals we analyzed related to their age and eye pathology.

Supporting Information

Figure S1 The FFT of recorder movement of the macula (red) and of the heart signal (green) is shown. The corresponding phase difference between the heart signal and macula movement is shown in blue. The arrows points to the corresponding y-axis.

Figure S2 A-Scans of the optic disc for the two extremes of the movement cycle.

Figure S3 A-Scans of the macula for the two extremes of the movement cycle.

Table S1

Acknowledgments

This paper is published posthumously following the untimely death of Carolyne Dion, who will be missed by her colleagues, family and friends.

Author Contributions

Conceived and designed the experiments: CD KS TO MRL SC. Performed the experiments: CD KS. Analyzed the data: CD SC. Contributed reagents/materials/analysis tools: TO MRL SC. Wrote the paper: CD KS MRL SC.

References

1. Wolfs RCW, Borger PH, Ramrattan RS, Klaver CCW, Hulsman CAA, et al. (2000) Changing Views on Open-Angle Glaucoma: Definitions and Prevalencesâ€"The Rotterdam Study. Investigative Ophthalmology & Visual Science 41: 3309–3321.
2. Lesk MR, Hafez AS, Descovich D (2006) Relationship between central corneal thickness and changes of optic nerve head topography and blood flow after intraocular pressure reduction in open-angle glaucoma and ocular hypertension. Archives of Ophthalmology 124: 1568–1572.
3. Downs JCP, Roberts MDP, Burgoyne CFM (2008) Mechanical Environment of the Optic Nerve Head in Glaucoma. Optometry & Vision Science 85: E425–E435.
4. Hommer A, Fuchsjager-Mayrl G, Resch H, Vass C, Garhofer G, et al. (2008) Estimation of ocular rigidity based on measurement of pulse amplitude using pneumotonometry and fundus pulse using laser interferometry in glaucoma. Investigative Ophthalmology & Visual Science 49: 4046–4050.
5. Mangouritsas G, Morphis G, Mourtzoukos S, Feretis E (2008) Association between corneal hysteresis and central corneal thickness in glaucomatous and non-glaucomatous eyes. Acta Ophthalmologica Articles online in advance of print.
6. Flammer J, Orgul S, Costa VP, Orzalesi N, Krieglstein GK, et al. (2002) The impact of ocular blood flow in glaucoma. Progress in Retinal and Eye Research 21: 359–393.
7. Garzozi HJ, Shoham N, Chung HS, Kagemann L, Harris A (2001) Ocular blood flow measurements and their importance in glaucoma and age-related macular degeneration. Israel Medical Association Journal 3: 443–448.
8. Silver DM, Farrell RA (1994) Validity of pulsatile ocular blood flow measurements. Survey of Ophthalmology 38: S72–S80.

9. James CB, Smith SE (1991) Pulsatile ocular blood-flow in patients with low tension glaucoma. British Journal of Ophthalmology 75: 466–470.
10. Kerr J, Nelson P, O'Brien C (1998) A comparison of ocular blood flow in untreated primary open-angle glaucoma and ocular hypertension. American Journal of Ophthalmology 126: 42–51.
11. Schmidt K-G, Von Ruckmann A, Mittag TW, Hessemer V, Pillunat LE (1997) Reduced ocular pulse amplitude in low tension glaucoma is independent of vasospasm. Eye 11: 485–488.
12. Evans DW, Hosking SL, Embleton SJ, Morgan AJ, Bartlett JD (2002) Spectral content of the intraocular pressure pulse wave: glaucoma patients versus normal subjects. Graefes Archive for Clinical and Experimental Ophthalmology 240: 475–480.
13. Bosley T, Cohen M, Gee W, Reed J, 3d, Sergott R, et al. (1993) Amplitude of the ocular pneumoplethysmography waveform is correlated with cardiac output. Stroke 24: 6–9.
14. Krakau CET, Lindberg S, Havelius U (1995) An instrument for recording the ocular pulse wave. Acta Ophthalmologica Scandinavica 73: 472–474.
15. Nichols W, Conti C, Walker W, Milnor W (1977) Input impedance of the systemic circulation in man. Circulation Research 40: 451–458.
16. Nichols WW, O'Rourke MF, Hartley C, McDonald DA (1998) Arnold; Oxford University Press.
17. Finkelstein SM, Collins VR, Cohn JN (1988) Arterial Vascular Compliance Response to Vasodilators by Fourier and Pulse Countour Analysis. Hypertension 12: 380–387.
18. Hu HH, Kuo T, Wong WJ, Luk YO, Chern CM, et al. (1999) Transfer function analysis of cerebral hemodynamics in patients with carotid stenosis. Journal of Cerebral Blood Flow and Metabolism 19: 460–465.
19. Kuo TBJ, Chern CM, Sheng WY, Wong WJ, Hu HH (1998) Frequency domain analysis of cerebral blood flow velocity and its correlation with arterial blood pressure. Journal of Cerebral Blood Flow and Metabolism 18: 311–318.
20. Findlay JM (1971) Frequency analysis of human involuntary eye movement. Kybernetik 8: 207–214.
21. Bolger C, Bojanic S, Sheahan NF, Coakley D, Malone JF (1999) Dominant frequency content of ocular microtremor from normal subjects. Vision Research 39: 1911–1915.
22. Kasprzak H, Iskander DR, Bajraszewski T, Kowalczyk A, Nowak-Szczepanowska W (2007) High accuracy measurement of spectral characteristics of movements of the eye elements. Optica Pura Y Aplicada 70: 7–11.
23. Nowak W, Hachol A, Kasprzak H (2008) Time-frequency analysis of spontaneous fluctuation of the pupil size of the human eye. Optica Applicata 38: 469–480.
24. Kowalska MA, Kasprzak HT, Iskander DR, Danielewska M, Mas D (2011) Ultrasonic In Vivo Measurement of Ocular Surface Expansion. Biomedical Engineering, IEEE Transactions on 58: 674–680.
25. Kasprzak HT, Iskander DR (2007) Spectral characteristics of longitudinal corneal apex velocities and their relation to the cardiopulmonary system. Eye 21: 1212–1219.
26. Singh K, Dion C, Costantino S, Wajszilber M, Lesk MR, et al. Development of a novel instrument to measure the pulsatile movement of ocular tissues. Experimental Eye Research 91: 63–68.
27. Singh K, Dion C, Wajszilber M, Ozaki T, Lesk MR, et al. Measurement of Ocular Fundus Pulsation in Healthy Subjects Using a Novel Fourier-Domain Optical Coherence Tomography. Investigative Ophthalmology & Visual Science 52: 8927–8932.
28. Plumb RD, Hamilton PK, Rea DJ, Wright SA, Hughes SM, et al. (2011) Wave reflection signatures: identifying early microvascular abnormalities in type 2 diabetes. The British Journal of Diabetes & Vascular Disease 11: 243–248.
29. Dragostinoff N, Werkmeister RM, Groschl M, Schmetterer L (2009) Depth-resolved measurement of ocular fundus pulsations by low-coherence tissue interferometry. Journal of Biomedical Optics 14: 054047.
30. Singh K, Dion C, Godin AG, Lorghaba F, Descovich D, et al. (2012) Pulsatile Movement of the Optic Nerve Head and the Peripapillary Retina in Normal Subjects and in Glaucoma. Investigative Ophthalmology & Visual Science.
31. Delori FC, Webb RH, Sliney DH (2007) Maximum permissible exposures for ocular safety (ANSI 2000), with emphasis on ophthalmic devices. Journal of the Optical Society of America A 24: 1250–1265.
32. Witte S, Baclayon M, Peterman EJ, Toonen RF, Mansvelder HD, et al. (2009) Single-shot two-dimensional full-range optical coherence tomography achieved by dispersion control. Optics Express 17: 11335–11349.
33. Hodapp E, Parrish RKI, Anderson DR (1993) Clinical decisions in glaucoma. St Louis: The CV Mosby Co.

18

Peripapillary Retinal Nerve Fiber Layer Assessment of Spectral Domain Optical Coherence Tomography and Scanning Laser Polarimetry to Diagnose Preperimetric Glaucoma

Harsha L. Rao*, Ravi K. Yadav, Uday K. Addepalli, Shashikant Chaudhary, Sirisha Senthil, Nikhil S. Choudhari, Chandra S. Garudadri

VST Glaucoma Center, L V Prasad Eye Institute, Banjara Hills, Hyderabad, India

Abstract

Purpose: To compare the abilities of peripapillary retinal nerve fiber layer (RNFL) parameters of spectral domain optical coherence tomograph (SDOCT) and scanning laser polarimeter (GDx enhanced corneal compensation; ECC) in detecting preperimetric glaucoma.

Methods: In a cross-sectional study, 35 preperimetric glaucoma eyes (32 subjects) and 94 control eyes (74 subjects) underwent digital optic disc photography and RNFL imaging with SDOCT and GDx ECC. Ability of RNFL parameters of SDOCT and GDx ECC to discriminate preperimetric glaucoma eyes from control eyes was compared using area under receiver operating characteristic curves (AUC), sensitivities at fixed specificities and likelihood ratios (LR).

Results: AUC of the global average RNFL thickness of SDOCT (0.786) was significantly greater ($p<0.001$) than that of GDx ECC (0.627). Sensitivities at 95% specificity of the corresponding parameters were 20% and 8.6% respectively. AUCs of the inferior, superior and temporal quadrant RNFL thickness parameters of SDOCT were also significantly ($p<0.05$) greater than the respective RNFL parameters of GDx ECC. LRs of outside normal limits category of SDOCT parameters ranged between 3.3 and 4.0 while the same of GDx ECC parameters ranged between 1.2 and 2.1. LRs of within normal limits category of SDOCT parameters ranged between 0.4 and 0.7 while the same of GDx ECC parameters ranged between 0.7 and 1.0.

Conclusions: Abilities of the RNFL parameters of SDOCT and GDx ECC to diagnose preperimetric glaucoma were only moderate. Diagnostic abilities of the RNFL parameters of SDOCT were significantly better than that of GDx ECC in preperimetric glaucoma.

Editor: Sanjoy Bhattacharya, Bascom Palmer Eye Institute, University of Miami School of Medicine, United States of America

Funding: The authors have no support or funding to report.

Competing Interests: The authors have declared that no competing interests exist.

* Email: harshalaxmanarao@gmail.com

Introduction

Spectral domain optical coherence tomography (SDOCT) and scanning laser polarimetry (SLP) are the two currently used common imaging techniques for peripapillary retinal nerve fiber layer (RNFL) evaluation in glaucoma. SDOCT is a recent technique which enables imaging the ocular structures with higher resolution and faster scan rate compared to the previous version of this technology (Stratus OCT, Carl Zeiss Meditec, Inc., Dublin, CA) [1,2]. GDx (Carl Zeiss Meditec Inc. Dublin, CA), the commonly used SLP device measures the RNFL birefringence in vivo and is based on the principle that polarized light passing through the birefringent RNFL undergoes a measurable phase shift, known as retardation, which is linearly related to the RNFL tissue thickness [3]. The current SLP protocol, called the enhanced corneal compensation (ECC), optimizes imaging by improving the signal-to-noise ratio compared to the previous version (GDx Variable Corneal Compensation) [4–6].

Though numerous studies have reported good diagnostic ability of both SDOCT [7–11] and GDx ECC [12–14] in glaucoma, there is limited literature on head to head comparison of these imaging techniques in the same population [15,16]. Also, most of these studies have employed a case-control design including glaucoma patients (cases), defined based on the presence of repeatable characteristic glaucomatous visual field (VF) defects; and normal subjects (controls), usually recruited from the general population and having normal intraocular pressures (IOP), healthy appearance of the optic nerve and normal VFs. However, in clinical practice, a diagnostic test is used to rule-in disease in very early stages (preferably in preperimetric stages of glaucoma) or rule-out disease in subjects suspected of having disease. In a previous study, we compared the diagnostic abilities of the RNFL parameters of SDOCT and GDx ECC in perimetric glaucoma and found them to be comparable [17]. However there were indications of SDOCT being better in early stages of perimetric glaucoma. With this background, the purpose of the current study was to compare the abilities of RNFL parameters of SDOCT and GDx ECC in detecting preperimetric glaucoma.

Methods

This was an observational, cross-sectional study of consecutive subjects referred by general ophthalmologists to a tertiary eye care facility between September 2010 and November 2012 as glaucoma suspects based on the optic disc appearance. Written informed consent was obtained from all participants and the Ethics Committee of L V Prasad Eye Institute approved the methodology. All methods adhered to the tenets of the Declaration of Helsinki for research involving human subjects.

Inclusion criteria were age ≥18 years, best corrected visual acuity of 20/40 or better and refractive error within ±5.0 D sphere and ±3 D cylinder. Exclusion criteria were presence of any media opacities that prevented good imaging and any retinal (including macular) or neurological diseases other than glaucoma which could confound the results of visual field examination and RNFL measurements with SDOCT or SLP. All participants underwent a comprehensive ocular examination which included a detailed medical history, best corrected visual acuity measurement, slit-lamp biomicroscopy, Goldmann applanation tonometry, gonioscopy, dilated fundus examination, digital optic disc photography, standard automated perimetry (SAP) and RNFL imaging with SDOCT and SLP.

SAP was performed using a Humphrey Field analyzer, model 750 (Zeiss Humphrey Systems, Dublin, CA), with the Swedish interactive threshold algorithm (SITA) standard 24-2 program. VFs with fixation losses, false positive and false negative response rates of less than 20% were considered reliable. VFs were considered glaucomatous if the pattern standard deviation had a P value of less than 5% and the glaucoma hemifield test result was outside normal limits [18]. VFs were considered normal if the above 2 criteria were not satisfied. For the study, we included all subjects with reliable and normal SAP results.

Digital optic disc photographs were obtained by trained technicians (FF 450plus, Carl Zeiss Meditec Systems GmbH, Pirmasens, Germany). Photographs consisted of a 50 degree image centered on the optic disc, a similar image centered on the macula, a 30 degree image centered on the optic disc and a 20 degree image centered on the disc. All these images also consisted of one colored and one red-free image each. The photographs were evaluated by two experts independently, who were masked to the clinical examination results of the subjects and also the results of visual field and imaging examinations. Experts classified the optic disc photographs into glaucomatous and non-glaucomatous based on the presence of focal or diffuse neuroretinal rim thinning, localized notching or nerve fiber layer defects. Discrepancies between the two experts were resolved by consensus. Eyes, where a classification to either glaucoma or control group was not possible by both the experts, were labeled as "suspects" and excluded from the analysis.

SDOCT examination was performed with the RTVue (software version 5.1.0.90). RTVue uses a scanning laser diode with a wavelength of 840±10 nm to provide images of ocular microstructures. The protocol used for RNFL imaging with RTVue in this study was ONH (optic nerve head) scan. This protocol has been explained earlier [19,20]. In brief, ONH protocol consists of 12 radial scans 3.4 mm in length and 6 concentric ring scans ranging from 2.5 to 4.0 mm in diameter all centered on the optic disc. ONH protocol calculates various parameters that describe the ONH and also generates a polar RNFL thickness map which is the RNFL thickness measured along a circle of 3.45 mm in diameter centered on the optic disc. The RNFL parameters generated and used in the study were temporal average (temporal 90 degree), superior average (superior 90 degree), nasal average (nasal 90 degree), inferior average (inferior 90 degree) and global average (over 360 degree). The RNFL parameters are also compared with the internal normative database of 861 eyes of different ethnicities within the software and one of the three diagnostic categorizations is provided. "Outside normal limits" categorization indicates that the value is lesser than the lower 99% confidence interval (CI) of the healthy, age-matched population. "Borderline" result indicates that the value is between the 95% and 99% CI, and a "within-normal-limits" indicates that the value is within the 95% CI. Only well-centered images with a signal strength index (SSI) of ≥30 were used for analysis. RNFL segmentation was inspected manually by one of the experts (HLR) and eyes in which the segmentation algorithm failed were excluded.

SLP examination was done using GDxPRO (version 1.1.1, Carl Zeiss Meditec Inc. Dublin, CA). The general principles of SLP and the algorithm used for ECC have been described in detail previously [3,5,12]. A corneal scan was obtained in all the participants before the RNFL scan to measure the corneal birefringence. Scan image was checked for focus, alignment and movement artifacts. All corneal scans had a quality score of ≥8. Following corneal scan acquisition, the macular ellipse was manually centered on the macular bow tie pattern. Macular bow tie pattern was well defined in all the eyes. RNFL was imaged using a single scan protocol. A fixed concentric measurement band centered on the optic disc with a 3.2-mm outer and a 2.4-mm inner diameter was used to generate the peripapillary retardation measurements. The parameters generated on the printout and used in this study were temporal average (temporal 50 degree), superior average (superior 120 degree), nasal average (nasal 70 degree), inferior average (inferior 120 degree), TSNIT (temporal superior nasal inferior and temporal) average (over 360 degree) and nerve fiber indicator (NFI). The NFI is a support vector machine score based on several RNFL measures and assigns a number from 0 to 100 to each eye. The higher the NFI, the greater is the likelihood of having glaucoma. NFI value of less than 30 is considered "within normal limits", 30 to 50 is considered "borderline" and more than 50 is considered "outside normal limits". The superior, inferior and TSNIT average are also compared with the internal normative database of 251 subjects within the software and one of the three diagnostic categorizations as with SDOCT is provided. Only well-focused, centered and illuminated images with a quality score of ≥7, typical scan score (TSS)>80 and a residual anterior segment retardation of ≤4 were included for analysis.

Participants had all examinations as well as RNFL imaging with SDOCT and SLP performed on the same day.

Statistical analysis

Descriptive statistics included mean and standard deviation for normally distributed variables and median and inter-quartile range (IQR) for non-normally distributed variables. Receiver operating characteristic (ROC) curves were used to describe the ability of RNFL parameters of both SDOCT and GDx ECC to discriminate glaucomatous eyes from control eyes. Sensitivities at

Table 1. Demographic and visual field characteristics of the patients.

	Control group (n = 94 eyes)	Glaucoma group (n = 35 eyes)	P value
Age (years)	51±13	53±12	0.61
Disc area (mm²)	2.21 (1.84, 2.55)	1.97 (1.45, 2.32)	0.02
Mean deviation (dB)	−1.68 (−2.71, −0.71)	−2.13 (−3.10, −0.84)	0.35
Pattern standard deviation (dB)	1.69 (1.53, 2.08)	1.74 (1.54, 2.25)	0.54
Visual field index (%)	99 (98, 99)	99 (97, 99)	0.33

dB: decibel. All values are median and inter-quartile ranges unless specified.

fixed specificities of 80% and 95% were determined for all the parameters. To obtain confidence intervals for area under the ROC curves (AUC) and sensitivities, a bootstrap re-sampling procedure was used (n = 1000 re-samples). As measurements from both eyes of the same subject are likely to be correlated, the standard statistical methods for parameter estimation lead to underestimation of standard errors and to confidence intervals that are too narrow [21]. Therefore, the cluster of data for the study subject was considered as the unit of resampling and bias corrected standard error was calculated during all estimations. This procedure has been used in literature to adjust for the presence of multiple correlated measurements from the same unit [22,23]. Likelihood ratios (LR) were reported for diagnostic categorization (outside normal limits, borderline, or within normal limits) provided after comparison with the instrument's internal normative database. LR is the probability of a given test result in those with disease divided by the probability of the same test result in those without the disease [24–26]. The LR for a given test result indicates how much that result will raise or lower the probability of disease. A LR of 1 or close to 1 would mean that the test provides no additional information about the post-test probability of the disease. LRs higher than 10 or lower than 0.1 would be associated with large effects on post-test probability, LRs from 5 to 10 or from 0.1 to 0.2 would be associated with moderate effects, LRs from 2 to 5 or from 0.2 to 0.5 would be associated with small effects [24]. The 95% CIs for LRs were calculated according to the method proposed by Simel et al. [27].

Statistical analyses were performed using commercial software (Stata ver. 12.1; StataCorp, College Station, TX). A p value of < 0.05 was considered statically significant.

Results

Three hundred and forty three eyes of 255 consecutive subjects referred for glaucoma evaluation to our center were analyzed. Twenty eight eyes with unreliable VFs, 2 eyes with poor quality disc photographs, 9 eyes with SSI of less than 30 on SDOCT and 28 eyes with either a quality score of <7, TSS value of <80 or residual anterior segment retardation of>4 on GDx ECC were excluded. Of the remaining, 121 eyes with glaucomatous VFs were excluded, leaving behind 155 eyes with normal VFs. Of these, 26 eyes classified as "disc suspects" by both glaucoma experts were excluded. Of the remaining 129 eyes, 35 eyes of 32 subjects with the optic disc classification as "glaucoma" formed the preperimetric glaucoma group and 94 eyes of 74 subjects with optic disc classification as "non-glaucoma" formed the control group. Table 1 shows that age and visual field parameters of the two groups were comparable. Glaucoma patients had significantly smaller optic discs than the control subjects. Figure 1 shows normal optic disc and RNFL on disc photograph (a), normal RNFL thickness on SDOCT (b) and normal RNFL birefringence on GDx ECC (c) in an eye in the control group. Figure 2 shows an eye in the preperimetric glaucoma group with glaucomatous optic disc and RNFL defects superiorly and inferiorly on disc photograph (a), corresponding RNFL thinning on SDOCT (b)

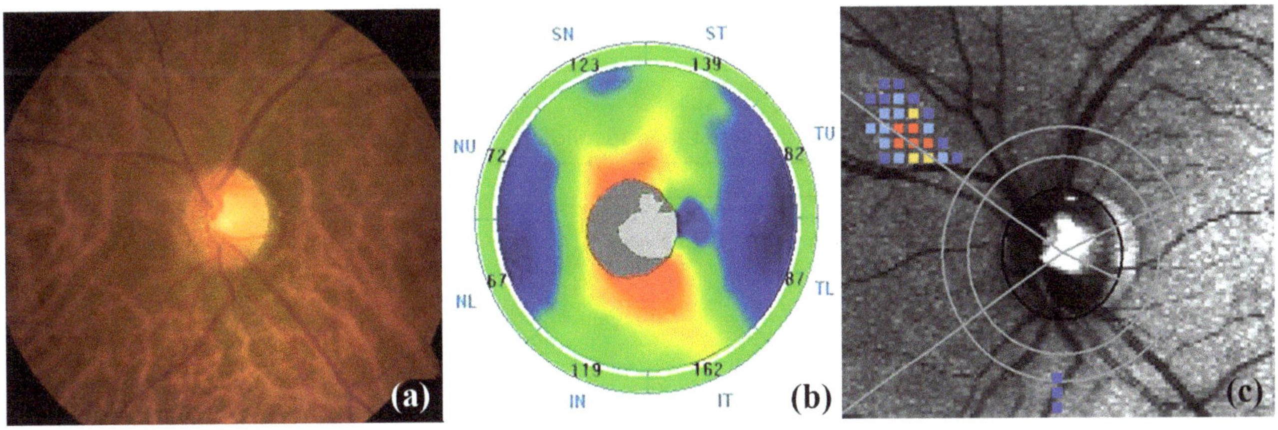

Figure 1. Representative image of an eye in the control group showing normal optic disc and retinal nerve fiber layer (RNFL) on disc photograph (a), normal RNFL thickness on spectral domain optic coherence tomography (b) and normal RNFL birefringence on GDx enhanced corneal compensation (c).

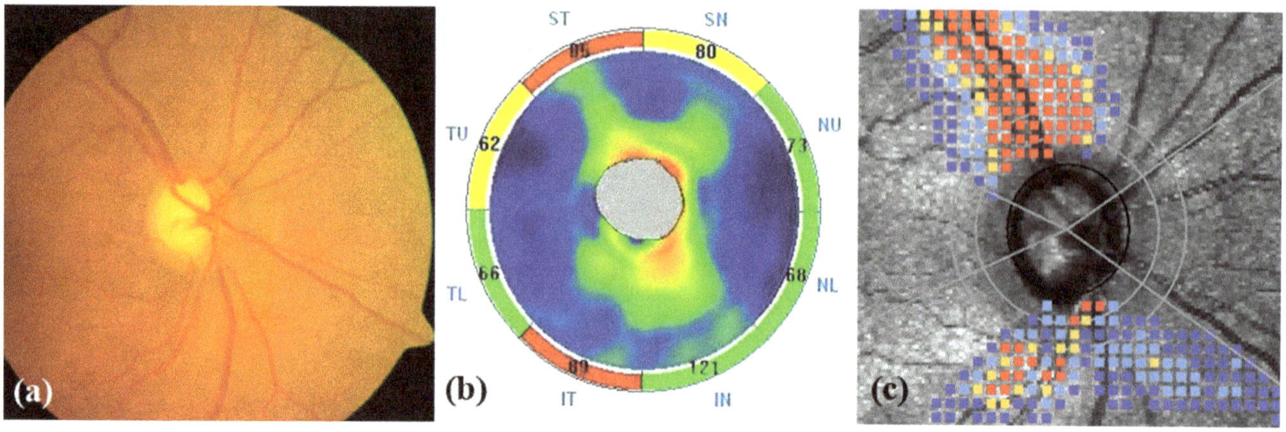

Figure 2. Representative image of an eye in the preperimetric glaucoma group showing glaucomatous optic disc with retinal nerve fiber layer (RNFL) defects superiorly and inferiorly (a), corresponding RNFL thickness abnormalities on spectral domain optic coherence tomography (b) and corresponding abnormal RNFL birefringence on GDx enhanced corneal compensation (c).

and corresponding RNFL birefringence abnormality on GDx ECC (c). VFs were normal in both the above eyes.

Table 2 shows the RNFL parameters of SDOCT in the two groups of participants. All RNFL parameters of SDOCT were significantly thinner in the glaucoma group compared to the control group. AUC and sensitivities at fixed specificities after adjusting for the differences in the disc area between the 2 groups using covariate-adjustment, as proposed by Pepe [28], are also shown in Table 2. Average, inferior and temporal RNFL thickness parameters showed the best AUCs and sensitivities at fixed specificities of 95% and 80%.

Table 3 shows the RNFL parameters of GDx ECC in the two groups of participants. Quality score and TSS were comparable between the groups, while residual anterior segment retardance was more in the glaucoma group. All RNFL parameters except the temporal and nasal quadrant RNFL measurements were significantly lesser in the glaucoma group. NFI value was significantly higher in the glaucoma group. AUC and sensitivities at fixed specificities after adjusting for the differences in the disc area between the 2 groups are also shown in Table 3. NFI and inferior quadrant RNFL parameter showed the best AUCs.

Except for the nasal quadrant measurements ($p = 0.77$), AUCs of all SDOCT RNFL measurements were significantly greater ($p < 0.05$) than the corresponding GDx ECC measurements in diagnosing preperimetric glaucoma. Figure 3 shows the ROC curves of the quadrant and overall average RNFL thickness parameters of SDOCT and GDx ECC.

Table 4 shows the LRs associated with the diagnostic categorization of the SDOCT and GDx ECC parameters after comparison with the respective instrument's internal normative database. Outside normal limits categories of SDOCT parameters were associated with small effects on the post-test probability of disease while that of GDx ECC parameters were associated with no effects. Within normal limits category of inferior quadrant RNFL average of SDOCT was associated with small effects on the post-test probability of disease. Within normal limits category of other SDOCT parameters and all GDx ECC parameters, and borderline categories of the RNFL parameters of both SDOCT and GDx ECC were associated with no effect on the post-test probability of glaucoma.

Discussion

In this study to compare the abilities of RNFL parameters of SDOCT and GDx ECC in diagnosing preperimetric glaucoma, we found that most of the SDOCT RNFL parameters were significantly better than the corresponding GDx ECC parameters.

Recent studies have compared the RNFL parameters of SDOCT and GDx ECC in perimetric glaucoma and have found that the diagnostic abilities were comparable [15–17]. Garas et

Table 2. Mean values of SDOCT retinal nerve fiber layer thickness parameters in glaucoma and control eyes with areas under the receiver operating characteristic curves and sensitivities at fixed specificities.

Retinal nerve fiber layer parameters (in microns)	Control (Mean ± SD)	Glaucoma (Mean ± SD)	P value	AUC	Sensitivity at 95% specificity	Sensitivity at 80% specificity
Signal strength index	51±10	51±9	0.98			
Temporal quadrant	79.0±10.8	69.8±9.7	<0.001	0.762 (0.631–0.851)	28.6% (2.6–53.2)	62.9% (43.8–80.5)
Superior quadrant	123.9±19.1	109.2±15.1	<0.001	0.701 (0.585–0.797)	22.9% (8.8–45.8)	45.7% (25.8–67.5)
Nasal quadrant	79.6±12.0	72.9±14.6	0.01	0.604 (0.486–0.731)	25.7% (12.8–44.7)	42.9% (26.4–62.1)
Inferior quadrant	128.2±20.1	108.9±17.4	<0.001	0.752 (0.634–0.842)	22.9% (7.7–45.7)	57.1% (30.4–80.5)
Average thickness	102.7±11.6	90.2±9.7	<0.001	0.786 (0.676–0.866)	20.0% (3.4–40.0)	45.7% (19.4–68.4)

SDOCT: spectral domain optical coherence tomograph; SD: standard deviation; AUC: area under the receiver operating characteristic curve; Figures in brackets are 95% confidence intervals. AUCs and sensitivities are adjusted for the difference in disc area between the control and glaucoma group.

Table 3. Mean values of GDx ECC retinal nerve fiber layer parameters in glaucoma and control eyes with areas under the receiver operating characteristic curves and sensitivities at fixed specificities.

Retinal nerve fiber layer parameters (in microns)	Control (Mean ± SD)	Glaucoma (Mean ± SD)	P value	AUC	Sensitivity at 95% specificity	Sensitivity at 80% specificity
Quality score*	9 (9, 9)	9 (9, 9)	0.77			
Typical scan score*	100 (99, 100)	100 (99, 100)	0.94			
Residual retardation*	1 (0, 2)	1 (1, 3)	0.03			
Temporal quadrant	19.8±6.6	19.9±7.9	0.88	0.521 (0.393–0.645)	11.4% (2.9-30.0)	28.6% (7.1–54.8)
Superior quadrant	56.7±10.2	52.1±10.0	0.02	0.598 (0.493–0.692)	11.4% (2.6-23.1)	22.9% (7.9–38.1)
Nasal quadrant	34.2±7.8	31.4±8.2	0.07	0.622 (0.517–0.743)	8.6% (2.4-19.2)	28.6% (8.0–54.8)
Inferior quadrant	57.7±9.9	52.2±10.4	0.01	0.632 (0.518–0.728)	8.6% (2.3-22.2)	28.6% (11.4–50.0)
Average	47.5±6.6	43.5±7.1	0.004	0.627 (0.513–0.728)	8.6% (2.0-18.5)	37.1% (22.2–54.8)
NFI*	27 (17, 42)	39 (28, 54)	0.001	0.671 (0.580–0.780)	14.3% (2.9-28.6)	34.3% (16.3–55.6)

ECC: enhanced corneal compensation; SD: standard deviation; AUC: area under the receiver operating characteristic curve; CI: confidence interval; NFI: nerve fiber indicator; *median with inter-quartile range. AUCs and sensitivities are adjusted for the difference in disc area between the control and glaucoma group.

al.[16] though had a group of preperimetric glaucoma subjects in their study, did not analyze the results separately in this subgroup.

It is important to note that the RNFL quadrants on the printouts of SDOCT and GDx ECC are not exactly similar. The 4 RNFL quadrants of SDOCT are 90 degrees each while the superior and inferior quadrants of GDx ECC are 120 degrees, temporal quadrant is 50 degrees and nasal quadrant is 70 degrees. This might have resulted in some bias during comparison. But considering the fact that the parameters are used in clinical practice as in the printout, we decided to analyze them as such.

There are no studies in literature evaluating the diagnostic ability of GDx ECC in preperimetric glaucoma. There are however, studies evaluating the diagnostic ability of RNFL parameters of SDOCT in preperimetric glaucoma and the AUCs and sensitivities reported in these studies are better than those found in our study [29–35]. This is probably because of the difference in the control group of our study compared to other studies. The control group in our study was selected from the group of subjects referred as glaucoma suspects based on their optic disc appearance by general ophthalmologists. These subjects were however diagnosed as normals based on the optic disc evaluation by glaucoma experts and the normal VFs. Therefore in true sense, optic discs included in the control group though were referred as suspects for glaucoma, were not true suspects but were the ones that caused a diagnostic uncertainty among general ophthalmologists. Significantly larger disc size in the control group suggests that these were the eyes with large discs and large physiologic cups, mislabeled as "glaucoma suspects" by general ophthalmologists. There was however no ambiguity in their classification by the glaucoma experts. In case of ambiguity, optic discs were called "suspects" and excluded from the analysis. We believe that including a control group which is likely to cause some amount of diagnostic uncertainty is more meaningful and mimics the real-life clinical situation than a control group with no suspicious findings of the disease as was used in the previous studies. We have earlier reported the effect of such a control group on the diagnostic ability of SDOCT in early glaucoma [20] and preperimetric glaucoma [36]. There was also no ambiguity in the classification of preperimetric glaucoma eyes as two glaucoma experts agreed upon the presence of glaucomatous structural changes. Also upon unmasking the eyes after analysis, of the 29 subjects who had contributed one eye to the preperimetric glaucoma group, 23 (79%) had perimetric glaucoma in the fellow eye.

We found that the AUC and sensitivity at fixed specificities of temporal quadrant RNFL thickness with SDOCT was comparable to that of the inferior quadrant and average RNFL thickness. All previous studies with SDOCT have reported the diagnostic ability of temporal RNFL thickness to be significantly lower than that of the inferior quadrant and average RNFL thickness [7–11]. Though the reason for this finding in our study is unclear, it may be related to the local change in the RNFL that happens in the papillomacular bundle in preperimetric glaucoma. Future studies correlating the temporal RNFL thickness change with the macular

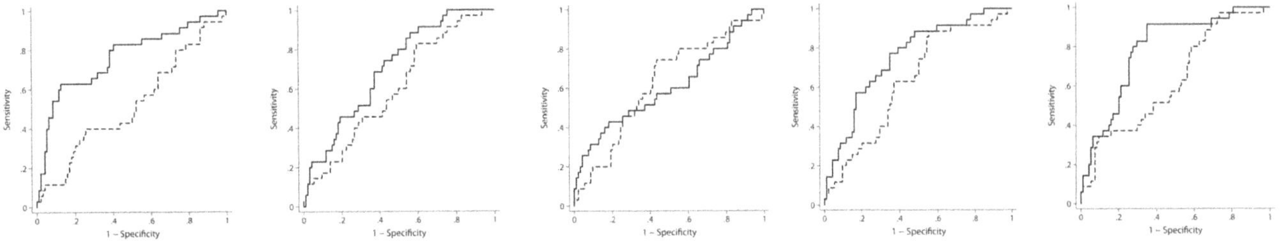

Figure 3. Receiver operating characteristic curves of the (a) temporal quadrant, (b) superior quadrant, (c) nasal quadrant, (d) inferior quadrant and (e) overall average retinal nerve fiber layer (RNFL) thickness parameters of spectral domain optical coherence tomography (solid line) and GDx enhanced corneal compensation (dashed line) in preperimetric glaucoma.

Table 4. Likelihood ratios (with 95% confidence interval)* of the normative database classification of SDOCT and GDx ECC parameters to discriminate glaucoma from control eyes.

RNFL Parameter	Within normal limits		Borderline		Outside normal limits	
	SDOCT	GDx ECC	SDOCT	GDx ECC	SDOCT	GDx ECC
Superior quadrant	0.68 (0.49–0.94)	0.95 (0.75–1.21)	1.05 (0.51–2.16)	1.04 (0.48–2.27)	3.26 (1.52–6.98)	1.19 (0.55–2.58)
Inferior quadrant	0.45 (0.27–0.74)	0.67 (0.45–1.00)	1.40 (0.65–3.01)	1.12 (0.60–2.10)	3.73 (2.10–6.62)	2.10 (1.16–3.80)
Average	0.66 (0.46–0.94)	0.71 (0.49–1.03)	2.44 (1.28–4.66)	0.81 (0.35–1.85)	3.99 (1.75–9.12)	1.79 (1.05–3.04)
Nerve fiber indicator		0.73 (0.52–1.04)		1.01 (0.52–1.96)		1.97 (1.05–3.72)

RNFL: retinal nerve fiber layer; SDOCT: spectral domain optical coherence tomograph; ECC: enhanced corneal compensation; SD: standard deviation.
* analysis based on number of eyes.

RNFL thickness change may be able to conclusively assess if this result is a true or a chance finding.

In addition to sensitivity, specificity and AUC, diagnostic tests can also be summarized in terms of LR. LR is higher than the other measures in hierarchy, as it expresses the magnitude by which the probability of a diagnosis in a given patient is modified by the results of the test [37–39]. In other words, the LR indicates how much a given diagnostic test result will change (increase or decrease) the pretest probability of the disease. We therefore evaluated the LRs associated with the diagnostic categorization of the RNFL parameter value, after comparison with the instrument's normative database. The magnitudes of the LRs associated with the outside normal limits category of SDOCT RNFL parameters were associated with small effects on the post-test probability of disease while that of GDx ECC parameters were associated with no effects. The "outside normal limits" category of SDOCT appeared to be better in "ruling in" glaucoma compared to that of GDX ECC. Within normal limits category of the inferior quadrant RNFL parameter of SDOCT was associated with small effects on the post-test probability of disease while that of all GDx ECC parameters were associated with no effects. This would mean that the "within normal limits" category of SDOCT may be better than GDx ECC in "ruling out" glaucoma. "Borderline" categories of both the devices were associated with no effects on the post-test probability of glaucoma, meaning that they were not useful either in "ruling in" or "ruling out" glaucoma. It should, however be noted that, in clinical practice even small effects on post-test probability may be relevant and useful, depending on the overall clinical picture and the pretest probability of disease.

A limitation of our study which might have inflated the diagnostic accuracy results, is the use of structural change on disc photographs as the gold standard while testing the technologies that once again evaluate the structural changes in glaucoma [40]. However, this is related to the lack of a good non-structural, reference standard for diagnosing glaucoma at this point in time in patients with normal SAP results. Though this might have affected the diagnostic accuracies, the effect on the comparison between devices may be minimal.

In conclusion, the abilities of RNFL parameters of SDOCT and GDx ECC to diagnose preperimetric glaucoma were only moderate. Diagnostic abilities of the RNFL parameters of SDOCT were significantly better than that of GDx ECC in preperimetric glaucoma.

Author Contributions

Conceived and designed the experiments: HLR RKY UKA SC SS NSC CSG. Performed the experiments: HLR RKY UKA SC SS NSC CSG. Analyzed the data: HLR. Contributed reagents/materials/analysis tools: HLR SS NSC CSG. Wrote the paper: HLR RKY UKA SC SS NSC CSG.

References

1. Nassif N, Cense B, Park B, Pierce M, Yun S, et al. (2004) In vivo high-resolution video-rate spectral-domain optical coherence tomography of the human retina and optic nerve. Opt Express 12: 367–376.
2. Wojtkowski M, Srinivasan V, Ko T, Fujimoto J, Kowalczyk A, et al. (2004) Ultrahigh-resolution, high-speed, Fourier domain optical coherence tomography and methods for dispersion compensation. Opt Express 12: 2404–2422.
3. Weinreb RN, Shakiba S, Zangwill L (1995) Scanning laser polarimetry to measure the nerve fiber layer of normal and glaucomatous eyes. Am J Ophthalmol 119: 627–636.
4. Toth M, Hollo G (2005) Enhanced corneal compensation for scanning laser polarimetry on eyes with atypical polarisation pattern. Br J Ophthalmol 89: 1139–1142.
5. Reus NJ, Zhou Q, Lemij HG (2006) Enhanced imaging algorithm for scanning laser polarimetry with variable corneal compensation. Invest Ophthalmol Vis Sci 47: 3870–3877.
6. Sehi M, Guaqueta DC, Greenfield DS (2006) An enhancement module to improve the atypical birefringence pattern using scanning laser polarimetry with variable corneal compensation. Br J Ophthalmol 90: 749–753.
7. Leung CK, Cheung CY, Weinreb RN, Qiu Q, Liu S, et al. (2009) Retinal nerve fiber layer imaging with spectral-domain optical coherence tomography: a variability and diagnostic performance study. Ophthalmology 116: 1257–1263, 1263 e1251–1252.
8. Knight OJ, Chang RT, Feuer WJ, Budenz DL (2009) Comparison of retinal nerve fiber layer measurements using time domain and spectral domain optical coherent tomography. Ophthalmology 116: 1271–1277.
9. Sung KR, Kim DY, Park SB, Kook MS (2009) Comparison of retinal nerve fiber layer thickness measured by Cirrus HD and Stratus optical coherence tomography. Ophthalmology 116: 1264–1270.
10. Rao HL, Zangwill LM, Weinreb RN, Sample PA, Alencar LM, et al. (2010) Comparison of different spectral domain optical coherence tomography scanning areas for glaucoma diagnosis. Ophthalmology 117: 1692–1699.
11. Rao HL, Babu JG, Addepalli UK, Senthil S, Garudadri CS (2012) Retinal nerve fiber layer and macular inner retina measurements by spectral domain optical coherence tomograph in Indian eyes with early glaucoma. Eye (Lond) 26: 133–139.
12. Medeiros FA, Bowd C, Zangwill LM, Patel C, Weinreb RN (2007) Detection of glaucoma using scanning laser polarimetry with enhanced corneal compensation. Invest Ophthalmol Vis Sci 48: 3146–3153.
13. Mai TA, Reus NJ, Lemij HG (2007) Diagnostic accuracy of scanning laser polarimetry with enhanced versus variable corneal compensation. Ophthalmology 114: 1988–1993.
14. Sehi M, Guaqueta DC, Feuer WJ, Greenfield DS, Advanced Imaging in Glaucoma Study Group (2007) Scanning laser polarimetry with variable and enhanced corneal compensation in normal and glaucomatous eyes. Am J Ophthalmol 143: 272–279.
15. Benitez-del-Castillo J, Martinez A, Regi T (2011) Diagnostic capability of scanning laser polarimetry with and without enhanced corneal compensation and optical coherence tomography. Eur J Ophthalmol 21: 228–236.
16. Garas A, Vargha P, Hollo G (2012) Comparison of diagnostic accuracy of the RTVue Fourier-domain OCT and the GDx-VCC/ECC polarimeter to detect glaucoma. Eur J Ophthalmol 22: 45–54.
17. Rao HL, Yadav RK, Addepalli UK, Chaudhary S, Senthil S, et al. (2014) Retinal nerve fiber layer evaluation of spectral domain optical coherence

tomograph and scanning laser polarimeter to diagnose glaucoma. Eye (Lond) 28: 654–661.

18. Anderson DR, Patella VM (1999) Automated Static Perimetry. St. Louis: Mosby. 152 p.
19. Rao HL, Kumar AU, Babu JG, Kumar A, Senthil S, et al. (2011) Predictors of normal optic nerve head, retinal nerve fiber layer, and macular parameters measured by spectral domain optical coherence tomography. Invest Ophthalmol Vis Sci 52: 1103–1110.
20. Rao HL, Kumbar T, Addepalli UK, Bharti N, Senthil S, et al. (2012) Effect of spectrum bias on the diagnostic accuracy of spectral-domain optical coherence tomography in glaucoma. Invest Ophthalmol Vis Sci 53: 1058–1065.
21. Glynn RJ, Rosner B (1992) Accounting for the correlation between fellow eyes in regression analysis. Arch Ophthalmol 110: 381–387.
22. Zhou XH, Obuchowski NA, McClish DK (2002) Analysis of correlated ROC data. In: Zhou XH, Obuchowski NA, McClish DK, eds. Statistical Methods in Diagnostic Medicine. New York: John Wiley & Sons, Inc. pp. 274–306.
23. Alonzo TA, Pepe MS (2002) Distribution-free ROC analysis using binary regression techniques. Biostatistics 3: 421–432.
24. Jaeschke R, Guyatt GH, Sackett DL (1994) Users' guides to the medical literature. III. How to use an article about a diagnostic test. B. What are the results and will they help me in caring for my patients? The Evidence-Based Medicine Working Group. JAMA 271: 703–707.
25. Radack KL, Rouan G, Hedges J (1986) The likelihood ratio. An improved measure for reporting and evaluating diagnostic test results. Arch Pathol Lab Med 110: 689–693.
26. Fagan TJ (1975) Letter: Nomogram for Bayes theorem. N Engl J Med 293: 257.
27. Simel DL, Samsa GP, Matchar DB (1991) Likelihood ratios with confidence: sample size estimation for diagnostic test studies. J Clin Epidemiol 44: 763–770.
28. Pepe MS (2003) The Statistical Evaluation of Medical Tests for Classification and Prediction. Oxford, UK: Oxford University Press. pp.130–67.
29. Jeoung JW, Park KH (2010) Comparison of Cirrus OCT and Stratus OCT on the ability to detect localized retinal nerve fiber layer defects in preperimetric glaucoma. Invest Ophthalmol Vis Sci 51: 938–945.
30. Hirashima T, Hangai M, Nukada M, Nakano N, Morooka S, et al. (2013) Frequency-doubling technology and retinal measurements with spectral-domain optical coherence tomography in preperimetric glaucoma. Graefes Arch Clin Exp Ophthalmol 251: 129–137.
31. Arintawati P, Sone T, Akita T, Tanaka J, Kiuchi Y (2013) The applicability of ganglion cell complex parameters determined from SD-OCT images to detect glaucomatous eyes. J Glaucoma 22: 713–718.
32. Nukada M, Hangai M, Mori S, Takayama K, Nakano N, et al. (2014) Imaging of Localized Retinal Nerve Fiber Layer Defects in Preperimetric Glaucoma Using Spectral-domain Optical Coherence Tomography. J Glaucoma 23: 150–159.
33. Rolle T, Briamonte C, Curto D, Grignolo FM (2011) Ganglion cell complex and retinal nerve fiber layer measured by fourier-domain optical coherence tomography for early detection of structural damage in patients with preperimetric glaucoma. Clin Ophthalmol 5: 961–969.
34. Tan O, Chopra V, Lu AT, Schuman JS, Ishikawa H, et al. (2009) Detection of macular ganglion cell loss in glaucoma by Fourier-domain optical coherence tomography. Ophthalmology 116: 2305–2314.
35. Lisboa R, Leite MT, Zangwill LM, Tafreshi A, Weinreb RN, et al. (2012) Diagnosing preperimetric glaucoma with spectral domain optical coherence tomography. Ophthalmology 119: 2261–2269.
36. Rao HL, Addepalli UK, Chaudhary S, Kumbar T, Senthil S, et al. (2013) Ability of different scanning protocols of spectral domain optical coherence tomography to diagnose preperimetric glaucoma. Invest Ophthalmol Vis Sci 54: 7252–7257.
37. Langlotz CP (2003) Fundamental measures of diagnostic examination performance: usefulness for clinical decision making and research. Radiology 228: 3–9.
38. Medeiros FA, Zangwill LM, Bowd C, Weinreb RN (2004) Comparison of the GDx VCC scanning laser polarimeter, HRT II confocal scanning laser ophthalmoscope, and stratus OCT optical coherence tomograph for the detection of glaucoma. Arch Ophthalmol 122: 827–837.
39. Zangwill LM, Jain S, Racette L, Ernstrom KB, Bowd C, et al. (2007) The effect of disc size and severity of disease on the diagnostic accuracy of the Heidelberg Retina Tomograph Glaucoma Probability Score. Invest Ophthalmol Vis Sci 48: 2653–2660.
40. Garway-Heath DF, Hitchings RA (1998) Sources of bias in studies of optic disc and retinal nerve fibre layer morphology. Br J Ophthalmol 82: 986.

19

Hepatocyte Growth Factor Genetic Variations and Primary Angle-Closure Glaucoma in the Han Chinese Population

Zhengxuan Jiang[1¶], Kun Liang[1¶], Biqing Ding[1¶], Wei Tan[2], Jing Wang[1], Yunxia Lu[3], Yuxin Xu[1], Liming Tao[1]*

1 Department of Ophthalmology, The Second Affiliated Hospital of Anhui Medical University, Hefei, Anhui, China, **2** Department of Ophthalmology, The First People's Hospital of Zunyi, the Third Affiliated Hospital of Zunyi Medical University, Zunyi, Guizhou, China, **3** Department of Biochemistry and Molecular Biology, Anhui Medical University, Hefei, Anhui, China

Abstract

Purpose: The aim of this study is to examine whether or not hepatocyte growth factor (HGF) genetic variations are associated with susceptibility to primary angle-closure glaucoma (PACG) in the Han Chinese population.

Methods: Three single-nucleotide polymorphisms (SNPs)–rs5745718, rs17427817, and rs3735520–in the HGF gene were genotyped in 238 adult patients with PACG and 287 age-, sex-, and ethnically matched healthy controls by using a polymerase chain reaction restriction fragment length polymorphism assay. Data was analyzed by χ^2 analysis.

Results: The three tested analyzed polymorphisms in the HGF gene were in Hardy-Weinberg equilibrium, in all the subjects. The frequencies of the genotype and allele of rs5745718 and rs1742817 in the HGF gene were significantly different between the PACG patients and the controls. On one hand, the frequencies of the CC genotype and C allele of rs5745718 were significantly decreased in PACG patients compared with controls ($P_c = 1.40\times10^{-3}$; $P_c = 3.21\times10^{-4}$, respectively); however, on the other hand, significantly decreased frequencies of the GG genotype and the G allele of rs17427817 were observed in PACG patients compared with the controls ($P_c = 0.006$,; $P_c = 6.06\times10^{-4}$, respectively). A comparison of the distributions of the genotypes and alleles of rs3735520 showed no statistically significant differences between the PACG patients and the controls ($p_c > 0.05$). The haplotype analysis results showed that the CGC haplotype frequency was significantly decreased in the patients with PACG compared with the controls ($p_c < 0.001$). No difference was detected between the patients and the controls with regard to the other haplotypes.

Conclusions: Our study suggests that rs5745718 and rs17427817 are associated with a decreased risk of PACG in the Chinese Han population. The CGC haplotype was demonstrated to possibly play a protective role against PACG in this population.

Editor: Richard Libby, University of Rochester, United States of America

Funding: This work was supported in part by the Anhui Provincial Natural Science Foundation (1208085MH178), the Natural Science Foundation of Higher Educational Bureau of Anhui Province (kj2011z189), the Talent Foundation of the Department of Personnel Anhui Province (2010-45), the Foundation of Anhui Medical University (2012xkj053) and Governor Foundation of Special Research of Clinical Application in Guizhou Province ([2012]131).The funders had no role in study design, data collection and analysis, decision to publish, or preparation of the manuscript.

Competing Interests: The authors have declared that no competing interests exist.

* E-mail: taolimingchina@yahoo.cn

¶ These authors contributed equally to this work.

Introduction

Glaucoma is the second largest cause of blindness worldwide after cataracts. It is estimated that 70 million people suffer from glaucoma globally, and there will be 79.6 million people with glaucoma and about 11.2 million patients with bilateral blindness by 2020 [1]. Primary angle-closure glaucoma (PACG) has relatively high visual morbidity rates and accounts for half of all blind glaucoma patients in the Chinese Han population [2]. Epidemiological studies have revealed that the majority of patients with PACG live in Asian regions, especially in China [3,4].

PACG is characterized by a diverse spectrum of clinical manifestations including a shallow anterior chamber [5], increased thickness of the lens [4], and a short axial length [6], often accompanied by hypermetropic refraction error [7,8]. The etiology of PACG remains largely unknown and is thought to be a multifactorial disease. It is assumed that a genetic predisposition as well as environmental elements are involved in the development of this disease [9]. Genetic factors play an important role in the occurrence of PACG. Previous studies have revealed that the risk of developing PACG is much higher in families in which first-degree relatives have the disease [10]. Several candidate genes are associated with PACG in different populations, including the matrix metalloproteinase-9 gene [11,12], myocilin [13], optineurin [14], and tumor necrosis factor-α [15]. However, these genes only partly explain the genetic predisposition to PACG, and more research is needed to determine the causative genes of this disease.

Hepatocyte growth factor (HGF) was thought to play an important role in the emmetropization process of the eye [16], and several single nucleotide polymorphisms (SNPs) of the HGF gene were firstly reported to be associated with hyperopia. As angle-closure glaucoma and hyperopia share the same feature of a short axial length, the HGF gene may be also a risk factor of PACG [17]. A recent study revealed that four SNPs of the HGF gene are associated with susceptibility to PACG in the Nepalese population [18]. There is much evidence to support the fact that genetic heterogeneity exists in different ethnic cohorts, even in the same population which comes from a different region. Therefore, this data prompted us to search for a relationship between SNPs of the HGF gene with a risk occurrence of PACG. We designed this case-control study and examined whether or not HGF polymorphisms were associated with susceptibility to PACG in the Han Chinese population.

Methods

Subjects

A total of 238 patients with PACG and 287 age-, sex-, and ethnically matched healthy controls were recruited from the Second Affiliated Hospital of Anhui Medical University (Anhui, People's Republic of China). Both the patients and healthy controls underwent a full ophthalmic examination, which included a visual acuity test, a slit-lamp examination of the anterior chamber, a gonioscopy, the measurement of central corneal thickness and intraocular pressure, a fundus examination with special attention to optic disc parameters, and a visual field test. A total of 238 patients were selected for the PACG group according to the following diagnostic criteria: the presence of glaucomatous optic neuropathy with a cup:disc ratio ≥0.7, peripheral visual loss, an intraocular pressure of more than 21 mmHg, and the presence of at least 180 degrees of closed angle in which the trabecular meshwork was not visible on a gonioscopy. Patients with secondary angle-closure glaucoma, which was caused by uveitis, trauma, or lens subluxation, were excluded. The healthy individuals came from the same geographical regions as the PACG patients, and the controls were age-, sex- and ethnically matched with the PACG patients. They were enrolled into the control group according to the following criteria: (1) none of the PACG symptoms or signs mentioned above; (2) no glaucoma history and familial glaucoma history; and (3) no ophthalmic diseases other than cataracts. The clinical characteristics of these subjects are shown in Table 1. The study was approved by the local institutional ethnics committee of the Second Affiliated Hospital of Anhui Medical University and met the tenets of the Declaration of Helsinki. Informed consent was obtained from all of the subjects. We obtained 5 ml of peripheral blood from each individual.

DNA Extraction and SNP Selection and Genotyping

Venous blood samples were obtained from the PACG patients and the controls in EDTA tubes and kept at −70°C until use. Genomic DNA was extracted from the peripheral venous blood using the QiaAmp DNA Blood Mini Kit (Qiagen, Hilden, Germany) according to the manufacturer's instructions.

As reported in earlier studies, since there is an association between HGF polymorphisms, and PACG and hyperopia in other ethnic groups [16,18], we selected rs17427817, rs5745718, and rs3735520 as candidate SNPs. Amplification of the target DNA in the HGF gene was analyzed by polymerase chain reaction (PCR) using the primers presented in Table 2. The PCR restriction fragments length polymorphism method was employed to determine the genotypes of the tested SNPs. Each PCR reactive solution consisted of the following: 5 μl Premix Taq (Ex Taq Version; TaKaRa Biotechnology Co. Ltd., Dalian, China), 20 pmol primers, and 0.2 μg genomic DNA. The conditions were as follows: initial denaturation at 95°C for 5 minutes followed by 38 cycles of denaturation at 94°C for 30 seconds, annealing at different temperatures (54°C for rs17427817 and rs5745718, 56°C for rs3735520) for 30 seconds, extension at 72°C for 30 seconds, and a final extension at 72°C for 5 minutes. The PCR products of the rs17427817, rs5745718, and rs3735520 polymorphisms were respectively digested with 2 U of NlaIV (MBI Fermentas, Burlington, ON, Canada), BssECI (MBI Fermentas), and BglII (Promega, Madison, WI, USA) restriction enzymes (Table 2) in a 10-μl reaction volume overnight. The digestion products were visualized on a 3.5% agarose gel and stained with GoldView (SBS Genetech, Beijing, China).

Table 1. Clinical characteristics of study participants.

Clinical features	PACG patients	Controls
Age (mean±SD)	56.2±10.7	58.4±11.2
Number	238	287
Sex (% male)	50.4%.	52.3%
IOP in mmHg (mean±SD)	24.6±8.7	12.3±7.2
C/D (mean±SD)	0.72±0.11	0.22±0.09

Statistical Analysis

The differences in age and gender between the cases and the controls were assessed by t-test and χ^2 test, respectively. The Hardy-Weinberg equilibrium was tested using the χ^2 test. The significance of the differences in the allele and genotype distribution between the patients and the controls was evaluated with the use of the χ^2 test performed by using SPSS (version 11.0, SPSS, Inc., Chicago, IL, USA). When the number of genotypes or alleles was fewer than 5 counts, the Fisher's exact test was used. The P-values were corrected (Pc) with the Bonferroni correction by multiple comparison with the number of analyses performed. A P-value of less than 0.05 was considered statistically significant.

Table 2. Primers of HGF SNPs and restriction enzymes used for FRLP analysis.

SNP	Primers	Restriction enzyme
rs17427817	5'-TCCCTCGGGATTGAGAACAGTG-3'	NlaIV
	5'-TTTGGAGGTCTTTACTACTT-3'	
rs5745718	5'-CTACAAAGAACCTACAACACAA-3'	BssECI
	5'-TCATCTTACTGAACTTGTTT-3'	
rs3735520	5'-ACCCTAATAAAGCACAAGA-3'	BglII
	5'-CCTGCCTGATAAGTCCCTGAG-3'	

Results

The patients in the PACG cohort numbered 238 and included 93 male and 114 female subjects. The average age of the PACG patients was 61.3±10.2 years. The healthy controls cohort included 287 subjects (150 male, 137 female) with a mean age of 64.7±8.7 years. The demographic characteristics between the PACG cases and the healthy controls were similar. There was no significant difference between the cases and the controls with respect to age and gender. The clinical features of the patients with PACG and the healthy controls are summarized in Table 2.

Three single-nucleotide polymorphisms of the HGF gene were successfully genotyped in the 238 PACG patients and 287 healthy controls. The observed genotype frequencies of the three tested SNPs in this study were in agreement with the Hardy-Weinberg equilibrium in both the cases and the controls. The genotype and allele frequency and odds ratio of the tested HGF polymorphisms in the study and control group are displayed in Table 3. The frequencies of the genotype and the allele of rs5745718 and rs1742817 in the HGF gene were significantly different between the PACG patients and the controls. On one hand, the frequencies of the CC genotype and C allele of rs5745718 were significantly decreased in patients with PACG compared with controls ($\chi^2 = 13.54$, $Pc = 1.40\times10^{-3}$, OR 0.46, 95% CI 0.30–0.69; $\chi^2 = 15.02$, $Pc = 3.21\times10^{-4}$, OR 0.48, 95% CI 0.33–0.69; respectively). On the other hand, significantly decreased frequencies of the GG genotype and the G allele of rs17427817 were observed in the PACG patients compared with the controls ($\chi^2 = 10.87$, $Pc = 0.006$, OR 0.52, 95% CI 0.35–0.77 and $\chi^2 = 13.81$, $Pc = 6.06\times10^{-4}$, OR 0.52, 95% CI 0.37–0.74, respectively). A comparison of the distribution of genotypes and alleles of rs3735520 showed no statistically significant differences between the PACG patients and the controls (P>0.05).

A haplotype analysis was performed by SHEsis platform [19], and the results are shown in Table 4. The CGC haplotype frequency was significantly decreased in patients with PACG compared with the controls (Pc<0.001, OR 0.59, 95% CI 0.45–0.77). No differences were detected between the patients and the controls with regard to the other haplotypes.

Discussion

Glaucoma is a neurodegenerative disease, which causes a progressive degeneration of the retinal ganglion cells in the optic disc or retinal nerve fiber. In this study, our results showed that the two analysed SNPs of HGF, rs17427817 and rs5745718, were associated with a decreased risk for PACG. A haplotype analysis revealed that people with the CGC haplotype are less susceptible to PACG. Additionally, the SNP rs3733520 in the HGF gene was not associated with PACG in this study.

The HGF protein has been shown to be involved in causing disruption to the emmetropization process within the eye and stimulating the growth and migration of many tissues of the eye [20–22]. Recent studies have found that some SNPs of the HGF gene were associated with susceptibility to hyperopia [16]. Several SNPs of the HGF gene were also identified as being associated with PACG in the Nepalese population [18].

Several strategies can be used to select a candidate gene in the study of genetic susceptibility to a certain disease. For example, one gene can be selected for study according to the functions that are involved in the pathogenesis of the relevant disease [23]. In this study, we selected the HGF gene as a candidate gene based on number of factors. First, earlier studies revealed that the mRNA level of HGF is higher in the rabbit lacrimal gland after corneal injury [24], and the level of HGF protein is significantly increased in the aqueous humour of glaucomatous eyes [25]. These results suggested that the HGF protein might have functional effects in the development of PACG. Second, it has been suggested that the upregulated expression of a certain gene may be associated with certain SNP alleles in its gene. The polymorphisms of the HGF gene have been widely studied in hyperopia in different populations. There is evidence to support the hypothesis that PACG and hyperopia have potentially similar cellular events in the pathogenesis of the two diseases [17]. Third, primary angle-closure glaucoma is one of the leading causes of visual morbidity in

Table 3. Frequencies of alleles and genotypes of HGF polymorphisms in PACG patients and controls.

SNP	Genotype/Allele	PACG(N = 238)	Controls(N = 287)	χ^2	P-value	Pc	OR(95% CI)
rs5745718	AA	9 (3.8%)	4 (1.4%)	3.072	0.095	NS	2.78 (0.85–9.14)
	AC	61 (25.6%)	42 (14.6%)	9.976	0.002	0.012	2.01 (1.30–3.12)
	CC	168 (70.6%)	241 (84.0%)	13.539	2.34×10^{-4}	1.40×10^{-3}	0.46 (0.30–0.69)
	A	79 (16.6%)	50 (8.7%)	15.016	1.07×10^{-4}	3.21×10^{-4}	2.09 (1.43–3.04)
	C	397 (83.4%)	524 (91.3%)	15.016	1.07×10^{-4}	3.21×10^{-4}	0.48 (0.33–0.69)
rs17427817	CC	11 (4.6%)	4 (1.4%)	5.082	0.024	NS	3.51 (1.10–11.2)
	CG	68 (28.6%)	54 (18.8%)	6.942	0.009	NS	1.73 (1.15–2.60)
	GG	159 (66.8%)	229 (79.8%)	10.873	0.001	0.006	0.52 (0.35–0.77)
	C	90 (18.9%)	62 (10.8%)	13.811	2.02×10^{-4}	6.06×10^{-4}	1.93 (1.36–2.73)
	G	386 (81.1%)	512 (89.2%)	13.811	2.02×10^{-4}	6.06×10^{-4}	0.52 (0.37–0.74)
rs3735520	TT	92 (38.7%)	95 (33.1%)	1.750	0.186	NS	1.27 (0.89–1.82)
	TC	112 (47.1%)	139 (48.4%)	0.098	0.754	NS	0.95 (0.67–1.34)
	CC	34 (14.2%)	53 (18.5%)	1.645	0.200	NS	0.74 (0.46–1.18)
	T	296 (62.2%)	329 (57.3%)	2.559	0.110	NS	1.23 (0.96–1.57)
	C	180(37.8%)	245(42.7%)	2.559	0.110	NS	0.82 (0.64–1.05)

PACG = primary angle-closure glaucoma; OR = odds ratio; 95% CI = 95% confidence interval; Pc = Bonferroni corrected P-value; NS = not significant.

China. Based on the functional studies of HGF, the genetic factor in this disease, and the association between the HGF gene and PACG in other populations [18], we designed a case-control association study to clarify whether or not polymorphisms of the HGF gene were associated with PACG in the Chinese Han population. As with the other association studies, many factors may influence the association results. We strictly selected patients who had been diagnosed with PACG according to international criteria. The subjects in the study were all from the Chinese Han population, and the healthy controls were age- and sex-matched with the PACG patients in order to avoid ethnic confounding.

Since one candidate gene has numerous SNPs and only a few of them may be involved in the development of the disease, it is extremely important to select the appropriate SNPs [26]. We selected rs17427817, rs5745718, and rs3735520 as the candidate SNPs based on the fact that these SNPs in the HGF gene were reported to be associated with hyperopia in the Chinese Han population and PACG in other populations [16,18]. On one hand, our study found two SNPs in the HGF gene were significantly associated with PACG in the Chinese Han population. The rs17427817 G allele and GG genotype were associated with decreased susceptibility to PACG in the Chinese Han population, CC genotype and C allele of the rs5745718 was also associated with a reduction in the risk of PACG. These results were consistent with previous studies which reported that rs17427817 and rs5745718 were associated with PACG in the Nepalese population and which reported that rs5745718 was associated with hyperopia in Caucasians [16,18]. This data revealed that the HGF gene may be a common susceptibility gene of PACG in the different populations [18]. On the other hand,this study failed to find an association between the rs3735520 SNP and PACG, which is consistent with previous findings regarding PACG in the Nepalese population and hyperopia in the Han Chinese population [16,18]. However, the rs3735520 was reported to be associated with mild to moderate myopia in Caucasian population and keratoconus in Australian. Interesting [27,28], the SNP was identified to be associated with longer vitreous chamber depth in Chinese population [29]. Taken together, these results indicate that PACG and hyperopia possibly share a common pathway in the development of these diseases.

A haplotype analysis revealed that the haplotype CGC conferred a reduced risk of PACG. It is clear from analysing the results of Table 4 that the CG haplotype formed by the C allele of rs5745718 and the G allele of rs17427817 is a protective haplotype. This result revealed that the C allele of rs5745718 and the G allele of rs17427817 were associated with reducing the risk of PACG, which is consistent with the results in Table 3. The patterns of linkage disequilibrium (LD) of the tested SNPs in this studied samples were compared with that available in the Nepalese population [18], and the results showed no significant difference among them. The LD results of the studies were similar with that in the international HapMap for the Han Chinese population.

Table 4. Results of haplotypes formed by rs5745718, rs17427817, and rs3735520 at HGF locus in PACG patients and controls in the Chinese Han population.

Haplotype	Case, Control Ratios	Pc	OR (95% CI)
AGC	0.058, 0.027	NS	-
AGT	0.105, 0.060	NS	-
CCC	0.037, 0.017	NS	-
CCT	0.148, 0.113	NS	-
CGC	0.283, 0.383	0.006	0.64 (0.49–0.83)
CGT	0.365, 0.403	NS	-

Pc = Bonferroni corrected P; OR = odds ratio; 95% CI = 95% confidence interval.

Like other candidate gene association studies, there are some limitations in our study. First, the ability to plausibly detect disease susceptibility genes is influenced by the sample group. The size of the patient sample group in our study was relatively small, and the patients were recruited only from the Han Chinese population. The results observed in this study need to be confirmed using larger sample sizes and other ethnic populations. Second, as rs5745718 and rs17427817 polymorphisms are in non-coding regions, their functional roles are unknown, and they may be in a linkage disequilibrium with the causative variants in the HGF gene. Some other SNPs need to be further investigated.

In conclusion, to the best of our knowledge, this is the first association study between HGF gene and PACG in the Chinese Han population. This study has revealed that the CC genotype and C allele of rs5745718 and the GG genotype and G allele of rs174278717 may be associated with a decreased risk of PACG in the Chinese Han population. The CGC haplotype has been demonstrated to possibly play a protective role against PACG in this population.

Acknowledgments

The authors are very grateful to everyone who participated in this study.

Author Contributions

Contributed to the final paper: ZJ KL BD WT JW YL YX LT. Conceived and designed the experiments: LT ZJ. Performed the experiments: ZJ KL BD. Analyzed the data: WT. Contributed reagents/materials/analysis tools: JE YX YL. Wrote the paper: ZJ.

References

1. Quigley HA, Broman AT (2006) The number of people with glaucoma worldwide in 2010 and 2020. Br J Ophthalmol 90: 262–267.
2. Casson RJ (2008) Anterior chamber depth and primary angle-closure glaucoma: an evolutionary perspective. Clin Experiment Ophthalmol 36: 70–77.
3. Congdon N, Wang F, Tielsch JM (1992) Issues in the epidemiology and population-based screening of primary angle-closure glaucoma. Surv Ophthalmol 36: 411–423.
4. Foster PJ, Baasanhu J, Alsbirk PH, Munkhbayar D, Uranchimeg D, et al. (1996) Glaucoma in Mongolia. A population-based survey in Hovsgol province, northern Mongolia. Arch Ophthalmol 114: 1235–1241.
5. Lin YW, Wang TH, Hung PT (1997) Biometric study of acute primary angle-closure glaucoma. J Formos Med Assoc 96: 908–912.
6. Abu-Amero KK, Morales J, Osman MN, Bosley TM (2007) Nuclear and mitochondrial analysis of patients with primary angle-closure glaucoma. Invest Ophthalmol Vis Sci 48: 5591–5596.
7. Congdon NG, Quigley HA, Hung PT, Wang TH, Ho TC (1996) Screening techniques for angle-closure glaucoma in rural Taiwan. Acta Ophthalmol Scand 74: 113–119.
8. Dai X, Nie S, Ke T, Liu J, Wang Q, et al. (2008) Two variants in MYOC and CYP1B1 genes in a Chinese family with primary angle-closure glaucoma. Zhonghua Yi Xue Yi Chuan Xue Za Zhi 25: 493–496.
9. Amerasinghe N, Zhang J, Thalamuthu A, He M, Vithana EN, et al. (2011) The heritability and sibling risk of angle closure in Asians. Ophthalmology118: 480–485.
10. Wang N, Wu H, Fan Z (2002) Primary angle closure glaucoma in Chinese and Western populations. Chin Med J (Engl) 115: 1706–1715.
11. Cong Y, Guo X, Liu X, Cao D, Jia X, et al. (2009) Association of the single nucleotide polymorphisms in the extracellular matrix metalloprotease-9 gene with PACG in southern China. Mol Vis 15: 1412–1417.

12. Awadalla MS, Burdon KP, Kuot A, Hewitt AW, Craig JE (2011) Matrix metalloproteinase-9 genetic variation and primary angle closure glaucoma in a Caucasian population. Mol Vis 17: 1420–1424.
13. Mengkegale M, Fuse N, Miyazawa A, Takahashi K, Seimiya M, et al. (2008) Presence of myocilin sequence variants in Japanese patients with open-angle glaucoma. Mol Vis 14: 413–417.
14. Rezaie T, Child A, Hitchings R, Brice G, Miller L, et al. (2002) Adult-onset primary open-angle glaucoma caused by mutations in optineurin. Science 295: 1077–1079.
15. Wang CY, Shen YC, Wei LC, Lin KH, Feng SC, et al. (2012) Polymorphism in the TNF-alpha(-863) locus associated with reduced risk of primary open angle glaucoma. Mol Vis 18: 779–785.
16. Veerappan S, Pertile KK, Islam AF, Schache M, Chen CY, et al. (2010) Role of the hepatocyte growth factor gene in refractive error. Ophthalmology 117: 239–245 e231–232.
17. Sihota R, Lakshmaiah NC, Agarwal HC, Pandey RM, Titiyal JS (2000) Ocular parameters in the subgroups of angle closure glaucoma. Clin Experiment Ophthalmol 28: 253–258.
18. Awadalla MS, Thapa SS, Burdon KP, Hewitt AW, Craig JE (2011) The association of hepatocyte growth factor (HGF) gene with primary angle closure glaucoma in the Nepalese population. Mol Vis 17: 2248–2254.
19. Shi YY, He L (2005) SHEsis, a powerful software platform for analyses of linkage disequilibrium, haplotype construction, and genetic association at polymorphism loci. Cell Res 15: 97–98.
20. Wordinger RJ, Clark AF, Agarwal R, Lambert W, McNatt L, et al. (1998) Cultured human trabecular meshwork cells express functional growth factor receptors. Invest Ophthalmol Vis Sci 39: 1575–1589.
21. Li Q, Weng J, Mohan RR, Bennett GL, Schwall R, et al. (1996) Hepatocyte growth factor and hepatocyte growth factor receptor in the lacrimal gland, tears, and cornea. Invest Ophthalmol Vis Sci 37: 727–739.
22. He PM, He S, Garner JA, Ryan SJ, Hinton DR (1998) Retinal pigment epithelial cells secrete and respond to hepatocyte growth factor. Biochem Biophys Res Commun 249: 253–257.
23. Jiang Z, Yang P, Hou S, Li F, Zhou H (2010) Polymorphisms of IL23R and Vogt-Koyanagi-Harada syndrome in a Chinese Han population. Hum Immunol 71: 414–417.
24. Wilson SE, Chen L, Mohan RR, Liang Q, Liu J (1999) Expression of HGF, KGF, EGF and receptor messenger RNAs following corneal epithelial wounding. Exp Eye Res 68: 377–397.
25. Hu DN, Ritch R (2001) Hepatocyte growth factor is increased in the aqueous humor of glaucomatous eyes. J Glaucoma 10: 152–157.
26. Zhou H, Jiang Z, Yang P, Hou S, Li F, et al. (2010) Polymorphisms of IL23R and Fuchs' syndrome in a Chinese Han population. Mol Vis 16: 2585–2589.
27. Yanovitch T, Li YJ, Metlapally R, Abbott D, Viet KN, et al. (2009) Hepatocyte growth factor and myopia: genetic association analyses in a Caucasian population. Mol Vis 15: 1028–1035.
28. Burdon KP, Macgregor S, Bykhovskaya Y, Javadiyan S, Li X, et al. (2011) Association of polymorphisms in the hepatocyte growth factor gene promoter with keratoconus. Invest Ophthalmol Vis Sci 52: 8514–8519.
29. Chen JH, Chen H, Huang S, Lin J, Zheng Y, et al. (2012) Endophenotyping reveals differential phenotype-genotype correlations between myopia-associated polymorphisms and eye biometric parameters. Mol Vis 18: 765–778.

20

Ex-PRESS Implantation versus Trabeculectomy in Open-Angle Glaucoma

Guohai Chen[1], Wensheng Li[2]*, Fangzheng Jiang[1], Sihong Mao[1], Yuhua Tong[1]

1 Department of Ophthalmology, Quzhou People's Hospital, Quzhou, Zhejiang, PR China, **2** Xiamen Eye Center of Xiamen University, Xiamen, Fujian, PR China

Abstract

Objective: To evaluate the efficacy and safety of Ex-PRESS implantation (Ex-PRESS) compared to trabeculectomy in the treatment of patients with open-angle glaucoma (OAG).

Methods: A comprehensive literature search using the Cochrane Methodology Register to identify randomized controlled clinical trials (RCCTs) comparing Ex-PRESS to trabeculectomy in patients with OAG. Efficacy estimates were measured by weighted mean difference (WMD) for the percentage intraocular pressure reduction (IOPR%) from baseline to end-point, and odds ratios (OR) for the complete success rate and postoperative interventions. Safety estimates were measured by OR for postoperative complications. Statistical analysis was performed using the RevMan 5.1 software.

Results: A total of four RCCTs were selected for this meta-analysis, including 215 eyes of 200 patients (110 eyes in the Ex-PRESS group, 105 eyes in the trabeculectomy group). There was no significant difference between Ex-PRESS and trabeculectomy in the IOPR% (WMD = 3.15; 95% confidence interval (CI), −6.17–12.47; P = 0.51). The pooled OR comparing Ex-PRESS to trabeculectomy for the complete success rate at one year after surgery were in favor of Ex-PRESS (OR = 2.93; 95% CI, 1.39–6.16; P = 0.005). The Ex-PRESS procedure was found to be associated with lower number of postoperative interventions (OR = 0.23; 95% CI, 0.07–0.81; P = 0.02) and with a significantly lower frequency of hyphema than trabeculectomy (OR = 0.21; 95% CI, 0.05–0.85; P = 0.03), whereas other complications did not differ statistically.

Conclusion: In OAG, Ex-PRESS and trabeculectomy provided similar IOP control, but Ex-PRESS was more likely to achieve complete success, with fewer postoperative interventions. Complication rates were similar for the two types of surgery, except for a lower frequency of hyphema in the Ex-PRESS group.

Editor: Margaret M. DeAngelis, University of Utah, United States of America

Funding: The authors have no support or funding to report.

Competing Interests: The authors have declared that no competing interests exist.

* E-mail: drlws@vip.tom.com

Introduction

Glaucoma is a leading cause of blindness. It has been estimated that over 5.9 million people worldwide will be bilaterally blind with open-angle glaucoma (OAG) by 2020, which is more prevalent in Europe and China compared to other parts of the world [1]. OAG is a progressive optic neuropathy, resulting in loss of retinal ganglion cells leading to progressive damage of the visual field. Glaucoma treatments are directed at reducing intraocular pressure (IOP), either pharmacologically or surgically. Glaucoma filtering surgery is required when IOP can no longer be controlled with medication or laser treatment.

Trabeculectomy has been the standard IOP-lowering procedure for OAG. Its success rate and complications are well established [2,3]. The Ex-PRESS miniature glaucoma device implantation (Ex-PRESS) has been developed as an alternative filtration procedure to trabeculectomy. Initially, the Ex-PRESS device was designed to be implanted at the limbus directly under the conjunctiva. However, it was found that this mehtod leads to high rate of complications, such as hypotony and conjunctival erosion [4,5]. The procedure was modified for the device to be placed under a partial thickness scleral flap [6]. Ex-PRESS has the potential advantage of being less traumatic than trabeculectomy as there is no need for an iridectomy and no removal of scleral tissue.

The efficacy and safety of the Ex-PRESS compared to trabeculectomy has been studied before, with the majority of reports suggesting similar efficacy and complication rates for the two types of surgery [7–9]. A recent meta-analysis of controlled clinical trials indicated that Ex-PRESS was recommended for uncontrolled glaucoma [10]. To our knowledge, there has been no meta-analysis of randomized controlled clinical trials (RCCTs) comparing the outcomes of Ex-PRESS versus trabeculectomy in patients with OAG. Therefore, we undertook a meta-analysis of all available RCCTs to assess the efficacy and safety of these two surgical procedures for the management of OAG.

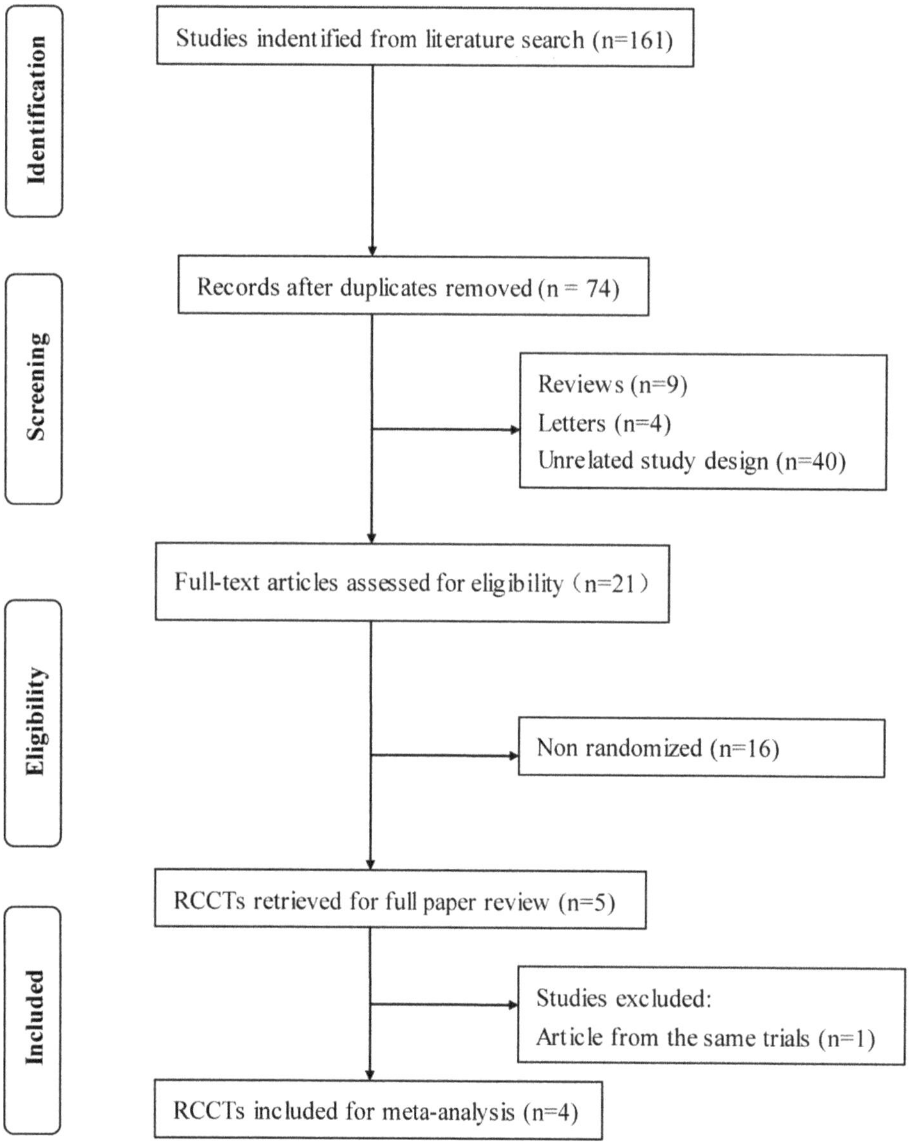

Figure 1. Flow diagram of studies included in this meta-analysis. RCCT = randomized controlled clinical trial.

Materials and Methods

Search Strategy

We conducted searches of PUBMED, EMBASE, ISI Web of Science, and the Cochrane Library, using the terms *Ex-PRESS*, *glaucoma* and *trabeculectomy*. A manual search was performed by checking the reference lists of original reports and review articles to identify studies not yet included in the computerized databases. The final search was carried out on August 2013, without restrictions regarding publication year or language.

Table 1. Characteristics and quality scores of included studies.

First author (year)	Design	Location	Follow-up(mo)	No. eyes*	Age (year)*	Quality score(%)
Beltran-Agullo (2013)	RCCT	Canada	6	33/31	65.9/61.9	68.75
Dahan (2012)	RCCT	South Africa	30	15/15	65.4/65.4	75.00
de Jong (2011)	RCCT	The Netherlands	60	39/39	62.4/68.6	75.00
Patel (2013)	RCCT	Canada	12	23/20	18~85**	65.63

*Ex-PRESS implantation group/Trabeculectomy group;
**Without mean age records; RCCT = randomized controlled clinical trial.

	Ex-PRESS			Trabeculectomy				Mean Difference
Study or Subgroup	Mean	SD	Total	Mean	SD	Total	Weight	IV, Fixed, 95% CI
Beltran-Agullo 2013	54.87	39.34	33	53.64	26.91	31	32.2%	1.23 [-15.20, 17.66]
Dahan 2012	44.13	29.35	15	47.91	43.45	15	12.3%	-3.78 [-30.31, 22.75]
de Jong 2011	51.69	26.27	39	45.89	29.95	39	55.5%	5.80 [-6.70, 18.30]
Total (95% CI)			**87**			**85**	**100.0%**	**3.15 [-6.17, 12.47]**

Heterogeneity: Chi² = 0.49, df = 2 (P = 0.78); I² = 0%

Test for overall effect: Z = 0.66 (P = 0.51)

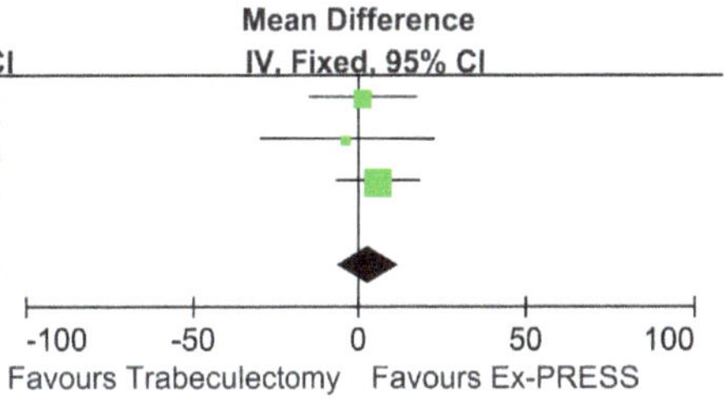

Figure 2. Percent intraocular pressure reduction from baseline comparing Ex-PRESS to trabeculectomy. SD = standard deviation; IV = inverse variance; CI = confidence interval; Ex-PRESS = Ex-PRESS implantation.

Inclusion and Exclusion Criteria

Articles were considered eligible for inclusion in the meta-analysis if the studies met the following inclusion criteria: (i) study design: RCCT; (ii) population: OAG patients (minimum age of 18 years with OAG that could not be controlled with maximal tolerated medical therapy and without history of uveitis or other ocular abnormality); (iii) intervention: Ex-PRESS versus trabeculectomy; (iv) outcome variables: at least one of the outcomes of interest discussed below was included. Abstracts from conferences and full texts without raw data available for retrieval, duplicate publications, letters, and reviews were excluded. For sequential reports on the same cohort of patients, only the most recent report was included, and data that could not be obtained from this last publication were obtained from the previous reports.

Outcome Measures

For efficacy, the primary outcome measure was the percentage of the IOP reduction (IOPR%). When authors reported the mean value and the standard deviation (SD) of the IOPR%, we used these values directly. For studies that only reported absolute values for the IOP at baseline and at end-point, the IOP reduction (IOPR) and the SD of the IOPR (SD_{IOPR}) were calculated as follows: $IOPR = IOP_{baseline} - IOP_{end\text{-}point}$, $SD_{IOPR} = (SD_{baseline}{}^2 + SD_{end\text{-}point}{}^2 - SD_{baseline} \times SD_{end\text{-}point})^{1/2}$, then the IOPR% and the SD of the IOPR% ($SD_{IOPR}\%$) were estimated by $IOPR\% = IOPR/IOP_{baseline}$, $SD_{IOPR}\% = SD_{IOPR}/IOP_{baseline}$ [11]. The secondary outcome measure was the proportion of patients with complete success at one year after surgery, which was defined as target end-point IOP (<18 mmHg) without anti-glaucoma medication. The tertiary outcome was the proportion of patients with postoperative interventions (e.g., bleb needing). We assessed safety by considering the proportions of patients with postoperative complications, including hypotony, shallow or flat anterior chamber, choroidal effusion, hyphema, and encapsulated bleb.

Data Extraction

The data were extracted independently by two reviewers (G.H.C. and W.S.L.). Disagreement was resolved by discussion. The information extracted from each study included the authors of each study, the year of publication, information on study design, location of the trial, duration of the study, number of subjects, IOP measurements, and success rate. The proportion of patients with postoperative interventions and complications was also recorded.

Qualitative Assessment

The qualities of RCCTs were assessed by two independent observers (F.Z.J. and S.H.M.) using a system reported by Downs and Blacks [12]. The system comprises 27 items distributed between 5 subscales regarding reporting (10 items), external validity (3 items), bias (7 items), confounding (6 items), and power (1 item). Any discrepancy in the qualitative assessment between the two observers was discussed and a consensus was reached. The total score of each trial was expressed as a percentage of the maximum achievable score. The studies with a quality score>50% were considered to have adequate quality.

Statistical Analysis

The quantitative data were entered into Cochrane Review Manager (RevMan, software version 5.1, Copenhagen, Denmark: The Nordic Cochrane Center, The Cochrane Collaboration, 2011). For continuous variables (e.g., IOPR%), the weighted mean difference (WMD) was measured, while the odds ratios (OR) were measured for dichotomous variables (e.g., number of eyes). Both outcomes were reported with a 95% confidence interval (CI). $P<0.05$ was considered statistically significant on the test for overall effect. The I^2 statistic was calculated to assess heterogeneity between studies ($P<0.05$ was considered representative of significant statistical heterogeneity). If there was heterogeneity between studies, a random-effects model was applied to the data.

	Ex-PRESS		Trabeculectomy			Odds Ratio
Study or Subgroup	Events	Total	Events	Total	Weight	M-H, Fixed, 95% CI
Dahan 2012	14	15	9	15	7.2%	9.33 [0.96, 90.94]
de Jong 2011	33	39	24	39	44.0%	3.44 [1.16, 10.15]
Patel 2012	15	23	11	20	48.8%	1.53 [0.45, 5.25]
Total (95% CI)		**77**		**74**	**100.0%**	**2.93 [1.39, 6.16]**
Total events	62		44			

Heterogeneity: Chi² = 2.14, df = 2 (P = 0.34); I² = 7%

Test for overall effect: Z = 2.83 (P = 0.005)

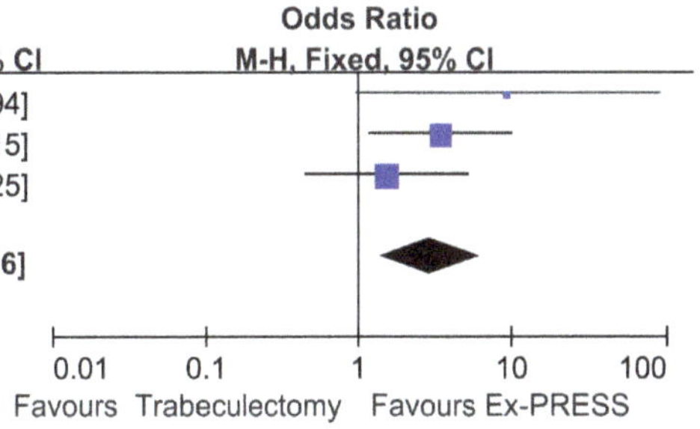

Figure 3. Complete success at one year after surgery comparing Ex-PRESS to trabeculectomy. M-H = Mantel-Haenszel; CI = confidence interval; Ex-PRESS = Ex-PRESS implantation.

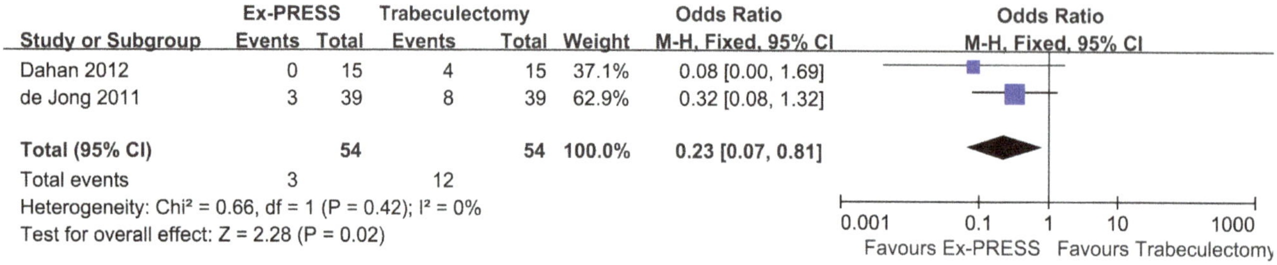

Figure 4. Postoperative interventions comparing Ex-PRESS to trabeculectomy. M-H = Mantel-Haenszel; CI = confidence interval; Ex-PRESS = Ex-PRESS implantation.

Alternatively, a fixed effects model was used for pooling the data. Begg's rank correlation test and Egger's linear regression test were employed to quantitatively assess publication bias ($P<0.05$ was considered representative of significant statistical publication bias).

Results

Overall Characteristics of Selected Trials and Quality Assessment

A total of 74 articles were initially identified. Of these, 69 were rejected according to the exclusion criteria listed above. The five remaining articles with full texts that met the inclusion criteria were assessed [13–17]. Two articles were from the same clinical trial, and the most recent article was selected [13,14]. Hence, a total of 4 studies were included in this meta-analysis. Figure 1 provides a flow diagram of the search results. In total, there were 215 eyes of 200 patients included in this meta-analysis. 110 eyes were included in the Ex-PPESS group, and 105 eyes were included in the trabeculectomy group. All studies fulfilled the quality criteria (Downs and Blacks score) of over 50%. The characteristics of the studies included and quality scores are summarized in Table 1.

Efficacy Analysis

Three studies involving 172 eyes compared Ex-PRESS to trabeculectomy in terms of the IOPR%. The combined results showed that both surgical procedures significantly decreased the IOP. There was no significant difference between Ex-PRESS and trabeculectomy in the IOPR% (WMD = 3.15; 95%CI, −6.17–12.47; P = 0.51), with no heterogeneity identified ($I^2 = 0\%$; P = 0.78) (Figure 2). Complete success at one year after surgery was achieved in 62 of 77 patients in the Ex-PRESS group compared with 44 of 74 patients in the trabeculectomy group. The pooled OR comparing Ex-PRESS to trabeculectomy for the complete success rate at one year were in favor of Ex-PRESS (OR = 2.93; 95% CI, 1.39–6.16; P = 0.005), with no heterogeneity identified ($I^2 = 7\%$; P = 0.34) (Figure 3). Of the two studies that reported postoperative interventions, a significant difference was found between Ex-PRESS and trabeculectomy (OR = 0.23; 95% CI, 0.07–0.81; P = 0.02), with no heterogeneity identified ($I^2 = 0\%$; P = 0.42) (Figure 4). Begg's rank correlation test and Egger's linear regression test indicated no publication bias for any of the parameters.

Safety Analysis

Postoperative complications comparing Ex-PRESS to trabeculectomy are shown in Figure 5. The three most common postoperative complications were hypotony, shallow or flat anterior chamber, and choroidal effusion. There were no significant differences between Ex-PRESS and trabeculectomy with respect to the incidence of hypotony, shallow or flat anterior chamber, or choroidal effusion (OR = 0.98; 95%CI, 0.49–1.95; P = 0.95; OR = 1.69; 95%CI, 0.76–3.74; P = 0.20 and OR = 0.93; 95%CI, 0.31–2.76; P = 0.90, respectively), and no statistical heterogeneity was observed between the studies (P = 0.14, P = 0.67, and P = 0.41, respectively). The Ex-PRESS was associated with a significantly lower frequency of hyphema than trabeculectomy (OR = 0.21; 95% CI, 0.05–0.85; P = 0.03), with no heterogeneity identified (P = 0.99). The Ex-PRESS was associated with a lower frequency of encapsulated bleb, but a difference that was not statistically significant (OR = 0.24; 95%CI, 0.04–1.51; P = 0.13), with no statistical heterogeneity (P = 0.97).

Discussion

Glaucoma treatments are directed at reducing IOP. Traditionally, trabeculectomy is considered the standard IOP-lowering procedure for OAG. Ideally, any procedure seeking to replace trabeculectomy should offer at least the same success rate, without increasing the level of complications. In recent years, Ex-PRESS has been introduced as an alternative to trabeculectomy. Numerous studies have reported on the biocompatibility, safety, and efficacy of Ex-PRESS during its evolution over the last decade [18–20]. However, trials have usually shown conflicting results, making it difficult to draw conclusions.

In this meta-analysis, we reviewed four RCCTs, including 215 eyes of 200 patients (110 eyes in the Ex-PRESS group, 105 eyes in the trabeculectomy group). In assessing the IOP, Ex-PRESS was associated with IOP-lowering efficacy comparable to that of trabeculectomy, demonstrating slightly bigger IOPR% reduction from baseline, but this difference that was not statistically significant(WMD = 3.15; 95%CI, −6.17–12.47; P = 0.51). Our analysis of the IOPR% was based on data pooled from trials of different durations, ranging from six months to five years. The longest follow up was five years by de Jong et al [14], which reported Ex-PRESS with better IOP control during the first three years, matching the trabeculectomy IOR lowering effect at four and five years. It was a compromise proposal to choose the data from the end-point, owing to the lack of data reported in all phases of follow-up and trials with different durations. With respect to the complete success rate at one year, Ex-PRESS was more likely to achieve complete success (OR = 2.93; 95% CI, 1.39–6.16; P = 0.005), with fewer postoperative interventions (OR = 0.23; 95% CI, 0.07–0.81; P = 0.02). The success rate during the first three years after Ex-PRESS was significantly higher, differences did not reach statistical significance up to year 3 reported by de Jong et al [14], which was the longest follow up. As only one year follow up results were available in three of the four trials included, our meta-analysis was focused on success rate at one year post surgery. For safety, Ex-PRESS was associated with a significantly

Study or Subgroup	Ex-PRESS Events	Ex-PRESS Total	Trabeculectomy Events	Trabeculectomy Total	Weight	Odds Ratio M-H, Fixed, 95% CI
3.1.1 Hypotony						
Beltran-Agullo 2013	15	33	14	31	48.4%	1.01 [0.38, 2.71]
Dahan 2012	1	15	5	15	28.7%	0.14 [0.01, 1.42]
Patel 2012	13	23	8	20	22.9%	1.95 [0.58, 6.58]
Subtotal (95% CI)		**71**		**66**	**100.0%**	**0.98 [0.49, 1.95]**
Total events	29		27			
Heterogeneity: Chi² = 3.94, df = 2 (P = 0.14); I² = 49%						
Test for overall effect: Z = 0.07 (P = 0.95)						
3.1.2 Shallow or flat anterior chamber						
Beltran-Agullo 2013	5	33	3	31	27.5%	1.67 [0.36, 7.65]
Dahan 2012	2	15	3	15	27.2%	0.62 [0.09, 4.34]
de Jong 2011	9	39	5	39	40.3%	2.04 [0.62, 6.76]
Patel 2012	2	23	0	20	5.0%	4.77 [0.22, 105.41]
Subtotal (95% CI)		**110**		**105**	**100.0%**	**1.69 [0.76, 3.74]**
Total events	18		11			
Heterogeneity: Chi² = 1.55, df = 3 (P = 0.67); I² = 0%						
Test for overall effect: Z = 1.29 (P = 0.20)						
3.1.3 Choroidal effusion						
Beltran-Agullo 2013	2	33	4	31	57.4%	0.44 [0.07, 2.57]
de Jong 2011	3	39	1	39	13.7%	3.17 [0.31, 31.86]
Patel 2012	2	23	2	20	28.9%	0.86 [0.11, 6.72]
Subtotal (95% CI)		**95**		**90**	**100.0%**	**0.93 [0.31, 2.76]**
Total events	7		7			
Heterogeneity: Chi² = 1.79, df = 2 (P = 0.41); I² = 0%						
Test for overall effect: Z = 0.13 (P = 0.90)						
3.1.4 Hyphema						
Beltran-Agullo 2013	1	33	5	31	47.7%	0.16 [0.02, 1.48]
Dahan 2012	0	15	1	15	13.9%	0.31 [0.01, 8.28]
de Jong 2011	0	39	2	39	23.5%	0.19 [0.01, 4.09]
Patel 2012	0	23	1	20	14.9%	0.28 [0.01, 7.18]
Subtotal (95% CI)		**110**		**105**	**100.0%**	**0.21 [0.05, 0.85]**
Total events	1		9			
Heterogeneity: Chi² = 0.14, df = 3 (P = 0.99); I² = 0%						
Test for overall effect: Z = 2.19 (P = 0.03)						
3.1.5 Encapsulated bleb						
Beltran-Agullo 2013	0	33	2	31	45.7%	0.18 [0.01, 3.82]
Dahan 2012	0	15	1	15	26.1%	0.31 [0.01, 8.28]
Patel 2012	0	23	1	20	28.2%	0.28 [0.01, 7.18]
Subtotal (95% CI)		**71**		**66**	**100.0%**	**0.24 [0.04, 1.51]**
Total events	0		4			
Heterogeneity: Chi² = 0.07, df = 2 (P = 0.97); I² = 0%						
Test for overall effect: Z = 1.52 (P = 0.13)						

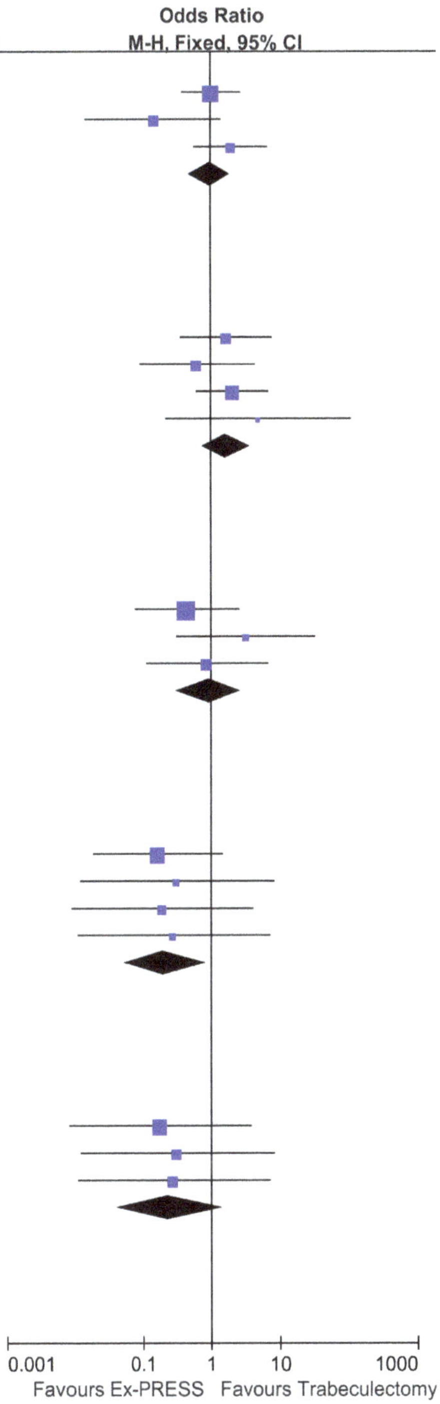

Figure 5. Postoperative complications comparing Ex-PRESS to trabeculectomy. M-H = Mantel-Haenszel; CI = confidence interval; Ex-PRESS = Ex-PRESS implantation.

lower frequency of hyphema than trabeculectomy (OR = 0.21; 95% CI, 0.05–0.85; P = 0.03), whereas other complications did not differ statistically. The Ex-PRESS procedure did not require an iridectomy, which is commonly performed with trabeculectomy, possibly resulting in an increased likelihood of inflammation and hyphema [21].

This meta-analysis may have some limitations. First, we cannot fully exclude publication bias. Although the Begg's and Egger's tests demonstrated no evidence of publication bias, the results should be interpreted with caution. Second, the studies were carried out with small or very small sample sizes and it is impossible to mask the surgical technique as trabeculectomy is easily differentiated from Ex-PRESS during postoperative follow-ups. These factors can affect the interpretation of the results. Third, a potential source of heterogeneity is trials duration and lack of data reported in all phases of follow-up.

Our findings indicate that Ex-PRESS and trabeculectomy provide similar IOP control, but Ex-PRESS is more likely to achieve complete success, with fewer postoperative interventions. Complication rates were similar for the two types of surgery, except for a lower frequency of hyphema noted in the Ex-PRESS group. RCCTs with longer duration and larger sample size are needed to provide more definitive information indicating whether Ex-PRESS is an effective and safe procedure for the treatment of OAG.

Acknowledgments

We would like to thank Radouil Tzekov for his work as a voluntary copy editor of the manuscript.

Author Contributions

Conceived and designed the experiments: GhC WsL FzJ. Performed the experiments: GhC ShM YhT. Analyzed the data: GhC WsL YhT. Wrote the paper: GhC WsL.

References

1. Quigley HA, Broman AT (2006) The number of people with glaucoma worldwide in 2010 and 2020. Br J Ophthalmol 90: 262–267.
2. Borisuth NS, Phillips B, Krupin T (1999) The risk profile of glaucoma filtration surgery. Curr Opin Ophthalmol 10: 112–116.
3. Gedde SJ, Herndon LW, Brandt JD, Budenz DL, Feuer WJ, et al. (2007) Surgical complications in the Tube Versus Trabeculectomy Study during the first year of follow-up. Am J Ophthalmol 143: 23–31.
4. Stewart RM, Diamond JG, Ashmore ED, Ayyala RS (2005) Complications following Ex-PRESS glaucoma shunt implantation. Am J Ophthalmol 140: 340–341.
5. Tavolato M, Babighian S, Galan A (2006) Spontaneous extrusion of a stainless steel glaucoma drainage implant (Ex-PRESS). Eur J Ophthalmol 16: 753–755.
6. Dahan E, Carmichael TR (2005) Implantation of a miniature glaucoma device under a scleral flap. J Glaucoma 14: 98–102.
7. Maris PJ, Ishida K, Netland PA (2007) Comparison of trabeculectomy with Ex-PRESS miniature glaucoma device implanted under a scleral flap. J Glaucoma 16: 14–19.
8. Sugiyama T, Shibata M, Kojita S, Ueki M, Ikeda T (2011) The first report on intermediate-term outcome of Ex-PRESS glaucoma filtration device implanted under a scleral flap in Japanese patients. Clin Ophthalmol 5: 1063–1066.
9. Seider MI, Rofangha S, Lin SC (2012) Resident-performed Ex-PRESS shunt implantation versus trabeculectomy. J Glaucoma 21: 469–474.
10. Wang W, Zhou M, Huang W, Zhang X (2013) Ex-PRESS implantation versus trabeculectomy in uncontrolled glaucoma: a meta-analysis. PloS One 8: e63591.
11. Cheng JW, Cai JP, Li Y, Wei RL (2011) Intraoperative mitomycin C for nonpenetrating glaucoma surgery: a systematic review and meta-analysis. J Glaucoma 20: 322–326.
12. Downs SH, Black N (1998) The feasibility of creating a checklist for the assessment of the methodological quality both of randomised and non-randomised studies of health care interventions. J Epidemiol Community Health 52: 377–384.
13. de Jong LA (2009) The Ex-PRESS glaucoma shunt versus trabeculectomy in open-angle glaucoma: a prospective randomized study. Adv Ther 26: 336–345.
14. de Jong L, Lafuma A, Aguade AS, Berdeaux G (2011) Five-year extension of a clinical trial comparing the EX-PRESS glaucoma filtration device and trabeculectomy in primary open-angle glaucoma. Clin Ophthalmol 5: 527–533.
15. Dahan E, Ben SG, Lafuma A (2012) Comparison of trabeculectomy and Ex-PRESS implantation in fellow eyes of the same patient: a prospective, randomised study. Eye (Lond) 26: 703–710.
16. Patel HY, Wagschal LD, Trope GE, Buys YM (2012) Economic analysis of the Ex-PRESS miniature glaucoma device versus trabeculectomy. J Glaucoma DOI: 10.1097/IJG.0b013e31827a06f4.
17. Beltran-Agullo L, Trope GE, Jin Y, Wagschal LD, Jinapriya D, et al. (2013) Comparison of visual recovery following Ex-PRESS versus trabeculectomy: results of a prospective randomized controlled trial. J Glaucoma DOI: 10.1097/IJG.0b013e31829e1b68.
18. Nyska A, Glovinsky Y, Belkin M, Epstein Y (2003) Biocompatibility of the Ex-PRESS miniature glaucoma drainage implant. J Glaucoma 12: 275–280.
19. Hendrick AM, Kahook MY (2008) Ex-PRESS min glaucoma shunt: surgical technique and review of clinical experience. Expert Rev Med Devices 5: 673–678.
20. De Feo F, Jacobson S, Nyska A, Pagani P, Tracerso CE (2009) Histological biocompatibility of a stainless steel miniature glaucoma drainage device in humans: a case report. Toxicol Pathol 37: 512–516.
21. Good TJ, Kahook MY (2011) Assessment of bleb morphologic features and postoperative outcomes after Ex-PRESS drainage device implantation versus trabeculectomy. Am J Ophthalmol 151: 507–513.

Anatomical Attributes of the Optic Nerve Head in Eyes with Parafoveal Scotoma in Normal Tension Glaucoma

Aparna Rao[1]*, Sujoy Mukherjee[2]

1 Glaucoma Services, LV Prasad Eye Institute, Patia, Bhubaneswar, India, 2 Diagnostic and Imaging Services, LV Prasad Eye Institute, Patia, Bhubaneswar, India

Abstract

Purpose: To evaluate optic nerve characteristics independent of systemic factors predisposing to parafoveal scotoma in normal tension glaucoma.

Methods: We included 40 patients with bilateral normal tension glaucoma with parafoveal scotoma (visual field defect in one hemifield within 10° of fixation with at least one point at $p<1\%$ lying at the two innermost paracentral points) in only one eye (Parafoveal group, PF, $n=40$) identified from the hospital database in this observational cross sectional study. The other eye with no parafoveal scotoma constituted the control group ($n=32$). Red free fundus photographs were evaluated using Image J software analyzing parameters including vertical and horizontal disc diameter, disc haemorrhage, location and angular width of the retinal nerve fibre layer depth and displacement of the central vessel trunk, CVT (vertical and horizontal). Clinical characteristics and disc parameters were compared in the two groups.

Results: The PF group had lower mean deviation(MD) and visual field index (VFI) and higher pattern standard deviation (PSD) than control group ($p\leq0.001$) for similar untreated IOP, ($p=0.9$). Disc haemorrhages were more frequent in the PF group, $p=0.01$. The PF group had greater width of nerve fibre layer defects, $p=0.05$ and greater vertical displacement of the central vessel trunk, $p=0.001$. On multivariate logistic regression, parafoveal scotoma was significantly associated with increased vertical distance of the CVT, $p=0.0001$.

Conclusion: Increased vertical displacement of the CVT is associated with parafoveal scotoma in normal tension glaucoma. Localising the vessel trunk may help clinicians in identifying patients at risk for parafoveal involvement.

Editor: Marta Agudo-Barriuso, Hospital Universitario Virgen de la Arrixaca. Fundación para la Formación e Investigación Sanitarias de la Región de Murcia. Instituto Murciano de Investigaciones Biosanitarias, Spain

Funding: These authors have no support or funding to report.

Competing Interests: The authors have declared that no competing interests exist.

* E-mail: aparna@lvpei.org

Introduction

Glaucomatous optic nerve damage is the end point of pressure dependent and independent glaucoma. [1,2] Factors leading to glaucomatous cupping in high tension glaucoma are well described in literature with mechanical compression and vascular factors being some postulated mechanisms for glaucomatous optic nerve damage. (1) Such descriptive mechanisms fail to explain the mechanism of glaucomatous cupping in low or normal tension glaucoma (NTG) patients where vascular factors are believed to predominate among many other risk factors [2,3].

Several studies have tried to identify possible systemic risk factors which include vascular abnormalities like migraine, Raynaud's phenomenon, cardiovascular insufficiency and female gender. [3] Local ocular factors like differential pressures across the optic nerve, now termed a translaminar pressure gradient and low cerebrospinal fluid pressure are now increasingly recognised as predominant risk factors for optic nerve damage at "normal" intraocular pressure (IOP). [4] Presumably, optic nerve head response to different pressure differentials across the lamina cribrosa may partly explain presence of visual field (VF) defects which are deeper and closer to fixation in NTG as compared to high pressure glaucoma or primary open angle glaucoma (POAG) eyes. A recent study demonstrated that eyes with initial parafoveal scotoma have baseline characteristics which are significantly different as compared to eyes with peripheral scotomas. [5] Studies have also reported difference in area of peripapillary atrophy among NTG eyes with IOP<15 or >15 mm Hg, suggesting IOP dependent mechanisms also actively playing a role in glaucomatous cupping. [6] Kim et al reported localized retinal nerve fiber layer defects (RNFLD) being closer to the center of the macula in the low IOP group than that in a relatively high IOP group, while no differences in angular width of RNFLD or field indices were noted between the 2 groups. [7] Anatomic differences in the optic nerve head which confer stress bearing function to different optic nerves as also to its different regions may be responsible for such observations and also late involvement of the central visual field till advanced stage of glaucoma in most eyes. Since central field is affected in advanced stages, evaluating causes of central involvement in earlier stages in some eyes with NTG would be useful. To identify these local optic nerve head parameters determining the stress response, we attempted to study differences in bilateral NTG eyes with involvement of parafoveal area in one eye only despite similar systemic risk factors (like hypertension, cardiovascular disease) influencing both eyes. This makes it easier to evaluate disc related factors responsible for early central involvement in one eye in a patient with NTG with similar systemic factors at play in both eyes.

Methods

Participants

Medical records of NTG patients who had undergone visual fields at our tertiary centre from 2007–2012 were reviewed and those with bilateral visual field defects were selected. Data that were retrieved included the best corrected visual acuity, family history of glaucoma, spherical equivalent, gonioscopy, slit lamp biomicroscopy, baseline untreated IOP by Goldmann applanation tonometry, central corneal thickness, dilated non-stereoscopic color optic disc photographs, Humphrey visual fields (Carl Zeiss Meditec, 24-2, 10-2 and macular program). All procedures adhered to the tenets of the Declaration of Helsinki and the study was approved by the institutional review board of LV Prasad Eye Institute. As routine protocol, a written informed consent is taken for all patients at our institute for detailed ophthalmic examination and all required diagnostic procedures. Patients with associated retinal or neurological problems with associated visual field defects were excluded.

Below are the routine protocols followed at our institute for the following investigations-.

Fundus photography protocol. All images were acquired by one examiner (SM) blinded to the diagnosis or details of the patient using the Visupac version 4.4.4 (FF 450 plus IR Carl Zeiss Ltd USA). Pupils were dilated by one drop of 1% tropicamide and 2.5% phenyephrine. Only images with good quality were selected for the study while those with motion artefacts, poor contrast, clarity or inability to distinguish disc margins were excluded from the study. Photographs were taken in color and red free frames.

Those with hazy media, refractive errors ≥ -3 dioptre (D), associated posterior segment lesions like diabetic retinopathy, ARMD, vascular occlusions) or anomalous insertion or tilted disc were excluded.

(c) Visual field testing. Only reliable fields with defects either in the superior **or** inferior quadrant were included which included fixation losses, false-positive errors, and false-negative errors were less than 20% while those with advanced biarcuate defects were excluded. A glaucomatous visual field (VF) defect was defined by a glaucoma hemifield test outside normal limits, the presence of at least three non-edge test points in the same hemifield on the pattern deviation probability plot at $p<5\%$ with at least one point at $p<1\%$ and excluding points directly above or below the blind spot. Parafoveal (PF) scotoma was defined as a VF defect in one hemifield within 10° of fixation with at least one point at P less than 1% lying at the two innermost paracentral points, with or without defects outside the central 10° in the superior or inferior arcuate area (**Figure 1**). All patients with PF scotoma in only one eye were included (eye with PF involvement henceforth termed as **PF group**). One eyed patients with PF involvement in one eye (therefore belonging to PF group) and absolute glaucoma in the other eye were also included. In all patients, the other eye with non-parafoveal defects served as control (henceforth **control group**). The visual field indices including mean deviation (MD), pattern standard deviation (PSD) and visual field index (VFI) as well as details like number of points with $p<1\%$, defects depth on pattern deviation and foveal threshold were compared in both groups.

Image analysis

To avoid magnification errors, only red free images showing disc, macula and posterior pole were selected for

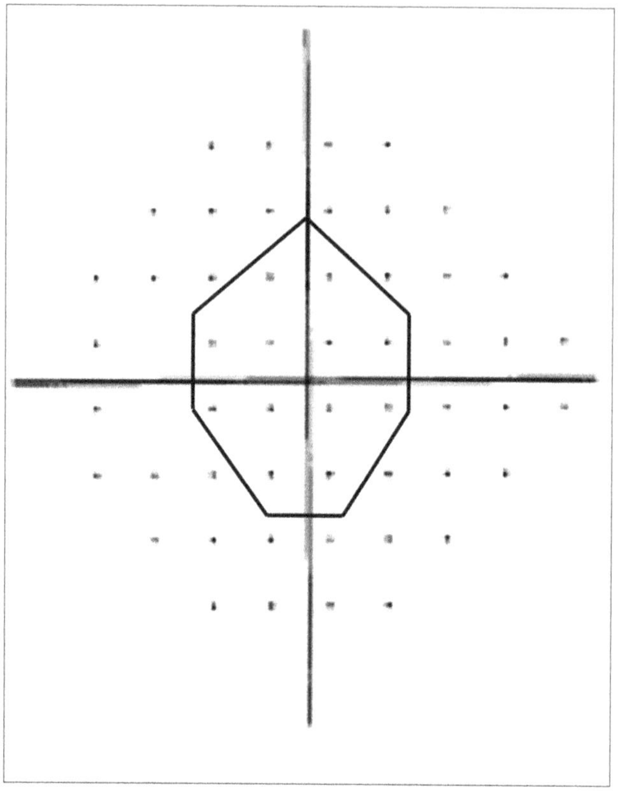

Figure 1. Pattern deviation plot to identify parafoveal scotoma defined by abnormal points within 12 points (shown by the dashed-line). The visual field defect would include those within 10° of fixation with at least one point at $p<1\%$ lying at the two innermost paracentral points.

analysis while magnified images capturing the disc alone were excluded. All images were exported to Image J software (http://rsbweb.nih.gov/ij/; www.nih.gov, National Institutes of Health, Bethesda, MD).for analysis and rescaled to a unified scale. Distances between two points of interest were measured in millimetre scale after rescaling in each of the images. All included photographs were analysed by two independent examiners (APR & SM) blinded to clinical details and an average of 3 measurements were used for analysis. Each image was then analysed using the following protocol:

a) Disc characteristics. The optic disc was evaluated using Image J measuring the vertical and horizontal disc diameter using the callipers function. The presence and location of disc haemorrhage was noted. The angular locations and widths of the RNFLD were measured as previously described with some modifications. [8] Briefly, a line from the centre of the optic disc to the foveal centre (the reference line), was drawn on the red free photographs. After identifying the reference line, the number of defects and the location of the defects (superotemporal, inferotemporal or PMB superior or inferior) were noted. The angular width of the defect was measured in degrees measured by the angle measurement tool in the image J software as the angle formed by the two border lines of the RNFL defect as shown, **Figure 2**. For multiple defects, the total width was calculated by summing the angular widths of all defects in that eye.

b) Position of Central Vessel Trunk (CVT). The disc was divided into 4 quadrants by two lines passing through its centre into superotemporal, superonasal, superonasal and inferonasal

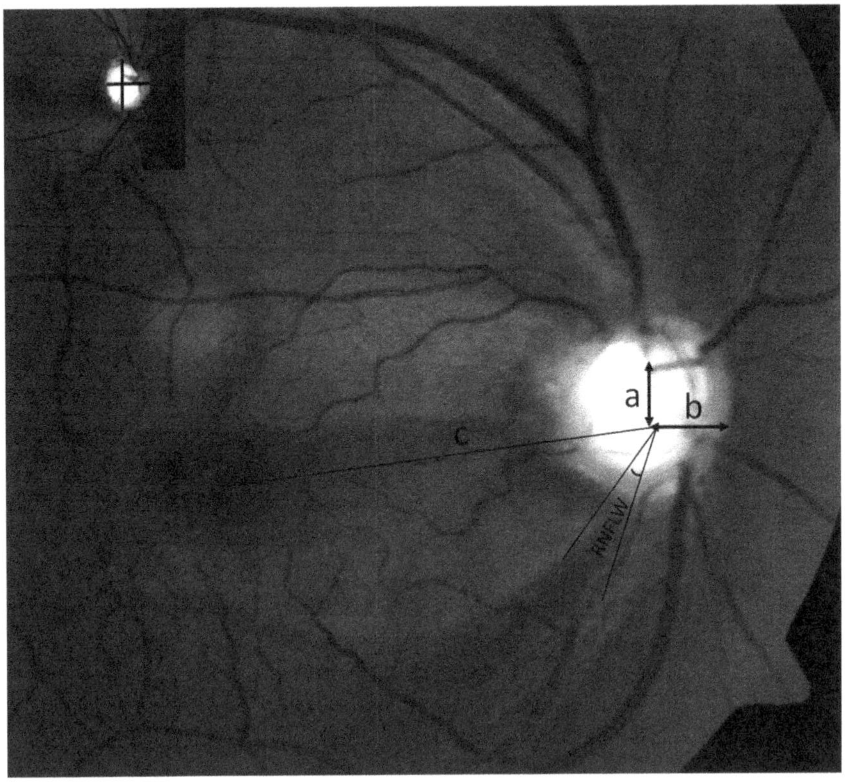

Figure 2. Parameters obtained from the red free fundus photograph. Reference line "c" is a line from the center of the optic disc to the center of the macula. The vertical distance of the central vessel trunk "a" and horizontal distance "b" was measured from the reference line and retinal nerve fibre layer width (RNFLW) using Image J software. Inset shows the division of the disc by two lines into 4 quadrants for determining the exit quadrant of the central vessel trunk.

quadrants (**Figure 2**). The exit quadrant of the CVT on the lamina cribrosa surface was then noted. The distance of the CVT was measured horizontally from the nasal disc border and vertically from the reference line by callipers in the image J software.

Statistical Analysis

An average of 3 readings obtained by Image J software was used for final analysis. Intraclass co-efficient was used to evaluate inter-examiner reproducibility for all measurements. For assessing repeatability, 10 consecutive images were examined by each examiner and repeatability coefficients evaluated for each of the horizontal and vertical CVT distance measurements (each being measured 10 times on each image by the same examiner at the same session, Table S1). Normality was analysed using Kolmogrov-Smirnov test while descriptive data were described as means (±SD) for normally distributed and median (and range) for non-parametric variables with alpha error set at <0.05. Comparisons between the PF and control group were done using student "t" test (or Mann-Whitney) while categorical variables were evaluated using chisquare tests. Separate analysis was done to evaluate differences between eyes with untreated IOP of <15 or >15 mm Hg. Association of parafoveal involvement with independent clinical variables including age, untreated IOP, corneal thickness and optic disc characteristics as defined earlier (disc diameter, horizontal and vertical distance of CVT, width of RNFLD) and visual field indices were analysed using univariate and multivariate logistic regression. Since visual field indices including MD, PSD and VFI were observed to be collinear variables evidenced by variance inflation factor >10, they were included in three separate models. All statistical analysis was done using Stata (Stata ver. 10.0; StataCorp, College Station, TX).

Results

We included 72 eyes of 40 patients with a mean age of 53 ± 10.8 years (range 34–76 years). This included 8 one eyed patients (male:female = 6:2) and 32 bilateral normal tension glaucoma (male:female = 20:12).

The average MD and VFI in the PF group was -11 ± 6.8 dB and 71 ± 20.9, respectively with a mean untreated IOP of 15 ± 2.8 mm Hg **(Table 1)**. There was no statistical difference in age (52 ± 10.09 vs 55 ± 11.9) or treated IOP (12 ± 2.5 vs11 ± 1.5), female gender (8 vs 6) or spherical equivalent (-1 ± 0.3 vs -0.3 ± 0.2 dioptres) between the two study groups (PF group vs control). Disc haemorrhages were more frequent in the PF group (18 of 40 eyes, 45%) than control group (6 of 32 eyes, 18.7%), $p = 0.01$.

All indices including MD, PSD and VFI were significantly better in the control group than the PF group with lower MD and VFI and higher PSD in the latter group for similar untreated IOP in the two groups. Visual field defects in the PF group included superior (n = 29) or inferior (n = 5) arcuate defects involving parafoveal area in 35 (of 40) eyes and isolated defects involving the parafoveal area in 6 eyes, **Table 2**. The control group has superior arcuate defect in 20 eyes and peripheral nasal step in12 eyes. Eyes in the PF group had a lower mean threshold of all points in the involved quadrant (superior or inferior) on the pattern deviation plot (17.2 ± 2.4 dB) as compared to controls

Table 1. Characteristics of eyes with parafoveal involvement (PF group) and other eye without parafoveal involvement (control) in bilateral normal tension glaucoma.

	PF group (n = 40)	Control (n = 32)	P value
Age (years)	52±10	55±11.9	0.8
Male/Female	19:8	7:6	0.05
Spherical equivalent(Dioptres)	−1±0.3	−0.8±0.2	0.2
Untreated intraocular pressure(mm Hg)	15±2.8	15±1.5	0.9
Central corneal thickness(μm)	532±22.4	524±24.6	0.6
Mean deviation(dB)	−11±6.8	−7±4.6	0.001
Pattern standard deviation(dB)	10±5.5		0.001
Visual field index (%)	71±20.9	85±14.6	<0.001
Disc haemorrhages	18, 45%	6, 18.7%	0.02
Intraocular pressure <15 mm Hg	16,40%	12, 37.5%	0.6

(25.4±4.1 dB) despite similar foveal thresholds (24 dB vs 31 dB,p = 0.06). The lowest defect depth on pattern deviation plot was also significantly worse for the PF group than control group (−31 dB vs −16 dB), p = 0.008 though the number of points with p<1% were not statistically different in the two groups, p = 0.3.

Mean deviation correlated negatively with width of RNFLD (r = −0.4, p = 0.008) and with vertical distance of CVT (r = −0.8, p = 0.01) while PSD correlated with positively with RNFLD width (r = 0.3, p = 0.02) and vertical CVT distance (r = 0.4, p<0.001).

Disc Measurements

The ICC for all disc measurements was good 0.91(vertical disc diameter), 0.89 (vertical CVT distance. 0.83 (horizontal CVT distance) and 0.92(width of RNFLD) while repeatability for horizontal and vertical CVT distance for the first examiner (APR) was 0.06–0.12 (Table S1).

Vertical disc diameter was greater in the PF group (2±0.8 vs 1±.0.2, p = 0.02) though horizontal disc diameter and cup disc ratio were not statistically significant, **Table 3**.

There were a mean of 1±0.6 RNFL defects per eye with 6 having papillomacular bundle defects all of which were situated in the inferior quadrant, **Figure 2**. There were more isolated RNFLD in the inferior quadrant in the PF group (25 eyes of 40 eyes, 62.5% vs 16 of 32 eyes, 50% in control group, p = 0.03) with combined defects in inferior and superior quadrant seen in the rest of eyes among both groups. The mean angular width of the RNFLD was 58±39.8 degrees (16–190°) with significantly greater width of the defects seen in the PF group (63±40.02 vs 47±39.2 degrees, p = 0.05). Comparing eyes with baseline IOP of <15 mm Hg and >15 mm Hg, we found a greater width in eyes with IOP>15 mm Hg (61±23.5 vs 54±38.4, p = 0.6). No other disc variables were found to be different among eyes with IOP< or > 15 mm Hg, **Table 4**.

Table 3. Disc characteristics of eyes with parafoveal involvement (PF group) and control group.

	PF group (n = 40)	Control (n = 32)	P value
Vertical disc diameter (mm)	2±0.8	1±.0.2	**0.02**
Horizontal disc diameter (mm)	1.5±0.2	1.6±0.2	0.1
RNFL defect width (degrees)	63±40.02	47±39.2	0.05
Vertical CVT distance (mm)	0.2±0.02	0.07±0.04	**0.001**
Horizontal CVT distance(mm)	0.7±0.2	0.8±0.2	0.8
Inferior RNFL defects	62.5%	50%	**0.03**
Superior CVT exit location	22	15	0.06

Table 2. Comparison of Visual field characteristics of eyes with parafoveal involvement (PF group) and control group.

	PF group (n = 40)	Control(n = 32)	P value
Superior/inferior defects	29:5	20:12	0.06
Mean threshold in involved quadrant (dB)	17.2±2.4	25.4±4.1	**0.04**
No of points <1%	11±7.3	−10±6.8	0.3
Foveal threshold (dB)	24±4.2	31±2.1	0.06
Visual field index (%)	71±20.9	85±14.6	
Lowest defect depth (dB)	−31±5.2	−16±6.2	**0.008**

Table 4. Comparison of disc characteristics in bilateral normal tension glaucoma with low or high untreated intraocular pressure (IOP).

	IOP<15 mm Hg	IOP>15 mm Hg	P value
Vertical disc diameter (mm)	1.9±1.2	1.8±0.7	0.7
Horizontal disc diameter (mm)	1.2±0.1	1.3±0.08	0.2
RNFL defect width (degrees)	61±23.5	54±38.4	0.6
Vertical CVT distance (mm)	1±0.9	1±0.5	0.2
Horizontal CVT distance (mm)	0.7±0.2	0.6±0.2	0.6
Mean deviation (dB)	−9±3.4	−6±5.8	0.9
Pattern standard deviation (dB)	7±4.6	8±4.3	0.7

The CVT was situated in the superior quadrant in 43 eyes (superonasal-46, superotemporal-7) and was inferiorly placed in 29 eyes (inferotemporal-20, inferonasal-9), p = 0.02. The horizontal distance of the CVT did not differ between the two groups (0.7±0.2 mm in PF group vs 0.8±0.2 mm in control group, p = 0.8). However the vertical distance of the CVT from the reference line was found to be significantly greater in PF group (0.2±0.02 mm) than control (0.07±0.04 mm), p = 0.001, signifying a greater displacement of the CVT from the central reference line in the PF group. Eyes with inferior RNFL defects had superonasal displacement of the CVT (except 3 eyes with combined superior RNFLD having CVT exit in inferonasal quadrant). All eyes with defects in the papillomacular bundle in the inferior quadrant had superonasally placed CVT (**Figure 3**). There was no significant difference in the CVT exit in eyes with IOP< or >15 mm Hg, **Table 4**. **Figure 4 and 5** shows some representative cases included in this study.

Comparing eyes with disc haemorrhage in both groups, eyes with haemorrhages in each of PF and control group had greater vertical CVT distance (0.18±0.08 vs in PF and 0.08±0.04 in control) than those without (0.13±0.07 mm in PF group and 0.06±0.02 in control group), p = 0.06 and 0.08, respectively. The mean deviation and VFI were better in the eyes without disc haemorrhages in both groups though this was also not statistically significant in any group, **Table 5**.

On univariate regression, greater age, lower untreated IOP, increased vertical disc diameter, greater width of RNFLD, worse visual field indices and vertical distance of CVT from the reference line were significantly associated with PF scotoma. On multivariate logistic regression using MD, PSD and VFI in three different models, parafoveal scotoma was significantly associated with increased vertical distance of the CVT from the disc margin, p = 0.0001 while age, untreated IOP, disc diameter (horizontal or vertical), visual field indices including MD/PSD & VFI or width of the RNFL defects did not significantly influence the involvement of parafovel area on visual fields. We repeated the same analysis excluding 8 one eyed patients and obtained similar results with vertical distance of CVT influencing parafoveal involvement of visual fields, **Figure 4**.

Discussion

This study observed large discs with greater vertical displacement of the central vessel trunk and worse visual field indices in eyes with parafoveal visual field defects in one eye of bilateral NTG patients. Disc haemorrhage was more frequent in eyes with PF involvement. The PF group also was observed to have greater width of RNFL defects with most the RNFLD appearing in the inferior quadrant, with corresponding displacement of the CVT to the quadrant diametrically opposite quadrant in all except 3 eyes. Since we evaluated the differences between two eyes of the same patient, influence of systemic associations like nocturnal hypotension or systemic vascular imbalance affecting both eyes were obviated and local anatomic/topographic differences in the two eyes predisposing to PF scotoma in NTG could be evaluated. Since we included eyes with involvement of superior or inferior fields, we could determine 'disc specific" characteristics responsible for early paracentral involvement in one eye of bilateral NTG patients.

Previous investigations have demonstrated a relationship between the CVT exit on the lamina cribrosa and the extent of neuroretinal rim loss, location of visual field defects and peripapillary atrophy. [9–11] Neuroretinal rim loss and visual field defects follow a specific pattern related to regional susceptibilities of different disc regions. The superotemporal and inferotemporal area are the most commonly affected in early glaucoma while the nasal rim remnants may be the last to be affected in advanced glaucoma. Visual field defects follow the pattern of rim loss with the temporal island being the last to be involved in glaucoma [1,2,12–14].

This is partly explained by regional differences in lamina cribrosa with the superior and inferior regions having larger pores and higher pore-interpore tissue ratio, the lower susceptibility of thin fibres from the macula called the papillomacular bundle as compared to thicker fibres from the periphery, and also prominent backward bowing of the lamina in the superior and inferior disc regions with less connective tissue [1,12].

Although the central field is spared till late stages of glaucoma, some eyes develop defects threatening fixation in the earlier stages of glaucoma with consequent greater risk for reduced quality of life. [5,15,16] Ritch and colleagues demonstrated that eyes with parafoveal defects differ significantly from those with peripheral scotomas and demonstrated a specific pattern of progression in the former group. [5] Their results supported the notion that eyes with parafoveal scotoma early in the disease process are associated with IOP independent risk factors as compared to those with peripheral scotoma. They postulated that IOP-independent factors associated with decreased or unstable ocular perfusion may preferentially damage the neuroretinal rim or RNFL closer to the papillomacular bundle in the inferior half of the optic nerve head or retina, compared with elevated IOP, though the mechanism behind the preferential involvement of the inferior part of the optic nerve head was not clear. Jung et al evaluating ocular factors like disc morphology reported narrower rim and larger cup in eyes with paracentral scotoma with thinner RNFL thickness inferiorly. [17] They postulated that these eyes may be associated with more ganglion cell death than those with peripheral scotoma despite similar level of visual field defect. Yet these studies included both eyes of the same patient which makes it difficult to segregate effect of systemic factors in central field involvement.

In our study we observed increased displacement of the CVT exit into the superonasal quadrant in eyes with parafoveal involvement in one eye of bilateral normal tension glaucoma thereby obviating the effects of systemic vascular factors. This

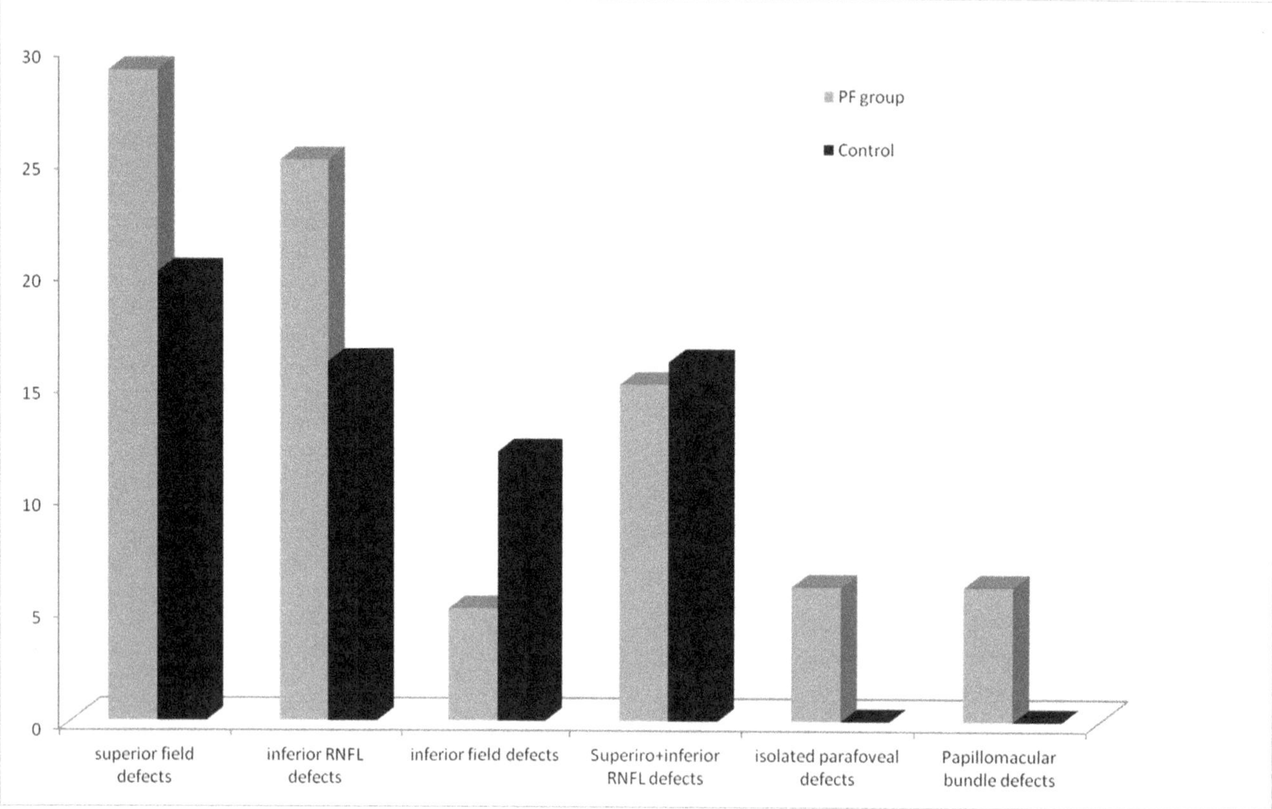

Figure 3. The parafoveal scotoma group showed a predominance of superior field defects (29 of 40 eyes) and inferior retinal nerve fibre layer defects (25 of 40 eyes).

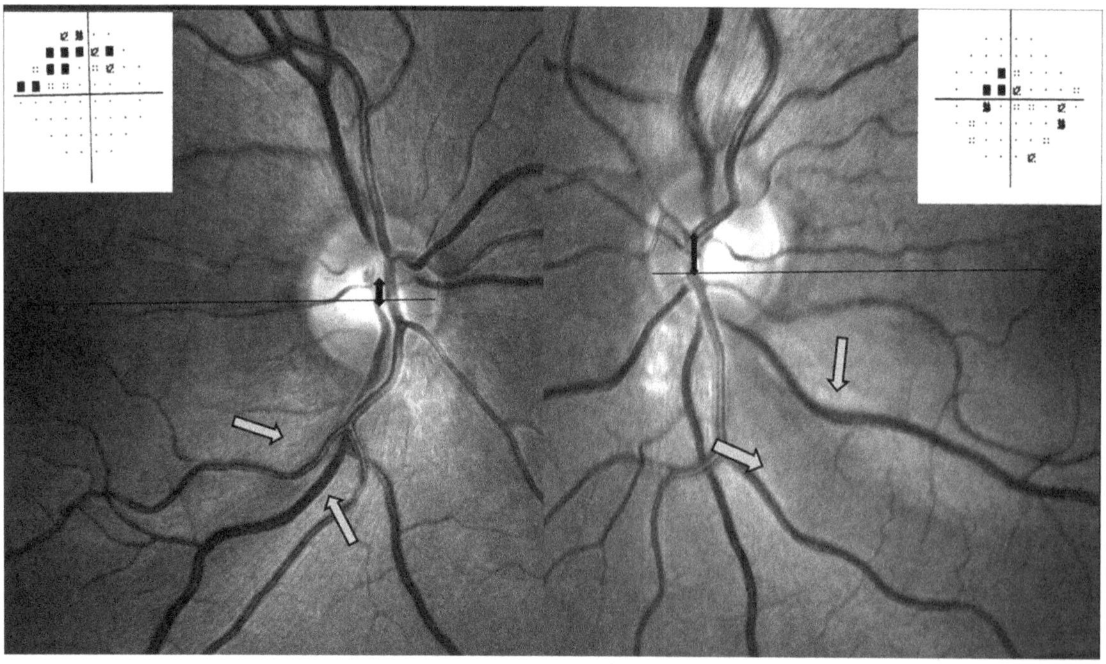

Figure 4. Red free Fundus photographs showing greater vertical displacement of the central vessel trunk (black solid arrows) into the superonasal quadrant away from the retinal nerve fibre layer defect inferotemporally (gray arrows) in the left eye with parafoveal scotoma (inset) as compared to the right eye with no parafoveal involvement (inset).

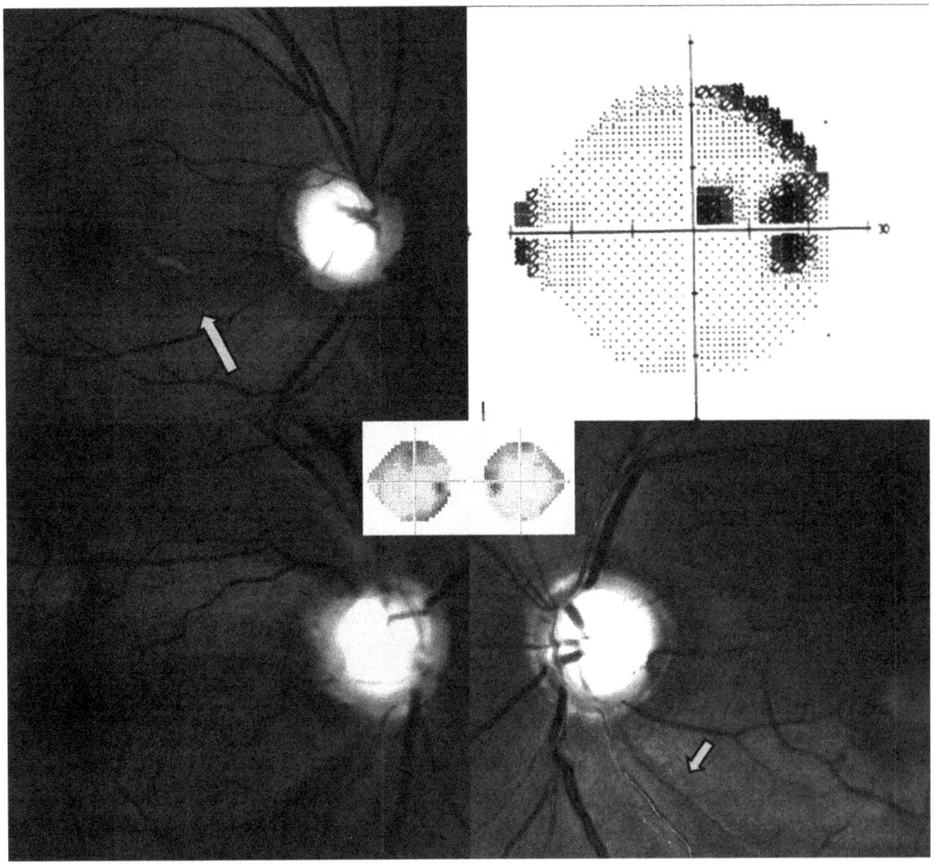

Figure 5. Red free photograph showing large disc in a patient with inferior papillomacular bundle defect (gray arrows) with superonasal displacement of the central vessel trunk (upper left) associated with parafoveal scotoma (upper right). Lower panel shows the red free photographs of case 6 with wedge shaped retinal nerve fibre layer defects involving superior, inferior and inferior papillomacular area, superonasally displaced central vessel trunk in the right eye and inferior defect (gray arrow) and centrally placed central vessel trunk in the left eye with parafoveal involvement in the right eye (inset).

suggests that involvement of the inferior optic nerve head, which is farthest from the central vessel trunk, is possibly due to increased distance of the inferior region from the central vessel trunk. This observation has been reported to be responsible for increased area of peripapillary atrophy and greater extent of neuroretinal rim loss in the area farthest from the location of CVT exit [10,11].

Jonas et al has postulated that the retinal vessel trunk may act as a stabilising element which would resist a more backward bowing of the lamina and also confer greater vicinity to a richer vascular supply making it more resistant to insult by vascular dysfunction. [10] Our study results support the theory that the CVT confers a mechanical support as well as provides a source of vascular supply to areas in its vicinity in normal eyes with increased displacement away from the centre being a risk for central field involvement early in the disease process.

Disc haemorrhage was more frequent in the PF group than in control eyes in this study. This concurs with previous studies of disc haemorrhages more frequent in eyes with parafoveal involvement. [3,5,17] However previous studies attributed systemic hypotension, vascular abnormalities like Raynaud's phenomenon as risk factors for disc haemorrhages. [2,3] The reported frequency of DH detection ranges from 0% to 0.4% in normal patients, 2% to 37% in patients with primary open-angle glaucoma, 11% to 42% in patients with NTG, and 0.4% to

Table 5. Comparison of disc characteristics in eyes with parafoveal involvement with or without disc haemorrhage.

	Disc haemorrhage	No disc haemorrhage	P value
Vertical disc diameter (mm)	1.7±0.4	1.6±0.7	0.8
Horizontal disc diameter (mm)	1.3±0.2	1.4±0.2	0.4
RNFL defect width (degrees)	42±30.4	39±23.6	0.3
Vertical CVT distance (mm)	0.18±0.08	0.13±0.07	0:06
Horizontal CVT distance (mm)	0.6±0.2	0.6±0.1	0.9

10% in patients with ocular hypertension. [18,19] Disc haemorrhage was found to be a risk factor for visual field progression in NTG eyes with IOP<15 mm Hg. [20] While the debate continues if disc haemorrhage is a risk factor or sign of progression, it is proved beyond doubt that disc haemorrhages are associated with greater visual field loss and signify vascular dysfunction at the level of the optic nerve. Our study did not find any significant difference in disc variables in eyes with and without disc haemorrhages in both groups. This may support the theory that these are more related to systemic vascular abnormalities rather than the influence of local factors.

Visual field indices were worse in PF groups with the latter group having lower defect depth despite similar foveal threshold and number of points with p<1% signifying deeper and more localised visual field defects as evidenced by a greater pattern standard deviation. This is in agreement with previous studies which have demonstrated similar results. [5] Ganglion cells are mostly concentrated in the central or paracentral area with the greatest density 1 mm from the fovea, most them being midget ganglion cells. [21–23] The ratio of midget to parasol ganglion cells increases from 30:1 in the centre to 3:1 in the periphery with larger receptive field radii of the cells in the periphery. This may mean that the ganglion cells at the centre with smaller receptive field may be more susceptible to regional differences in supply of nutritional factors or blood supply than in the periphery. It may be postulated that displacement of the central vessel trunk away snaps off vascular supply to areas in its immediate vicinity; such a vascular imbalance would induce more localised damage to the ganglion cells in that specified area in NTG despite similar systemic factors say blood pressure or optic nerve blood flow or local factors like intraocular pressure. This may in part explain involvement of central area in only one eye or greater defect depth in PF group despite similar number of points with p<1% in patients with similar systemic risk factors and further studies exploring this theory would be desirable. The visual field index is more centrally weighted highlighting the importance of central visual field. The extent of displacement of the CVT exit with respect to the VFI in different areas may be interesting to evaluate in future studies.

While the role of IOP independent factors has been established earlier, several studies are focussing on IOP dependent factors in NTG eyes. [6,7,20] Lee et al found significantly higher mean IOP and greater IOP fluctuations in eyes with baseline untreated IOP>15 mm Hg thought the rate of progression was similar to those with untreated IOP<15 mm Hg. Wang et al reported greater area of inferior peripapillary atrophy in eyes with IOP< 15 mm while Yamagami et al found IOP dependent VF damage in patients with an IOP of between 15 and 21 mm Hg. [15,24] Similarly, RNFL defects were found to be more central in location in eyes with lower IOP while the angular width of the defects did not depend on the IOP. [6,7] In our study, we found a greater width of RNFLD in the PF group, though on multivariate analysis, this was not however a significant association. Similar observations have been reported in a study evaluating disc morphology in eyes with and without PF involvement. [17] It may be speculated that structural changes like RNFL thickness are more dependent on the mechanical factors like loss of support connective tissues at the level of the optic nerve while functional changes like those in visual field are more related to vascular factors like proximity to the CVT or autoregulation. Further studies are warranted which explores the differences in regional structure and their association to functional changes in NTG eyes.

This study observed a difference in vertical disc diameter between two eyes of the same patient. Inter-eye asymmetry is a strong indicator of glaucoma. While most studies have studied asymmetric cup disc ratio, few studies like Blue Mountains study have evaluated the asymmetry in disc parameters including vertical disc diameter. [25] This study found a median value for disc diameter asymmetry of 0.07–0.08 mm in glaucoma patients. They however observed that this asymmetry may not be useful for differentiating patients from normals. This observation has caused a major shift in focus from disc asymmetry to asymmetry in cup disc ratio, which is currently the most important determinant for defining glaucoma. Yet, we believe that disc diameter (determining cup size asymmetry) differences in glaucomatous eyes may actually explain differential extent of involvement of both eyes in the same patient. The importance of disc diameter in predisposing an eye to any particular insult may possibly be determined by anatomical differences responsible for disc asymmetry which may also be responsible for anatomical differences in vascular supply. Further studies probing the asymmetry in disc parameters with anatomical differences in vascular supply in glaucoma patients are required to investigate and confirm this possibility.

One of the limitations of our study was that we cannot extrapolate this observation to high myopic eyes since those with high refractive errors or tilted disc (which are potential confounders) were excluded. Also it is unclear if different disc phenotypes like tilted discs would have different CVT exits and therefore alter the susceptibilities of the optic nerve head. We cannot explain why the CVT exit is seen more into the superonasal quadrant in NTG and whether this phenomenon plays a major role in other types of high pressure glaucoma as well.

In conclusion, a greater displacement of the CVT exit from the centre may suggest a higher risk of involvement the central visual field warranting closer follow up and possibly aggressive treatment in bilateral NTG eyes. Further studies evaluating its role in other types of glaucoma and progression of glaucoma is warranted in the future.

Author Contributions

Conceived and designed the experiments: APR SM. Performed the experiments: APR SM. Analyzed the data: APR. Contributed reagents/materials/analysis tools: APR SM. Wrote the paper: APR SM.

References

1. Fechtner RD, Weinreb RN (1994) Mechanisms of optic nerve damage in primary open angle glaucoma. Surv Ophthalmol. 39: 23–42.
2. Drance S, Anderson DR, Schulzer M, Collaborative Normal-Tension Glaucoma Study Group (2001) Risk factors for progression of visual field abnormalities in normal-tension glaucoma. Am J Ophthalmol. 131: 699–708.
3. Ishida K, Yamamoto T, Sugiyama K, Kitazawa Y (2000). Disk hemorrhage is a significantly negative prognostic factor in normal-tension glaucoma. Am J Ophthalmol. 129: 707–714.
4. Ren R, Jonas JB, Tian G, Zhen Y, Ma K, et al (2010) Cerebrospinal fluid pressure in glaucoma: a prospective study. Ophthalmology. 117: 259–66.

5. Park SC, De Moraes CG, Teng CC, Tello C, Liebmann JM, et al (2011) Initial parafoveal versus peripheral scotomas in glaucoma: risk factors and visual field characteristics. Ophthalmology. 118: 1782–9.
6. Wang XH, Stewart WC, Jackson GJ (1996) Differences in optic discs in low-tension glaucoma patients with relatively low or high pressures. Acta Ophthalmol Scand. 74: 364–367.
7. Kim DM, Seo JH, Kim SH, Hwang SS (2007) Comparison of localized retinal nerve fiber layer defects between a low-teen intraocular pressure group and a high-teen intraocular pressure group in normal-tension glaucoma patients. J Glaucoma. 16: 293–296.
8. Kim TW, Park UC, Park KH, Kim DM (2007) Ability of Stratus OCT to identify localized retinal nerve fiber layer defects in patients with normal standard automated perimetry results. InvestOphthalmol Vis Sci. 48: 1635–1641.
9. Huang H, Jonas JB, Dai Y, Hong J, Wang M, et al (2013) Position of the central retinal vessel trunk and pattern of remaining visual field in advanced glaucoma. Br J Ophthalmol. 97: 96–100.
10. Jonas JB, Budde WM, Nemeth J, Gründler AE, Mistlberger A, et al (2001) Central retinal vessel trunk exit and location of glaucomatous parapapillary atrophy in glaucoma. Ophthalmology. 108: 1059–1064.
11. Jonas JB, Fernández MC (1994) Shape of the neuroretinal rim and position of the central retinal vessels in glaucoma. Br J Ophthalmol. 78: 99–102.
12. Lee SS, Schwartz B (1992) Role of the temporal cilioretinal artery in retaining central visual field in open-angle glaucoma. Ophthalmology 99: 696–9.
13. Hitchings RA, Anderton SA (1983) A comparative study of visual field defects seen in patients with low-tension glaucoma and chronic simple glaucoma. Br J Ophthalmol. 67: 818–821.
14. Curcio CA, Allen KA (1990) Topography of ganglion cells in human retina. J Comp Neurol. 1990; 300: 5–25.
15. Hood DC, Raza AS, de Moraes CG, Odel JG, Greenstein VC, et al (2011) Initial arcuate defects within the central 10 degrees in glaucoma. Invest Ophthalmol Vis Sci. 52: 940–946.
16. Su D, Park SC, Simonson JL, Liebmann JM, Ritch R (2013) Progression pattern of initial parafoveal scotomas in glaucoma. Ophthalmology. 120: 520–7.
17. Jung KI, Park HY, Park CK (2012) Characteristics of optic disc morphology in glaucoma patients with parafoveal scotoma compared to peripheral scotoma. Invest Ophthalmol Vis Sci. 53: 4813–20.
18. Grieshaber MC, Terhorst T, Flammer J (2006) The pathogenesis of optic disc splinter haemorrhages: a new hypothesis. Acta Ophthalmol Scand. 84: 62–68.
19. Hendrickx KH, van den Enden A, Rasker MT, Hoyng PF (1994) Cumulative incidence of patients with disc hemorrhages in glaucoma and the effect of therapy. Ophthalmology. 101: 1165–72.
20. Lee J, Kong M, Kim J, Kee C (2013) Comparison of Visual Field Progression Between Relatively Low and High Intraocular Pressure Groups in Normal Tension Glaucoma Patients. J Glaucoma.Jun 6. [in press].
21. Dacey DM, Petersen MR (1992) Dendritic field size and morphology of midget and parasol ganglion cells of the human retina. Proc Natl Acad Sci U S A. 89: 9666–9670.
22. De Monasterio FM, Gouras P (1975) Functional properties of ganglion cells of the rhesus monkey retina. J Physiol. 251: 167–195.
23. Walsh N, Fitzgibbon T, Ghosh KK (1999) Intraretinal axon diameter: a single cell analysis in the marmoset (Callithrix jacchus). J Neurocytol. 28: 989–998.
24. Yamagami J, Shirato S, Araie M (1990) The influence of the intraocular pressure on the visual field of low tension glaucoma. Nihon Ganka Gakkai Zasshi. 94: 514–518.
25. Ong LS, Mitchell P, Healey PR, Cumming RG (1999) Asymmetry in optic disc parameters: the Blue Mountains Eye Study. Invest Ophthalmol Vis Sci.;40: 849–57.

22

Soluble Guanylate Cyclase α_1–Deficient Mice: A Novel Murine Model for Primary Open Angle Glaucoma

Emmanuel S. Buys[1]*, Yu-Chieh Ko[2,3], Clemens Alt[4], Sarah R. Hayton[1], Alexander Jones[2], Laurel T. Tainsh[1], Ruiyi Ren[5], Andrea Giani[6], Maeva Clerté[7], Emma Abernathy[2], Robert E. T. Tainsh[1], Dong-Jin Oh[6], Rajeev Malhotra[7], Pankaj Arora[7], Nadine de Waard[2], Binglan Yu[1], Raphael Turcotte[4,8], Daniel Nathan[1], Marielle Scherrer-Crosbie[7], Stephanie J. Loomis[6], Jae H. Kang[9], Charles P. Lin[4], Haiyan Gong[5], Douglas J. Rhee[6], Peter Brouckaert[10], Janey L. Wiggs[6], Meredith S. Gregory[2,6], Louis R. Pasquale[2,6,9], Kenneth D. Bloch[1,7], Bruce R. Ksander[2,6]

1 Anesthesia Center for Critical Care Research, Department of Anesthesia, Critical Care, and Pain Medicine, Massachusetts General Hospital, Harvard Medical School, Boston, Massachusetts, United States of America, **2** Department of Ophthalmology, Schepens Eye Research Institute, Harvard Medical School, Boston, Massachusetts, United States of America, **3** Department of Ophthalmology, School of Medicine, National Yang-Ming University, Taipei, Taiwan, **4** Wellman Center for Photomedicine and Center for Systems Biology, Massachusetts General Hospital, Harvard Medical School, Boston, Massachusetts, United States of America, **5** Department of Ophthalmology, Boston University School of Medicine, Boston, Massachusetts, United States of America, **6** Department of Ophthalmology, Massachusetts Eye and Ear Infirmary, Harvard Medical School, Boston, Massachusetts, United States of America, **7** Cardiology Division, Department of Medicine, Massachusetts General Hospital, Harvard Medical School, Boston, Massachusetts, United States of America, **8** Department of Biomedical Engineering, Boston University, Boston, Massachusetts, United States of America, **9** Channing Division of Network Medicine, Brigham and Women's Hospital, Harvard Medical School, Boston, Massachusetts, United States of America, **10** VIB Department of Molecular Biomedical Research, Ghent University, Ghent, Belgium

Abstract

Primary open angle glaucoma (POAG) is a leading cause of blindness worldwide. The molecular signaling involved in the pathogenesis of POAG remains unknown. Here, we report that mice lacking the α_1 subunit of the nitric oxide receptor soluble guanylate cyclase represent a novel and translatable animal model of POAG, characterized by thinning of the retinal nerve fiber layer and loss of optic nerve axons in the context of an open iridocorneal angle. The optic neuropathy associated with soluble guanylate cyclase α_1–deficiency was accompanied by modestly increased intraocular pressure and retinal vascular dysfunction. Moreover, data from a candidate gene association study suggests that a variant in the locus containing the genes encoding for the α_1 and β_1 subunits of soluble guanylate cyclase is associated with POAG in patients presenting with initial paracentral vision loss, a disease subtype thought to be associated with vascular dysregulation. These findings provide new insights into the pathogenesis and genetics of POAG and suggest new therapeutic strategies for POAG.

Editor: Richard Libby, University of Rochester, United States of America

Funding: This work was conducted with support from Harvard Catalyst-the Harvard Clinical and Translational Science Center (NIH Award #UL1 RR 025758, and financial contributions from Harvard University and its affiliated academic health care centers) (ESB, BRK); a Shaffer Fund Grant from the Glaucoma Research Foundation (ESB); NEI R21 EY020987 (ESB, BRK); NEI R01 EY022746-01 (ESB); an American Heart Association Fellow-to-Faculty Transition Award #11FTF7290032 (RM); NCRR 1S10RR022586 (MSC); NIH CA87969, CA49449, EY09611, CA055075 (JHK); the Massachusetts Lions Eye Research Fund (HG, RR); the FWO-Flanders and UGent-GOA funds (PB); NEI R01 EY015872 (JLW); the Harvard Glaucoma Center of Excellence (LRP and JLW); a Harvard Ophthalmology Scholar award (LRP); a Physician-Scientist award from Research to Prevent Blindness in NYC (LRP); an Allergan Horizon grant (LRP); NEI R01 EY015473 (LRP); and NHGRI 5U01HG004728 (LRP). The funders had no role in study design, data collection and analysis, decision to publish, or preparation of the manuscript.

Competing Interests: Peter Brouckaert: The Flemish Institute for Biotechnology receives a fee from a nonexclusive license of sGCα1−/− mice to the pharmaceutical industry. This study was partly funded by an Allergan Horizon grant. There are no further patents, products in development or marketed products to declare. This does not alter the authors' adherence to all the PLOS ONE policies on sharing data and materials, as detailed online in the guide for authors.

* E-mail: Ebuys@partners.org

Introduction

Glaucoma is a progressive eye disease that ultimately leads to blindness due to the irreversible loss of retinal ganglion cells (RGCs) with concomitant optic nerve degeneration [1]. Over 4 million Americans and 65 million people worldwide have glaucoma, making it the leading cause of blindness in the US and the second leading cause of blindness worldwide. Although available therapies delay disease progression [1], protection remains incomplete and vision loss due to glaucoma cannot be regained, highlighting the need for novel therapeutic approaches and drug targets [2]. In primary open-angle glaucoma (POAG), one of the most common glaucoma subtypes, there is variable elevation of intraocular pressure (IOP) associated with impaired aqueous outflow that occurs despite normal anterior segment anatomy and an open iridocorneal angle [1].

Although multiple POAG risk factors have been identified [2], the etiology of POAG remains to be elucidated, likely because the disease can be stratified into various subtypes defined by discrete but yet unknown biochemical pathways. Two major pathophysiologic mechanisms for POAG have been proposed. In the "mechanical theory" [1,2,3,4] optic neuropathy is caused by increased IOP, an important risk factor for glaucoma [5,6]. While elevated IOP is currently the only risk factor amenable to treatment, some patients with high IOP do not develop POAG and other patients with low or normal IOP do, suggesting that other pathologies may contribute to the etiology of POAG [2,6]. Alternatively, a vascular component has been hypothesized to contribute to POAG pathophysiology. Intravenous administration of the endothelial and NO-dependent vasodilator acetylcholine, fails to mediate brachial artery vasodilation in untreated POAG [7]. Also, flow-mediated vasodilation [8] and retinal vascular autoregulation [9] are impaired in POAG. Furthermore, POAG patients with initial paracentral visual field loss tend to have more frequent systemic vascular risk factors such as migraines and hypotension [10], and low ocular perfusion pressure (mean arterial blood pressure – IOP) is a risk factor for POAG [11,12]. However, the extent to which vascular dysfunction contributes to glaucomatous optic neuropathy remains to be elucidated and is controversial [3,4].

Nitric oxide (NO) is an attractive candidate as a factor that could modify both mechanical and vascular events in POAG pathogenesis. NO, an important modulator of smooth muscle function, is synthesized by a family of three enzymes referred to as NO synthases (NOSs), all of which are expressed in the eye [13,14,15]. NO activates the cGMP-generating heterodimeric enzyme soluble guanylate cyclase (sGC). sGC consists of one α and one β subunit and mediates many of the physiological effects of NO, including the ability of NO to relax smooth muscle cells [16,17]. Two isoforms of each sGC subunit have been identified (α_1, α_2, β_1, and β_2), but only the sGC$\alpha_1\beta_1$ and sGC$\alpha_2\beta_1$ heterodimers appear to function in vivo [18].

NO-cGMP signaling has been suggested to participate in the regulation of aqueous humor (AqH) outflow and IOP [19,20]. Preclinical studies have demonstrated the ability of NO-donor compounds to lower IOP [21,22] and enhance tissue oxygenation of the optic nerve head [23]. Importantly, NO metabolites and cGMP levels are decreased in plasma and AqH samples from POAG patients [24,25]. Moreover, two independent studies have identified NOS3 gene variants that are associated with POAG in women [26,27]. A third study that did not find an association between NOS3 variants and POAG had a small sample size and did not provide gender specific results [28]. Together, these findings suggest that impaired NO-cGMP signaling can contribute to the etiology of POAG [29,30]. Several mechanisms, including genetic variation and oxidative stress can regulate NO-cGMP signaling. However, the mechanisms by which NO-cGMP signaling modulates POAG risk and whether impaired NO-cGMP signaling can result in POAG remain unclear.

Here, we identify mice deficient in sGCα_1 (sGC$\alpha_1^{-/-}$ mice) as a new murine model of POAG characterized by age-related optic neuropathy, an age-related increase in IOP, and retinal vascular dysfunction. Moreover, in a nested case-control study, we identified a genetic association between the locus containing the genes encoding the α_1 and β_1 subunits of sGC and a subtype of POAG characterized by paracentral vision loss and vascular dysregulation.

Materials and Methods

Ethics statement

This study was carried out in strict accordance with the recommendations in the Guide for the Care and Use of Laboratory Animals of the National Institutes of Health. Housing and all procedures involving experimental animals (mice) described in this study were specifically approved by the Institutional Animal Care and Use Committees (IACUC) of Massachusetts General Hospital (Subcommittee on Research Animal Care), and the Schepens Eye Research Institute. All procedures were performed under adequate anesthesia, and all efforts were made to minimize suffering. The Institutional Review Board of the Massachusetts Eye and Ear Infirmary, Harvard School of Public Health, and Brigham and Women's Hospital approved the gene association studies described. All participants provided written informed consent. The Human Research Committees of Massachusetts Eye and Ear Infirmary, Partners Healthcare System, and the Harvard School of Public Health approved the consent procedure.

Animals

Age-matched, one- to 17-month-old female sGC$\alpha_1^{-/-}$ mice and WT mice on a 129S6 background were studied [31]. Mice were anesthetized (for AqH outflow measurements and SD-OCT) by intraperitoneal (IP) injection of ketamine (100 mg/kg) and xylazine (9 mg/kg) or (for IOP measurements and SLO experiments) with isoflurane (2%). Mice were euthanized (for tissue harvest) using pentobarbital (10 mg IP). Observers masked as to animal genotype performed all data acquisition and analyses described.

Histology and immunohistochemistry

Human eyes (obtained from the New England Eye Bank (Newton, MA)) and mouse eyes were fixed in paraformaldehyde, embedded in paraffin, sectioned and incubated with antibodies specific for sGCα1, sGCβ1, or α-smooth muscle actin (1:100 dilution; Abcam), followed by reaction with AlexaFluor goat anti-rabbit or anti-mouse IgG (1:1000, Invitrogen), Dylight donkey anti-rabbit IgG (1:100, Stratech Scientific), or biotinylated secondary antibodies.

Retinal flatmounts were prepared from paraformaldehyde-fixed eyes and stained with anti-βIII-tubulin (1:150 dilution; Millipore) or anti-SMI32 (1:500 dilution; Covance) antibodies. Stained RGCs were detected with biotin-, rhodamine-labeled secondary antibodies using confocal microscopy (Leica-TCS-SP5). For RGC counting, retinal flat mounts were divided into quadrants: superior, temporal, nasal, and inferior. Using the optic nerve head (ONH) as the origin, 3 standard regions that were distributed at a 1-mm interval along the radius (0.09 mm^2) were selected from each quadrant: two from the peripheral region (2 mm from the ONH) and one from the intermediate region (1 mm from the ONH). 12 rectangular regions of each eye were photographed at 40× magnification with a confocal microscope (Leica TSC SPS confocal microscope).

For Toluidine Blue staining, mouse eyes were fixed in 2.5% glutaraldehyde and 2% paraformaldehyde, post-fixed in 2% osmium tetroxide in 1.5% potassium ferrocyanide, dehydrated, mid-sagittally sectioned, embedded in Epon-Araldite, and stained.

Spectral domain optical coherence tomography

Retinal nerve fiber layer (RNFL) thickness was measured using a SD-OCT system (Bioptigen, NC). Pupils of anesthetized mice were dilated with topical application of 1% tropicamide. SD-OCT was performed using 100 horizontal raster and consecutive B-scan lines composed of 1200 A-scans. Total retinal thickness and RNFL thickness were analyzed using InVivoVue Diver 2.0 software (Bioptigen). Data were post-processed using a custom-made algorithm allowing additional filtering to only include RNFL thickness values between 5.4 and 24 microns in thickness. The 5.4–24 micron range was selected based on the average RNFL thickness ± 3 times the standard deviation described previously

[32] for RNFL thickness of control mice. To validate the automated segmentation analysis, RNFL thickness was measured in 24 points of a 5×5 grid using the caliper tool provided by the Bioptigen software (fig. S1B).

Paraphenylenediamine staining

Optic nerve cross-sections were prepared and axons were counted as previously described [33]. The myelin sheath of all axons, and the axoplasma of damaged axons were stained with paraphenylenediamine (PPD) and examined for glaucomatous damage. Sections of nerve between the orbit and chiasm were dissected, processed, embedded in resin, sectioned, and stained with PPD. To count axons, the optic nerve was outlined at 100× magnification and its cross-sectional area was automatically calculated (METAMORPH, Version 4.6r9, Universal Imaging, Downingtown, PA). Axons were counted manually and marked on images using the technique described previously [33]. The program tracked the total area counted and the total axon count for all images. The total counted area was 10% of the total nerve area. The final count was calculated and expressed as number of axons per optic nerve.

IOP measurement

IOP measurements were acquired in anesthetized mice using a rebound tonometer (Tonolab) as described previously [34]. Five TonoLab readouts were averaged to obtain a single IOP value per eye.

Ultrasound bio-microscopy (UBM)

UBM images were acquired and analyzed with a Vevo 770 scanner (VisualSonics), as previously described [35].

Assessment of aqueous humor turnover

AqH turnover was measured noninvasively, using a previously published fluorophotometric technique [36]. Benzalkonium chloride (10 µl of a 0.02% solution in saline) was applied to the eye of anesthetized mice to permeabilize the cornea to fluorescein. After 5 minutes, 10 µl of a 0.02% fluoresce in saline solution was applied to the eye for 5 minutes. Images were captured from a focal plane intermediate between the iris and cornea using a microscope (SZX16, Olympus) equipped with an Olympus DP72 camera, a GFP filter, and acquisition software (cellSens Standard 1.2, Olympus). Average pixel intensity in the green channel was determined in an area of interest free of corneal defects using ImageJ. AqH clearance was determined by the decay constant calculated from the relative fluorescent intensity measured at 10-minute intervals for 60 minutes after a single fluorescein treatment.

Scanning laser ophthalmoscopy

We previously developed a scanning laser ophthalmoscope (SLO) for confocal imaging of the mouse retina [37]. The SLO was used to record, at video rate, the width of the retinal arteries, visualized by intravenous (I.V.) injection of fluorescein sodium prior to, during, and after injection of 0.8 mg/kg sodium nitroprusside. To compute the width of the retinal arterioles, short segments (approximately 10 pixels in length) of the retinal arterioles were isolated from the recorded and re-aligned movies at fixed distances (measurements at 150 µm and 250 µm were averaged to yield one value/arteriole) from the optic nerve head. The width of each blood vessel segment was determined in MatLab as the width at which the pixel intensity dropped to 50% of the maximum (full width at half maximum, FWHM). The diameter of retinal arterioles (each 50 frame averages) was measured at baseline and after I.V. injection of 0.8 mg/kg sodium nitroprusside (in 50 µl of saline), a dose that was selected because it was associated with a similar drop in systemic blood pressure in WT and $sGC\alpha_1^{-/-}$ mice. The relative change in diameter was calculated for each blood vessel. Injecting 50 µl of vehicle did not alter blood pressure or retinal arteriole diameter.

In vivo hemodynamics

Mice were anaesthetized by IP injection with ketamine (100 mg/kg), fentanyl (50 µg/kg), and pancuronium (2 mg/kg); intubated; and mechanically ventilated ($FiO_2 = 1$, 10 µl/g, 120 breaths per minute). A saline-filled catheter was inserted into the left carotid artery for infusion of saline (2 ml/h) and for measurement of mean arterial blood pressure (MAP) before, during and after I.V. injection of 0.8 mg/kg sodium nitroprusside. The sodium nitroprusside-induced decrease in MAP is expressed as % decrease from baseline.

Statistical analysis for animal data

Statistical analyses (other than for the targeted gene association study, see below) were performed using Microsoft Excel or Stata 8.0. Normality of data was confirmed using the Shapiro-Wilk test. IOP, SLO, and MAP comparisons were performed using either student's t test when comparing 2 groups, 1-way ANOVA with Bonferroni post-hoc pairwise testing when groups were stratified by age, or multivariate linear regression to assess the ability of age to predict IOP. Least-squares regression analysis for exponential decay ($Y = Ae^{-kt}$) was performed when assessing the change in aqueous fluorescein concentration (Y) over time (t), and exponential decay constants were compared using linear regression. Aqueous fluorescein concentrations and SD-OCT thickness were analyzed using 2-way repeated measures ANOVA, with post-hoc comparisons using 1-way ANOVA in circumstances of significant interaction *p*-values (e.g. for aqueous humor outflow rate measurements in 57-week-old mice). Data are presented as mean ± SD in the text and mean ± SEM in the figures. $P<0.05$ was considered significant.

Association between GUCY1A3/GUCY1B3 single nucleotide polymorphisms (SNPs) and POAG in the Glaucoma Gene and Environment (GLAUGEN) study

The GWAS methods have been described previously [38]. Briefly, the GLAUGEN (**Glau**coma **g**enes and **en**vironment, dbGaP Study Accession #: phs000308.v1.p1) cohort included 976 POAG cases, defined as individuals with reproducible visual field defects correlating with clinical evidence of ON degeneration, and 1140 controls drawn from two longitudinal studies (the Nurses Health Study and the Health Professionals Follow-up study) and one clinic-based cohort from the Massachusetts Eye and Ear Infirmary. All participants were residents of the continental United States and were of European ancestry, confirmed by both self-identification and genetic markers. Genotyping was performed using the Illumina 660W-Quad-v1 platform at the Broad Institute and appropriate quality filters were applied to ensure a clean dataset. 495,132 SNPs passed quality control filters. POAG-SNP association in two soluble guanylate cyclase genes (GUCY1A3 and GUCY1B3) was analyzed. As these genes are adjacent, a list of SNPs within, between, and in a 50 kb window on either side of the genes was obtained using the UCSC Genome Browser [39]. These SNPs were entered into the SNAP proxy search to generate a list of all genotyped and tagging SNPs on the Illumina 660W-Quad platform, giving a total of 51 SNPs. Logistic regression for each gene to assess the association between individual SNPs and POAG was preformed using PLINK v1.07. The regression model included age, gender, race, study site, DNA source, DNA extraction method, and three eigenvectors. A sub-analysis was restricted to patients with paracentral visual field loss only (defined as having one or more paracentral scotomas and no peripheral visual field loss) leaving 175 cases and 1140 controls, and subsequently stratified according to gender (leaving 106 female cases and 682 female controls). SAS software was used to sort the results. To control for multiple comparisons (3 subgroups were analyzed: 1: POAG vs. control; 2: type of visual field loss; 3: gender), a Bonferroni correction of 3.3×10^{-4} (51 GUCY SNPs tested in 3 subsets of patients: $0.05/153 = 3.3\times10^{-4}$) was applied to define statistical significance.

Results

Expression of sGC in the mouse and human eye

Although expression of sGC has been detected in ocular tissue, including cultured human trabecular meshwork (TM) cells [20], human ciliary body and TM [40], drosophila photoreceptors [41], as well as rabbit [42], rat [43], and turtle [44] retina, detailed knowledge of spatial expression of the $sGC\alpha_1\beta_1$ isoform in the eye is still lacking. Therefore, ocular $sGC\alpha_1$ and $sGC\beta_1$ localization was determined histologically in tissue sections of enucleated human and mouse eyes. $sGC\alpha_1$ and $sGC\beta_1$ are expressed in three anatomical sites that may be important for glaucoma. $sGC\alpha_1$ and $sGC\beta_1$ are abundantly expressed in the ciliary muscle (CM, fig. 1A and 1D), suggesting that sGC might modulate CM contractility and AqH outflow. sGC is also present in the smooth muscle cell layer of retinal blood vessels in the human and mouse eye (fig. 1B and 1E), implying that sGC regulates blood flow in the retina, just as it does in the systemic vasculature. Finally, $sGC\alpha_1$ and $sGC\beta_1$ are expressed in RGCs (fig. 1C and 1F), suggesting that sGC may directly regulate RGC function and/or viability.

Retinal and optic nerve damage in $sGC\alpha_1^{-/-}$ mice

To avoid the potentially confounding effects of systemic hypertension (a risk factor for POAG [1]) observed in male but not female $sGC\alpha_1^{-/-}$ mice [31,45], we included only female mice in our study that do not develop hypertension, even as they age [31]. Thickness of the retina and of the RNFL was measured using spectral-domain optical coherence tomography (SD-OCT), a technique previously shown to provide reproducible non-invasive measurements of RNFL thickness in mice [46]. Total retinal thickness was similar in $sGC\alpha_1^{-/-}$ and age-matched wild-type (WT) mice, regardless of their age (fig. 2A and fig. S1). However, the RNFL was thinner in old $sGC\alpha_1^{-/-}$ mice than in age-matched WT mice (fig. 2A and fig. S1). RNFL thickness did not differ in young, age-matched $sGC\alpha_1^{-/-}$ and WT mice (fig. 2A and fig. S1), suggesting that abnormal embryonic development does not contribute to the observed RNFL thinning associated with $sGC\alpha_1$-deficiency.

To further characterize RNFL thinning in $sGC\alpha_1^{-/-}$ mice, retinal whole mounts from WT and $sGC\alpha_1^{-/-}$ mice were stained with either an anti-SMI32 antibody that stains nerve fibers or an anti-βIII tubulin antibody that stains both ganglion cells and nerve fibers. SMI32 staining revealed a loss of nerve fibers in whole-mount retinas isolated from old but not young $sGC\alpha_1^{-/-}$ mice (fig. 2B). Moreover, a lower number of RGCs were detected in old $sGC\alpha_1^{-/-}$ mice than in age-matched WT mice, a finding that was confirmed by immunohistochemistry in retinal flat-mounts (fig. 2C).

Because POAG is typically characterized by optic nerve damage, we investigated the impact of $sGC\alpha_1$-deficiency on total axon counts in the optic nerve, visualized using paraphenylene-diamine staining. The number of axons in twelve-month-old $sGC\alpha_1^{-/-}$ mice was less than in age-matched WT mice (fig. 2D). Together, these results indicate that, in mice, impaired NO-cGMP signaling results in optic neuropathy, an important feature of POAG.

Age-related intraocular pressure elevation in $sGC\alpha_1^{-/-}$ mice

Because IOP is considered the most important risk factor for POAG, IOP was measured non-invasively in young and old WT and $sGC\alpha_1^{-/-}$ mice. No difference in IOP was detected between young $sGC\alpha_1^{-/-}$ and age-matched WT mice. In contrast, IOP was higher in old $sGC\alpha_1^{-/-}$ mice than in age-matched WT mice (fig. S2A).

To further investigate the age-dependency of increased IOP associated with $sGC\alpha_1$-deficiency, we performed longitudinal measurements of IOP in age-matched $sGC\alpha_1^{-/-}$ and WT mice. IOP increased in $sGC\alpha_1^{-/-}$ but not in WT mice as they aged from 19 to 37 weeks (fig. 3). Similar results were obtained in separate validation cohorts of WT and $sGC\alpha_1^{-/-}$ mice (fig. S2B and C). Together, these results demonstrate that $sGC\alpha_1$-deficiency is associated with a subtle age-dependent IOP increase in mice.

$sGC\alpha_1$ deficiency does not alter anterior segment morphology

Central corneal thickness (CCT) is a risk factor for the conversion from ocular hypertension to POAG, making CCT measurements an integral component in the management of patients diagnosed with glaucoma [5]. In addition, CCT influences the measurement of IOP via rebound tonometry [47]. CCT, measured histologically, did not differ in age-matched 38±3-week-old WT and $sGC\alpha_1^{-/-}$ mice (87±7 and 87±9 μm, respectively; $n = 8$ each; $P = 0.90$) with normal and elevated IOP, respectively (14±1 versus 21±1 mmHg; $P = 5.9\times10^{-7}$). Therefore, $sGC\alpha_1$-deficiency does not affect CCT and abnormal CCT is not responsible for the elevated IOPs seen in old $sGC\alpha_1^{-/-}$ mice (fig. 4A).

To exclude the possibility that anatomical abnormalities impairing AqH drainage, such as those observed in DBA/2J mice [48] or in mice deficient in cytochrome P4501B1 ($Cyp1b1^{-/-}$ mice) [49], underlie the elevated IOP observed in older $sGC\alpha_1^{-/-}$ mice, we examined the morphology of the iridocorneal angle in 12-month-old WT and $sGC\alpha_1^{-/-}$ mice with normal and elevated IOP, respectively (15.8±1.2 and 19.1±1.7 mmHg; $n = 3$ each; $P = 0.041$). Morphologically, eyes of $sGC\alpha_1^{-/-}$ mice appeared normal, with a clear anterior chamber revealing complex iris detail and small round pupils. Depth of the anterior chamber (DAC) was assessed using *in vivo* ultrasound biomicroscopy. DAC did not differ in 56±3-week-old WT and $sGC\alpha_1^{-/-}$ mice (0.34±0.01 and 0.33±0.01 mm in $n = 4$ and 6, respectively; $P = 0.26$) with IOPs of 16±2 and 19±2 mmHg, respectively ($P = 4.3\times10^{-2}$, fig. 4B). In addition, ultrasound biomicroscopy revealed no morphological abnormalities in $sGC\alpha_1^{-/-}$ mice that could account for the elevated IOP measurements. Histological analyses revealed no apparent iridocorneal abnormalities in 12-month-old $sGC\alpha_1^{-/-}$ mice, including a normal ciliary body, a well-defined trabecular meshwork, and a patent Schlemm's canal (fig. 4C and D). Importantly, SD-OCT analysis of the iridocorneal angle, capable of distinguishing between an open and a closed angle (as in old DBA2/J mice), did not reveal any evidence for angle-closure in 12-

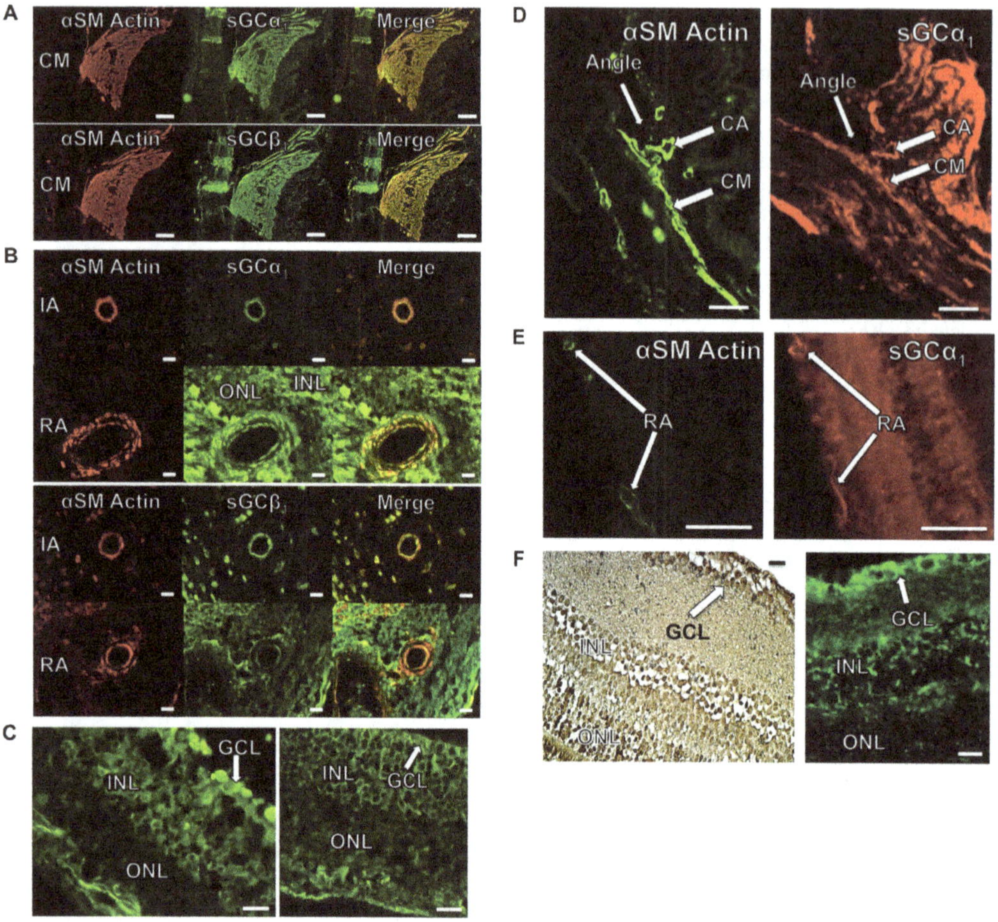

Figure 1. Localization of sGC α_1 and β_1 subunits in the human and murine eye. Panels **A–C** depict tissue sections from human eyes. Panels **D–F** depict tissue sections from mouse eyes. **A**: Ciliary muscle (CM), stained for α-smooth muscle actin (red), sGCα_1 (green, **upper panel**), or sGCβ_1 (green, **lower panel**). Both sGCα_1 and sGCβ_1 co-localized with α-smooth muscle actin in CM (yellow in merged images). Scale bars: 100 μm. **B**: An arteriole in the iris (IA) and an arteriole in the retina (RA) were stained for α-smooth muscle actin (red), sGCα_1 (green, **upper panels**), or sGCβ_1 (green, **lower panels**). Both sGCα_1 and sGCβ_1 co-localized with α-smooth muscle actin in the smooth muscle cell layer of arterioles in the iris and retina (yellow in merged images). ONL: outer nuclear layer, INL: inner nuclear layer. Scale bars: 20 μm. **C**: sGCα_1 (**left panel**) and sGCβ_1 (**right panel**) expression was detected histologically in the outer nuclear layer (ONL), inner nuclear layer (INL), and ganglion cell layer (GCL, white arrow) of the retina. sGCα_1 and sGCβ_1 are visualized by green fluorescence. Scale bars: 20 μm. **D**: Adjacent sections of a wild-type (WT) murine eye were stained for α-smooth muscle actin (green, **left panel**) or sGCα_1 (red, **right panel**). sGCα_1 co-localized with α-smooth muscle actin in ciliary muscle (CM) and in arterioles in the ciliary body (CA). The iridocorneal angle is indicated. Scale bars: 50 μm. **E**: Adjacent sections of a WT murine eye were stained for α-smooth muscle actin (green, **left panel**) or sGCα_1 (red, **right panel**). sGCα_1 co-localized with α-smooth muscle actin in retinal arterioles (RA). Scale bars: 50 μm. **F**: sGCα_1 (**left panel**) and sGCβ_1 (**right panel**) expression was detected histologically in the outer nuclear layer (ONL), inner nuclear layer (INL), and ganglion cell layer (GCL, white arrow) of the mouse retina. sGCα_1 is visualized by brown peroxidase stain and sGCβ_1 is visualized by green fluorescence. Scale bars: 20 μm.

month-old sGC$\alpha_1^{-/-}$ mice (fig. 4E and movies S1, S2, S3). Taken together, these data suggest that sGCα_1-deficiency does not alter the morphology of the anterior segment of the eye and that angle closure does not underlie the elevated IOP observed in old sGC$\alpha_1^{-/-}$ mice.

Decreased aqueous humor turnover in sGC$\alpha_1^{-/-}$ mice

IOP is determined by the balance between AqH production by the ciliary body and the rate of AqH outflow through the filtration angle. The AqH outflow rate was assessed using a fluorophotometric technique in age-matched WT and sGC$\alpha_1^{-/-}$ mice (fig. 5A). Monitoring decay of fluorescence provides a noninvasive index of AqH dynamics in the mouse eye [36]. Twelve-week-old WT and sGC$\alpha_1^{-/-}$ mice had similar IOPs and no difference in the rate of AqH outflow (fig. 5B). In contrast, AqH clearance was less in 57-week-old sGC$\alpha_1^{-/-}$ mice with elevated IOP than in age-matched WT mice (fig. 5C). These data indicate that there is an age-related decrease in AqH outflow in sGC$\alpha_1^{-/-}$ mice.

Retinal arterial dysfunction in sGC$\alpha_1^{-/-}$ mice

We previously reported that systemic vascular dysfunction, a potential etiologic factor for POAG [7,8,9], is manifest in the aorta [16], femoral arteries [16], carotid arteries [50], and mesenteric arteries [45] of both male and female sGC$\alpha_1^{-/-}$ mice. To assess retinal vascular function [9], we measured retinal arterial diameter using in vivo laser ophthalmoscopy (SLO, fig. S3A and B). Treatment with an NO-donor compound decreased blood pressure similarly in female WT and sGC$\alpha_1^{-/-}$ mice (59±2% and 60±3%, respectively, $n=5$ each; $P=0.37$). However, retinal arterial diameter decreased more in female WT than in sGC$\alpha_1^{-/-}$ mice (fig. 6 and fig. S3C). An altered retinal hemodynamic response to a decrease in blood pressure indicates

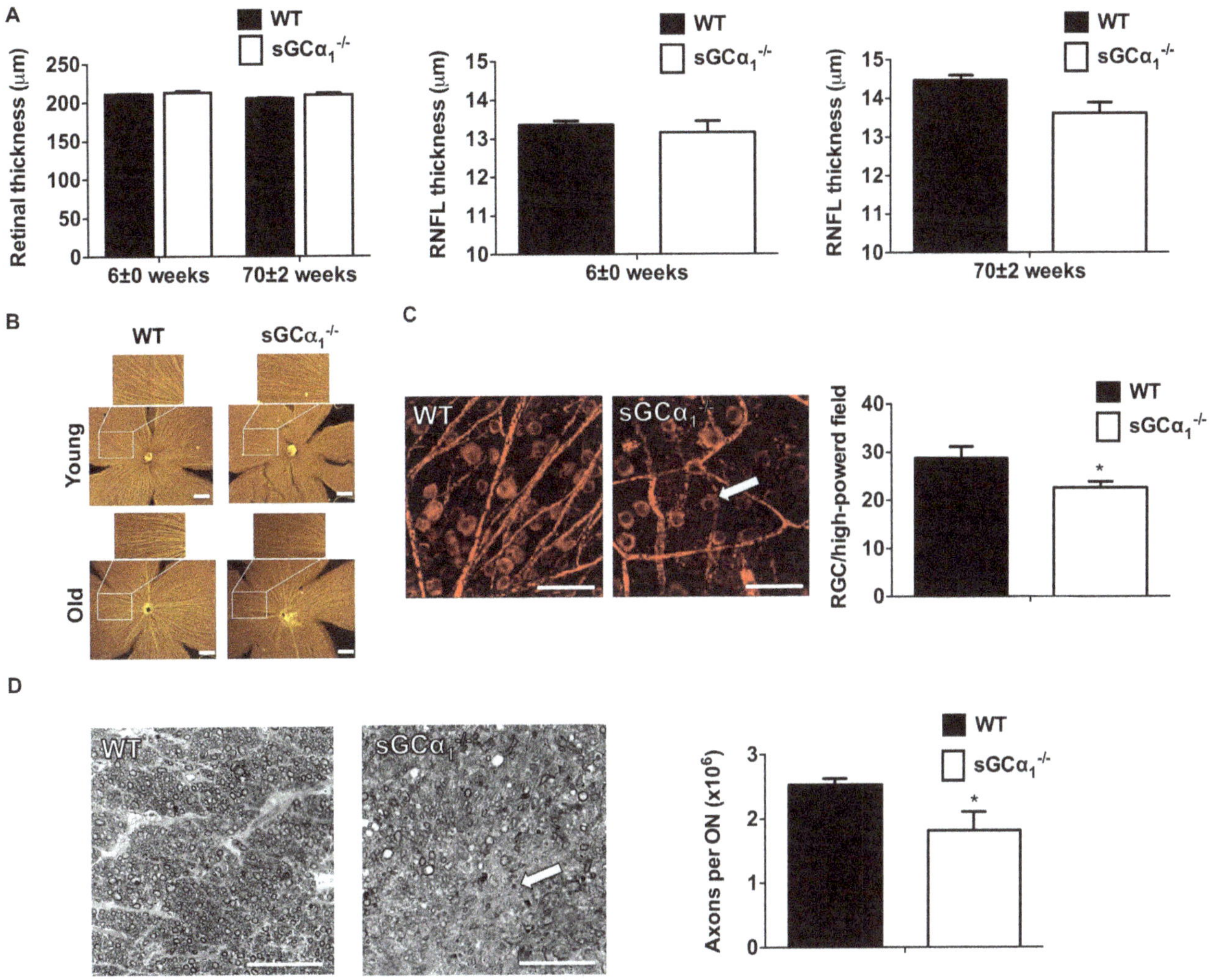

Figure 2. Retinal nerve fiber layer (RNFL) thinning and glaucomatous optic neuropathy in sGCα$_1$$^{-/-}$ mice. A: Quantitative analysis, assessed by SD-OCT (see also fig. S1), of total retinal thickness (**left panel**) and RNFL thickness, in young (6-week-old, **middle panel**) and old (70-week-old, **right panel**) wild-type (WT, $n=19$ and 13, respectively) and soluble guanylate cyclase α$_1$-deficient (sGCα$_1$$^{-/-}$) mice ($n=15$ and 14, respectively; $*P=1.2\times10^{-2}$). **B**: Representative whole-mount retinas from age-matched young (20-week-old) and old (56-week-old) WT and sGCα$_1$$^{-/-}$ mice, reacted with antibodies directed against SMI32, staining retinal nerve fibers yellow. Scale bars: 500 μm. **C**: Representative confocal images, taken at a similar distance from the optic nerve, of flat-mounted retinas isolated from age-matched 52-week-old WT and sGCα$_1$$^{-/-}$ mice that were reacted with antibodies directed against βIII Tubulin, and quantitative analysis of the number of RGCs/high-powered field ($n=8$ and 7, respectively; $*P=3.6\times10^{-2}$). A retinal ganglion cell (red) is indicated by an arrow. Scale bars: 20 μm. **D**: Representative cross sections through the optic nerve of 52-week-old WT and sGCα$_1$$^{-/-}$ mice stained with paraphenylenediamine, and quantitative analysis of the calculated number of axons/optic nerve (ON). The arrow indicates an injured area in the optic nerve, characterized by the absence of well-formed myelinated axons ($n=7$ and 6, respectively; $*P=4.9\times10^{-2}$). Scale bars: 25 μm.

that vascular reactivity in the retinal vasculature is abnormal in sGCα$_1$$^{-/-}$ mice.

Association between a genetic locus containing the genes encoding the α$_1$ and β$_1$ subunits of sGC and POAG

To explore the contribution of sGC to human POAG pathogenesis, we evaluated 51 single nucleotide SNP located throughout the genomic region that includes *GUCY1A3* and *GUCY1B3* for their association with POAG in humans. *GUCY1A3* and *GUCY1B3* encode the sGCα$_1$ (inactivated in sGCα$_1$$^{-/-}$ mice) and sGCβ$_1$ subunits, respectively, that constitute the predominant sGC isoform in most types of tissues [51]. We performed a gene association study among POAG cases and controls from the Glaucoma Genes and Environment (GLAUGEN) study [38]. None of the tested SNPs were associated with POAG overall (table 1).

We next hypothesized that POAG in sGCα$_1$$^{-/-}$ mice (with systemic and retinal vascular dysfunction) shares a common etiology with POAG in patients with paracentral visual field loss, a subtype of POAG previously suggested to be associated with vascular dysregulation [10]. Therefore, we focused our analysis on a subpopulation of POAG patients with initial paracentral scotomas and no peripheral visual field loss. Given the previously described interactions between NOS3 and female gender [26] in POAG, we analyzed men and women separately. The SNP rs11722059, located in the *GUCY1A3/GUCY1B3* intergenic region, was significantly associated with POAG characterized by paracentral visual field loss in women ($P=3.1\times10^{-4}$, $OR=1.90$, $CI=1.34$–2.69; table 1). Replication of the candidate gene

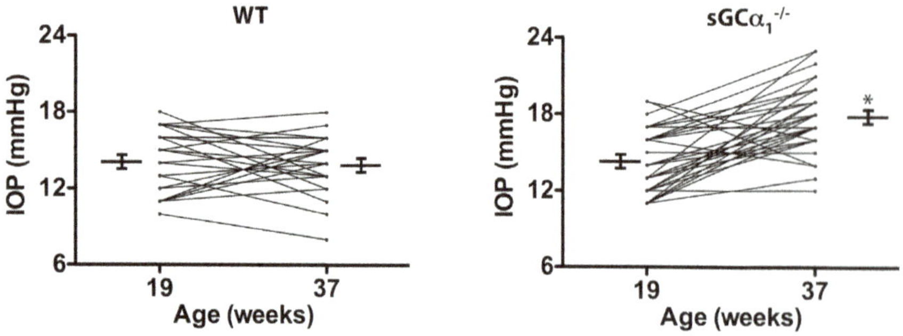

Figure 3. Intraocular pressure (IOP) increases with age in sGC$\alpha_1^{-/-}$ mice. IOP, measured serially at 2 time points (19±1 and 37±3 weeks) in eyes from age-matched wild-type (WT, **left panel**) and soluble guanylate cyclase α_1-deficient (sGC$\alpha_1^{-/-}$) mice (**right panel**). While IOP remained stable in WT mice as they aged from 19 to 37 weeks (14±2 to 14±2 mmHg; $n=25$; $P=0.67$), IOP increased in sGC$\alpha_1^{-/-}$ mice (14±2 to 18±3 mmHg; $n=37$; $^*P=1.9\times10^{-8}$).

association study is required to confirm the result from this candidate gene association study. Nevertheless, tentative identification of a risk variant located in the locus encoding sGCα_1 and sGCβ_1, both expressed in ocular tissue (fig. 1), highlights the potential relevance of sGC in the pathogenesis of POAG.

Discussion

In this study, we report that sGC$\alpha_1^{-/-}$ mice develop POAG, characterized by RNFL thinning, loss of RGC's, and optic neuropathy in the setting of an open iridocorneal angle. An age-dependent decrease in AqH turnover suggests that an increase in outflow resistance underlies the elevated IOP observed in old sGC$\alpha_1^{-/-}$ mice. In addition, our findings suggest that impaired NO-cGMP signaling results in retinal vascular dysfunction, a possible contributor to the pathophysiology of POAG. Importantly, the relevance of sGC$\alpha_1^{-/-}$ mice as a new animal model for POAG is highlighted by the tentative identification of a genetic association between the genetic locus encoding the α_1 and β_1 subunits of sGC and a POAG subtype thought to be associated with vascular dysregulation.

The RNFL contains the RGC axons that converge to form the optic nerve. Glaucoma is characterized by loss of axons and death

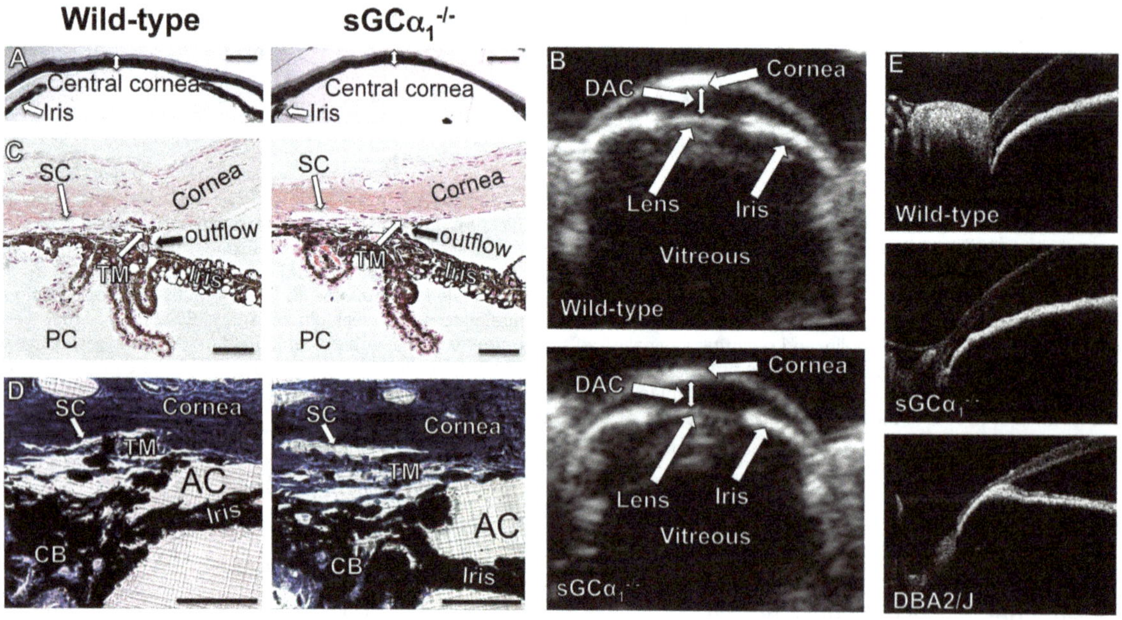

Figure 4. Morphology of the cornea and anterior segment does not differ in WT and sGC$\alpha_1^{-/-}$ mice. A: Representative light microscopic images of the central cornea in wild-type (WT, left) and soluble guanylate cyclase α_1-deficient mice (sGC$\alpha_1^{-/-}$, right). Central corneal thickness (CCT) was similar in age-matched WT and sGC$\alpha_1^{-/-}$ mice. Double arrows: CCT. Scale bar: 200 µm. **B**: Representative ultrasound biomicroscopy images of the ocular anterior segment, obtained in WT (**upper panel**) and sGC$\alpha_1^{-/-}$ mice (**lower panel**). The cornea, iris, vitreous, and lens are evident. Depth of the anterior chamber (DAC, double arrow) did not differ in WT and sGC$\alpha_1^{-/-}$ mice. **C** and **D**: Representative light microscopic images of paraffin sections stained with hematoxylin and eosin (C, scale bar: 100 µm) or Toluidine Blue (D, scale bar: 50 µm) containing the iridocorneal angles of 12-month-old WT (**left panels**) and sGC$\alpha_1^{-/-}$ mice (**right panels**). Location of the cornea, iris root, ciliary body (CB), anterior chamber (AC), and posterior chamber (PC) are indicated. **E**: Representative SD-OCT images of the ocular anterior segment, obtained in a 12-month-old wild-type mouse (**upper panel**), a 12-month-old sGC$\alpha_1^{-/-}$ mouse (**middle panel**), and a 12-month-old DBA2/J mouse in which the angle is closed (**lower panel**). SD-OCT revealed no morphological abnormalities in sGC$\alpha1^{-/-}$ mice that would suggest a closed angle as detected in old DBA2/J mice. See also **Movies S1, S2, S3.**

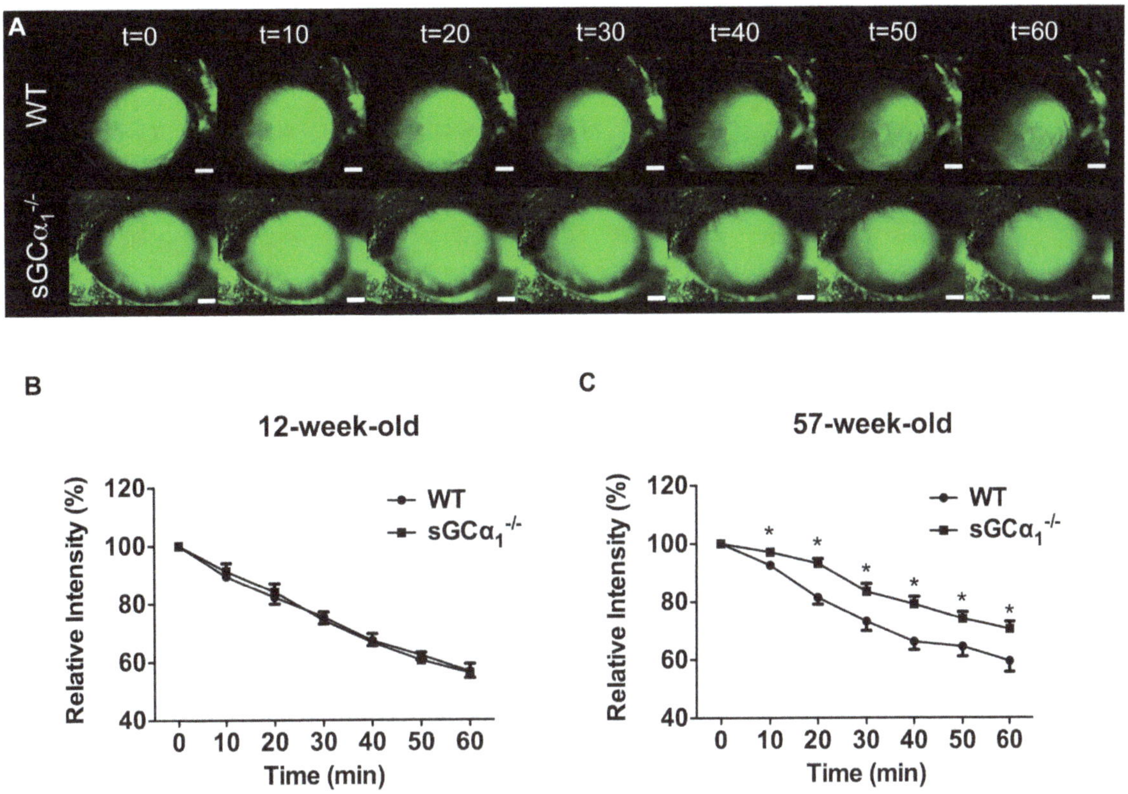

Figure 5. Decreased aqueous humor outflow rate in sGC$\alpha_1{}^{-/-}$ mice. A: Shown is a representative series of images captured from 57-week-old wild-type (WT) and soluble guanylate cyclase α_1-deficient (sGC$\alpha_1{}^{-/-}$) mice at 10-minute intervals after application of fluorescein. Scale bars: 2 mm. **B**: In 12-week-old WT and sGC$\alpha1^{-/-}$ mice with similar IOPs (16±2 and 16±1 mmHg in $n=9$ and 8, respectively; $P=0.91$) the rate of AqH outflow did not differ, as shown by similar relative fluorescent intensities at all time points measured ($P=0.99$) and similar exponential decay constants (0.0098 min^{-1} ($r^2=0.997$) and 0.0096 min^{-1} ($r^2=0.998$), respectively; $P=0.12$). **C**: IOP was greater in 57-week-old sGC$\alpha1^{-/-}$ mice than in age-matched WT mice (18±2 mmHg and 16±1, respectively; $n=10$ each; $P=0.043$), and AqH clearance was delayed in sGC$\alpha1^{-/-}$ mice, as shown by a lower exponential decay constant (0.0058 min^{-1} ($r^2=0.972$) versus 0.0092 min^{-1} ($r^2=0.976$), respectively; $P=0.0056$) and higher fluorescent intensities at all time points measured. *$P=0.033$, 0.0006, 0.024, 0.0029, 0.035, 0.025, between WT and sGC$\alpha_1{}^{-/-}$ mice at 10, 20, 30, 40, 50, and 60 minutes, respectively.

of RGCs, which can be detected as thinning of the RNFL. Retinal damage, characterized by thinning of the RNFL and loss of RGCs in old sGC$\alpha_1{}^{-/-}$ but not age-matched WT mice was demonstrated via SD-OCT and histologic examination. In addition, the number of optic nerve axons was significantly lower in twelve-month-old sGC$\alpha_1{}^{-/-}$ mice than in age-matched WT mice, indicating optic neuropathy associated with sGCα_1-deficiency. The observation that RNFL thickness did not differ in young WT and sGC$\alpha_1{}^{-/-}$ mice, neither of which had high IOPs, suggests that lack of sGCα_1 does not directly affect ganglion cell viability during embryonic development or during the first weeks after birth.

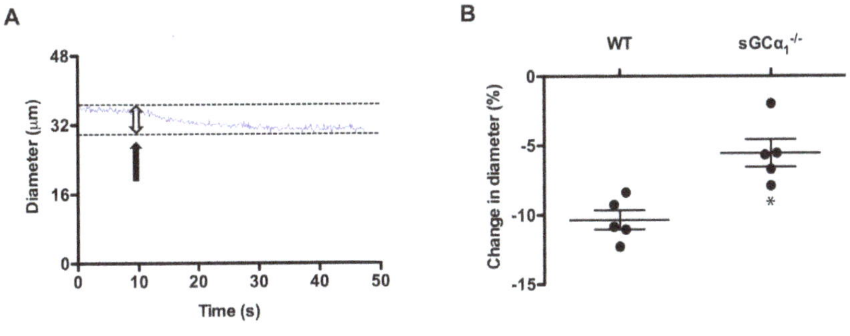

Figure 6. Retinal vascular dysfunction in sGC$\alpha_1{}^{-/-}$ mice. A: Representative trace depicting the diameter in one segment of a retinal arteriole in a wild-type (WT) mouse before, during (arrow), and after injection of the NO-donor compound sodium nitroprusside. Dashed lines indicate the diameter before and after sodium nitroprusside injection. **B**: Quantitative analysis of the change in diameter (double arrow in fig. 6A) induced by injection of 0.8 mg/kg sodium nitroprusside in WT and sGC$\alpha_1{}^{-/-}$ mice. $n=5$ mice (3–4 arterioles per mouse were assessed, see also fig. S3). *$P=4.1\times10^{-3}$.

Table 1. Association between *GUCY1A3/GUCY1B3* single nucleotide polymorphisms (SNPs) and POAG in the Glaucoma Gene and Environment (GLAUGEN) study.

Gender	VF loss	MA	Top SNP	P value	OR	95% CI	Chr	N cases	N controls
all	any	A	rs9992550	0.04271	1.43	(1.01, 2.02)	4	976	1140
women	any	A	rs11722059	0.02734	1.29	(1.03,1.61)	4	570	682
men	any	G	rs13115024	0.05038	0.61	(0.38, 1.00)	4	406	458
all	paracentral	A	rs11722059	0.00406	1.50	(1.14, 1.98)	4	175	1140
women	***paracentral***	***A***	***rs11722059***	***0.00031***	***1.90***	***(1.34, 2.69)***	***4***	***106***	***682***
men	paracentral	A	rs4691842	0.01468	1.62	(1.10, 2.40)	4	69	458

Most significant single nucleotide polymorphisms (SNPs) stratified by gender and type of visual field (VF) loss. 51 SNPs were analyzed within the GUCY1A3/GUCY1B3 locus and 50 kb upstream and downstream of the region. A Bonferroni correction of 3.3×10^{-4}, correcting for analyzing 51 SNPs and 3 subgroups, was applied to define statistical significance. The top SNP (rs11722059) reached significance in women with paracentral visual field (VF) loss (P value of 3.1×10^{-4}, bold and italicized). MA: minor allele; OR: multivariable odds ratio associated with each minor allele dose, generated by multiple logistic regression analyses adjusting for age, gender, study site, DNA source, DNA extraction method, and three eigenvectors; CI: confidence interval; Chr: chromosome; N: number.

Several risk factors for POAG have been suggested [2]. Elevated IOP is the best characterized risk factor but may not explain all POAG risk. It is becoming increasingly clear that compounds that do not lower IOP dramatically but that have properties that address the underlying glaucomatous disease process may be suitable therapeutic agents [52,53]. For example, brimonidine, an α_2-adrenergic receptor agonist postulated to modulate vascular reactivity in an NO-dependent manner [54], corrected the retinal vasculopathy in patients with normotensive glaucoma and retinal vascular dysregulation [55]. A randomized clinical trial revealed that brimonidine was superior to timolol in stabilizing visual field deterioration despite producing only a modest IOP-lowering effect (~1 mmHg) similar to that of timolol [56]. Together, these data suggest that strategies, other than lowering IOP, such as those targeting vascular dysfunction, may be efficacious treatments for glaucoma [57]. It is important to emphasize that, even though in the majority of glaucoma clinical drug trials reduction of IOP is the primary efficacy endpoint, the United States Food and Drug Administration has expressed interest in drugs that prevent progression of glaucomatous damage without necessarily lowering IOP [52,53]. Nonetheless, benefit-to-risk ratio will likely continue to be determined by drug efficacy and health risk assessment from clinical trials in comparison to the benchmark, IOP lowering drugs [52].

Our data demonstrates that impaired NO-cGMP signaling results in elevated IOP. The observation that IOPs are similar in young WT and sGC$\alpha_1^{-/-}$ mice but increase with age in sGC$\alpha_1^{-/-}$ but not WT mice indicates that elevated IOP seen in sGC$\alpha_1^{-/-}$ mice depends on age, an important risk factor for POAG [1]. Similarly modest changes in IOP impact POAG risk in humans, highlighting the potential biological significance of the increase in IOP in sGC$\alpha_1^{-/-}$ mice [58]. For example, a 2 mmHg difference in IOP distinguished between progression and non-progression in glaucoma patients [58,59,60]. Additional longitudinal studies are required to further characterize the exact timeframe of the increase in IOP associated with sGCα_1-deficiency. Examination (by histology, ultrasound, and SD-OCT) of the iridocorneal angle and anterior chamber of sGC$\alpha_1^{-/-}$ mice with elevated IOP did not reveal any evidence of morphological abnormalities of the peripheral cornea or outflow pathway illustrating that the outflow pathway was not physically obstructed (a characteristic of closed-angle glaucoma). The rate of AqH outflow dynamics, assessed via a previously reported non-invasive method [36] that will require validation using a more reliable method [61], was similar in young WT and sGC$\alpha_1^{-/-}$ mice but impaired in old sGC$\alpha_1^{-/-}$ mice with elevated IOPs suggesting that an increase in outflow resistance (indicative of POAG) may contribute to the IOP increase in sGC$\alpha_1^{-/-}$ mice. The mechanism underlying the age-dependency of the effect of sGC-deficiency on AqH outflow dynamics remains to be determined.

The abundant expression of sGCα_1 and sGCβ_1 in the CM, together with the established role of sGC in mediating smooth muscle cell relaxation [16,17], suggests that sGC can alter outflow by regulating smooth muscle-like contractility of the longitudinal fibers of the CM. The contractile state of smooth muscle tissue is the target of Rho-kinase inhibitors, currently being tested in clinical trials for glaucoma and ocular hypertension [62]. It is conceivable that AqH drainage is similarly influenced by impaired NO-cGMP signaling and enhanced RhoA-signaling: both could result in augmented contractility of the longitudinal fibers of the CM, thereby potentially decreasing AqH drainage and increasing IOP [63]. However, the possibility remains that sGCα_1-deficiency affects AqH production or that changes in Schlemm's canal cell or TM cell volume, previously reported to be modulated by NO-cGMP signaling [64], contribute to the altered AqH dynamics in sGC$\alpha_1^{-/-}$ mice.

The hypothesis that retinal vascular dysfunction contributes to the glaucomatous phenotype in sGC$\alpha_1^{-/-}$ mice was based on the observed peripheral vascular dysfunction in sGC$\alpha_1^{-/-}$ mice and on the association of a genetic variant in the locus containing the sGCα_1 and sGCβ_1 genes with glaucomatous paracentral vision loss in women, a subtype of POAG previously postulated to be associated with ocular vascular dysregulation [10]. To test whether retinal vascular function is affected by sGCα_1-deficiency, the retinal vasculature was visualized via SLO and the diameter of retinal arteries was measured at baseline and after treatment with the NO donor sodium nitroprusside. We previously demonstrated that the ability of a low dose of sodium nitroprusside to reduce blood pressure was attenuated in sGC$\alpha_1^{-/-}$ mice, reflecting the systemic vascular dysfunction associated with impaired NO-cGMP signaling [31]. In contrast, a high dose of sodium nitroprusside reduced blood pressure similarly in sGC$\alpha_1^{-/-}$ and WT mice [31], a mechanism that involves activation of sGC$\alpha_2\beta_1$ [17]. Systemic administration of sodium nitroprusside at a dose that decreased blood pressure similarly in WT and sGC$\alpha_1^{-/-}$ mice, thereby avoiding the potential confounding impact on retinal vascular diameter of differences in systemic blood pressure between WT and sGC$\alpha_1^{-/-}$ mice, induced vasoconstriction of the retinal vasculature in both WT and sGC$\alpha_1^{-/-}$ mice. Vasoconstriction likely results from baroreflex activation in response to an acute drop in blood pressure or may be mediated by the renin-angiotensin system, as previously described in other vascular beds in response to circulatory shock [65]. Importantly, the decrease in retinal arterial diameter upon NO administration was less apparent in sGC$\alpha_1^{-/-}$ than in WT mice. The observation that the retinal hemodynamic response to a decrease in blood pressure is abnormal in sGC$\alpha_1^{-/-}$ mice, suggests that impaired NO-cGMP signaling is associated with retinal vascular dysfunction, just as it is with systemic vascular dysfunction. In summary, sGCα_1-deficiency may result in optic neuropathy via a variety of mechanisms, either by increasing IOP and/or by impairing retinal blood flow. In addition, we cannot exclude the possibility that impaired NO-sGC signaling sensitizes RGCs to small increases in IOP that may not injure WT RGCs [66]. Also, we recognize that additional work is necessary to examine the impact of gender on the development of POAG in sGC$\alpha_1^{-/-}$ mice, especially in light of observations suggesting that gender may play an important role in the pathogenesis of POAG [26].

Although several mechanically- and chemically-induced models of ganglion cell death and glaucoma have been developed in mice [67,68] to date, only a few spontaneously-occurring murine models of glaucoma that do not involve ocular manipulation have been described. As they age, DBA/2J mice develop a progressive form of secondary angle closure glaucoma [48]. TG-MYOC^{Y437H} mice that overexpress a mutant form of the human myocilin (MYOC) gene mimics human juvenile open-angle glaucoma and is considered a model of POAG [69]. However, mutations in MYOC account for only a minority of POAG cases. Cyp1b1$^{-/-}$ mice develop angle dysgenesis that mimics the congenital version of open-angle glaucoma but these mice do not develop elevated IOP [49]. More recently, transiently elevated IOP [70], optic nerve damage [71], and decreased AqH outflow [72] were described in mice with a targeted mutation in the type I collagen gene. Our data suggests that sGC$\alpha_1^{-/-}$ mice are an additional model of POAG that may be useful to study mechanisms of IOP regulation and the role of vascular dysfunction in the etiology of POAG.

Linkage analysis and genome-wide association studies have identified several genes associated with POAG, a disease with significant heritability [73,74]. Our identification, in an exploratory genetic analysis aimed at investigating the relevance of our mouse model in human POAG, of a variant (rs11722059) in the *GUCY1A3/GUCY1B3 locus* significantly associated with a subpopulation of POAG patients characterized by paracentral scotomas, is a step towards understanding the contribution of sGC to the etiology of this important subtype of POAG. Interestingly, rs11722059 is in linkage disequilibrium ($D' = 0.86$; $r^2 = 0.67$) with another *GUCY1A3/GUCY1B3* SNP (rs13139571) that was recently associated with blood pressure in 200,000 individuals of European decent from the International Consortium for blood pressure [75]. Overall, these results identify a role for sGC$\alpha_1\beta_1$ in the POAG phenotype characterized by vascular dysregulation and paracentral visual field loss, and suggest a possible mechanistic link between blood pressure and POAG. Together with the previously reported association between vascular dysfunction and POAG [8,55], and with the finding that sGCα_1-deficiency is associated with both systemic and retinal vascular dysfunction, the results of our candidate gene association study raises the possibility that retinal vascular dysfunction contributes to the development of POAG associated with impaired NO-cGMP signaling.

While the focus of this study was to categorize a new murine model of POAG and identify a well-characterized signaling mechanism (NO-cGMP signaling) as centrally involved in the etiology of POAG, rather than to formally report on a new genetic association, we recognize that the human genetic association described requires confirmation in a replication cohort. Because recruitment ascertainment typically targets patients more likely to have peripheral visual field defects, there are currently no other available POAG cohorts of sufficient size with paracentral scotoma information that could be used for replication. For example, only 26 of 2170 cases in the NEI Glaucoma Human Genetics Collaboration presented with initial paracentral loss [76]. In spite of this limitation, we believe the genetic association data provided highlights the significance of sGC-signaling in the etiology of POAG and will motivate investigators to identify cohorts to replicate the GLAUGEN finding.

In humans, several mechanisms have been identified that can impair NO-cGMP signaling, potentially contributing to the development of POAG. For example, a candidate gene association study in 527 incident cases and 1543 controls revealed interactions between NOS3 gene variants, potentially affecting expression and/or activity of NOS3 (and, ultimately, sGC enzyme activity), and high tension POAG in females [26]. Alternatively, the mechanism by which increased oxidative stress results in POAG [77] may involve direct oxidation and inactivation of sGC [78]. NO- and heme-independent sGC activators, capable of activating oxidized sGC, such as cinaciguat [79], are available and are being tested in the clinic for a variety of cardiovascular diseases [80]. Other potential therapeutic targets include proteins that control GMP levels and which are abundantly present in the eye (including cGMP-catabolizing phosphodiesterases [81] and particulate guanylate cyclases [82]). Pharmacological modulation of the activity of these proteins may increase outflow, attenuate retinal arterial dysfunction, and prevent disease progression.

Conclusions

Our results demonstrate that impairing a well-characterized signaling pathway (NO-cGMP signaling) results in optic neuropathy, possibly by modulating IOP and retinal vascular function. Our data identify sGC$\alpha_1^{-/-}$ mice as a novel translational animal model for POAG, providing a tool for investigators to study the pathogenesis of POAG and to test new strategies for disease prevention. Furthermore, we identified a genomic locus containing the sGCα_1 and sGCβ_1 genes that is associated with glaucoma with paracentral visual field loss in women. Together, these findings identify sGC as a potential therapeutic target to treat POAG and may inform the clinical development of existing cGMP-elevating therapeutic compounds for treating glaucomatous retinal injury.

Supporting Information

Figure S1 SD-OCT analysis of retinal nerve fiber layer thickness in sGC$\alpha_1^{-/-}$ mice. A: Representative heat maps of absolute total retinal thickness and RNFL thickness in 12 month-old wild-type (WT) and soluble guanylate cyclase α_1-deficient (sGC$\alpha_1^{-/-}$) mice. No differences in total retinal thickness were detected between sGC$\alpha_1^{-/-}$ and WT mice (fig. 2A). RNFL thickness was thinner in sGC$\alpha_1^{-/-}$ mice than in WT mice, as demonstrated by the darker blue colors in the sGC$\alpha_1^{-/-}$ RNFL heat map (see also fig. 2A). Color scale varies between 1.53 (black) and 247.93 (white) μm. See fig. 2A for quantitative data. **B**: Validation of the automated segmentation analysis. The manually determined RNFL thickness data recapitulated the automated segmentation analysis and confirmed that the RNFL is thinner in old in sGC$\alpha_1^{-/-}$ mice than in old WT mice. **Left panel**: Representative en-face image of the retina acquired using SD-

OCT imaging (left), showing the 24 points (marked by X) of a 5×5 grid at which RNFL thickness was measured, and B-scans (right, A-E) showing placement of the 24 calipers used to measure RNFL thickness. **Middle panel**: mean RNFL thickness measured in all 24 pre-defined points in WT (upper number) and $sGC\alpha_1^{-/-}$ mice (lower number). **Right panel**: mean RNFL thickness (as averages of RNFL thickness measured manually in 24 points), assessed using a 2-way repeated measures ANOVA, did not differ in 6-week-old $sGC\alpha_1^{-/-}$ and age-matched WT mice ($n = 15$ and 20, respectively; $P = 0.29$), but was thinner in 70-week-old $sGC\alpha_1^{-/-}$ mice than in age-matched WT mice ($n = 17$ each; $^*P = 1.4 \times 10^{-2}$).

Figure S2 Intraocular pressure (IOP) increases with age in $sGC\alpha_1^{-/-}$ mice. A: IOP in young (15±6-week-old) and old (39±14-week-old) wild-type (WT) and soluble guanylate cyclase α_1-deficient ($sGC\alpha_1^{-/-}$) mice. No statistically significant difference in IOP was detected between young $sGC\alpha_1^{-/-}$ and age-matched WT mice ($n = 61$ and 112, respectively; $P = 0.08$). In contrast, IOP was higher in old $sGC\alpha_1^{-/-}$ mice than in age-matched WT mice ($n = 468$ and 140, respectively). $^*P = 2.9 \times 10^{-7}$ vs. 39±14-week-old WT. **B**: IOP in a second independent cohort of WT eyes ($n = 27$) measured serially at 2 time points. IOP was 15±2 and 15±1 mmHg in 30±0 and 62±0-week-old WT mice, respectively. $P = 0.93$. **C**: IOP in a second independent cohort of $sGC\alpha_1^{-/-}$ eyes ($n = 41$) measured serially at 2 time points. IOP increased from 15±2 to 19±2 mmHg in 26±4 and 73±5-week-old $sGC\alpha_1^{-/-}$ mice, respectively. $^*P = 4.8 \times 10^{-16}$.

Figure S3 Fluorescein angiography in WT and $sGC\alpha_1^{-/-}$ mice. A: Serial images (A–G) of fluorescein angiography between 1 and 3 seconds after I.V. injection of fluorescein. Retinal arterioles (arrows in **panel A**) were identified based on earlier filling with fluorescein than veins (arrows in **panel E**). **B**: Image of fluorescein angiography. The width of the arterioles was determined (boxes) at fixed distances from the optic nerve head (inner dashed ring = 150 µm; outer dashed ring = 250 µm). **C**: Quantitative analysis of the diameter of retinal arterioles in wild type (WT, **left panel**) and soluble guanylate cyclase α_1-deficient mice ($sGC\alpha_1^{-/-}$, **middle panel**) before and after a challenge with 0.8 mg/kg sodium nitroprusside. Baseline diameter of retinal arterioles was similar in WT and $sGC\alpha_1^{-/-}$ mice ($P = 0.40$). Injection of 0.8 mg/kg sodium nitroprusside reduced the diameter of retinal arterioles in both WT ($^*P = 7.8 \times 10^{-12}$) and $sGC\alpha_1^{-/-}$ mice ($^*P = 1.7 \times 10^{-6}$). The change in diameter induced by injection of sodium nitroprusside was more pronounced in WT than in $sGC\alpha_1^{-/-}$ mice (**right panel**, $^*P = 9.0 \times 10^{-6}$). $n = 17$ and 15 WT and $sGC\alpha_1^{-/-}$ arterioles, respectively; 3–4 arterioles/mouse from 5 mice, each. See also fig. 6B for data analysis per mouse.

Movie S1 Representative movies of SD-OCT analyses of the iridocorneal angle in age matched 12-month old wild-type (WT, **movie S1**) and soluble guanylate cyclase α_1-deficient mice (**movie S2**). To demonstrate the ability of SD-OCT to discriminate between open and closed angles we imaged a closed angle in a 12-month-old DBA/2J mouse with elevated IOP (**movie S3**). Movies are representative examples of images observed in at least five mice per group in two replicate experiments.

Movie S2 Representative movies of SD-OCT analyses of the iridocorneal angle in age matched 12-month old wild-type (WT, **movie S1**) and soluble guanylate cyclase α_1-deficient mice (**movie S2**). To demonstrate the ability of SD-OCT to discriminate between open and closed angles we imaged a closed angle in a 12-month-old DBA/2J mouse with elevated IOP (**movie S3**). Movies are representative examples of images observed in at least five mice per group in two replicate experiments.

Movie S3 Representative movies of SD-OCT analyses of the iridocorneal angle in age matched 12-month old wild-type (WT, **movie S1**) and soluble guanylate cyclase α_1-deficient mice (**movie S2**). To demonstrate the ability of SD-OCT to discriminate between open and closed angles we imaged a closed angle in a 12-month-old DBA/2J mouse with elevated IOP (**movie S3**). Movies are representative examples of images observed in at least five mice per group in two replicate experiments.

Acknowledgments

The authors thank Dr. P. T. Ellinor for use of the SZX16 scope equipped with DP72-camera and Dr. J. Miller for use of the SD-OCT Bioptigen system.

Author Contributions

Performed statistical analyses: RM. Conceived and designed the experiments: ESB YCK CA MSC CPL HG DJR PB JLW MSG LRP KDB BRK. Performed the experiments: ESB YCK CA SRH AJ LTT RR AG MC EA RETT DJO NdW BY RT DN MSC SJL JHK MSG. Analyzed the data: ESB YCK CA AJ LTT RR AG MC PA RT DN MSC SJL JHK HG JLW MSG LRP KDB BRK. Contributed reagents/materials/analysis tools: PB. Wrote the paper: ESB RM PA MSC HG DJR PB JLW MSG LRP KDB BRK.

References

1. Weinreb RN, Khaw PT (2004) Primary open-angle glaucoma. Lancet 363: 1711–1720.
2. Quigley HA (2011) Glaucoma. Lancet 377: 1367–1377.
3. Vajaranant TS, Pasquale LR (2012) Estrogen deficiency accelerates aging of the optic nerve. Menopause 19: 942–947.
4. Flammer J, Orgul S, Costa VP, Orzalesi N, Krieglstein GK, et al. (2002) The impact of ocular blood flow in glaucoma. Prog Retin Eye Res 21: 359–393.
5. Kass MA, Gordon MO, Gao F, Heuer DK, Higginbotham EJ, et al. (2010) Delaying Treatment of Ocular Hypertension: The Ocular Hypertension Treatment Study. Arch Ophthalmol 128: 276–287.
6. Leske MC, Connell AM, Wu SY, Nemesure B, Li X, et al. (2001) Incidence of open-angle glaucoma: the Barbados Eye Studies. The Barbados Eye Studies Group. Arch Ophthalmol 119: 89–95.
7. Henry E, Newby DE, Webb DJ, O'Brien C (1999) Peripheral endothelial dysfunction in normal pressure glaucoma. Invest Ophthalmol Vis Sci 40: 1710–1714.
8. Su WW, Cheng ST, Ho WJ, Tsay PK, Wu SC, et al. (2008) Glaucoma is associated with peripheral vascular endothelial dysfunction. Ophthalmology 115: 1173–1178 e1171.
9. Feke GT, Pasquale LR (2008) Retinal blood flow response to posture change in glaucoma patients compared with healthy subjects. Ophthalmology 115: 246–252.
10. Park SC, De Moraes CG, Teng CC, Tello C, Liebmann JM, et al. (2011) Initial parafoveal versus peripheral scotomas in glaucoma: risk factors and visual field characteristics. Ophthalmology 118: 1782–1789.
11. Leske MC (2009) Ocular perfusion pressure and glaucoma: clinical trial and epidemiologic findings. Curr Opin Ophthalmol 20: 73–78.
12. Cherecheanu AP, Garhofer G, Schmidl D, Werkmeister R, Schmetterer L (2013) Ocular perfusion pressure and ocular blood flow in glaucoma. Curr Opin Pharmacol 13: 36–42.
13. Nathanson JA, McKee M (1995) Identification of an extensive system of nitric oxide-producing cells in the ciliary muscle and outflow pathway of the human eye. Invest Ophthalmol Vis Sci 36: 1765–1773.

14. Fernandez-Durango R, Fernandez-Martinez A, Garcia-Feijoo J, Castillo A, de la Casa JM, et al. (2008) Expression of nitrotyrosine and oxidative consequences in the trabecular meshwork of patients with primary open-angle glaucoma. Invest Ophthalmol Vis Sci 49: 2506–2511.
15. Neufeld AH, Hernandez MR, Gonzalez M (1997) Nitric oxide synthase in the human glaucomatous optic nerve head. Arch Ophthalmol 115: 497–503.
16. Nimmegeers S, Sips P, Buys E, Brouckaert P, Van de Voorde J (2007) Functional role of the soluble guanylyl cyclase alpha(1) subunit in vascular smooth muscle relaxation. Cardiovasc Res 76: 149–159.
17. Friebe A, Mergia E, Dangel O, Lange A, Koesling D (2007) Fatal gastrointestinal obstruction and hypertension in mice lacking nitric oxide-sensitive guanylyl cyclase. Proc Natl Acad Sci U S A 104: 7699–7704.
18. Russwurm M, Behrends S, Harteneck C, Koesling D (1998) Functional properties of a naturally occurring isoform of soluble guanylyl cyclase. Biochem J 335: 125–130.
19. Kotikoski H, Vapaatalo H, Oksala O (2003) Nitric oxide and cyclic GMP enhance aqueous humor outflow facility in rabbits. Curr Eye Res 26: 119–123.
20. Ellis DZ, Dismuke WM, Chokshi BM (2009) Characterization of soluble guanylate cyclase in NO-induced increases in aqueous humor outflow facility and in the trabecular meshwork. Invest Ophthalmol Vis Sci 50: 1808–1813.
21. Krauss AH, Impagnatiello F, Toris CB, Gale DC, Prasanna G, et al. (2011) Ocular hypotensive activity of BOL-303259-X, a nitric oxide donating prostaglandin F2alpha agonist, in preclinical models. Exp Eye Res 93: 250–255.
22. Nathanson JA (1992) Nitrovasodilators as a new class of ocular hypotensive agents. J Pharmacol Exp Ther 260: 956–965.
23. Khoobehi B, Chiroli V, Ronchetti D, Miglietta D, Thompson H, et al. (2011) Enhanced oxygen saturation in optic nerve head of non-human primate eyes following the intravitreal injection of NCX 434, an innovative nitric oxide-donating glucocorticoid. J Ocul Pharmacol Ther 27: 115–121.
24. Galassi F, Renieri G, Sodi A, Ucci F, Vannozzi L, et al. (2004) Nitric oxide proxies and ocular perfusion pressure in primary open angle glaucoma. Br J Ophthalmol 88: 757–760.
25. Chang CJ, Chiang CH, Chow JC, Lu DW (2000) Aqueous humor nitric oxide levels differ in patients with different types of glaucoma. J Ocul Pharmacol Ther 16: 399–406.
26. Kang JH, Wiggs JL, Rosner BA, Hankinson SE, Abdrabou W, et al. (2010) Endothelial nitric oxide synthase gene variants and primary open-angle glaucoma: interactions with sex and postmenopausal hormone use. Invest Ophthalmol Vis Sci 51: 971–979.
27. Magalhaes da Silva T, Rocha AV, Lacchini R, Marques CR, Silva ES, et al. (2012) Association of polymorphisms of endothelial nitric oxide synthase (eNOS) gene with the risk of primary open angle glaucoma in a Brazilian population. Gene 502: 142–146.
28. Weiss J, Frankl SA, Flammer J, Grieshaber MC, Hollo G, et al. (2012) No difference in genotype frequencies of polymorphisms of the nitric oxide pathway between Caucasian normal and high tension glaucoma patients. Mol Vis 18: 2174–2181.
29. Polak K, Luksch A, Berisha F, Fuchsjaeger-Mayrl G, Dallinger S, et al. (2007) Altered nitric oxide system in patients with open-angle glaucoma. Arch Ophthalmol 125: 494–498.
30. Nathanson JA, McKee M (1995) Alterations of ocular nitric oxide synthase in human glaucoma. Invest Ophthalmol Vis Sci 36: 1774–1784.
31. Buys ES, Sips P, Vermeersch P, Raher MJ, Rogge E, et al. (2008) Gender-specific hypertension and responsiveness to nitric oxide in sGC{alpha}1 knockout mice. Cardiovasc Res 79: 179–186.
32. Sandbach JM, Coscun PE, Grossniklaus HE, Kokoszka JE, Newman NJ, et al. (2001) Ocular pathology in mitochondrial superoxide dismutase (Sod2)-deficient mice. Invest Ophthalmol Vis Sci 42: 2173–2178.
33. Anderson MG, Libby RT, Gould DB, Smith RS, John SW (2005) High-dose radiation with bone marrow transfer prevents neurodegeneration in an inherited glaucoma. Proc Natl Acad Sci U S A 102: 4566–4571.
34. Haddadin RI, Oh DJ, Kang MH, Filippopoulos T, Gupta M, et al. (2009) SPARC-null mice exhibit lower intraocular pressures. Invest Ophthalmol Vis Sci 50: 3771–3777.
35. Brown AS, Zhang M, Cucevic V, Pavlin CJ, Foster FS (2005) In vivo assessment of postnatal murine ocular development by ultrasound biomicroscopy. Curr Eye Res 30: 45–51.
36. Avila MY, Mitchell CH, Stone RA, Civan MM (2003) Noninvasive assessment of aqueous humor turnover in the mouse eye. Invest Ophthalmol Vis Sci 44: 722–727.
37. Alt C, Lin CP (2012) In vivo quantification of microglia dynamics with a scanning laser ophthalmoscope in a mouse model of focal laser injury. Proceedings of SPIE 8209: 820907.
38. Wiggs JL, Kang JH, Yaspan BL, Mirel DB, Laurie C, et al. (2011) Common variants near CAV1 and CAV2 are associated with primary open-angle glaucoma in Caucasians from the USA. Hum Mol Genet 20: 4707–4713.
39. Kent WJ, Sugnet CW, Furey TS, Roskin KM, Pringle TH, et al. (2002) The human genome browser at UCSC. Genome Res 12: 996–1006.
40. Wu RY, Ma N (2012) Expression of nitric oxide synthase and guanylate cyclase in the human ciliary body and trabecular meshwork. Chin Med J (Engl) 125: 129–133.
41. Gibbs SM, Becker A, Hardy RW, Truman JW (2001) Soluble guanylate cyclase is required during development for visual system function in Drosophila. J Neurosci 21: 7705–7714.
42. Haberecht MF, Schmidt HH, Mills SL, Massey SC, Nakane M, et al. (1998) Localization of nitric oxide synthase, NADPH diaphorase and soluble guanylyl cyclase in adult rabbit retina. Vis Neurosci 15: 881–890.
43. Kajimura M, Shimoyama M, Tsuyama S, Suzuki T, Kozaki S, et al. (2003) Visualization of gaseous monoxide reception by soluble guanylate cyclase in the rat retina. Faseb J 17: 506–508.
44. Blute TA, Velasco P, Eldred WD (1998) Functional localization of soluble guanylate cyclase in turtle retina: modulation of cGMP by nitric oxide donors. Vis Neurosci 15: 485–498.
45. Buys ES, Raher MJ, Kirby A, Mohd S, Baron DM, et al. (2012) Genetic modifiers of hypertension in soluble guanylate cyclase alpha1-deficient mice. J Clin Invest 122: 2316–2325.
46. Gabriele ML, Ishikawa H, Schuman JS, Bilonick RA, Kim J, et al. (2010) Reproducibility of spectral-domain optical coherence tomography total retinal thickness measurements in mice. Invest Ophthalmol Vis Sci 51: 6519–6523.
47. Marini M, Da Pozzo S, Accardo A, Canziani T (2011) Comparing applanation tonometry and rebound tonometry in glaucomatous and ocular hypertensive eyes. Eur J Ophthalmol 21: 258–263.
48. John SW, Smith RS, Savinova OV, Hawes NL, Chang B, et al. (1998) Essential iris atrophy, pigment dispersion, and glaucoma in DBA/2J mice. Invest Ophthalmol Vis Sci 39: 951–962.
49. Libby RT, Smith RS, Savinova OV, Zabaleta A, Martin JE, et al. (2003) Modification of ocular defects in mouse developmental glaucoma models by tyrosinase. Science 299: 1578–1581.
50. Atochin DN, Yuzawa I, Li Q, Rauwerdink KM, Malhotra R, et al. (2010) Soluble guanylate cyclase alpha1beta1 limits stroke size and attenuates neurological injury. Stroke 41: 1815–1819.
51. Mergia E, Russwurm M, Zoidl G, Koesling D (2003) Major occurrence of the new alpha(2)beta(1) isoform of NO-sensitive guanylyl cyclase in brain. Cell Signal 15: 189–195.
52. Chen J, Runyan SA, Robinson MR (2011) Novel ocular antihypertensive compounds in clinical trials. Clin Ophthalmol 5: 667–677.
53. Weinreb RN, Kaufman PL (2009) The glaucoma research community and FDA look to the future: a report from the NEI/FDA CDER Glaucoma Clinical Trial Design and Endpoints Symposium. Invest Ophthalmol Vis Sci 50: 1497–1505.
54. Rosa RH Jr., Hein TW, Yuan Z, Xu W, Pechal MI, et al. (2006) Brimonidine evokes heterogeneous vasomotor response of retinal arterioles: diminished nitric oxide-mediated vasodilation when size goes small. Am J Physiol Heart Circ Physiol 291: H231–238.
55. Feke GT, Hazin R, Grosskreutz CL, Pasquale LR (2011) Effect of brimonidine on retinal blood flow autoregulation in primary open-angle glaucoma. J Ocul Pharmacol Ther 27: 347–352.
56. Krupin T, Liebmann JM, Greenfield DS, Ritch R, Gardiner S (2011) A randomized trial of brimonidine versus timolol in preserving visual function: results from the Low-Pressure Glaucoma Treatment Study. Am J Ophthalmol 151: 671–681.
57. Pasquale LR, Feke GT, Harris A (2012) Why the low-pressure glaucoma treatment study makes sense. Expert Rev Ophthalmology 7: 295–297.
58. Konstas AG, Quaranta L, Mikropoulos DG, Nasr MB, Russo A, et al. (2012) Peak intraocular pressure and glaucomatous progression in primary open-angle glaucoma. J Ocul Pharmacol Ther 28: 26–32.
59. Glaucoma Laser Trial Research Group (1995) The Glaucoma Laser Trial (GLT) and glaucoma laser trial follow-up study: 7. Results. Am J Ophthalmol 120: 718–731.
60. Leske MC, Heijl A, Hyman L, Bengtsson B, Dong L, et al. (2007) Predictors of long-term progression in the early manifest glaucoma trial. Ophthalmology 114: 1965–1972.
61. Aihara M, Lindsey JD, Weinreb RN (2003) Aqueous humor dynamics in mice. Invest Ophthalmol Vis Sci 44: 5168–5173.
62. Rao VP, Epstein DL (2007) Rho GTPase/Rho kinase inhibition as a novel target for the treatment of glaucoma. BioDrugs 21: 167–177.
63. Honjo M, Tanihara H, Inatani M, Kido N, Sawamura T, et al. (2001) Effects of rho-associated protein kinase inhibitor Y-27632 on intraocular pressure and outflow facility. Invest Ophthalmol Vis Sci 42: 137–144.
64. Ellis DZ, Sharif NA, Dismuke WM (2010) Endogenous regulation of human Schlemm's canal cell volume by nitric oxide signaling. Invest Ophthalmol Vis Sci 51: 5817–5824.
65. Reilly PM, Bulkley GB (1993) Vasoactive mediators and splanchnic perfusion. Crit Care Med 21: S55–68.
66. Cone FE, Gelman SE, Son JL, Pease ME, Quigley HA (2010) Differential susceptibility to experimental glaucoma among 3 mouse strains using bead and viscoelastic injection. Exp Eye Res 91: 415–424.
67. McKinnon SJ, Schlamp CL, Nickells RW (2009) Mouse models of retinal ganglion cell death and glaucoma. Exp Eye Res 88: 816–824.
68. Weinreb RN, Lindsey JD (2005) The importance of models in glaucoma research. J Glaucoma 14: 302–304.
69. Zode GS, Kuehn MH, Nishimura DY, Searby CC, Mohan K, et al. (2011) Reduction of ER stress via a chemical chaperone prevents disease phenotypes in a mouse model of primary open angle glaucoma. J Clin Invest 121: 3542–3553.
70. Aihara M, Lindsey JD, Weinreb RN (2003) Ocular hypertension in mice with a targeted type I collagen mutation. Invest Ophthalmol Vis Sci 44: 1581–1585.
71. Mabuchi F, Lindsey JD, Aihara M, Mackey MR, Weinreb RN (2004) Optic nerve damage in mice with a targeted type I collagen mutation. Invest Ophthalmol Vis Sci 45: 1841–1845.

72. Dai Y, Lindsey JD, Duong-Polk X, Nguyen D, Hofer A, et al. (2009) Outflow facility in mice with a targeted type I collagen mutation. Invest Ophthalmol Vis Sci 50: 5749–5753.

73. Fan BJ, Wiggs JL (2010) Glaucoma: genes, phenotypes, and new directions for therapy. J Clin Invest 120: 3064–3072.

74. Burdon KP (2012) Genome-wide association studies in the hunt for genes causing primary open-angle glaucoma: a review. Clin Experiment Ophthalmol 40: 358–363.

75. Ehret GB, Munroe PB, Rice KM, Bochud M, Johnson AD, et al. (2011) Genetic variants in novel pathways influence blood pressure and cardiovascular disease risk. Nature 478: 103–109.

76. Wiggs JL, Hauser MA, Abdrabou W, Allingham RR, Budenz DL, et al. (2012) The NEIGHBOR Consortium Primary Open-Angle Glaucoma Genome-wide Association Study: Rationale, Study Design, and Clinical Variables. J Glaucoma. Epub Date: 2012/07/26.

77. Majsterek I, Malinowska K, Stanczyk M, Kowalski M, Blaszczyk J, et al. (2011) Evaluation of oxidative stress markers in pathogenesis of primary open-angle glaucoma. Exp Mol Pathol 90: 231–237.

78. Stasch JP, Schmidt PM, Nedvetsky PI, Nedvetskaya TY, H SA, et al. (2006) Targeting the heme-oxidized nitric oxide receptor for selective vasodilatation of diseased blood vessels. J Clin Invest 116: 2552–2561.

79. Evgenov OV, Pacher P, Schmidt PM, Hasko G, Schmidt HH, et al. (2006) NO-independent stimulators and activators of soluble guanylate cyclase: discovery and therapeutic potential. Nat Rev Drug Discov 5: 755–768.

80. Stasch JP, Pacher P, Evgenov OV (2011) Soluble guanylate cyclase as an emerging therapeutic target in cardiopulmonary disease. Circulation 123: 2263–2273.

81. Francis SH, Blount MA, Corbin JD (2011) Mammalian cyclic nucleotide phosphodiesterases: molecular mechanisms and physiological functions. Physiol Rev 91: 651–690.

82. McKie PM, Sangaralingham SJ, Burnett JC Jr. (2010) CD-NP: an innovative designer natriuretic peptide activator of particulate guanylyl cyclase receptors for cardiorenal disease. Curr Heart Fail Rep 7: 93–99.

23

Cross-Talk between Ciliary Epithelium and Trabecular Meshwork Cells In-Vitro: A New Insight into Glaucoma

Natalie Lerner, Elie Beit-Yannai*

Department of Clinical Biochemistry and Pharmacology, Ben-Gurion University of the Negev, Beer-Sheva, Israel

Abstract

Purpose: It is assumed that the non-pigmented ciliary epithelium plays a role in regulating intraocular pressure via its neuroendocrine activities. To test this hypothesis, we investigated the effect on a human trabecular meshwork (TM) cell line (NTM) of co-culture with a human non-pigmented ciliary epithelium cell line (ODM-2).

Methods: The cellular cross-talk between ODM-2 and NTM cells was studied in a co-culture system in which the two cell types were co-cultured for 5 to 60 min or 2, 4 and 8 h and then removed from the co-culture and analyzed. Analyses of the ERK and p38 mitogen-activated protein kinase (MAPK) pathways and of the activity of TM phosphatases and matrix metalloproteins (MMPs) were performed. Acid and alkaline phosphatase activity was determined by the DiFMUP (6, 8-difluoro-4-methylumbelliferyl phosphate) assay. MMP levels were determined by gelatin zymography.

Results: Exposure of NTM cells to ODM-2 cells led to the activation of the MAPK signal transduction pathways in NTM cells within 5 min of co-culture. Phosphorylation of ERK1/ERK2 and p38 peaked at 10 and 15 min and then decreased over time. Interaction between ODM-2 and NTM cells promoted the expression of MMP-9 in the NTM cells after 4 h of co-culture.

Conclusions: Our findings provide support for the hypothesis that crosstalk does indeed take place between ODM-2 and NTM cells. Future studies should be designed to determine the relationship between the MMP system, MAPK kinases and phosphatases. Manipulation of these signaling molecules and the related NTM signal transduction pathways may provide targets for developing improved treatments for glaucoma.

Editor: Wayne Iwan Lee Davies, University of Western Australia, Australia

Funding: The authors have no support or funding to report.

Competing Interests: The authors have declared that no competing interests exist.

* Email: bye@bgu.ac.il

Introduction

According to the prediction of a general increase in age-related diseases in the coming years, it is expected that the number of glaucoma patients worldwide will reach 80 million by 2020, despite current advances in therapy [1]. Glaucoma is characterized by the ongoing deterioration of the retinal ganglion layer and worsening of visual field defects, accompanied by changes in the optic nerve head. High intraocular pressure (IOP) has long been considered the most important risk factor for the onset and progression of glaucoma, and therefore pharmacological and surgical treatments have focused on lowering the IOP. However, while IOP management is the only effective glaucoma treatment, it cannot always prevent ongoing nerve damage, and it is still unclear which aspect of IOP (mean, peak, or diurnal) is the factor most relevant to the disease progression. Even normal tension glaucoma patients [2] benefit from IOP lowering-therapy, thus suggesting that relative, rather than absolute, metrics (peak/mean/diurnal) affect the progression of the disease.

Since the FDA approval of prostaglandin analogues in 1996, no new drug families for the treatment of glaucoma have been introduced into clinical practice, despite increasing awareness of the need for new approaches to glaucoma therapy [3–6], with emphasis on neuroprotection. One current avenue of research focuses on the aqueous humor (AH) drainage system [7]. AH produced and released by the ciliary epithelium to the posterior chamber travels through the pupil to the anterior chamber, finally leaving the eye through the trabecular meshwork (TM) tissue to Schlem's canal or through the uveo-sclera outflow system. The Rho-associated kinase (ROCK) inhibitors that are currently in clinical trials [8] actby relaxing the TM through inhibition of the actin cytoskeleton contractile tone of smooth muscle. This relaxation results in increased aqueous outflow directly through the TM, resulting in a lowering of the IOP [9].

In addition to its role in pressure maintenance, the AH was previously considered to be responsible for nutrient supply and waste product clearance, but it is now realized that the AH is also a rich source of dozens of active protein nucleotide and messenger molecules and vesicles [10–15]. However, the exact roles of these components remain, at least partially, obscure. In 2007, Coca-Prados and Escribano hypothesized that the ciliary epithelium acts in a paracrine manner by releasing active factors capable of affecting the TM [16]. In keeping with this hypothesis, we set out to demonstrate the possible AH-mediated influence of the ciliary epithelium on the TM. We suggest that active components released by the non-pigmented ciliary epithelium are transferred by the AH to the TM cells, where they exert their influence.

The active proteins of the AH whose levels and activity are affected by elevated IOP include kinases [17] and phosphatases [11]. The kinases act to phosphorylate either tyrosine or serine/threonine residues, which affects the function of many signal transduction proteins. The regulation of phosphorylated proteins is then directed by three main families of phosphatases–protein-tyrosine phosphatases (PTP), serine/threonine phosphatases (PP) and dual-specificity phosphatases that cleave both PTP and PP. There is a delicate balance between kinase and phosphatase activity, which plays a role in signaling pathway outcome Dephosphorylation of specific phosphorylated sites can inhibit kinase activity. Several human diseases have been attributed to disturbances in Kinase-phosphatases balance, including cancer, diabetes and inflammation [18]. It has been suggested that in the eye increased phosphatase activity in the TM and/or the ciliary muscles could contribute to lowering of the IOP, thus making the TM a possible target for new anti-glaucoma therapies [19].

Among the known targets of oxidant-mediated signaling is the mitogen-activated protein kinase (MAPK) cascade, which comprises highly conserved serine/threonine kinases, connecting cell surface receptors to regulatory targets in response to various stimuli [20]. The MAPK pathway can be stimulated by a number of factors contributing to the pathophysiology of primary open-angle glaucoma, including different types of mechanical [21–23] and oxidative [24] stress. In addition, there is accumulating evidence that members of the MAPK family play a critical role in TM cell apoptosis [25]. Among the MAPK proteins, p38 has been shown to mediate TGF-β2 up-regulation via the gene *SPARC*, one of the most highly transcribed and ubiquitous genes in the TM, especially in the juxtacanalicular region–the region believed to be the anatomic location of outflow regulation and the part of the AH where outflow resistance is maximal [26].

Matrix metalloproteinase (MMP) has been shown to be one of the most important activated proteins downstream of the MAPK activation and its activity is regulated by the kinase-phosphatases balance. The promoter regions of inducible MMP genes are regulated by MAPKs. This MAPK regulation depends on the nature of the extracellular stimuli, namely, the presence of different growth factors, cytokines, and IFγ [27,28]. MMPs play a powerful role in the resistance of the drainage system to AH outflow [21] and, as such, have also been suggested as a potential intervention site for glaucoma therapy [29]. A number of studies have provided evidence for the direct influence of MAPK signaling on the activity of MMPs within the TM [13,30]. In the present study, we examined in vitro the presence of soluble factors involved in cross talk of between non-pigmented ciliary epithelium and TM cells with the aim to shed light on the MAPK-phosphatases balance and its consequences for the activity of the MMPs.

Materials and Methods

Cell lines

A human normal trabecular meshwork (NTM) cell line [31] was generously donated by Alcon Laboratories, Texas, USA. A human non-pigmented ciliary epithelial cell line (ODM-2) [32,33] and a ciliary muscle cell line (HCM) [34] were kindly supplied by Prof. Miguel Coca Prados, Yale University, MA, USA. All cell lines were cultured at 37°C and 5% CO_2 in Dulbecco's modified Eagle's medium (DMEM) supplemented with fetal bovine serum, penicillin, streptomycin, and glutamate, as previously described [31,35].

Establishment of co-cultures

Sterile round glass cover slips (Marienfeld, 22 mm) were placed in six-well plates, and 3 ml of NTM cell suspension was pipetted onto each coverslip (1 million cells/well; ~100,000 cells/cm^2). The cultures were incubated in DMEM at 37°C in 5% CO_2/95% air for 24 h to allow the NTM cells to attach to the cover slips. In parallel, HCM, ODM-2, and NTM cells were seeded in 60-mm cell culture dishes (2.5 million cells in 5 ml per dish; ~90,000 cells/cm^2). After 24 h, two cover slips with their adhered NTM cells, but free of conditioning medium, were introduced into each cell culture dish with the cell-coated side of the coverslip facing upwards (Figure 1). Since the study focused on cell-cell communication, it was not necessary to determine the basal levels of the TM cells or the base-line activity of the tested proteins. As a control for the possible ODM-2:NTM signaling effects, we used the following co-cultures: ODM-2:HCM to verify the specificity of the signaling, and NTM:NTM to exclude contact effects. All the co-cultures were incubated for various periods of time, as indicated below. At the end of the incubation, the coverslips with the attached cells were removed, and analyzed as described below. The experiments were performed in duplicate and repeated independently three times.

Gelatin zymography and western blot analysis

Following co-incubation with ODM-2 cells, the NTM cells were lysed with buffer containing 20 mM Hepes (pH 7.4), 150 mM NaCl, 1 mM EGTA, 1 mM EDTA, 10% glycerol, 1 mM $MgCl_2$, 25 mM NaF, 1 mM Na_3VO_4, and protease inhibitors. After incubation on ice for 30 min, the lysates were sonicated for 10 centrifuged at 12,000 g at 4°C, and the supernatant was collected. The supernatant was analyzed for protein concentration by using the Bradford method [36]. For gelatin zymography, 20 μg of total protein from the lysates were electrophoresed through a 10% SDS-PAGE gel polymerized with 0.1% gelatin. Gels were washed twice, each time for 1 h in 2.5% Triton X-100, to remove SDS. Gels were then incubated for 16 h at 37°C in a developing buffer containing 50 mM Tris, 200 mM NaCl, 5 mM $CaCl_2$, and 0.02% Brij-35. Gels were stained with 30% methanol, 10% acetic acid, and 0.5% w/v Coomassie Brilliant Blue for 30 min, followed by distaining and then, dried between sheets of cellophane (Gel drying frames, Sigma). Gelatinolytic activity was manifested as horizontal white bands on a blue background. The proteolytic digestion of gelatin was quantified using an EZQuant-Gel 2.1, EZQuant Biology Solution. Three independent experiments were performed in duplicate.

For Western blot analysis, 20 μg of protein extracted from NTM cells were mixed with Laemmli buffer (Bio-Rad) containing 0.1% β-mercaptoethanol, boiled for 5 min, and separated on a10% SDS-PAGE gel. Proteins were transferred to nitrocellulose membranes and probed with primary antibodies against phospho-specific ERK1/2 (Sigma M9692, mouse monoclonal; 1:3,000 dilution), total ERK1/2 (Sigma M5670, rabbit polyclonal; 1:20,000 dilution), anti-phospho-p38 (Sigma M8177, mouse monoclonal; 1:2,000 dilution), and total p38 (Sigma M0800, rabbit polyclonal; 1:10,000 dilution). β-actin was determined using anti β-actin (Sigma A2228, mouse monoclonal 1:4000 dilution). The membranes were then incubated with secondary antibodies (anti-rabbit GE Health life sciences Na934v or anti-mouse Jackson 112035062) for 1 h at room temperature, and the immunocomplexes were detected with an enhanced chemiluminescence reagent (Amersham Pharmacia Biotech, Buckinghamshire, Eng-

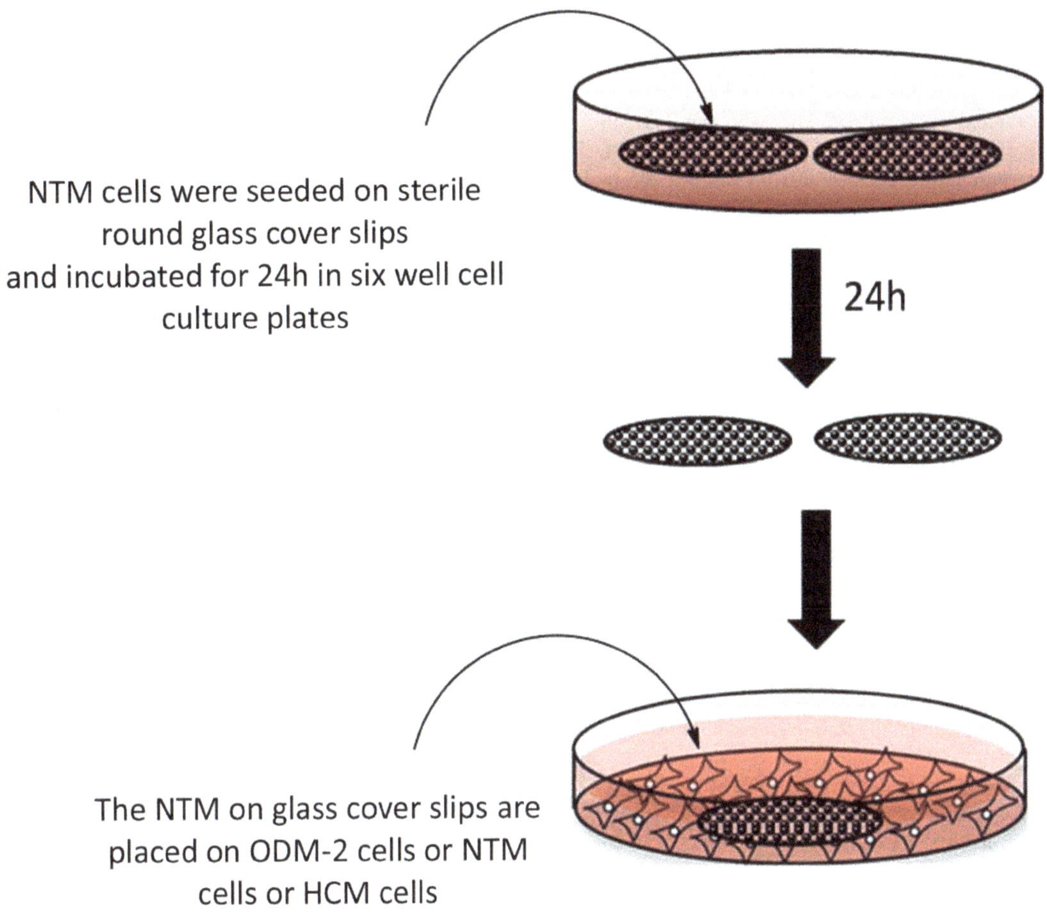

Figure 1. Schematic description of the co-culture model. Sterile round glass cover slips were placed in six-well plates, and seeded with NTM cell. The cultures were incubated for 24 h to allow the NTM cells to attach to the cover slips. In parallel, ODM-2 as the tested cells, HCM and NTM cells as controls were seeded in 60-mm cell culture dishes. After 24 h, two cover slips with their adhered NTM cells were introduced into each cell type culture dish.

land) for 1 min, followed by exposure to Kodak X-ray film (Rochester, NY). The films were scanned, and densitometry was analyzed by EZQuant-Gel software (EZQuant Biology Solution). The results from replicate experiments, expressed as percentages of the control, were pooled and averaged. Three independent experiments were performed in triplicate.

Phosphatase assays

Fluorogenic substrates based on 4-methylumbelliferone (4-MU) have been widely used for the detection of glycosidase and phosphatase activities, especially alkaline phosphatases. 6, 8-Difluoro-4-methylumbelliferyl phosphate (DiFMUP) is a fluorinated derivative of 4-MU with a lower pKa value, which makes it suitable for the detection of both alkaline and acid phosphatases. Hydrolysis of DiFMUP by a phosphatase results in the release of fluorescent DiFMU, which can be easily followed in continuous mode by a fluorescence reader.

NTM cells adheed to coverslips were co-incubated with ODM-2 cells for 5, 10, 15, 30, or 60 min. The NTM cell cultures on the coverslips were then removed from the co-culture and washed in PBS. Cells were lysed in a buffer containing 20 mM Tris (pH 7.5), 6 mM $MgCl_2$, 100 mM NaCl, 0.1 mM EGTA, 1 m EDTA, and 0.5 mM dithiothreitol. Lysates were centrifuged, and the supernatants were retained. The assay was carried out in black flat-bottomed 96-well plates in a total reaction volume of 100 µl. The total 100 µl of reaction mixture included 5 µl of sample, 25 µl of DiFMUP (Biorad) 200 µM diluted in DMSO, 70 µl of acidic buffer (sodium acetate 50 mM, EDTA 1 mM, DTT 21 mM, NaCl 100 mM; doubly distilled water to 10 mL, pH 5.5) or alkaline buffer (Hepes 50 mM, EDTA 1 mM, DTT 2 mM, NaCl 150 mm, doubly distilled water to 50 mL; pH 6.9). Blanks included wells without samples and wells without DiFMUP. The supernatants were incubated with 10 µM of DiFMUP, for 10 min at 37°C with intermittent mixing in a fluorescence plate reader, infinite microplate reader (M200; Tecan Group Ltd.) and the data capture software (Bio-Lynx) with 360 nm excitation and 460 nm emission filters. Three independent experiments were performed in triplicate.

Statistics

All the data acquired in the study was compared to that for NTM:NTM cells at the shorter incubation time tested (5 min or 4 h) as the reference point. Analysis of data was performed using a one-way ANOVA (InState 3.0, Graphpad Software).

Results

MAPK

To evaluate the cross-talk between the ciliary epithelium and the TM, the two cell lines were co-cultured in Petri dishes. A co-culture of NTM cells grown on cover slips introduced to NTM cells was used as control. After removal of the NTM cells on the cover slips at different time points following initiation of the co-culture, NTM proteins were analyzed for total Erk (tErk) and its active phosphorylated form (pErk). The ratio between the two represents the activity of the Erk branched pathway of the MAPK. A significant increase (ANOVA $p<0.001$) in Erk activation vis-à-vis the control treatment was found from 10 min following co-culture up to 30 min (Figure 2). This increase in Erk activation peaked at 10 min, demonstrating a transient activation with a bell shape. The phosphorylated Erk/total Erk ratio did not change with time in HCM cells exposed to ODM-2 cells (Figure S1).

To evaluate the communication between the ciliary epithelium and the TM, the two cell lines were co-cultured in petri dishes. A co-culture of NTM cells with NTM cells was used as control. The degree of activation of the p38 pathway of the MAPK was significantly elevated (ANOVA $p<0.01$ for 10 min) in the ODM-2:NTM co-culture vis-à-vis the NTM:NTM control (Figure 3). A trend of elevated activation can be seen from 5 min of co-culture through 60 min. The ratio of phosphorylated p38/total p38 did not change with time in HCM cells exposed to ODM-2 cells (Figure S2).

Acid and alkaline phosphatase activity following co-culture of NTM cells with ODM-2 cells

We determined the activity of alkaline and acid phosphatases as indicative of serine/threonine phosphatases and tyrosine phosphatases, respectively, by the fluorescent DIMFUP method. The activity of the two families of phosphatases peaked at 10 min and then dropped markedly at 15 min (ANOVA $p<0.001$) (Figure 4). At 30 min post co-culture, the activity of the NTM cells exposed to ODM-2 cells was similar to that of the control, namely, NTM cells co-cultured with NTM cells. While the phosphatase activities of the ODM-2:NTM co-cultures remained steady between 30 and 60 min, a continuous non-significant decline in phosphatase activity was found in the control group.

Activity of MMPs following co-culture of NTM cells with ODM-2

MAPK activation is known to regulate the expression of different MMPs, which contribute to the AH outflow by decreasing the resistance of the extracellular matrix to AH drainage. To verify the specific response of NTM cells to co-culture with ODM-2 cells, two controls were used in these experiments, the NTM:NTM co-culture to control for contact effects and the HCM:NTM co-culture to control for the specificity of the signaling effects. The method facilitates the detection of the non-active form of the enzymes (pro-enzymes) and the post-cleavage active enzymes with gelatinolytic activity. The NTM cell lysate obtained after the co-culture contained MMP-9 and MMP-2. These two MMPs, which have previously been reported in TM cells, were identified according to their molecular weights and migration distance on the zymography gel. MMP-2 activity was barely measurable, but MMP-9 activity was easily quantified (Figure 5). A significant increase (ANOVA $p<0.001$) in MMP-9 activity following NTM exposure to ODM-2 cells was found at 8 h post co-culture. Although the activity of MMP-9 was higher for the HCM:NTM control co-culture than for the NTM:NTM control co-culture, the difference was not significant and the activity in both controls was lower than that in the ODM-2:NTM co-culture. MMP-9 activity in the NTM cells following ODM-2:NTM co-culture exhibited a bell-shaped curve with a peak at 8 h.

Discussion

Elevated IOP, known to be the main risk factor for the development of primary open-angle glaucoma, can be controlled by medication targeting the production and/or drainage of the AH. The role of MMPs within the drainage system was demonstrated in the study of Bradley et al. [37]. These authors concluded that the balance of MMPs and their tissue inhibitors, TIMMPs, that controls the endogenous extracellular matrix turnover, is responsible for the maintenance of TM outflow resistance. However at present, there areno drugs that target the balance of MMPs and TIMMPs within the TM, the main AH drainage pathway (although some currently available prostaglandin analogues that are effective IOP lowering agents exert their pharmacological action by targeting the MMPs involved mainly in the uveo-scleral AH drainage).

In the present study, the gelatinolytic activity of MMPs following TM signaling activation by ciliary epithelium cells was evaluated. We focused on MAPK and phosphatase pathways, although other pathways such as Wnt [38] or Akt [39] might be involved. We report here for the first time that, in a co-culture model of ODM-2 and NTM cell lines, cross-talk between ODM-2 cells and NTM cells appears to promote MMP-9 activity. To date, the mechanism governing the up-regulation of MMPs as the result of interaction between ODM-2 and NTM cells has been hypothesized but not demonstrated [16]. We therefore focused on the elucidation of the signaling pathways that are modulated by the co-culture. Bearing in mind that pigmented epithelium cells, synchronized in vivo with non-pigmented epithelium cells, in the production of AH. This synchronization might make a significant contribution to the signaling release of non-pigmented ciliary epithelial cells. Our study focused solely on effects of the latter. However, possible contribution of pigmented epithelial cells in the present model will require further research. Although this, study was performed in quite well characterized cell lines [31–34], the relevance and the importance of the present findings would be strengthened by their replication in a primary culture.

It is known that the promoter regions of inducible MMP genes are regulated by MAPKs in a manner that depends on the nature of the extracellular stimuli [40]. Our results revealed that interaction of ODM-2 with NTM cells leads to increased phosphorylation of the ERK1/2 pathway and to increased p38 signaling in NTM cells. Taken together, these results suggest that cross-talk between ODM-2 and NTM cells results in signal activation, signifying, in turn, that these pathways may be intimately involved in the regulation of levels of MMPs in the co-culture of NTMs and ODM-2 cells. Recent reports suggest that targeting of MAPKs, in particular ERK1/2 and JNK, may be a potent approach to reduce MMP expression in a variety of cells [41]. Downstream MAPK signaling pathway active molecules, such as c-Jun and C-Fos, translocate to the nucleus to promote transcription directly or indirectly. Indeed, in our preliminary, unpublished data in our laboratory indicated that, c-Jun expression in NTM cells increased in response to the stimuli induced by ODM-2:NTM co-culture. We still do not have a clear picture of the putative soluble transcription regulators of the ERK1/2 and p38 signaling pathways in the ODM-2:NTM co-culture vis-à-vis the NTM:NTM co-culture. The MAPK-MMP pathways appear to be regulated transcrip-tionally by classic mediators, such TNF-α [42], VGEF [43], TGF-β [44] and interleukins [42], all of which, in turn, activate a pleotropic cascade of signaling pathways.

A number of studies have demonstrated the role of neuropeptides in mediating the levels of MMPs [45,46]. Transcripts (mRNA) for neuropeptides have been found in both dissected

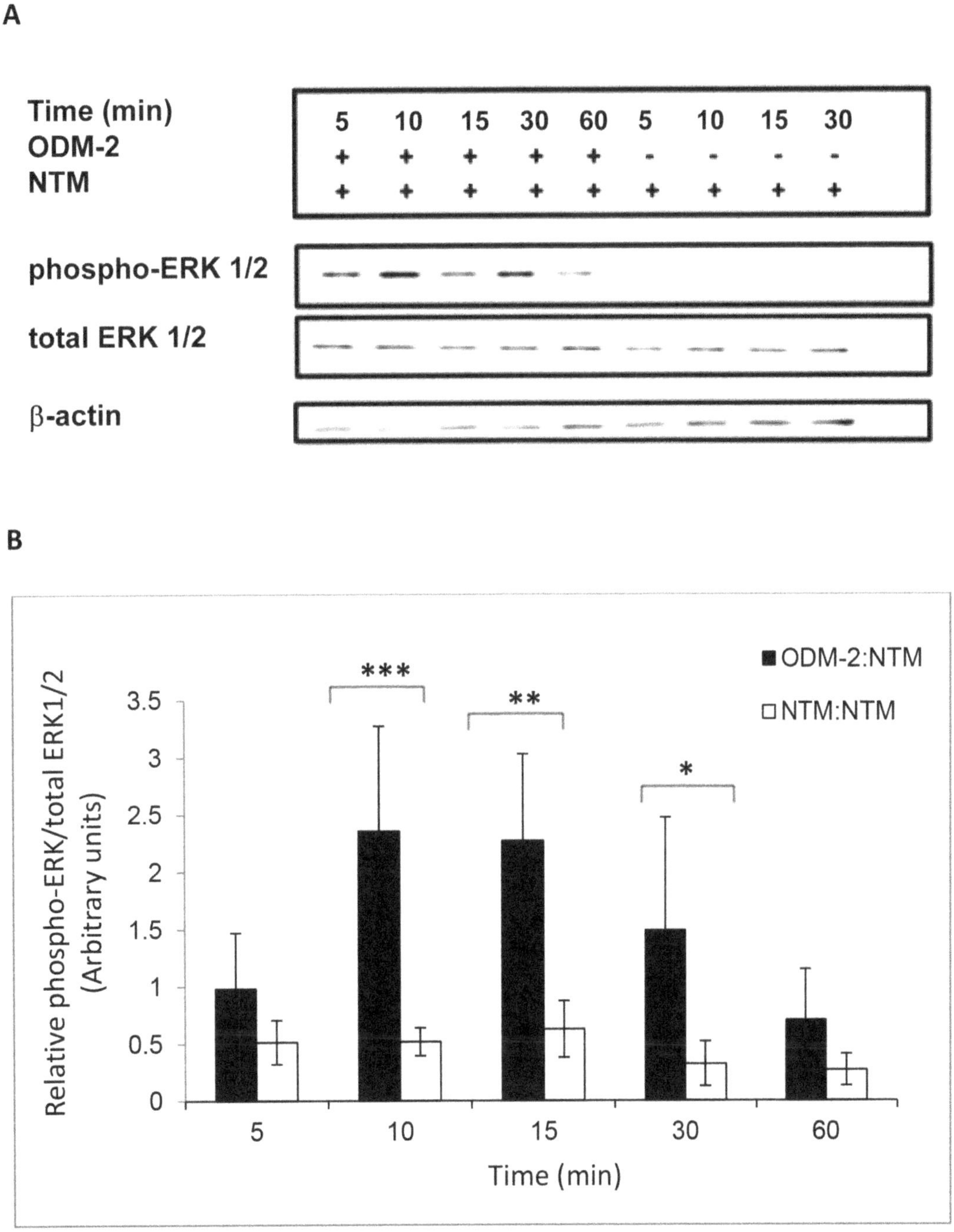

Figure 2. ERK1/2 activation in NTM cells co-cultured with ODM-2 cells for 5, 10, 15, 30, 60 min. Total protein was extracted from NTM cells. Phosphorylated and total ERK1/2 proteins were analyzed by Western blot. (A) Representative western blot film. (B) A significant increases in ERK activation in NTM cells following co-culture with ODM-2 cells. The bar graph represents the means ± SD of three independent experiments performed in duplicates. One-way ANOVA (***$p<0.001$, **$p<0.01$,*$p<0.05$).

ciliary processes and cultured ciliary epithelial cells by Northern blot analysis and RT-PCR. The secreted products of ciliary epithelial cells either in the AH or in the culture medium of cultured ciliary epithelial cells have been detected by radioimmunoassay, suggesting that communication occurs between these two types of tissue. Furthermore, it has been found that neuroendocrine processing enzymes are co-expressed with the neuroendocrine peptides, suggesting that the neuropeptides synthesized in the ciliary epithelium undergo endoproteolytic processing and storage before they are secreted [16]. Coca-Prados [16] proposed that the neuropeptides released by the ciliary epithelium in the AH can serve as messengers to communicate with surrounding tissues in the anterior segment of the eye, particularly, in the TM. It is therefore possible that one or more of the factors described above or some unknown neuropeptide are induced in the ODM-2:NTM co-culture, thereby giving rise to a positive feedback to the ERK1/2 and p38 pathways, which leads to the MMP-mediated degenerative changes in the NTM cells.

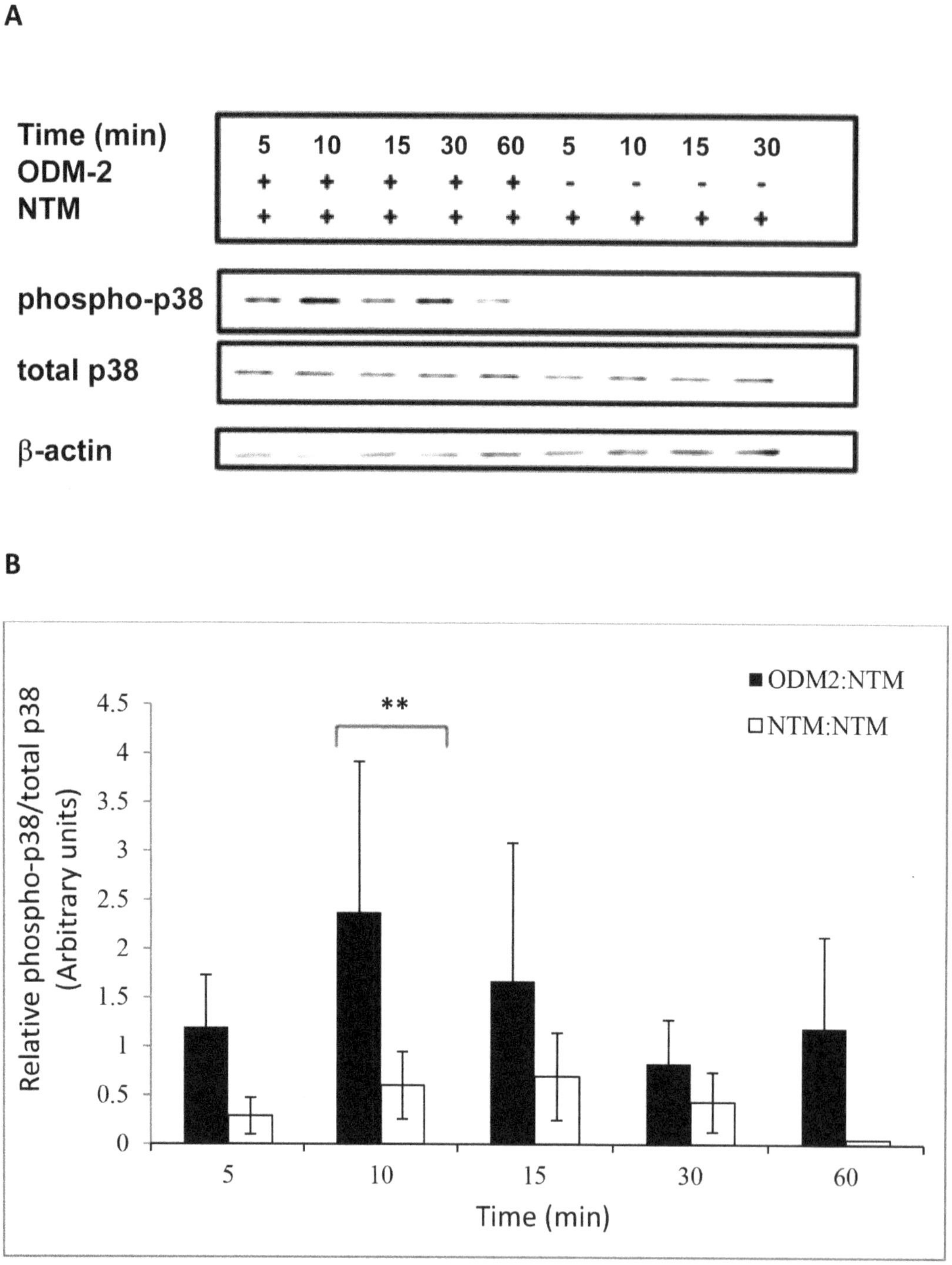

Figure 3. p38 activation in NTM cells co-cultured with ODM-2 cells for 5, 10, 15, 30, 60 min. Total protein was extracted from NTM cells. Phosphorylated and total p38 proteins were analyzed by Western blot. (A) Representative western blot film. (B) A significant increases in p38 activation in NTM cells following co-culture with ODM-2 cells. The bar graph represents the means ± SD of three independent experiments performed in duplicates. One-way ANOVA (**$p<0.01$).

While the role of kinases in the regulation of MMPs has been extensively studied, the role of phosphatases in the homeostasis of MMPs remains obscure. Nonetheless, it is now apparent that they are equally important in mediating cell signaling, apoptosis, growth, migration and adhesion. The early report of Holladay et al. that okadaic acid, a protein phosphatase 1 and 2A inhibitor, increases MMP-3 (stromelysin-1) expression in murine keratinocytes [47,48] has been confirmed and extended by other researchers [49]. The specific mechanisms that contribute to the increase in MMP abundance following phosphatase inhibition remain largely unexplored. It is possible that the increased MMP presence following phosphatase inhibition may simply reflect maintenance of the phosphorylation and hence the activation state of signaling pathways upstream of the transcriptional regulation of the MMPs. For instance, PP2A mediates the dephosphorylation of MAPK kinase 1 and the ERK family kinases [50], which are

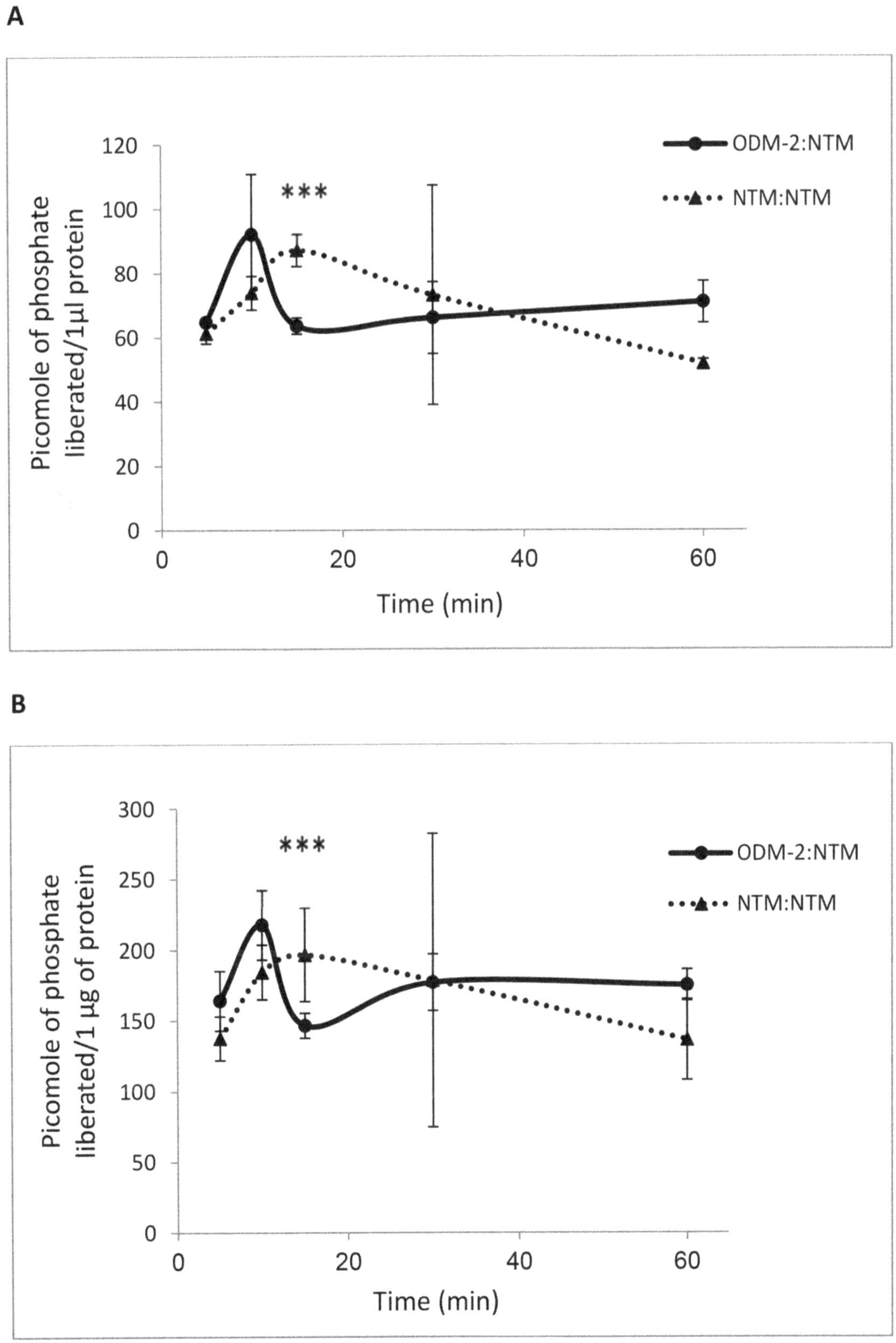

Figure 4. Alkaline and acid phosphatase activity of NTM cells following co-culture with ODM-2 cells for 5, 10, 15, 30 or 60 min. NTM:NTM co-culuure was used as controls. (A) Alkaline phosphatase and (B) acid phosphatase activity determined by the DiFMUP assay. The quantity of DiFMU is expressed as phosphate liberated, since equivalent amounts of DiFMU and phosphate are generated in the reaction. Means of two independent experiments performed in triplicate; one-way ANOVA (***$p<0.001$).

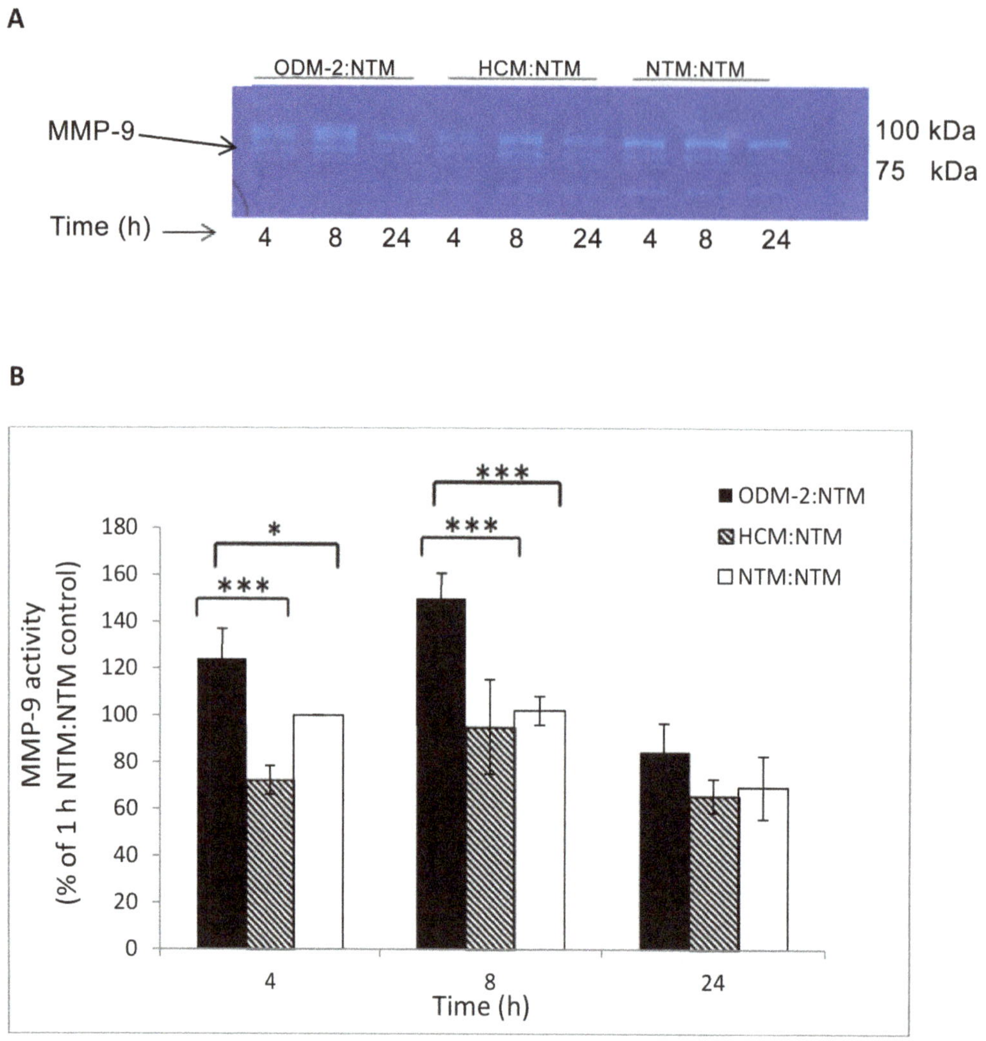

Figure 5. MMP-9 activity following ODM-2 and NTM cells co-culture. Gelatinolytic activity of MMP-9 (92 kDa) in NTM cells was examined by gelatin zymography after 4, 8, and 24 h of co-culture with ODM-2 cells. As controls, NTM cells were co-cultured with HCM or NTM cells. (A) Zymogram of co-culture groups. (B) MMP-9 quantitative analysis of NTM cells co-cultured with ODM, NTM or HCM cells for 4, 8 and 24 h. The bar graph represents the means ± SD of three independent experiments performed in duplicate; one-way ANOVA (*$p<0.05$, ***$p<0.001$).

associated with MMP and TIMMP regulation. More specifically, Westermarck's group found that okadaic acid-induced expression of MMP-3 is mediated through transactivation of AP-1 complexes containing c-Jun and JunB in HT-1080 cells [47]. However, the process may be more complex than previously thought, as the recent work of Rietz et al. shows that okadaic acid increases the abundance of MMP-9 in fibroblasts through p38-MAPK and is inhibited by isoprenaline via a pathway involving β-arrestin 2, PP2A and an NF-κB binding motif [49].

In the current study, it was observed that within 10–15 min of co-culture with ODM-2 cells, NTM cells revealed increase levels of MAPKs, whereas a complex activity/time response exist in the alkaline and acid phosphatases activity as compared to control. In ODM-2:NTM and the control cells a quick and short up-regulation of general phosphatase activity was found, followed by down-regulation. The changes were more marked in the ODM:NTM co-culture, with different kinetics relative to the control NTM:NTM cells, indicating that processes occurring beyond simple contact stress do exist. The involvement of phosphatases in the ocular drainage system was demonstrated partially in our previous research in AH [11]. The phosphatases response detected is a general analysis reflecting probably several phosphatases activity, and further research clarifying the specific phosphatases involved is required. The changes in phosphatases kinetics may support the crosstalk between MAPK kinases, MMPs and phosphatases. However, more detailed experiments are needed designed to determine the relationship between the MMP system, MAPK kinases and phosphatases, with focus on PP2A phosphatase.

Supporting Information

Figure S1 Effect on ERK1/2 activation in NTM cells of interaction between NTM and HCM cells co-cultured for 5, 10, 15, 30, or 60 min. Following co-culture of the cells, total protein was extracted from NTM cells. Changes in ERK activation in normal TM cells following co-culture with HCM cells. Phosphorylated ERK1/2 proteins were analyzed by Western blot. The bar graph represents the means ± SD of two independent experiments performed in triplicate. One-way

ANOVA (NS p>0.05). Phosphorylated Erk/total Erk ratio did not change with time in HCM cells exposed to ODM-2 cells.

Figure S2 Effect on p38 activation in NTM cells of interaction between NTM and HCM cells co-cultured for 5, 10, 15, 30, or 60 min. Following co-culture of the cells, total protein was then extracted from NTM cells. Changes in p38 activation in normal TM cells following co-culture with HCM cells. Phosphorylated p38 proteins were analyzed by Western blot. The bar graph represents the means ± SD of three independent experiments performed in duplicate. One-way ANOVA (NS p> 0.05). Phosphorylated p38/total p38 ratio did not change with time in HCM cells exposed to ODM-2 cells.

Acknowledgments

The authors thank Professor Coca-Prados for the human ODM-2 cell line originally established in his lab, Alcon Research Ltd. for providing the NTM5 cell line, and Ms Mazal Rubin for excellent technical assistance. The authors also thanks Professor Sofia Schriaber-Avisar and Ms Inez Mureinik for careful languish auditing the manuscript.

Author Contributions

Conceived and designed the experiments: EB NL. Performed the experiments: NL. Analyzed the data: EB NL. Contributed reagents/materials/analysis tools: EB NL. Contributed to the writing of the manuscript: EB NL.

References

1. Quigley HA, Broman AT (2006) The number of people with glaucoma worldwide in 2010 and 2020. Br J Ophthalmol 90: 262–267.
2. McKinnon SJ, Goldberg LD, Peeples P, Walt JG, Bramley TJ (2008) Current Management of Glaucoma and the Need for Complete Therapy-Page 2. Am J Manag Care 14: S20–S27.
3. Dahlmann-Noor AH, Vijay S, Limb GA, Khaw PT (2010) Strategies for optic nerve rescue and regeneration in glaucoma and other optic neuropathies. Drug Discov Today 15: 287–299.
4. Chang EE, Goldberg JL (2012) Glaucoma 2.0: neuroprotection, neuroregeneration, neuroenhancement. Ophthalmology 119: 979–986.
5. Johnson TV, Martin KR (2013) Cell transplantation approaches to retinal ganglion cell neuroprotection in glaucoma. Curr Opin Pharmacol 13: 78–82.
6. Strouthidis NG, Girard MJA (2013) Altering the way the optic nerve head responds to intraocular pressure–a potential approach to glaucoma therapy. Curr Opin Pharmacol 13: 83–89.
7. Goel M, Picciani RG, Lee RK, Bhattacharya SK (2010) Aqueous humor dynamics: a review. The Open Ophthalmol J 4: 52.
8. Inoue T, Tanihara H (2013) Rho-associated kinase inhibitors: A novel glaucoma therapy. Prog Ret Eye Res 37: 1–12.
9. Wang SK, Chang RT (2014) An emerging treatment option for glaucoma: Rho kinase inhibitors. Clin Ophthalmol 8: 883.
10. Borkenstein A, Faschinger C, Maier R, Weger M, Theisl A, et al. (2013) Measurement of tumor necrosis factor-alpha, interleukin-6, Fas ligand, interleukin-1α, and interleukin-1β in the aqueous humor of patients with open angle glaucoma using multiplex bead analysis. Mol Vis 19: 2306.
11. Latarya G, Mansour A, Epstein I, Cotlear D, Pikkel J, et al. (2012) Human Aqueous Humor Phosphatase Activity in Cataract and Glaucoma. Invest ophthalmol Vis Sci 53: 1679–1684.
12. Rao PV (2014) Bioactive lysophospholipids: role in regulation of aqueous humor outflow and intraocular pressure in the context of pathobiology and therapy of glaucoma. J Ocul Pharmacol Ther 30: 181–190.
13. Sawada H, Fukuchi T, Tanaka T, Abe H (2010) Tumor necrosis factor-alpha concentrations in the aqueous humor of patients with glaucoma. Invest Ophthalmol Vis Sci 51: 903–906.
14. Stamer WD, Hoffman EA, Luther JM, Hachey DL, Schey KL (2011) Protein profile of exosomes from trabecular meshwork cells. J Proteomics 74: 796–804.
15. Takai Y, Tanito M, Ohira A (2012) Multiplex cytokine analysis of aqueous humor in eyes with primary open-angle glaucoma, exfoliation glaucoma, and cataract. Invest ophthalmol Vis Sci 53: 241–247.
16. Coca-Prados M, Escribano J (2007) New perspectives in aqueous humor secretion and in glaucoma: the ciliary body as a multifunctional neuroendocrine gland. Prog Ret Eye Res 26: 239–262.
17. Shmulevich A, Beit-Yannai E (2009) Differential modulation of MAPKs in relation to increased intraocular pressure in the aqueous humor of rat eye injected with hyaluronic acid. Curr Eye Res 34: 466–475.
18. Halliwell B (2011) Free radicals and antioxidants - quo vadis? Trends Pharmacol Sci 32: 125–130.
19. Wiederholt M, Groth J, Strauss O (1998) Role of protein tyrosine kinase on regulation of trabecular meshwork and ciliary muscle contractility. Invest Ophthalmol Vis Sci 39: 1012–1020.
20. Beit-Yannai E, Shmulevich A (2007) Does the aqueous humor have a role in mitogen-activated protein kinase (MAPK) intracellular signaling in Glaucoma? Med Hypotheses 68: 299–302.
21. Alexander J, Samples J, Van Buskirk E, Acott T (1991) Expression of matrix metalloproteinases and inhibitor by human trabecular meshwork. Invest ophthalmol Vis Sci 32: 172–180.
22. Hashimoto A, Yoshikawa M, Niwa A, Konno R (2005) Mice lacking D-amino acid oxidase activity display marked attenuation of stereotypy and ataxia induced by MK-801. Brain Res 1033: 210–215.
23. Li DQ, Luo L, Chen Z, Kim HS, Song XJ, et al. (2006) JNK and ERK MAP kinases mediate induction of IL-1beta, TNF-alpha and IL-8 following hyperosmolar stress in human limbal epithelial cells. Exp Eye Res 82: 588–596.
24. Aslan M, Cort A, Yucel I (2008) Oxidative and nitrative stress markers in glaucoma. Free Rad Biol Med 45: 367–376.
25. Zhang X, Schroeder A, Callahan EM, Coyle BM, Wang N, et al. (2006) Constitutive signalling pathway activity in trabecular meshwork cells from glaucomatous eyes. Exp Eye Res 82: 968–973.
26. Oh DJ, Kang MH, Ooi YH, Choi KR, Sage EH, et al. (2013) Overexpression of SPARC in human trabecular meshwork increases intraocular pressure and alters extracellular matrix. Invest Ophthalmol Vis Sci 54: 3309–3319.
27. Vandooren J, Van den Steen PE, Opdenakker G (2013) Biochemistry and molecular biology of gelatinase B or matrix metalloproteinase-9 (MMP-9): the next decade. Crit Rev Biochem Mol Biol 48: 222–272.
28. Hosseini M, Rose AY, Song K, Bohan C, Alexander JP, et al. (2006) IL-1 and TNF induction of matrix metalloproteinase-3 by c-Jun N-terminal kinase in trabecular meshwork. I Invest ophthalmol Vis Sci 47: 1469–1476.
29. De Groef L, Van Hove I, Dekeyster E, Stalmans I, Moons L (2013) MMPs in the Trabecular Meshwork: Promising Targets for Future Glaucoma Therapies? Invest ophthalmol Vis Sci 54: 7756–7763.
30. Sanka K, Maddala R, Epstein DL, Rao PV (2007) Influence of actin cytoskeletal integrity on matrix metalloproteinase-2 activation in cultured human trabecular meshwork cells. Invest Ophthalmol Vis Sci 48: 2105–2114.
31. Pang I-H, Shade DL, Clark AF, Steely HT, DeSantis L (1994) Preliminary characterization of a transformed cell strain derived from human trabecular meshwork. Current eye Res 13: 51–63.
32. Coca-Prados M, Wax MB (1986) Transformation of human ciliary epithelial cells by simian virus 40: induction of cell proliferation and retention of beta 2-adrenergic receptors. P Natl Acad USA 83: 8754–8758.
33. Ghosh S, Hernando N, Martín-Alonso JM, Martin-Vasallo P, Coca-Prados M (1991) Expression of multiple Na+, K+-ATPase genes reveals a gradient of isoforms along the nonpigmented ciliary epithelium: Functional implications in aqueous humor secretion. J Cel Physiol 149: 184–194.
34. Sánchez-Sánchez F, Martínez-Redondo F, Aroca-Aguilar JD, Coca-Prados M, Escribano J (2007) Characterization of the intracellular proteolytic cleavage of myocilin and identification of calpain II as a myocilin-processing protease. J Biol Chem 282: 27810–27824.
35. Martin-Vasallo P, Ghosh S, Coca-Prados M (1989) Expression of Na, K-ATPase alpha subunit isoforms in the human ciliary body and cultured ciliary epithelial cells. J Cel Physiol 141: 243–252.
36. Bradford MM (1976) A rapid and sensitive method for the quantitation of microgram quantities of protein utilizing the principle of protein-dye binding. Anal Biochem 72: 248–254.
37. Bradley JM, Vranka J, Colvis CM, Conger DM, Alexander JP, et al. (1998) Effect of matrix metalloproteinases activity on outflow in perfused human organ culture. Invest Ophthalmol Vis Sci 39: 2649–2658.
38. Marchenko ND, Marchenko GN, Weinreb RN, Lindsey JD, Kyshtoobayeva A, et al. (2004) β-Catenin regulates the gene of MMP-26, a novel matrix metalloproteinase expressed both in carcinomas and normal epithelial cells. The international J Bioche Cell Biol 36: 942–956.
39. Huang P, Zhang SS-M, Zhang C (2009) The two sides of cytokine signaling and glaucomatous optic neuropathy. J Ocul Biol Dis Inform 2: 98–103.
40. Chakraborti S, Mandal M, Das S, Mandal A, Chakraborti T (2003) Regulation of matrix metalloproteinases: an overview. Mol Cell Biochem 253: 269–285.
41. Loeser RF, Erickson EA, Long DL (2008) Mitogen-activated protein kinases as therapeutic targets in osteoarthritis. Curr Opin Rheumatol 20: 581–586.
42. Liacini A, Sylvester J, Li WQ, Zafarullah M (2002) Inhibition of interleukin-1-stimulated MAP kinases, activating protein-1 (AP-1) and nuclear factor kappa B (NF-kappa B) transcription factors down-regulates matrix metalloproteinase gene expression in articular chondrocytes. Matrix Biol 21: 251–262.
43. Pufe T, Harde V, Petersen W, Goldring MB, Tillmann B, et al. (2004) Vascular endothelial growth factor (VEGF) induces matrix metalloproteinase expression in immortalized chondrocytes. J Pathol 202: 367–374.
44. Kumar M, Makonchuk DY, Li H, Mittal A, Kumar A (2009) TNF-like weak inducer of apoptosis (TWEAK) activates proinflammatory signaling pathways

and gene expression through the activation of TGF-beta-activated kinase 1. J Immunol 182: 2439–2448.
45. Rhim E-M, Park S-H, Kim D-S, Kim S-Y, Choi K-K, et al. (2011) The effect of tumor necrosis factor (TNF)-α to induce matrix metalloproteinase (MMPs) from the human dental pulp, gingival, and periodontal ligament cells. J Korean Acad Conservative Dentistry 36: 26–36.
46. Sehgal I, Thompson TC (1998) Neuropeptides induce Mr 92,000 type IV collagenase (matrix metalloprotease-9) activity in human prostate cancer cell lines. Cancer Res 58: 4288–4291.
47. Westermarck J, Lohi J, Keski-Oja J, Kähäri V-M (1994) Okadaic acid-elicited transcriptional activation of collagenase gene expression in HT-1080 fibrosarcoma cells is mediated by JunB. Cell growth & differentiation: the molecular biology journal of the American Association for Cancer Res 5: 1205–1213.
48. Holladay K, Fujiki H, Bowden GT (1992) Okadaic acid induces the expression of both early and secondary response genes in mouse keratinocytes. Mol Carcinogen 5: 16–24.
49. Rietz A, Spiers J (2012) The relationship between the MMP system, adrenoceptors and phosphoprotein phosphatases. Brit J Pharmacol 166: 1225–1243.
50. Garcia L, Garcia F, Llorens F, Unzeta M, Itarte E, et al. (2002) PP1/PP2A phosphatases inhibitors okadaic acid and calyculin A block ERK5 activation by growth factors and oxidative stress. FEBS Lett 523: 90–94.

24

Anti-VEGF Agents with or without Antimetabolites in Trabeculectomy for Glaucoma

Qi Xiong[1], Zhiliang Li[2], Zhaohui Li[1], Yi Zhu[1], Sancar Abdulhalim[1], Ping Wang[1], Xiaojun Cai[1]*

1 Department of Ophthalmology, Zhongnan Hospital of Wuhan University, Wuhan, Hubei, P.R. China, 2 Department of Orthpedics, Union Hospital of Tongji Medical College, Huazhong University of Science and Technology, Wuhan, Hubei, P.R. China

Abstract

Purpose: We aimed to evaluate the intraoperative application of antimetabolites compared with anti-vascular endothelial growth factor (VEGF) agents with or without antimetabolites in trabeculectomy (Trab) for glaucoma.

Methods: Relevant studies were selected through extensive search using PubMed, EMBASE, the Cochrane Library, and Web of Science databases in August 2013. The primary efficacy estimate was measured using weighted mean difference of the percentage of intraocular pressure reduction (IOPR%) from baseline to end-point, and the secondary efficacy estimates were odds ratio (OR) and 95% confidence interval (CI) for complete success rate and qualified success rate. ORs were also used to measure the tolerability estimate for adverse events. Meta-analyses of fixed or random effects models were conducted using RevMan software 5.2 to pool the results of the studies included. Heterogeneity was assessed using Chi^2 test and the I^2 measure.

Results: Nine studies enrolling a total of 349 patients were included. The weighted mean difference of IOPR% from baseline was 7.23 (95% CI: 2.57–11.89) for antimetabolites vs. anti-VEGF agents and 3.96 (95% CI: −4.18–12.10) for antimetabolites vs. anti-VEGF agents plus antimetabolites. The pooled ORs comparing antimetabolites with anti-VEGF agents were 2.37 (95% CI: 0.78, 7.21) for the complete success rate and 1.93 (95% CI: 0.52, 7.16) for qualified success rate. The pooled ORs comparing antimetabolites with anti-VEGF agents plus antimetabolites were 1.43 (95% CI: 0.48, 4.29) for the complete success rate and 2.11 (95% CI: 0.12, 37.72) for qualified success rate. The rates of adverse events did not significantly differ between antimetabolites and anti-VEGF agents, with pooled ORs of 0.86 (0.28–2.69) for bleb leakage, 3.01 (0.45–20.10) for choroidal effusion, 0.96 (0.23–3.98) for flat anterior chamber, and 0.90 (0.12–6.60) for hypotony. Further, the rates of adverse events were similar between antimetabolites and anti-VEGF agents plus antimetabolites, with pooled ORs of 0.40 (0.08–2.00) and 8.00 (0.93–68.59) for bleb leakage and hypotony, respectively.

Conclusions: In comparison with anti-VEGF agents, antimetabolites were more effective in lowering IOP in Trab, while the intraoperative application of these two types of agents did not indicate statistically significant differences in the complete success rate, qualified success rate, or incidence of adverse events.

Editor: Pedro Gonzalez, Duke University, United States of America

Funding: No current funding sources for this study.

Competing Interests: The authors have declared that no competing interests exist.

* E-mail: xiaojuncai168@163.com

Introduction

Glaucoma is characterized by optic nerve atrophy and visual field defects, which is one of the many clinically common irreversible blinding eye diseases, seriously threatening the optic nerve function. There were 60.5 million people with glaucoma worldwide in 2010, and it is predicted that glaucoma will affect more than 79.6 million people by 2020 [1]. Glaucoma treatments, either pharmacologically or surgically, are directed toward reducing intraocular pressure (IOP). Since it was first introduced in 1968, trabeculectomy (Trab) has been the most effective therapy in reducing IOP in patients with medically uncontrollable glaucoma [2–4]. Unlike most other surgical procedures, this filtrating surgery can be successfully performed by inhibiting the wound healing process [5]. Excessive postoperative scarring of the conjunctiva and Tenon's capsule, resulting in new water channels being blocked and poor postoperative control of IOP, has been reported to be the major reason for the failure of Trab [6,7].

Antimetabolites, such as mitomycin C (MMC) and 5-fluorouracil (5-FU), which have been used in Trab to delay the wound healing process, can improve the success rate of surgery by inhibiting both inflammation and fibroblastic activity. Due to their nonspecific effects on cell biology, their application may lead to cell damage, followed by persistent low postoperative IOP with decreased vision, bleb leakage, corneal epithelium defect, and endophthalmitis [8,9]. Thus, to minimize the risk of these potential adverse events, novel effective therapies involving wound healing processes, are currently undergoing experimental and clinical study.

Vascular endothelial growth factor (VEGF) is a cytokine with multiple effects on wound healing [10,11]. In a study conducted by Li et al [12], VEGF expression was observed in aqueous humor samples of postoperative glaucoma patients and rabbits, which accelerated the proliferation of Tenon's fibroblasts in vitro. Bevacizumab and ranibizumab, which are monoclonal antibodies against VEGF, showed promising results as a potent means to lessen scarring after filtration surgery. Several studies have demonstrated that either subconjunctival or intravitreal anti-VEGF agents may function as a potential adjuvant therapy to reduce the incidence of fibroblast proliferation and scar formation after Trab [13,14].

Several studies have recently compared the efficacy of antimetabolites with anti-VEGF agents in inhibiting scarring after Trab. Some of these studies found antimetabolites to be more effective, while others showed anti-VEGF agents as being more effective. These inconsistent results have made it difficult to draw evidence-based conclusions that could be applied in clinical practice. To the best of our knowledge, relevant data has not yet been systematically evaluated and reported. Therefore, here we performed a meta-analysis of controlled clinical trials to assess the efficacy and tolerability of antimetabolites and anti-VEGF agents in Trab for glaucoma.

Materials and Methods

Meta-analysis was performed according to a predetermined protocol described in the following paragraph. As outlined by the Cochrane Handbook for Systematic Reviews of Interventions [15] and PRISMA statement [16], standard systematic review techniques were followed throughout the entire process.

Literature search

Two investigators (Q.X. and Z.L.L.) searched PubMed, EMBASE, the Cochrane Library, and Web of Science databases systematically for relevant studies in August 2013. The following search terms were used: (1) mitomycin C, or 5-fluorouracil; (2) bevacizumab, Avastin, ranibizumab, or Lucentis; and (3) trabeculectomy. A manual search was performed by checking the reference lists of the original reports and review articles in order to identify studies that were not yet included in the computerized databases. No language restriction was set.

Inclusion and exclusion criteria

Published studies were included on the basis of the following criteria: (i) study design: controlled clinical study; (ii) population: glaucoma patients who underwent Trab or phacotrabeculectomy; (iii) intervention: intraoperative application of antimetabolites vs. anti-VEGF agents with or without antimetabolites at any concentration and dose in Trab; and (iv) outcome variables: at least one of the following: percentage of IOP reduction (IOPR%), complete success rate, and qualified success rate. Letters, reviews, duplicate publications, abstracts from conferences, unqualified control group, and full texts without raw data were excluded from this study.

Data extraction

Two investigators (Q.X. and Z.H.L.) independently extracted data using standardized data abstraction forms. Differences were resolved by discussion with a third independent expert (X.J.C.) in ophthalmology. Information collected from these publications included the included the following: author name, publication year, study design, country or region, study duration, sample size, age and sex of the study population, IOP measurements, success rate, and incidence of adverse events.

Assessment of study quality

The quality of clinical trials included in this study was assessed by two authors (Q.X and Z.L.L.) using a previously reported system by Downs and Blacks [17] that can assess both randomized and nonrandomized studies. The system comprises 27 items distributed among 5 subscales with regard to reporting (10 items), external validity (3 items), bias (7 items), confounding (6 items), and power (1 item). Any discrepancy in the qualitative assessment was discussed with a third investigator (Y.Z.) until a consensus was reached. The total score of each trial was expressed as a percentage of the maximum achievable score. Studies with a quality score of >50% were considered to have high quality.

Outcome measures

The primary outcome for efficacy was IOPR%. When mean and standard deviation (SD) of IOP and IOPR were reported, we used them directly. When these were unavailable, they were calculated according to the methods described in the Cochrane Handbook for Systematic Reviews of Interventions: $IOPR = IOP_{baseline} - IOP_{end\ point}$, $SD_{IOPR} = (SD_{baseline}{}^2 + SD_{end\ point}{}^2 - SD_{baseline} \times SD_{end\ point})^{1/2}$. IOPR% and SD of IOPR% ($SD_{IOPR\%}$) were estimated by $IOPR\% = IOPR/IOP_{baseline}$ and $SD_{IOPR\%} = SD_{IOPR}/IOP_{baseline}$, respectively. For efficacy, the proportions of qualified success and complete success were used. Complete success was defined as target end point IOP without medications, and qualified success was defined as target end point IOP with or without medications. The third outcome was the incidence of adverse events, including bleb leakage, choroidal effusion, flat anterior chamber, and hypotony.

Statistical analysis

Statistical analyses were performed using RevMan 5.2 software. We calculated pooled odds ratio (OR) for dichotomous outcomes, and weighted mean difference (WMD) or standard mean difference (SMD) for continuous outcomes. Heterogeneity among trials was assessed by inspection of graphical presentations and using Chi^2 test and the I^2 measure [18]. Significant heterogeneity was defined as $P < 0.05$ for chi-square or the I^2 measure >50%. We used a fixed effects model to pool results when there was no significant heterogeneity; otherwise, a random effects model was used (inverse of variance method and DerSimonian and Laird method). $P < 0.05$ indicated statistical significance on the test for overall effect. Subgroup analysis was performed to evaluate the effect of methodological characteristics in terms of study designs, which were differentiated as retrospective (Retro), prospective (Pro) nonrandomized, and randomized.

Results

Literature search

In total, 146 papers were identified by our literature search. Of 146, 84 papers were duplicates; thus, these were excluded. Based on the content of the titles and abstracts of the remaining 62 papers, we excluded 44 papers for reasons outlined in Figure 1. Further 9 papers were excluded owing to unqualified control groups and lack of required outcomes. Finally, 9 eligible controlled clinical trials that met our inclusion criteria were included in this systematic review [19–27].

Characteristics and quality of the included studies

Of the 9 included studies, 5 reported the use of antimetabolites vs. anti-VEGF agents, whereas the other 4 reported the use of antimetabolites vs. anti-VEGF agents with antimetabolites. The baseline characteristics of the included studies are summarized in

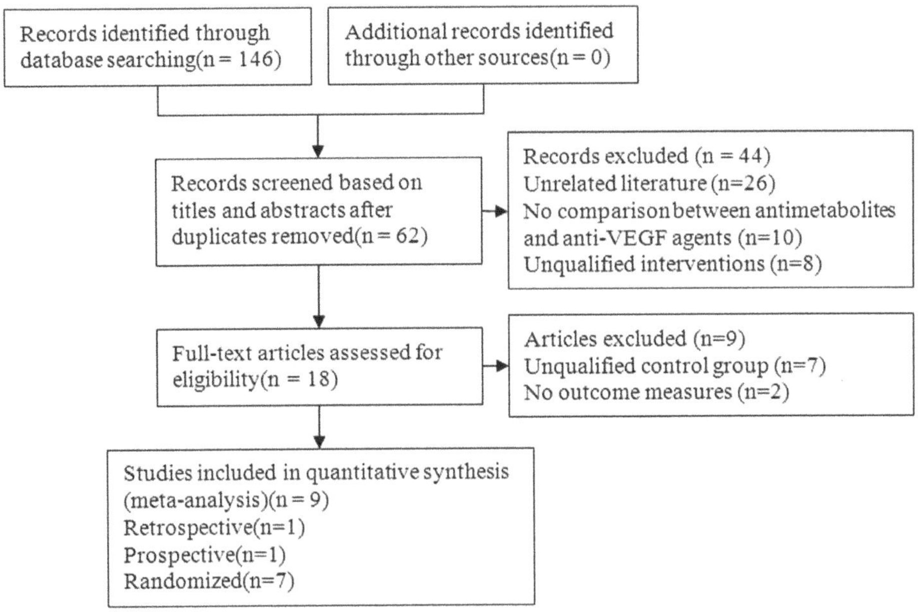

Figure 1. Flow chart of literature search and study selection.

Table 1. Seven studies were randomized controlled trials (RCTs), which were undertaken in Iran, India, Turkey, Aurora, Korea, and Australia, whereas the other 2 were prospective (Pro) nonrandomized [19] and retrospective (Retro) [27]. A total of 355 eyes of 349 patients were enrolled. The duration of follow-up ranged from 6 to 25 months. The mean ages of patients ranged from 58 to 71.7 years. With regard to quality assessment, Downs and Blacks scores of all the included studies were >16 (50%). Quality assessment details are summarized in Table 2

Main results of meta-analysis

IOPR% (antimetabolites vs. anti-VEGF agents). Five studies involving 187 eyes compared antimetabolites with anti-VEGF agents in terms of IOPR%. Mild heterogeneity was observed between these studies ($p = 0.28$, $I^2 = 21\%$). The combined results showed that both the agents significantly decreased IOP. Antimetabolites were found to achieve a numerically greater IOPR% from baseline, and the differences in IOPR% were statistically significant (WMD = 7.23, 95% CI: 2.57–11.89) (Table 3). We then divided the studies into 2 subgroups according to study design (Pro nonrandomized and randomized). A statistically significant result was observed in RCTs but not in the Pro nonrandomized trial (Table 4).

IOPR% (antimetabolites vs. anti-VEGF agents plus antimetabolites). Four studies involving 107 eyes compared antimetabolites with anti-VEGF agents plus antimetabolites in terms of IOPR%. No statistical heterogeneity was observed between studies ($p = 0.50$, $I^2 = 0\%$). The combined results showed that both the agents significantly decreased IOP. The differences in IOPR% were not all statistically significant (WMD = 3.96, 95% CI: −4.18–12.10) (Table 3). We then divided the studies into 2 subgroups according to study design (Retro and randomized). The two subgroups showed different results (Table 4).

Complete and qualified success (antimetabolites vs. anti-VEGF agents). All studies reported the probability of complete success, no significant difference was observed between the two groups [pooled OR = 2.37 (95% CI: 0.78, 7.21)] (Table 5). Further, there was no significant difference between antimetabolites and anti-VEGF agents in the subgroup analyses according to study design [pooled OR = 2.49 (0.54, 11.47) for randomized and 1.82 (0.47, 6.99) for Pro nonrandomized]. Five studies also reported the proportion of patients achieving target end point IOP with or without medications at follow-up endpoint; the difference in qualified success rate between the 2 groups was not statistically significant [pooled OR = 1.93 (0.52, 7.16)]. For the subgroup analysis according to study design, the difference between groups was not statistically significant [pooled OR = 2.04 (0.35, 11.91) for randomized and 1.20 (0.29, 4.98) for Pro nonrandomized] (Table 5).

Complete and qualified success (antimetabolites vs. anti-VEGF agents plus antimetabolites). In the 2 studies that reported the probability of complete success, no significant difference was found between the two groups [pooled OR = 1.43 (0.48, 4.29); Table 6]. There was also no significant difference between the two groups in the sensitivity analyses according to study design [pooled OR = 1.33 (0.29, 6.06) for Retro and 1.56 (0.32, 7.60) for randomized]. Two studies also reported the proportion of patients achieving target end point IOP with or without medications at follow-up endpoint; the difference in qualified success rate between the two groups was not statistically significant [pooled OR = 2.11 (0.12, 37.72)]. For the subgroup analysis according to design, there was no statistically significant in RCT trial [pooled OR = 2.11 (0.12, 37.72); Table 6].

Adverse events

No significant differences in the incidence of bleb leakage, choroidal effusion, flat anterior chamber, and hypotony were found between antimetabolites and anti-VEGF agents, with the pooled ORs being 0.86 (0.28–2.69), 3.01 (0.45–20.10), 0.96 (0.23–3.98), and 0.90 (0.12–6.60), respectively (Table 7). Moreover, the rates of adverse events did not significantly differ between antimetabolites and anti-VEGF agents plus antimetabolites, with pooled ORs of 0.40 (0.08–2.00) and 8.00 (0.93–68.59) for bleb leakage and hypotony, respectively.

Table 1. Characteristics of included studies.

First Author(year)	Design	Location	Numbers of patients	Numbers of eyes	Mean age	Sex(male/female)		Intervention regimen	Follow-up (month)
						Antimetabolites	Anti-VEGF agents		
Jurkowska (2011)	Pro	Caucasion	62	62	71.1/70.6	11/19	16/16	5-FU/4min vs.Bevacizumab	12/12
Niflorushan (2012)	RCT	Iran	34	36	58.6/60.7	11/6	11/6	MMC/3min vs. Bevacizumab	7.8/7.4
Sengupta (2012)	RCT	India	38	38	62.1/64.1	6/4	5/5	MMC/2–3min vs. Bevacizumab	6/6
Simsek (2012)	RCT	Turkey	27	27	58/61	7/8	6/6	5-FU vs. Bevacizumab	17/17
Akkan (2012)	RCT	Turkey	42	42	64.1/64.3	11/10	13/8	MMC/ 2min vs. Bevacizumab	12/12
KAHOOK (2010)	RCT	Aurora	10	10	64.2/70.6	---	---	MMC/2min vs. Ranibizumab +MMC	6/6
Suh (2013)	RCT	Korea	36	36	60.5/64.1	21/3	10/2	5-FU/5min vs. 5-FU+ Bevacizumab	24/24
Chua (2012)	RCT	Australia	39	43	64.5/66.8	21/8	11/11	5-FU vs. 5-FU+ Bevacizumab	18/18
Freiberg (2013)	Retro	Germany	61	61	67	25/36	---	5-FU vs. 5FU+ Bevacizumab	25

RCT = prospective randomized controlled trial; Retro = retrospective; Pro = prospective non-randomized; 5-FU = 5-fluorouracil; MMC = mitomycin C.

Discussion

Trab is an effective surgical treatment for glaucoma. The primary factor that can lead to successful Trab is preventing exaggerated wound healing responses, which are primarily mediated by fibroblast migration and proliferation [7,28]. Current antifibrotic drugs, such as MMC and 5-FU, can optimize surgical outcomes by avoiding conjunctival healing [29]. While these agents are associated with widespread nonselective cell death and apoptosis, resulting in severe adverse events and complications [30,31], their application is limited and the search for an ideal pharmacological agent to modulate the wound-healing response with a safer profile is urgently needed. A multicenter study recently failed to demonstrate that subconjunctival applications of CAT-152, a humanized monoclonal antibody to TGFβ2, could prevent scar formation [32]. Several other agents, such as paclitaxel, interferon, ribozymes, p21 (WAF-1/Cip-1), and MMP inhibitors have been studied, but they have not yet been completely satisfactory [33–36]. VEGF, a critical component of the wound healing process, has been proved to promote angiogenesis and enhance scar formation [37]. Some studies have reported increased VEGF expression in aqueous humor samples of both human and rabbits after Trab [12]. For this reason, anti-VEGF agents may display effective action during Trab. Researchers have recently also suggested that the application of anti-VEGF agents in Trab can effectively reduce the expression of VEGF and formation of new blood vessels of the bleb, resulting in less scarring and better bleb formation, thus achieving a long-term effect of IOP control [38,39]. There are, at present, a large number of studies comparing the effectiveness and safety of antimetabolites with anti-VEGF agents in Trab. However, there is a lack of reliable evidence-based conclusions that could be applied in clinical practice. Therefore, the present meta-analysis was undertaken to assess the clinical safety and tolerability of the aforementioned agents in Trab for glaucoma.

In the current meta-analysis, we reviewed 9 controlled clinical trials using a wide range of clinically relevant outcome measures. With regard to IOP assessment, this study found that both the agents significantly decreased IOP, but in comparison with anti-VEGF agents, antimetabolites were associated with better IOP-lowering efficacy, leading to a numerically higher percentage of IOP reduction. For the outcomes of Trab in combination with anti-VEGF agents plus antimetabolites vs. with antimetabolites alone, the differences in IOPR% were not all statistically significant. One possible reason for the finding may be that antimetabolites have widespread nonselective cell death and apoptosis effects in comparison with anti-VEGF agents. Antimetabolites not only inhibit fibroblast proliferation of the sclera and conjunctiva but also, via different pharmacological mechanisms, result in a better IOP control [23]. No significant difference was found in complete and qualified success rates between the two groups. This may be a potential reason for the different definitions of complete and qualified success. For example, complete success of Trab was defined as a 30% decline in baseline IOP in some studies [19,24], and 20% in others studies [20,21,27]. Another possible reason is the small sample size and short duration of follow-up, making it difficult to draw stable and credible conclusions. There was a similar result with regard to in adverse events of the two types of agents. This may also be due to a small sample size and short duration of follow-up. As is known, the objective of antimetabolites and anti-VEGF agents as an adjuvant to Trab is to not only lower IOP but also to promote an improved and less scarred bleb formation. Anti-VEGF agents can reduce vascularization in the bleb and make it bleb more durable, thereby

Table 2. Quality scoring components for 9 clinical trials included.

First Author(year)	Quality Score component					Score	
	I	II	II	IV	V	Over all	Percentage (%)
KAHOOK (2010)	11	2	4	5	3	25	78.13%
Jurkowska (2011)	10	2	4	3	1	20	62.50%
Niflorushan (2012)	11	2	4	4	3	24	75.00%
Sengupta (2012)	11	2	7	5	4	29	90.63%
Simsek (2012)	10	2	4	3	3	22	68.75%
Akkan (2012)	11	2	4	4	3	24	75.00%
Chua (2012)	11	2	4	3	1	21	65.63%
Suh (2013)	11	2	4	4	1	22	68.75%
Freiberg (2013)	9	2	4	3	1	19	59.38%

increasing the success rate of the surgery [24]. Here, in the included studies, characteristics and morphological features of the bleb were not evaluated. Therefore, our conclusions should be interpreted with caution.

Our study had a number of strengths. First, we strictly followed the Cochrane Handbook for Systematic Reviews of Interventions and PRISMA statement, including the literature search, data extraction, quality assessment, and statistical analysis. This makes our conclusions more scientific and reliable. Second, the subgroup analysis was performed according to study design, indicating that the conclusions from this analysis are robust.

There were also several limitations: (1) Randomization: Among the 9 included studies, 7 were RCTs, 1 was Pro nonrandomized, and 1 was Retro. Only 4 of the 7 studies provided sufficient information on how to specifically implement RCTs and described the implementation of allocation concealment. Inappropriate methods of RCTs may result in potential selection bias in the conclusion. (2) Masking: Only 1 of the 7 studies performed masking, while others did not mention masking, which may result in implementation and measurement bias in the conclusion. (3) Placebo controlled: Trials should be ideally devised as placebo-controlled studies; however, none of the trials were designed to be placebo or sham controlled, which may exaggerate the treatment effect in Trab and result in bias. (4) Publication bias: We not only performed electronic searches but also conducted a manual search to identify all potential relevant papers, including published and non-published ones, to avoid publication bias. Unfortunately, we may have failed to include some papers, particularly those published in languages other than Chinese or English. In addition, the test for publication bias was not conducted due to a limited

Table 3. Percentage IOP reduction from baseline comparing antimetabolites with anti-VEGF agents with or without antimetabolites.

Trials	Antimetabolites		Anti-VEGF agents		WMD(Fixed)(95%CI)
	No.of Eyes	IOPR%[Mean(SD)]	No. of Eyes	IOPR%[Mean(SD)]	
Antimetabolites vs. Anti-VEGF agents					
Jurkowska (2011)	30	52.94(28.48)	32	49.83(27.78)	3.11[−10.91, 17.13]
Niflorushan (2012)	18	58.28(18.20)	18	41.64(31.51)	16.64[−0.17, 33.45]
Sengupta (2012)	10	41.94(20.54)	10	46.36(17.22)	−4.42[−21.03, 12.19]
Simsek (2012)	15	61.25(12.44)	12	49.36(8.94)	11.89[3.81, 19.97]
Akkan (2012)	21	46.93(12.83)	21	41.96(11.48)	4.97[−2.39, 12.33]
Total	94		93		7.23[2.57, 11.89]
Test for heterogeneity Ch $I^2 = 5.07$, df = 4(p = 0.28); $I^2 = 21\%$					
Test for overall effect: z = 3.04, p = 0.002					
Antimetabolites vs. Anti-VEGF agents + Antimetabolites					
Kahook MY(2010)	5	55(40.3)	5	36.47(16.12)	18.53[−19.51, 56.57]
Suh W(2013)	24	54.5(18.7)	12	46.9(18.2)	7.60[−5.13, 20.33]
Freiberg FJ(2013)	34	50(22.04)	27	50(21.67)	0.00[−11.03, 11.03]
Total	63		44		3.96[−4.18, 12.10]
Test for heterogeneity Ch $I^2 = 1.37$, df = 2(p = 0.50); $I^2 = 0\%$					
Test for overall effect: z = 0.95, p = 0.34					

CI = confidence interval; IOP = intraocular pressure; IOPR% = percentage intraocular pressure reduction; WMD = weighted mean difference.

Table 4. Subgroup analysis evaluating the effect of trial design on percentage IOP reduction.

subgroup	Numbers of studies	WMD(Fixed)(95%CI)	Heterogeneity			Overall effect	
			CHI^2	P	I^2(%)	Z	P
Antimetabolites vs. Anti-VEGF agents							
All trials	5	7.23[2.57, 11.89]	5.07	0.28	21%	3.04	0.002
Pro	1	3.11[−10.91, 17.13]	----	----	----	0.43	0.66
RCTs	4	7.74[2.80,12.68]	4.69	0.20	36%	3.07	0.002
Antimetabolites vs. Anti-VEGF agents + Antimetabolites							
All trials	3	3.96[−4.18, 12.10]	1.37	0.50	0	0.95	0.34
Retro	1	0.00[−11.03, 11.03]	----	----	----	0.00	1.00
RCT	2	8.70[−3.37,20.77]	0.29	0.59	0	1.41	0.16

RCT = prospective randomized controlled trial; Retro = retrospective; Pro = prospective non-randomized.

Table 5. Complete success and qualified success comparing antimetabolites with anti-VEGF agents.

Trial	Studies(n)	Success rate, n/N(%)		OR(95%CI)	Heterogeneity			Overall effect	
		Antimetabolites	Anti-VEGF agents		CHI^2	P	I^2(%)	Z	P
Complete success									
All trials	5	71/94	56/93	2.37[0.78, 7.21]	8.03	0.09	50%	1.53	0.13
Pro	1	26/30	25/32	1.82[0.47, 6.99]	----	----	----	0.87	0.38
RCT	4	45/64	31/61	2.49[0.54,11.47]	7.70	0.05	61%	1.17	0.24
Qualified success									
All trials	5	79/94	67/93	1.93[0.52, 7.16]	8.97	0.06	55%	0.98	0.32
Pro	1	26/30	27/32	1.20[0.29, 4.98]	----	----	----	0.26	0.80
RCT	4	53/64	40/61	2.04[0.35,11.91]	7.73	0.05	61%	0.79	0.43

RCT = prospective randomized controlled trial; Pro = prospective non-randomized.

Table 6. Complete success and qualified success comparing antimetabolites with anti-VEGF agents combined with antimetabolites.

Trial	Studies(n)	Success rate, n/N(%)		OR(95%CI)	Heterogeneity			Overall effect	
		Antimetabolites	Antimetabolites +Anti-VEGF agents		CHI^2	P	I^2(%)	Z	P
Complete success									
All trials	2	38/48	24/32	1.43 [0.48, 4.29]	0.02	0.89	0%	0.65	0.52
Pro	1	24/28	18/22	1.33 [0.29, 6.06]	----	----	----	0.37	0.71
RCT	1	14/20	6/10	1.56 [0.32,7.60]	----	----	----	0.55	0.59
Qualified success									
All trials	2	53/54	36/37	2.11 [0.12, 37.72]	----	----	----	0.51	0.61
Pro	1	34/34	27/27	----	----	----	----	----	----
RCT	1	19/20	9/10	2.11 [0.12, 37.72]	----	----	----	0.51	0.61

RCT = prospective randomized controlled trial; Pro = prospective non-randomized.

Table 7. Adverse events.

Adverse events	Studies(n)	Crude event rate, n/N		OR(95%CI)	Heterogeneity			Overall effect	
		Antimetabolites	Antimetabolites /Antimetabolites +Anti-VEGF agents		CHI^2	P	I^2(%)	Z	P
Antimetabolites vs. Anti-VEGF agents									
Bleb leak	4	5/79	6/81	0.86[0.28, 2.69]	1.14	0.77	0%	0.25	0.80
Choroidal offusion	3	3/43	0/40	3.01[0.45, 20.10]	0.01	0.99	0%	1.14	0.26
Flat anterior chamber	4	3/76	3/75	0.96[0.23,3.98]	1.00	0.80	0%	0.06	0.95
Hypatony	3	1/46	1/43	0.90[0.12, 6.60]	1.19	0.28	16%	0.11	0.92
Antimetabolites vs. Anti-VEGF agents + Antimetabolites									
Bleb leak	2	4/29	4/17	0.40[0.08, 2.00]	----	----	----	1.12	0.26
Hypatony	2	8/39	1/32	8.00[0.93, 68.59]	----	----	----	1.90	0.06

number of studies included in our meta-analysis. (5) Heterogeneity: There was significant heterogeneity in some studies, which may reflect differences in age, gender, sample size, differences in definition of complete and qualified success, and outcome of measurements. A random effects model was used when statistically significant heterogeneity was met. (6) Follow-up: The follow-up duration in two studies was only 6 months, which may affect the long-term results of our study.

In conclusion, this is the first meta-analysis specifically answering the question of whether anti-VEGF agents are more effective and safer than antimetabolites in Trab for glaucoma. The results of this meta-analysis suggest that antimetabolites are more effective in lowering IOP in Trab in comparison with anti-VEGF agents alone; however, antimetabolites are comparable with anti-VEGF agents with regard to qualified success rate, complete success rate, and incidence of adverse events. Although there were some limitations, we believe that the results of this meta-analysis possess sufficient credibility and are worth consideration in future clinical practice. We believe that more RCTs with larger sample sizes and systematic studies are required for further confirmation of the presented results.

Author Contributions

Conceived and designed the experiments: QX ZLL ZHL YZ SA PW XJC. Performed the experiments: QX ZLL ZHL XJC. Analyzed the data: QX ZLL ZHL PW XJC. Contributed reagents/materials/analysis tools: QX ZHL YZ SA PW XJC. Wrote the paper: QX ZLL YZ.

References

1. Quigley HA, Broman AT (2006) The number of people with glaucoma worldwide in 2010 and 2020. Br J Ophthalmol 90:262–267.
2. Burr J, Azuara-Blanco A, Avenell A, Tuulonen A (2012) Medical versus surgical interventions for open angle glaucoma. Cochrane Database Syst Rev 9:CD004399.
3. Hitchings R (1998) Initial Treatment for Open-Angle Glaucoma–Medical, Laser, or Surgical?: Surgery Is the Treatment of Choice for Open-Angle Glaucoma. Archives of Ophthalmology 116:241.
4. Cairns J (1968) Trabeculectomy. Preliminary report of a new method. Am J Ophthalmol 66:673–679.
5. Skuta GL, Parrish RK 2nd (1987) Wound healing in glaucoma filtering surgery. Surv Ophthalmol 32:149–170.
6. Lama PJ, Fechtner RD (2003) Antifibrotics and wound healing in glaucoma surgery. Surv Ophthalmol 48:314–346.
7. Addicks EM, Quigley HA, Green WR, Robin AL (1983) Histologic characteristics of filtering blebs in glaucomatous eyes. Archives of Ophthalmology 101:795–798.
8. Greenfield DS, Suner IJ, Miller MP, Kangas TA, Palmberg PF, et al. (1996) Endophthalmitis after filtering surgery with mitomycin. Arch Ophthalmol 114:943–949.
9. Seah SK, Prata JA Jr, Minckler DS, Baerveldt G, Lee PP, et al. (1995) Hypotony following trabeculectomy. J Glaucoma 4:73–79.
10. Bao P, Kodra A, Tomic-Canic M, Golinko MS, Ehrlich HP, et al. (2009) The role of vascular endothelial growth factor in wound healing. J Surg Res 153:347–358.
11. Nissen NN, Polverini PJ, Koch AE, Volin MV, Gamelli RL, et al. (1998) Vascular endothelial growth factor mediates angiogenic activity during the proliferative phase of wound healing. Am J Pathol 152:1445–1452.
12. Li Z, Van Bergen T, Van de Veire S, Van de Vel I, Moreau H, et al. (2009) Inhibition of vascular endothelial growth factor reduces scar formation after glaucoma filtration surgery. Invest Ophthalmol Vis Sci 50:5217–5225.
13. Grewal DS, Jain R, Kumar H, Grewal SPS (2008) Evaluation of subconjunctival bevacizumab as an adjunct to trabeculectomy: a pilot study. Ophthalmology 115:2141–2145. e2142.
14. Jonas JB, Spandau UH, Schlichtenbrede F (2007) Intravitreal bevacizumab for filtering surgery. Ophthalmic Research 39:121–122.
15. Higgins JP, Green S, Collaboration C (2008) Cochrane handbook for systematic reviews of interventions. Wiley Online Library 5.
16. Moher D, Liberati A, Tetzlaff J, Altman DG (2009) Preferred reporting items for systematic reviews and meta-analyses: the PRISMA statement. Annals of internal medicine 151:264–269.
17. Downs SH, Black N (1998) The feasibility of creating a checklist for the assessment of the methodological quality both of randomised and non-randomised studies of health care interventions. Journal of Epidemiology and Community Health 52:377–384.
18. Reck M, Von Pawel J, Zatloukal PV, Ramlau R, Gorbounova V, et al. (2010) Overall survival with cisplatin–gemcitabine and bevacizumab or placebo as first-line therapy for nonsquamous non-small-cell lung cancer: results from a randomised phase III trial (AVAiL). Annals of oncology 21:1804–1809.
19. Jurkowska-Dudzinska J, Kosior-Jarecka E, Zarnowski T (2012) Comparison of the use of 5-fluorouracil and bevacizumab in primary trabeculectomy: results at 1 year. Clin Experiment Ophthalmol 40:e135–142.
20. Nilforushan N, Yadgari M, Kish SK, Nassiri N (2012) Subconjunctival bevacizumab versus mitomycin C adjunctive to trabeculectomy. Am J Ophthalmol 153:352–357 e351.
21. Sengupta S, Venkatesh R, Ravindran RD (2012) Safety and efficacy of using off-label bevacizumab versus mitomycin C to prevent bleb failure in a single-site phacotrabeculectomy by a randomized controlled clinical trial. J Glaucoma 21:450–459.
22. Simsek T, Cankaya AB, Elgin U (2012) Comparison of needle revision with subconjunctival bevacizumab and 5-fluorouracil injection of failed trabeculectomy blebs. J Ocul Pharmacol Ther 28: 542–546.

23. Akkan JU, Cilsim S (2013) Role of Subconjunctival Bevacizumab as an Adjuvant to Primary Trabeculectomy: A Prospective Randomized Comparative 1-Year Follow-up Study. J Glaucoma 00:000-000.
24. Kahook MY (2010) Bleb morphology and vascularity after trabeculectomy with intravitreal ranibizumab: a pilot study. Am J Ophthalmol 150:399–403 e391.
25. Chua BE, Nguyen DQ, Qin Q, Ruddle JB, Wells AP, et al. (2012) Bleb vascularity following post-trabeculectomy subconjunctival bevacizumab: a pilot study. Clin Experiment Ophthalmol 40:773–779.
26. Suh W, Kee C (2013) The effect of bevacizumab on the outcome of trabeculectomy with 5-Fluorouracil. J Ocul Pharmacol Ther 29:646–651.
27. Freiberg FJ, Matlach J, Grehn F, Karl S, Klink T (2013) Postoperative subconjunctival bevacizumab injection as an adjunct to 5-fluorouracil in the management of scarring after trabeculectomy. Clin Ophthalmol 7:1211–1217.
28. Hitchings RA, Grierson I (1983) Clinico pathological correlation in eyes with failed fistulizing surgery. Trans Ophthalmol Soc U K 103:84–88.
29. Rulli E, Biagioli E, Riva I, Gambirasio G, De Simone I, et al. (2013) Efficacy and Safety of Trabeculectomy vs Nonpenetrating Surgical Procedures: A Systematic Review and Meta-analysis. JAMA Ophthalmol 131:1573–1582.
30. Parrish R, Minckler D (1996) "Late endophthalmitis"--filtering surgery time bomb? Ophthalmology 103:1167–1168.
31. Pakravan M, Miraftabi A, Yazdani S, Koohestani N, Yaseri M (2011) Topical mitomycin-C versus subconjunctival 5-fluorouracil for management of bleb failure. Journal of ophthalmic & vision research 6:78–86.
32. Khaw P, Grehn F, Holló G, Overton B, Wilson R, et al. (2007) CAT-152 0102 Trabeculectomy Study Group et al. A phase III study of subconjunctival human anti-transforming growth factor beta (2) monoclonal antibody (CAT-152) to prevent scarring after first-time trabeculectomy. Ophthalmology 114:1822–1830.
33. Heatley G, Kiland J, Faha B, Seeman J, Schlamp CL, et al. (2004) Gene therapy using p21WAF-1/Cip-1 to modulate wound healing after glaucoma trabeculectomy surgery in a primate model of ocular hypertension. Gene therapy 11:949–955.
34. Wang X, Crowston JG, White AJ, Zoellner H, Healey PR (2013) Interferon-alpha and Interferon-gamma modulate Fas-mediated apoptosis in Mitomycin-C resistant Human Tenon's Fibroblasts. Clin Experiment Ophthalmol 14: 000–000.
35. Nakamura-Shibasaki M, Ko J, Takenaka J, Chikama TI, Sonoda KH, et al. (2013) Matrix metalloproteinase and cytokine expression in Tenon fibroblasts during scar formation after glaucoma filtration or implant surgery in rats. Cell biochemistry and function 31:482–488.
36. Choritz L, Grub J, Wegner M, Pfeiffer N, Thieme H (2010) Paclitaxel inhibits growth, migration and collagen production of human Tenon's fibroblasts--potential use in drug-eluting glaucoma drainage devices. Graefes Arch Clin Exp Ophthalmol 248:197–206.
37. Kahook MY, Schuman JS, Noecker RJ (2005) Needle bleb revision of encapsulated filtering bleb with bevacizumab. Ophthalmic surgery, lasers & imaging: the official journal of the International Society for Imaging in the Eye 37:148–150.
38. Coote MA, Ruddle JB, Qin Q, Crowston JG (2008) Vascular changes after intra-bleb injection of bevacizumab. J Glaucoma 17:517–518.
39. Yu J, Kahook M, Schuman J (2007) Bevacizumab binding to human sclera post topical application [E-Abstract 4815]. Invest Ophthalmol Vis Sci 48:4815.

Permissions

All chapters in this book were first published in PLOS ONE, by The Public Library of Science; hereby published with permission under the Creative Commons Attribution License or equivalent. Every chapter published in this book has been scrutinized by our experts. Their significance has been extensively debated. The topics covered herein carry significant findings which will fuel the growth of the discipline. They may even be implemented as practical applications or may be referred to as a beginning point for another development.

The contributors of this book come from diverse backgrounds, making this book a truly international effort. This book will bring forth new frontiers with its revolutionizing research information and detailed analysis of the nascent developments around the world.

We would like to thank all the contributing authors for lending their expertise to make the book truly unique. They have played a crucial role in the development of this book. Without their invaluable contributions this book wouldn't have been possible. They have made vital efforts to compile up to date information on the varied aspects of this subject to make this book a valuable addition to the collection of many professionals and students.

This book was conceptualized with the vision of imparting up-to-date information and advanced data in this field. To ensure the same, a matchless editorial board was set up. Every individual on the board went through rigorous rounds of assessment to prove their worth. After which they invested a large part of their time researching and compiling the most relevant data for our readers.

The editorial board has been involved in producing this book since its inception. They have spent rigorous hours researching and exploring the diverse topics which have resulted in the successful publishing of this book. They have passed on their knowledge of decades through this book. To expedite this challenging task, the publisher supported the team at every step. A small team of assistant editors was also appointed to further simplify the editing procedure and attain best results for the readers.

Apart from the editorial board, the designing team has also invested a significant amount of their time in understanding the subject and creating the most relevant covers. They scrutinized every image to scout for the most suitable representation of the subject and create an appropriate cover for the book.

The publishing team has been an ardent support to the editorial, designing and production team. Their endless efforts to recruit the best for this project, has resulted in the accomplishment of this book. They are a veteran in the field of academics and their pool of knowledge is as vast as their experience in printing. Their expertise and guidance has proved useful at every step. Their uncompromising quality standards have made this book an exceptional effort. Their encouragement from time to time has been an inspiration for everyone.

The publisher and the editorial board hope that this book will prove to be a valuable piece of knowledge for researchers, students, practitioners and scholars across the globe.

List of Contributors

David P. Crabb, Nicholas D. Smith, Franziska G. Rauscher, John L. Barbur and David F. Edgar
Department of Optometry and Visual Science, City University London, London, United Kingdom

Catharine M. Chisholm
Bradford School of Optometry and Vision Science, University of Bradford, Bradford, United Kingdom

David F. Garway-Heath
NIHR Biomedical Research Centre for Ophthalmology, Moorfields Eye Hospital NHS Foundation Trust and UCL Institute of Ophthalmology, London, United Kingdom

Katharina Bell, Sebastian Funke, Norbert Pfeiffer and Franz H. Grus
Experimental Ophthalmology, Department of Ophthalmology, Medical Center of the Johannes Gutenberg University, Mainz, German

Michael W. Marcus and Rogier P. H. M. Müskens
Department of Ophthalmology, University Medical Center Groningen, University of Groningen, Groningen, The Netherlands

Nomdo M. Jansonius
Department of Ophthalmology, University Medical Center Groningen, University of Groningen, Groningen, The Netherlands
Department of Epidemiology, Erasmus Medical Center, Rotterdam, The Netherlands

Wishal D. Ramdas, Roger C. W. Wolfs and Johannes R. Vingerling
Department of Epidemiology, Erasmus Medical Center, Rotterdam, The Netherlands
Department of Ophthalmology, Erasmus Medical Center, Rotterdam, The Netherlands

Albert Hofman and Bruno H. Stricker
Department of Epidemiology, Erasmus Medical Center, Rotterdam, The Netherlands
Department of Internal Medicine, Erasmus Medical Center, Rotterdam, The Netherlands
Department of Medical Informatics, Erasmus Medical Center, Rotterdam, The Netherlands

Paulus T. V. M. De Jong
Department of Ophthalmogenetics, Netherlands Institute for Neuroscience, Amsterdam, The Netherlands
Department of Ophthalmology, Academic Medical Center, Amsterdam, The Netherlands

Jeff Min, Zachary L. Lukowski, Monica A. Levine, Craig A. Meyers, Ashley R. Beattie and Mark B. Sherwood
Department of Ophthalmology, College of Medicine, University of Florida, Gainesville, Florida, United States of America

Gregory S. Schultz
Department of Ob/Gyn and Institute of Wound Healing, College of Medicine, University of Florida, Gainesville, Florida, United States of America

Don A. Samuelson
College of Veterinary Medicine, University of Florida, Gainesville, Florida, United States of America

Padma Iyer, Robert Lalane III, Corey Morris, Pratap Challa and Robin Vann
Department of Ophthalmology, Duke University School of Medicine, Durham, North Carolina, United States of America

Ponugoti Vasantha Rao
Department of Ophthalmology, Duke University School of Medicine, Durham, North Carolina, United States of America
Department of Pharmacology and Cancer Biology, Duke University School of Medicine, Durham, North Carolina, United States of America

Susan D. Orwig and Raquel L. Lieberman
School of Chemistry and Biochemistry, Georgia Institute of Technology, Atlanta, Georgia, United States of America

Masaki Tanito, Sachiko Kaidzu, Yasuyuki Takai and Akihiro Ohira
Department of Ophthalmology, Shimane University Faculty of Medicine, Izumo, Shimane, Japan

Yatu Guo
Tianjin Medical University, Tianjin, China, Tianjin Eye Hospital, Tianjin Eye Institute, Tianjin Key Lab of Ophthalmology and Visual Science, Tianjin, China
Krieger Mind/Brain Institute, Johns Hopkins University, Baltimore, Maryland, United States of America

Wenbo Cheng
Tianjin Medical University, Tianjin, China
Department of Ophthalmology, the People's Hospital of Changzhi, Shanxi, China

Xia Chen, Ningdong Li and Kanxing Zhao
Tianjin Eye Hospital, Tianjin Eye Institute, Tianjin Key Lab of Ophthalmology and Visual Science, Tianjin, China

Hongtuan Zhang and Xiong Yang
Second Hospital of Tianjin Medical University, Tianjin, China

Laura G. Reinholdt, Anne M. Czechanski, Danilo G. Macalinao, Leah Rae Donahue and Katharine H. MacNicoll
The Jackson Laboratory, Bar Harbor, Maine, United States of America

Gareth R. Howell
The Jackson Laboratory, Bar Harbor, Maine, United States of America
The Howard Hughes Medical Institute, Bar Harbor, Maine, United States of America

Simon W. M. John
The Jackson Laboratory, Bar Harbor, Maine, United States of America
The Howard Hughes Medical Institute, Bar Harbor, Maine, United States of America
Department of Ophthalmology, Tufts University of Medicine, Boston, Massachusetts, United States of America

Chyuan-Sheng Lin
Department of Pathology and Cell Biology, Irving Cancer Research Center, Columbia University, New York, New York, United States of America

Masamitsu Shimazawa, Yasushi Ito, Yuta Inokuchi, Hideaki Hara and Tomohiro Nakanishi
Molecular Pharmacology, Department of Biofunctional Evaluation, Gifu Pharmaceutical University, Gifu, Japan

Hajime Yamanaka, Takuya Hayashi, Yasuyoshi Watanabe and Hirotaka Onoe
RIKEN Center for Molecular Imaging Science, Kobe, Japan

Bin Ji, Makoto Higuchi and Tetsuya Suhara
Molecular Imaging Center, National Institute of Radiological Sciences, Chiba, Japan

Kazuyuki Imamura
Department of Systems Life Engineering, Maebashi Institute of Technology, Maibashi, Japan

Makoto Araie
Department of Ophthalmology, University of Tokyo School of Medicine, Tokyo, Japan

Alberto Izzotti, Mariagrazia Longobardi and Cristina Cartiglia
Department of Health Sciences, University of Genoa, Genoa, Italy

Sergio Claudio Saccà
Department of Head/Neck Pathologies, Ophthalmology Unit, St. Martino Hospital, Genoa, Italy

Yoshimasa Takano, Ai Shimizu, Kotaro Yamamoto, MinGe Mengkegale, Akiko Miyazawa and Toru Nakazawa
Department of Ophthalmology, Tohoku University Graduate School of Medicine, Sendai, Miyagi, Japan

Dong Shi
Department of Ophthalmology, Tohoku University Graduate School of Medicine, Sendai, Miyagi, Japan
Department of Ophthalmology, the Fourth Affiliated Hospital, China Medical University, Shenyang, Liaoning, China

Nobuo Fuse
Department of Ophthalmology, Tohoku University Graduate School of Medicine, Sendai, Miyagi, Japan
Department of Integrative Genomics, Tohoku Medical Megabank Organization, Sendai, Miyagi, Japan

Tomoyo Funayama
Department of Chemistry, Faculty of Education, Bunkyo University, Koshigaya, Saitama, Japan

Yukihiko Mashima
Department of Ophthalmology, Keio University School of Medicine, Shinjuku-ku, Tokyo, Japan

Noriko Yasuda
Department of Ophthalmology, Tokyo Metropolitan Police Hospital, Tokyo, Japan

Takeo Fukuchi and Haruki Abe
Division of Ophthalmology and Visual Science, Graduate School of Medical and Dental Sciences, Niigata University, Niigata, Japan

Hidenao Ideta
Ideta Eye Hospital, Kumamoto, Japan

Kohji Nishida
Department of Ophthalmology, Osaka University Graduate School of Medicine, Suita, Osaka, Japan

Julia E. Richards
Department of Ophthalmology and Visual Sciences, W. K. Kellogg Eye Center, University of Michigan, Ann Arbor, Michigan, United States of America
Department of Epidemiology, University of Michigan, Ann Arbor, Michigan, United States of America

Masakazu Nakano, Yuichi Tokuda, Natsue Omi, Hiroko Adachi, Masahiro Fuwa and Kei Tashiro
Department of Genomic Medical Sciences, Kyoto Prefectural University of Medicine, Kyoto, Japan

Yoko Ikeda, Morio Ueno, Kojiro Imai, Kazuhiko Mori and Shigeru Kinoshita
Department of Ophthalmology, Kyoto Prefectural University of Medicine, Kyoto, Japan

Masaaki Kageyama
Research and Development Center, Santen Pharmaceutical Co. Ltd., Nara, Japan

Kristy R. Crooks, Xuejun Qin, Yutao Liu, Jason R. Gibson, Karen R. Larocque-Abramson and Silke Schmidt
Center for Human Genetics, Duke University Medical Center, Durham, North Carolina, United States of America

R. Rand Allingham and Michael A. Hauser
Center for Human Genetics, Duke University Medical Center, Durham, North Carolina, United States of America
Department of Ophthalmology, Duke University Eye Center, Duke University Medical Center, Durham, North Carolina, United States of America

Cecilia Santiago-Turla, Pratap Challa and Leon W. Herndon
Department of Ophthalmology, Duke University Eye Center, Duke University Medical Center, Durham, North Carolina, United States of America

Elizabeth Del Bono and Janey L. Wiggs
Department of Ophthalmology, Harvard Medical School and Massachusetts Eye and Ear Infirmary, Boston, Massachusetts, United States of America

Stephen Akafo
Unit of Ophthalmology, Department of Surgery, University of Ghana Medical School, Accra, Ghana

Alejandra Bosco, Monica L. Vetter, Michael R. Steele and Cesar O. Romero
Department of Neurobiology and Anatomy, University of Utah, Salt Lake City, Utah, United States of America

Samuel D. Crish and David J. Calkins
Department of Ophthalmology and Visual Sciences, Vanderbilt University, Nashville, Tennessee, United States of America

Denise M. Inman and Philip J. Horner
Department of Neurosurgery, University of Washington, Seattle, Washington, United States of America

Yutao Liu, Jason Gibson, Joshua Wheeler and Lydia Coulter Kwee
Center for Human Genetics, Duke University Medical Center, Durham, North Carolina, United States of America
Department of Medicine, Duke University Medical Center, Durham, North Carolina, United States of America

Michael A. Hauser
Center for Human Genetics, Duke University Medical Center, Durham, North Carolina, United States of America
Department of Medicine, Duke University Medical Center, Durham, North Carolina, United States of America
Duke University Eye Center, Duke University Medical Center, Durham, North Carolina, United States of America

Cecile M. Santiago-Turla, Pratap Challa, Leon W. Herndon and R. Rand Allingham
Duke University Eye Center, Duke University Medical Center, Durham, North Carolina, United States of America

Stephen K. Akafo
Unit of Ophthalmology, Department of Surgery, University of Ghana Medical School, Korle Bu, Ghana

Paul R. Lichter and Sayoko E. Moroi
Department of Ophthalmology and Visual Sciences, University of Michigan, Ann Arbor, Michigan, United States of America

Julia E. Richards
Department of Ophthalmology and Visual Sciences, University of Michigan, Ann Arbor, Michigan, United States of America
Department of Epidemiology, University of Michigan, Ann Arbor, Michigan, United States of America

Douglas E. Gaasterland
Eye Doctors of Washington, Chevy Chase, Maryland, United States of America

Christopher A. Girkin
Department of Ophthalmology, University of Alabama at Birmingham, Birmingham, Alabama, United States of America

Donald L. Budenz
Department of Ophthalmology, Bascom Palmer Eye Institute, Miami, Florida, United States of America

Carolyne Dion, Kanwarpal Singh and Tsuneyuki Ozaki
Institut National de la Recherche Scientifique - Énergie, Matériaux et Télécommunications, Varennes, Québec, Canada
Centre de Recherche de l'Hôpital Maisonneuve-Rosemont, Montréal, Québec, Canada

Mark R. Lesk
Centre de Recherche de l'Hôpital Maisonneuve-Rosemont, Montréal, Québec, Canada
Department of Ophthalmology, Faculty of Medicine, Université de Montréal, Montréal, Québec, Canada

Santiago Costantino
Centre de Recherche de l'Hôpital Maisonneuve-Rosemont, Montréal, Québec, Canada
Department of Ophthalmology, Faculty of Medicine, Université de Montréal, Montréal, Québec, Canada
Biomedical Engineering Institute, Université de Montré al, Montré al, Québec, Canada

Harsha L. Rao, Ravi K. Yadav, Uday K. Addepalli, Shashikant Chaudhary, Sirisha Senthil, Nikhil S. Choudhari and Chandra S. Garudadri
VST Glaucoma Center, L V Prasad Eye Institute, Banjara Hills, Hyderabad, India

Zhengxuan Jiang, Kun Liang, Biqing Ding, Jing Wang, Yuxin Xu and Liming Tao
Department of Ophthalmology, The Second Affiliated Hospital of Anhui Medical University, Hefei, Anhui, China

Wei Tan
Department of Ophthalmology, The First People's Hospital of Zunyi, the Third Affiliated Hospital of Zunyi Medical University, Zunyi, Guizhou, China

Yunxia Lu
Department of Biochemistry and Molecular Biology, Anhui Medical University, Hefei, Anhui, China

Guohai Chen, Fangzheng Jiang, Sihong Mao and Yuhua Tong
Department of Ophthalmology, Quzhou People's Hospital, Quzhou, Zhejiang, PR China

Wensheng Li
Xiamen Eye Center of Xiamen University, Xiamen, Fujian, PR China

Aparna Rao
Glaucoma Services, LV Prasad Eye Institute, Patia, Bhubaneswar, India

Sujoy Mukherjee
Diagnostic and Imaging Services, LV Prasad Eye Institute, Patia, Bhubaneswar, India

Emmanuel S. Buys, Sarah R. Hayton, Laurel T. Tainsh, Robert E. T. Tainsh, Binglan Yu and Daniel Nathan
Anesthesia Center for Critical Care Research, Department of Anesthesia, Critical Care, and Pain Medicine, Massachusetts General Hospital, Harvard Medical School, Boston, Massachusetts, United States of America

Kenneth D. Bloch
Anesthesia Center for Critical Care Research, Department of Anesthesia, Critical Care, and Pain Medicine, Massachusetts General Hospital, Harvard Medical School, Boston, Massachusetts, United States of America
Cardiology Division, Department of Medicine, Massachusetts General Hospital, Harvard Medical School, Boston, Massachusetts, United States of America

Alexander Jones, Emma Abernathy and Nadine de Waard
Department of Ophthalmology, Schepens Eye Research Institute, Harvard Medical School, Boston, Massachusetts, United States of America

Yu-Chieh Ko
Department of Ophthalmology, Schepens Eye Research Institute, Harvard Medical School, Boston, Massachusetts, United States of America
Department of Ophthalmology, School of Medicine, National Yang-Ming University, Taipei, Taiwan

Meredith S. Gregory and Bruce R. Ksander
Department of Ophthalmology, Schepens Eye Research Institute, Harvard Medical School, Boston, Massachusetts, United States of America
Department of Ophthalmology, Massachusetts Eye and Ear Infirmary, Harvard Medical School, Boston, Massachusetts, United States of America

Louis R. Pasquale
Department of Ophthalmology, Schepens Eye Research Institute, Harvard Medical School, Boston, Massachusetts, United States of America
Department of Ophthalmology, Massachusetts Eye and Ear Infirmary, Harvard Medical School, Boston, Massachusetts, United States of America
Channing Division of Network Medicine, Brigham and Women's Hospital, Harvard Medical School, Boston, Massachusetts, United States of America

Clemens Alt and Charles P. Lin
Wellman Center for Photomedicine and Center for Systems Biology, Massachusetts General Hospital, Harvard Medical School, Boston, Massachusetts, United States of America

Raphael Turcotte
Wellman Center for Photomedicine and Center for Systems Biology, Massachusetts General Hospital, Harvard Medical School, Boston, Massachusetts, United States of America
Department of Biomedical Engineering, Boston University, Boston, Massachusetts, United States of America

Ruiyi Ren and Haiyan Gong
Department of Ophthalmology, Boston University School of Medicine, Boston, Massachusetts, United States of America

Andrea Giani, Dong-Jin Oh, Stephanie J. Loomis, Douglas J. Rhee and Janey L. Wiggs
Department of Ophthalmology, Massachusetts Eye and Ear Infirmary, Harvard Medical School, Boston, Massachusetts, United States of America

Maeva Clerté, Rajeev Malhotra, Pankaj Arora and Marielle Scherrer-Crosbie
Cardiology Division, Department of Medicine, Massachusetts General Hospital, Harvard Medical School, Boston, Massachusetts, United States of America

Jae H. Kang
Channing Division of Network Medicine, Brigham and Women's Hospital, Harvard Medical School, Boston, Massachusetts, United States of America

Peter Brouckaert
VIB Department of Molecular Biomedical Research, Ghent University, Ghent, Belgium

Natalie Lerner and Elie Beit-Yannai
Department of Clinical Biochemistry and Pharmacology, Ben-Gurion University of the Negev, Beer-Sheva, Israel

Qi Xiong, Zhaohui Li, Yi Zhu, Sancar Abdulhalim, Ping Wang and Xiaojun Cai
Department of Ophthalmology, Zhongnan Hospital of Wuhan University, Wuhan, Hubei, P.R. China

Zhiliang Li
Department of Orthpedics, Union Hospital of Tongji Medical College, Huazhong University of Science and Technology, Wuhan, Hubei, P.R. China

Index

www.ingramcontent.com/pod-product-compliance
Lightning Source LLC
LaVergne TN
LVHW060559210926
848485LV00005B/1340

* 9 7 8 1 6 3 9 2 7 3 8 2 9 *